Home Health Administration

Home Health Administration

Marilyn D. Harris, RN, MSN, CNAA

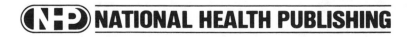

NHP NATIONAL HEALTH PUBLISHING

This book is dedicated to my husband, Charles,
and my colleagues who provided the support and encouragement
necessary to develop the idea for this book into a reality.

Contents

Part I Home Health Administration

Part II Standards for Home Health Agencies

Contributors

Carol Easley Allen, PhD, RN
Associate Professor
Department of Nursing
California State University
Los Angeles, California

Madalon O'Rawe Amenta, DrPH, RN
Associate Professor of Nursing
The Pennsylvania State University
McKeesport Campus
McKeesport, Pennsylvania

Emily Amerman, MSW
Deputy Director for Long Term Care
Philadelphia Corporation for Aging
Philadelphia, Pennsylvania

Pamela A. Andresen, MS, RN
Assistant Professor, Community and
    Mental Health Nursing
Niehoff School of Nursing
Loyola University of Chicago
Chicago, Illinois

Ida M. Androwich, MS, RNC
Assistant Professor, Community and
    Mental Health Nursing
Niehoff School of Nursing
Loyola University of Chicago
Chicago, Illinois

Lazelle E. Benefield, MSN, RN
President, L. Benefield Associates
Assistant Professor
School of Nursing, College of Health
    Sciences
Old Dominion University
Norfolk, Virginia

Carol Brocker, MA, RN
Nursing Education Outreach Staff
Maine Medical Center
Portland, Maine

Gregory J. Brown, BBA
Director of Financial Services
Visiting Nurse Association of Eastern
    Montgomery County
Abington, Pennsylvania

Lynda C. Brubaker, MSN, RN
Graduate Student
University of Pennsylvania
Philadelphia, Pennsylvania

Kathleen A. Carlson, CAE, RN
Legislative Program Director
Pennsylvania Nurses Association
Harrisburg, Pennsylvania

Ann H. Cary, PhD, MPH, RN
Project Director—Home Care Ad-
    ministration Program
School of Nursing, The Catholic Univer-
    sity of America
Washington, DC

Elizabeth Z. Cathcart, MPH, RN,
    CNAA
Chief Executive Officer
Home Health Services, Inc.
Wayne, Pennsylvania

Diane Chaloux, MS, RN
Home Care Supervisor
Androscoggin Home Health Services
Auburn, Maine

Sharon L. Colegrove, RN
Associate, Advanced Risk Management
    Techniques
Laguna Hills, California

Kathi Collins, BSN, RN
Nursing Supervisor
Moorestown Visiting Nurse Association
Moorestown, New Jersey

Joanne Tully Cossman, MPH, RN
Manager, Continuing Care
Community Health Care Plan
New Haven, Connecticut

Margaret J. Cushman, MSN
President
VNA Group, Hartford, Connecticut
Chairman, National Association for
    Home Care

Elizabeth A. Daubert, BSN, MPH,
    FAAN
Executive Director
Connecticut Association for Home
    Care, Inc.
Wallingford, Connecticut

Elissa Della Monica, MSN, RN
Director of Professional Services
Visiting Nurse Association of Eastern
    Montgomery County
Abington, Pennsylvania

Keith De Vantier
Corporate Vice President of Sales &
    Marketing
Foster Medical Corporation
Conshohocken, Pennsylvania

Janna Dieckmann, MSN, RN
Lecturer
University of Pennsylvania, School of
    Nursing
Philadelphia, Pennsylvania

Cheryl E. Easley, AM, RN
Assistant Professor
University of Michigan School of
    Nursing
Ann Arbor, Michigan

David M. Eisenberg, PhD
Director, Long Term Care
Philadelphia Corporation for Aging
Philadelphia, Pennsylvania

Maureen A. Eng, MA, RN
Executive Director
New Jersey Hospice Organization
Princeton, New Jersey

Joanne Kelly Erb, MSN, RN
Home Care Coordinator
Osteopathic Medical Center of Philadel-
    phia
Philadelphia, Pennsylvania

Clay Figard, Jr.
Vice President, Marketing
Delta Computer Systems, Inc.
Altoona, Pennsylvania

Charmaine McMaster Fitzig, DrPH,
    MPH, MS, RN
Associate Clinical Professor
Columbia University School of Nursing
New York, New York

E. Michael Flanagan, JD, BS
Arent, Fox, Kintner, Plotkin & Kahn
Washington, DC

William W. Fonner, BA
Executive Vice President
The Buckman Van Buren Group
Abington, Pennsylvania

Allan G. Ginsberg, RPh, BSc, FASCP
President
United Medical Services, Inc.
Philadelphia, Pennsylvania

E. Joyce Gould, MSN, RN
Assistant Administrator for Clinical Ser-
    vices
United Home Health Services
Philadelphia, Pennsylvania

Bette Groshens, MEd, RN
Home Care Director
Abington Memorial Hospital
Abington, Pennsylvania

Val J. Halamandaris, JD, BA
President
National Association for Home Care
Washington, DC

Marilyn D. Harris, MSN, RN, CNAA
Executive Director
Visiting Nurse Association of Eastern
    Montgomery County
Abington, Pennsylvania

Carol-Rae Green Hoffmann, MA, PhD
President, Wyndmoor Group, Inc.
Wyndmoor, Pennsylvania
Associate Professor
Montgomery County Community
    College
Blue Bell, Pennsylvania

Stephen Paul Holzemer, MSN, RNC
Consultant, Community Health Nursing
    Education and Care Delivery
Conservatory for Nursing
New York, New York

Jessie F. Igou, DrPH, RN
Assistant Professor of Nursing
Pennsylvania State University
State College, Pennsylvania

Terrance Keenan
Vice President for Special Programs
The Robert Wood Johnson Foundation
Princeton, New Jersey

Mary Ann Keirans, BSN, MA, MBA,
    CNAA
Administrator
Visiting Nurse Association/Home
    Health Service of Luzerne County
Kingston, Pennsylvania

Priscilla D. Kissick, MN, RN
Executive Director
Wissahickon Hospice
Philadelphia, Pennsylvania

Charlotte L. Kohler, CPA
Partner
Kohler & Company CPA & Consultants
Greenbelt, Maryland

Mary Jane Koren, MD
Associate Chief of Staff/Extended Care
Bronx Veterans Administration Medical
    Center
Bronx, New York

Robert F. Leduc
President, Visiting Nurse Associations
    of America
Denver, Colorado

Bernard R. Lorenz, CPA
President, Bernard R. Lorenz &
    Associates
Lutherville, Maryland

Michele Lucas, MSN, RN
Assistant Director
Jeanes Home Health
Philadelphia, Pennsylvania

Sharon Dezzani Martin, BS Ed, BSN,
    RN
Home Care Regional Manager
Androscoggin Home Health Services
Auburn, Maine

Barbara A. McCann, MA
Director, Accreditation Program for
    Hospice Care and Home Care
Joint Commission on Accreditation of
    Hospitals
Chicago, Illinois

Patricia Moulton, MSN, RNC
Long Term Home Care Coordinator
West Essex Community Health Services
Fairfield, New Jersey

Susan C. Nolt, MBA, RN
Director of Program and Staff Development
Visiting Nurse Home Care Association
Lancaster, Pennsylvania

Lynne D. Pancoast, MSN, RN
Executive Director
Jeanes Home Health
Philadelphia, Pennsylvania

Carol Ann Parente, MSN, RN, CRNP
Adult Nurse Practitioner
Hospice Coordinator
Visiting Nurse Association of Eastern
    Montgomery County
Abington, Pennsylvania

Mary Kay Pera
Executive Director
Pennsylvania Association of Home
    Health Agencies
Harrisburg, Pennsylvania

Donna Ambler Peters, MA, RN, CNAA
Director of Nursing Research and
    Quality Assurance
The Johns Hopkins Hospital
Baltimore, Maryland

Catherine H. Pignatello, MPH, RN
Administrator of Professional Services
West Essex Community Health Services,
    Inc.
Fairfield, New Jersey

Karen M. Polise, MSN, RN
Clinical Nurse Specialist, Ventilator Assisted Children Home
Program
Children's Hospital of Philadelphia
Philadelphia, Pennsylvania

Alan E. Reider, JD, MPH, AB
Partner
Arent, Fox, Kintner, Plotkin & Kahn
Washington, DC

Nancy L. Rhodes, BSN
Vice President, Planning and Program
    Development
Visiting Nurse Corporation
Milwaukee, Wisconsin

Nancy Day Robinson, DSW
Director of Accreditation Program
National Home Caring Council
Washington, DC

Nancy DiPasquale Ruane, MAN, RN
Consultant, Family and Community
    Health Nursing
Alliance Associates
Philadelphia, Pennsylvania

Marilyn Seiler, BSN, RNC
Quality Assurance Manager
Health Care Professionals
Oklahoma City, Oklahoma

Jerry L. Sellentin, PhD AEP
Director of Human Resources
Bryan Memorial Hospital
Lincoln, Nebraska

Lori R. Sherman, BSN, RN
Home Health Management Consultant
Clark, New Jersey

David Barton Smith, PhD
Professor and Chairman
Department of Health Administration
Temple University School of Business
Philadelphia, Pennsylvania

Judith Baigis Smith, PhD, RN
Director, Community Health Nursing
    Program
University of Pennsylvania, School of
    Nursing
Philadelphia, Pennsylvania

Judith Lloyd Storfjell, PhD Candidate,
MS, RN
Health Care Consultant, President
Health Care at Home Management Cor-
poration
Berrien Springs, Michigan

James Tehan, JD, MPH
Special Counsel for Hospital Home
Health Care Agency of California
Torrance, California

Elaine R. Volk, BSN, CRNI, CNSN, RN
Home Care Director
Hospital Home Care of Greater
Philadelphia
Philadelphia, Pennsylvania

Rebecca A. Walker, MA, BSN, RN
Director of Clinical Development
Visiting Nurse Association of Baltimore
Baltimore, Maryland

Peggie R. Webb, MSEd, BSN, RN
President
Home Health Development Corporation
Spring House, Pennsylvania

Linda Weinberg, MSN, RN
Graduate Student
University of Pennsylvania
Philadelphia, Pennsylvania

Kathleen Williams, MSN, RN
Director, Home Health Care
Saint Agnes Medical Center
Philadelphia, Pennsylvania

Rebecca Wolf
Administrative Assistant to the President
Visiting Nurse Associations of America
Denver, Colorado

Joan Reynolds Yuan, MSN, RNC
Nursing Supervisor
Visiting Nurse Association of Eastern
Montgomery County
Abington, Pennsylvania

Foreword

Although we tend to think of home health care as a modern phenomenon, care of people in the home has always been with us. In its most informal aspect, it was care given by one family member to another in their residence. Neighbors often assisted with the care of neighbors. Certain religious and social groups visited homes to assist with the care of the poor or aged.

The more formal approach, as we know it in the United States, began in the mid-1800s with the founding of the earliest visiting nurse association in Buffalo, New York in 1885; Boston, Massachusetts and Philadelphia, Pennsylvania in 1886; and Brooklyn, New York in 1888. Health departments had home care programs for the follow-up of people with infectious diseases.

Care was basic and focused on the entire family. The nurse was the major health care provider in the home. Often, home care was initiated because of one individual, but the nurse evaluated the health of the existing family unit, to assist all family members, as well as the patient to attain health goals.

Service was usually planned on a five-day week (Monday through Friday) during the usual working day. A skeleton staff worked on weekends to cover daily visits or emergencies.

Social problems--poverty, inadequate housing, unemployment--were major problems in many situations and assumed equal, if not primary importance, in planning for health care in the home. It became necessary to add various services to the agency staff to address adequately the complexity of problems evident in planning for the care of people at home. Physical and occupational therapists, social workers and nutritionists became important members of the home care team. The nurse was not only the provider of nursing service, but also the coordinator of care for patients.

Financial support for the agency came from fundraising, income from endowed funds and the United Way. Some insurance programs, such as Metropolitan Life, paid for service to their policy holders. Agencies charged the patient a fee "according to ability to pay," but the charge was often very modest and in many cases, service was "free" or at no charge to the patient or family.

The advent of Medicare in 1966 and Medicaid in 1967 brought drastic changes to the home care industry. Federal law required compliance with a stated set of regulations for administration, financial management, and patient care. Over the years these regulations have been changed and added to with more rigid requirements for compliance.

At the same time, the demand for home health care increased. With shortened hospital stays, people required a more sophisticated level of care at home. Technological developments permitted complex care to be given outside of institutions. Technology also lengthened the life-span, not only for the elderly, but also for younger individuals with debilitating chronic diseases.

Today's home health agency administrator functions in the midst of increasing regulatory surveillance of quality care, financial accountability, and documentation. Administrators must ensure that there is a competent clinical staff available 24 hours a day, seven days a week, who can cope with patient needs ranging from teaching infant care to new parents to apnea monitoring or parenteral nutrition therapy. Additionally, computer programs for billing services, strategic planning, and patient care are an inherent part of the administrator's day.

A difficulty for today's home health agency administrators is the availability of published material to assist them in the daily management of their agencies. They must turn to a variety of publications to find help in addressing the many issues and questions that surface in home care. Questions can arise on billing procedures, regulatory changes, ethical dilemmas, and new patient programs.

This book provides a resource for home health administrators. It is divided into parts, each one developing in detail a component of agency administration. With this format, the reader can select specific areas to review as necessary. The Table of Contents allows ready identification of the issues presented, as well as the specific supporting chapters. The bibliography provides additional resource material.

This book should provide easy reference for the administrator who must juggle the administrative, financial, and clinical complexities of home health care in a continually changing regulatory and technological climate.

Francis A. McVey
Former Executive Director
Visiting Nurse Association
of Brooklyn, Inc.
February, 1987

Introduction

Marilyn D. Harris

The idea for this textbook started when the need was recognized for an in-house manual to be used by the students attending the Visiting Nurse Association of Eastern Montgomery County for their practicum in home health administration. Supervisors and other staff often spend much time explaining to students what the agency is, what services are offered, where the agency gets its funding, and other important issues.

This book presents an overview of home health administration. Each chapter could be expanded into a book length publication. Authors have included bibliographies in addition to the reference lists so that interested readers can pursue particular topics in more detail.

All of the contributors to this textbook are involved in some aspect of home health care. The authors include staff, board members, nurse practitioners, consultants, accountants, lawyers, teachers, supervisors, administrators, and representatives from national and state organizations. They represent home health care agencies under governmental, institutional, proprietary, and voluntary auspices. Various geographical areas of the United States are also represented.

Part I provides a comprehensive perspective on home health administration. It includes brief histories and descriptions of the types of agencies. Individuals who are employed in each type of agency have shared their experiences and addressed the following areas: the purpose of the agency; mission/philosophy; governing body; case mix and staffing pattern; development of policies and procedures; capital requirements and cash flow. The writers also share their opinions on the advantages and disadvantages of their type of agency.

Part II addresses standards for home health agencies. Agency standards including certification, accreditation, certificate of need, and licensure are described. Professional standards concerning the licensure, certification, and educational requirements of the staff and administration are included. The benefits of membership in national and state organizations are explained by the staffs of these organizations.

Part III lists selected management issues that are important to home care administrators. Such issues as referral sources, staffing, productivity, labor relations, personnel, staff education, and long-term care are addressed.

Part IV explores a limited number of clinical issues that impact on service delivery or cost identification. Documentation, patient classification systems, nursing diagnoses, and high-tech issues are presented from the administrator's viewpoint. Case studies are included as illustrations.

Part V describes the components of quality assurance and program evaluation in home health agencies.

Part VI deals with financial issues. The current insurance climate is of concern to administrators. Other issues are budgets, reimbursement, and management information systems.

Part VII addresses legal, ethical, and political issues. Contracts, informed consent, and liability are discussed. Administrators must be aware of the many legislative and regulatory issues that impact on home care both at the state and national levels. The contributors review these issues at both levels and provide information on how personnel in home health agencies can become involved in the legislative or regulatory process.

Ethical concerns surface at both the clinical and administrative levels. These concerns are discussed from theoretical and practical viewpoints.

Part VIII includes strategic planning, marketing, and survival issues. Topics such as diversification, corporate restructure, mergers, acquisitions, and grantsmanship are included.

Part IX addresses areas of opportunity to serve as resource personnel and innovators. Student and volunteer programs may be two areas of administration that are not present in all agencies; but, these programs present multiple opportunities for collaborative relationships with other agencies or educational institutions. The physician's role in home care is presented by a physician. The role of the fiscal intermediary is also reviewed.

Part X attempts to put the administration of home health services into perspective. The editor shares her viewpoint on administration in today's economic and political climate, and one national leader shares his ideas on the future of home care.

In an effort to make this book a practical and useful "how-to" manual, in addition to a textbook, case studies have been included to illustrate how selected agencies have implemented specific concepts described in several sections.

Although issues are addressed on a chapter-by-chapter basis, many of the topics overlap one another. For example, ethical issues are mentioned in the chapter on discharge planning and high-tech procedures, and financial issues surface in reference to budgeting, reimbursement, and documentation. Productivity is common to staffing, budgeting, and ethical issues.

Today's home health care climate is ever changing. Information included in this book was current as of the Fall of 1986. Readers are encouraged to review current guidelines and regulations, specifically in such areas as reimbursement, documentation requirements, and Medicare forms, to keep informed of important changes that may have occurred since this book went to press.

It is my hope that each reader will find this publication to be a ready reference for the multifaceted aspects of home health care administration.

Part I

Home Health Administration

Chapter One

Home Health Administration: An Overview

Janna Dieckmann

Definition of Home Health Care

Home health care is the sensitive, active, and educational provision of professional nursing care and other health care services to people of any age in their homes or other noninstitutional setting. Emerging as a specialty within nursing with the development of the profession itself in the late nineteenth century, home care has evolved and changed in response to social, economic, political, and scientific changes in the society as a whole.

In its century of development, two key goals of home health care have remained constant--the provision of nursing services to those in the home and the education of the client and the family toward the goals of health. The form of home health care today especially reflects the development of the social insurance programs of the 1960s, Medicare and Medicaid. The type of services that are offered depends on patient, family, and community needs, nursing goals, and the payment sources available to nurses and home health care agencies.

A formal definition of home health care has been offered by four prominent national organizations involved in home health care provision: the Council of Home Health Agencies and Community Health Service, National League for Nursing; The National Home Care Council; The National Association of Home Health Agencies; and the Assembly of Outpatient and Home Care Institutions, American Hospital Association. This definition is:

> Home health service is that component of comprehensive health care whereby services are provided to individuals and families in their places of residence for the purpose of promoting, maintaining, or restoring health or minimizing the effects of illness and disability. Services appropriate to the needs of the individual patient and family are planned, coordinated and made available by an agency or institution, organized for the delivery of health care through the use of employed staff, contractual arrangements, or a combination of administrative patterns. (McNamara 1985, 61)*

---

* Adapted by permission from *Hospitals*, Vo. 56, No. 21, November 1, 1982. Copyright 1982, American Hospital Publishing, Inc.

Description of Home Health Care

Home health care begins with the client, the individual who requires nursing service. Contemporary requirements for care in the home are that the patient receiving services be "homebound." While the definition of homebound status has been flexible, it has generally been interpreted to mean that the patient's health is impaired to the extent that he could not seek services outside the home. Provision of nursing services is then offered in the home. Other groups of clients requiring services in the home are postpartum women and their infants who may be leaving the hospital earlier than usual, with the provision that their insuring agency will provide home care. Children who have failure to thrive syndrome, or who may be ventilator-dependent are other groups requiring home care services.

While there is almost always one identified individual who is the focus of the home health care services, the nursing goals for the patient's development must be implemented in the context of the individual's family and community. The family, neighbors, and other members of the patient's informal support system generally provide the 24-hour care and support to the patient throughout the time assistance is required. If this group is unable to provide adequate care, the patient may need more intensive services from the home health agency, or consideration of the possibility of nursing home placement.

For the home health care nurse, it is probably most useful to define the family in a very flexible manner. Traditional definitions may be quite strict in identifying only close biological relatives as "family." In practice, the definition of the family includes anyone the patient so identifies. Those included may vary from distant relatives, to a boarder who has lived in the home for years, to close friends, to neighbors who feel an obligation to the patient. The flexible definition of family increases the pool of available helpers for the dependent client. Nursing must consider not only the learning needs of the members of this support system in their provision of care, but also the concrete educational needs and psychosocial supports that these people will require in order to continue their role. It is not enough to simply instruct. Assuring that the needs of the support system are met usually requires nursing intervention as well.

The client's community may facilitate or detract from the provision of nursing care and the advancement of nursing service. Communities vary from densely concentrated urban neighborhoods, to sprawling suburban towns, to lonely rural back roads. While a client may be isolated from supports in any situation, the concentration of people and services, the availability of transportation and pharmacy services, and the proximity and diversity of grocery services, makes a real difference in the challenges confronted by the home health care patient.

The community and the membership of the patient and the family in it have further effects on the patient and family system and their needs for home health care. The patient and family socioeconomic background and class status influence their expectations of care. The family's cultural and ethnic background influences their expectations for health, health care services, and their ability to meet those needs in the wider American health care delivery system. Many religious groups have prohibitions of which nurses should be aware. Individuals, families, and communities may have particular ways of defining the discussion of health, illness, and dying which home health care nursing must recognize. Nursing must acquire the ability to practice within these parameters.

The nurse who moves from the hospital to home care will find differences at every step. The most prominent one is the difference in location, that the home in all its many variations has replaced the hospital. It is nurses themselves who must adapt to the family, rather than patients adapting to the hospital situation. The nurses serve as expert consultants in adapting treatment measures to the home setting. This may involve, for example, obtaining equipment, making referrals to other services, or negotiating with the physician to alter the medication program.

Initiation of Home Health Care Services

The home health patient is seen by the agency after a referral has been made for the patient's care. This referral may be from the patient, the family, a community social service agency, or a local physician. But many home care referrals are from the nurse or discharge planner attached to an acute care hospital. Referrals are made to the home health agencies from the hospital subsequent to patient needs being identified during the hospitalization or while under care at an ambulatory clinic or emergency department. The referral generally includes the name and address of the patient, family contacts, diagnoses, medications, and proposed treatment measures. It is often not overly complex, generally focusing on the basic needs of the patient.

The agencies that provide home health care may be voluntary agencies, such as visiting nurse associations, proprietary agencies, official health departments, or hospital-based home care departments. No matter what specific organizations exist, most agencies provide the first home care visit within 24 hours of the initial referral. This first visit is often the most complex of the entire service period. During this admission visit, the nurse conducts an evaluation of the patient and family, assesses the environment, analyzes the impact of the disease(s) on the patient, identifies functional impairments of the patient, determines the knowledge of and adherence to prescribed treatment for the disease, and ascertains patient and family desires for care and their eventual goals. The nurse provides initial interventions to establish the basis for the patient, the family, and the support system to continue providing needed care until the next nursing visit. The patient's and family's active participation in the goals of treatment and in the plans of care is sought and utilized to the fullest extent.

Ongoing services to the patient are provided for several weeks, but extend, under Medicare, until the skilled care needs of the situation are exhausted. This period is usually short. However, at times patients requiring technical treatments such as dressing changes or urinary catheter management may receive intermittent services over several years.

The nurse visits to provide nursing interventions based on the overall goals of the case, working toward incremental change at each visit. The home health care nurse utilizes many resources to facilitate patient and family progress. The services of the multidisciplinary team—the physical therapist, occupational therapist, social worker, speech therapist, and home health aide—may be utilized for the patient's benefit. The nurse will probably be in communication with the patient's physician to coordinate the treatment plan during the patient's rehabilitation from the acute phase of the illness. The home care nurse relies heavily on ongoing services within the formal and informal support networks of the family and community to prepare the client for discharge from home health care, and to provide ongoing support when skilled care is no longer required. The nurse will make appropriate referrals to these networks, or suggest that the patient do so.

Discharge of the case occurs usually when the patient has met the goals of care, although the achieved outcome varies significantly among patients. Some patients progress easily and completely to the goals of care, while others may achieve only a partial outcome. The patient is prepared for this discharge during the whole period of home health care provision through learning the skills needed by him to resume independent management of health care needs. At discharge, the nurse usually notifies the primary medical provider and other involved services that the case is closed.

Some home health services follow different sequences of care provision. If home health care services are offered under a long-term home care program, the Medicare requirements for short-term, intermittent, skilled care often do not apply. Instead, the goal of services is maintenance of the dependent patient outside of an institutional setting. Another model of care is provided under maternal-child programs in which pregnant women are seen in health clinics and through home health care. They are often seen through the first birthday of the infant. While the goal of service in both cases remains the maximization of patient and family independence in self-management of health concerns, the period of service is quite different.

Early Sources for Home Health Care

A recording of the dates and accomplishments of a practice area such as home health care is important in understanding the development toward current achievements in the field. But the history of home health care is also an ongoing case study in organizational styles and reimbursement patterns. Insight into this history teaches the implications of patterns of social and economic change for the provision of home health services in the 1980s and beyond.

In the early decades of this century, home health care held great promise to contribute to health education and service provision. While growth in home health care occurred, it was not as great as expected nor located within the voluntary agencies who had prepared for expansion (Buhler-Wilkerson 1983). Home health care has frequently changed direction, often suddenly and sharply, frequently as the direct result of changing reimbursement practices which mirror the contemporary experience. An opportunity to avoid the pitfalls of the past emerges when the similar patterns of the past are acknowledged in the present.

Until the twentieth century, most of the care for ill persons was given in the home informally by household members, almost always women. Historians today are aware of some early experiments in home health nursing which developed during the early nineteenth century in the United States. Reflecting then-contemporary ideas, these programs focused on moral elevation as well as illness interventions. The Ladies' Benevolent Society of Charleston, South Carolina, provided charitable works to the poor and ill beginning in 1813. In Philadelphia, lay nurses who attended a short training program were then sent out to care for the newborns and postpartum mothers of all social strata. Significant in time and place, these early programs did not spread, however, and their influence on the development of visiting nursing and organized home health care later in the century is unclear.

Florence Nightingale's innovations in training nurses, replacing the employment of lay nurses, strongly influenced the patterns of nursing education and service provision in the United States. Although William Rathbone established the first District Nursing Association in Liverpool, England, in 1859, it was not until 1877 that district nursing utilizing graduates of the new nurse training schools was introduced into the United States.

High incidence and mortality rates from communicable diseases such as tuberculosis, diphtheria, and typhoid fever affected the population as a whole. Increased urbanization and industrialization also increased human diseases. The late nineteenth century benefited from the new scientific explanations for disease, and the public health nurse became the agent for preventive education of the public. Nursing interventions, improved urban sanitation, economic improvements, and better nutrition laid the basis for a significant reduction in incidence of deadly communicable disease by 1910.

Early Home Health Care

Around 1900, nurses who had graduated from the early training programs worked either in private duty nursing or in the few positions as hospital administrators and teachers. The new field of public health nursing began to employ a few nurses, often adapting the model of service provision used by the private duty nurse in middle and upper class homes. Where private-duty nurses lived in with the patients and their families, the public health nurses visited several families in one day, providing personal care to the sick and health teaching to families.

The circumstances of the employment of visiting nurses at this time were different from the home health care nurses of today. Many agencies hired only one nurse. The administration of the agency and the supervision of the nurse were done by the board of the agency. The board members usually included wealthy or prominent women of the community, whose charitable community service was the direction of both nursing care and good works by the nurse.

Public health nursing at the turn of the century was defined as "primarily family health work of an educational and preventive character but including restorative work" (Dock and Stewart 1925,312), which utilized a large and comprehensive plan for uplifting the general health level through outreach to the community. The mission of the public health nurse was the poor and the immigrant.

Early visiting nurse agencies saw the goal of their voluntary organizations as the development of innovative services whose maintenance would eventually become the role of government. Lillian Wald and her co-workers at the Nurse's Settlement at Henry Street in New York City were responsible for many new services. From their public health nursing practice emerged other nursing specialties such as school nursing and occupational health nursing. In this period, these specialties were truly branches of home health care. Clients identified within the institutional setting were visited in the home, where health promotion and family education were the focus of the nurses' efforts.

Both the nurses and the lay people who participated in the new visiting nurse agencies recognized the need for exchange of ideas and development of a professional identity. The publication of the *Visiting Nurse Quarterly* in 1909 began to establish a professional medium of exchange on clinical and organizational concerns. The establishment of the National Organization for Public Health Nursing in 1912, with membership including lay members as well as nurses, provided an accessible network for the developing leadership in the field. Organizational focus of the NOPHN was "improving the educational and service standards of the public health nurse, and promoting public understanding of and respect for her work" (Rosen 1958,381). The NOPHN was almost immediately the dominant force in public health nursing and contributed to the direction and implementation of public health nursing until 1953, when it merged with other groups to form the National League for Nursing.

Rapid growth of the field of practice increased the importance of providing effective educational preparation of those nurses who would work in public health and was a concern to many. Education for public health nursing began to diverge from the established training school programs about 1906. Specialized programs given to graduates of the training schools provided significant amounts of both theory and practice in public health nursing. The coursework of these early certificate programs would be familiar to contemporary nurses. Public health nursing did not become a regular part of basic nursing education programs until much later.

With the growing complexity of public health nursing practice, recurring questions of what is, or what is not, public health and visiting nursing arose and were discussed at length. Even today there is confusion about what to title the practice and about how to define the boundaries of the field.

Specialization conflicted with the generalist practice. Early in the 1900s there was a trend toward specialization to accommodate the particular needs of such areas as tuberculosis nursing, working with children in the schools, and occupational health nursing. Health nursing, or preventive health education, also gained supporters. Practitioners realized gradually that this specialist model was too fragmented, and support turned again to the generalist model. Here, the nurse emphasized the preventive care role while providing bedside care.

While this remains a universal ideal, its institutional implementation has never been fully developed. By the end of the 1920s, the rapid expansion of public health nursing had stabilized, with more nurses employed in official agencies, under the direction of medical and public health professionals, than in the voluntary visiting nurse associations where nursing had always set the direction.

Mechanisms for reimbursement at the very beginning were simpler than they are today. The same board of trustees that provided administration to the agencies, also raised the funds, often through their social networks, to carry out the mission to the poor and needy. Those patients who were determined able to pay were charged a small fee, even a nickel, as the charitable interpretation was to promote individuals to stand on their own whenever possible.

Beginning in Los Angeles in 1898, municipalities, and eventually the federal government, took on the role for financial support of home health care. An innovation at its creation in 1909, the special nursing service provided by the Metropolitan Life Insurance Company for its policyholders served as a model for others. Nurses in existing agencies, or in agencies developed specifically by the company, provided home care services in a significant amount until the close of this service in 1953.

Agencies such as the American Red Cross provided home care in areas outside the larger cities. Through the Rural Nursing Service, later the Town and Country Nursing Service, the Red Cross developed and passed to local voluntary or public administration almost 3000 generalized programs of public health nursing services.

The impact of the Great Depression of the 1930s reduced both charitable and public funding for home health care resulting in cutbacks in personnel and services. New Deal legislation created new employment for some nurses in official health programs. As had the Sheppard-Towner Act of 1921 which targeted improvements in maternal and child health care, the impact of the Public Health Title VI of the 1935 Social Security Act was to focus available financial resources toward state and local official organizations rather than toward the nonofficial voluntary agencies. This marked a permanent change in emphasis away from the voluntaries.

Further development of home health care services was limited by World War II, but the war mobilization also brought significant advances in nursing education. An increasing emphasis on baccalaureate nursing programs saw the first inclusion of public health nursing in the required course work. By the mid-1950s, the National League for Nursing would require public health nursing courses, but only in baccalaureate level programs. This content is still absent from most diploma and associate degree programs and from the nursing licensure examinations.

The early 1950s were a time of deep and significant change in the public health nursing community. Early in the decade both Metropolitan Life Insurance Company and the American Red Cross discontinued their support of home health care and the voluntary agencies that had provided the services. Potential for program growth beyond the sponsoring agencies' abilities to support it, due to changing patterns of disease toward long-term chronic illnesses, may have been responsible for this shift.

The influence of the National Organization for Public Health Nursing on connecting different agencies and on increasing the spread of knowledge and information relating to practice had gradually decreased in the late 1940s. The lack of ability to financially support an effective agency and the popular trend in the nursing profession to centralize its professional organizations laid the groundwork for the merger of the NOPHN into the newly created National League for Nursing, joining several other specialty nursing organizations. The specialty journal, *Public Health Nursing* (formerly *The Visiting Nurse Quarterly*) also ceased publication.

Public health nurses participated in both national nursing organizations and in the American Public Health Association (APHA). Both the American Nurses Association and the APHA have made definitional statements regarding community health and public health nursing which have implications for home health practice. Continuing changes in the field, variations in definition of practice, and growing variety of reimbursement mechanisms have not eased the problem of defining this area of nursing care.

The 1950s also presented new organizational forms for service delivery. Concern over duplication and a desire for excellent, comprehensive service provision fueled a movement toward combination agencies, the merger of official and voluntary nursing service in one area to provide joint public health and home health care services. A prominent and innovative format in the 1960s, interest in this organizational style declined in the 1970s with consequent separation of the previously combined services into the traditional public and voluntary and private structures.

The initiation of Medicare and Medicaid health insurance benefits for the elderly and poor in July, 1966, is the single most important event in home health care delivery in recent years. Adequate funding for home health care was an infusion to voluntary organization and service provision. Where a few hospital-based programs had developed since the late 1940s, many more were implemented, and joined by increasing numbers of entrepreneurial groups drawn by the new profit-making opportunities. While in 1960, only 250 official health agencies provided nursing care of the sick on a regular basis; by 1968, 1328 public health nursing agencies--50% of all official agencies--provided this service (Roberts and Heinrich 1985,1168).

Chronology of Home Health Care in the United States

1796   Boston Dispensary organizes first home care program in the
        United States.

1813   Ladies Benevolent Society of Charleston, DC, founded to provide
        relief of distress and aid to the sick poor.

1832   The Nurse Society of Philadelphia provides care for sick poor in
        their homes.

1859   The first District Nursing Association established in Liverpool,
        England by William Rathbone.

1875   First United States training schools for nurses under Nightingale
        model established.

1877   New York City Mission sends trained nurses into homes of the
        sick poor.

1886   The Visiting Nurse Society of Philadelphia and the Boston Instructive
        District Nursing Association are established.

1893   Henry Street Nurses' Settlement founded in New York City by
        Lillian Wald and Mary Brewster.

1898   First municipal home care nurse employed in the United States at
        Los Angeles to visit the sick poor.

1901   Fifty-eight organizations doing public health nursing involving about
        130 nurses.

1905   Two hundred public health nursing organizations with about 440
        nurses.

1907   Alabama legally approves employment of public health nurses by local
        boards of health.

1909   Five hundred and sixty-six public health organizations providing care,
        with 1413 nurses.

1909   *The Visiting Nurse Quarterly,* first ongoing specialty journal in the field begins publication.

1909   The Metropolitan Life Insurance Company offers home nursing to its industrial policyholders.

1911   The Visiting Nurse Association of Cleveland and Western Reserve University organize first nursing course to include significant field work and collegiate lecture in public health nursing.

1912   The National Organization for Public Health Nursing (NOPHN) is founded.

1912   Rural Nursing Service of the American Red Cross is established which later becomes the Town and Country Nursing Service.

1916   1922 public health nursing organizations with 5,152 nurses.

1921   Until 1929, Sheppard-Towner Act provides federal matching funds for prenatal and infant care programs supporting home care by nurses.

1922   Four thousand and forty public health nursing organizations with 11,548 nurses.

1925   Kentucky Committee for Mothers and Babies, later to become the Frontier Nursing Service founded by Mary Breckenridge.

1925   First NOPHN statement of qualifications for public health nurses.

1931   Four thousand, two hundred and fifty-five public health nursing agencies with 15,865 nurses.

1935   Government funding of public health nursing emphasizes health departments over nonofficial agencies.

1944   First basic nursing program accredited as including sufficient public health nursing content.

1947   First hospital-based home care program at Montefiore Hospital in New York City.

1950   Twenty-five thousand and ninety-one nurses employed in public health field.

1950   Red Cross rural nursing service is discontinued.

1953   NOPHN merges with other organizations to form the National League for Nursing; publication of *Public Health Nurse* ceases.

1953   Metropolitan Life Insurance ends its support of home nursing services.

1955   Twenty-seven thousand, one hundred and twelve health nurses employed.

1966   Home health services under Medicare and Medicaid begin providing support for official and nonofficial agencies in caring for the sick and an assist to proprietary home health agencies.

1983   Medicare implements a prospective payment system leading to changes in hospital discharge patterns.

Reasons for the Growth in Home Health Care

This analysis of the history of home health care provides the basis for looking at the reasons for the current growth in home health care. Provision of services in the home has grown in numbers of visits, in numbers of involved professionals, and in numbers of home health care agencies.

The rise in home health care and the potential for further expansion of the field are due to the many changes in the contemporary sociopolitical situation and in economic forces which together provide the environment for home health care. Changing patterns of disease and population, emerging economic reimbursement mechanisms, and changing social values draw together to construct the contemporary home health care delivery system.

The change in the distribution of disease since the turn of the century provides the first factor in the growth of home health care. Improved scientific knowledge of disease agents, regular immunizations, and the availability of antibiotics, provision of basic nutrition to most people, pasteurization of milk, and other factors have decreased the risk of developing and dying from nineteenth century disease threats such as tuberculosis, severe diarrheal illnesses, cholera, and many others. In place of these acute illnesses, chronic illnesses are now the primary causes of death in the United States. These illnesses, such as hypertension, cardiac disease, pulmonary disease, and diabetes, have a long period of development leading to irreversible changes in the body and frequently permanent impairment of the individual's functional abilities. While early intervention may limit the effect of the chronic disease exacerbations, affected individuals generally experience long periods of debility necessitating rehabilitation during which they may fail to regain their previous abilities. The health care delivery system is faced with making policy decisions about people for whom illness and disease is irreversible, degenerative, and function-impairing. Long-term chronic illness reduces individual and family resources, and decreases the financial ability to pay privately for needed services. It will be a challenge to society both to develop systems that are efficient in meeting patient needs and effective in controlling overall costs. Home care has shown promise in being the alternative with the chance of success to meet this large and growing need.

A second and related change affecting the growth of home health care are the changes in the distribution of the population of the United States. This nation is growing older as a whole. While in 1900 only 4.1% of Americans were over 65 years, by 1984 this had tripled to 11.9% of the population, a change in real numbers from 3.1 million to 28.0 million (American Association of Retired Persons 1985). This change in the over-65 population is interrelated with the changes in the distribution of disease toward increased prevalence of chronic illnesses. With decreased mortality in the younger population due to acute illnesses, more individuals are living into their later years, the time in which chronic illness is more likely to appear. Additionally, better treatment of complications of older age and chronic illness mean that even with serious diseases, people tend to live longer than previously.

Complicating this population trend toward longer life have been changes in social behavior of families. Changing distribution of employment, economic recession, and improved transportation has dispersed families across the country more than ever before. Fewer relatives may be available living close by when elderly individuals require assistance. Changing patterns of female employment which has increased the percentage of women in the workforce has simultaneously reduced the number of female family members available for full-time care of the chronically ill. As a result of all these structural changes in the family, care of the impaired elderly may need to be increasingly a social and governmental responsibility.

A third factor in the growth of home health care, also an effect of the increase in chronic illness prevalence, has been the expansion of rehabilitative services for those at home with chronic illnesses. Rehabilitation is a long-term process requiring adaptation of the impaired individual back into the home environment. This adaptation may require diverse professional services. Home health care has expanded its utilization of the therapies—physical therapy, occupational therapy, and speech therapy—in home rehabilitation efforts. Social work also has a place in the care of the homebound individual. When individuals require a diversity of services, overall utilization of home health care increases.

Changing reimbursement patterns have had such a profound effect on the outline of services provided under home health care that reimbursement is said to set the direction for home health care. While a look at the history of the practice field substantiates this position, this fourth reason for the rise in home health care has had an especially strong impact since the passage of Medicare and Medicaid home care coverage with the Social Security Amendments of 1965, with the first services being offered in 1966. Medicare focus on short-term, intermittent interventions has limited access and funding to innovate and develop new concepts for long-term home care management. Further, Medicare reimbursement has made home health care a profitable venture for proprietary agencies and hospitals. This has multiplied the number of functioning agencies in areas both with and without certificate of need. This competition has thus far led to growth, but it has also opened questions of quality assurance due to the lack of specific training in home health care skills in the new agencies.

Hopes for cost containment in the health care delivery system have also encouraged the growth of home health care, a fifth reason for its expansion. Changes in Medicare reimbursement for hospitalization toward prospective payment popularly known as the DRG system (for Diagnostic Related Groups), have given fiscal encouragement to limit the length of acute hospitalizations. A result has been the discharge to nursing home or private home of individuals who, in other times, may have remained in the acute care institution. "Sicker and quicker" has been used to describe the situation of those released to home care under this program. Increased acuity of home care patients implies more frequent skilled visits, more time-consuming visits due to increased complexity, and patients at greater risk for decompensation and rehospitalization. A shift of care from acute institution to the home can provide the beginnings for still further changes in home health care.

The optimism that cost containment motives will increase home health care utilization is tempered by at least two different problems. On the one hand, the desire for overall cost containment in health services is, instead of increasing reimbursement to encourage hospital discharge, paradoxically curtailing the home care services offered the client. Medicare intermediaries in particular have attempted to limit strictly the categories of those clients reimbursed under Medicare regulations of skilled care, intermittent services, and homebound status. On the other hand, some experts have questioned whether the real total cost of care for the client has been identified to compare with costs of acute hospital care. Lost income to the family caregiver, cost of physical maintenance of the home, and other informal costs have not usually been figured into the comparison equations.

These trends toward early discharge combined with the availability in home care of increasingly sophisticated biomedical equipment leads to the sixth factor increasing home care. Complex services once rarely seen in the home — renal dialysis, ventilators, intravenous antibiotics, and many more — are now in frequent use providing a home-going option for patients previously enduring long-term hospital stays. Simplified technology, effective teaching of the patients' support systems, and efficient supplier networks providing the diversity of required equipment have fit complex care into the needs of the home environment.

A seventh and last area affecting the growth in home health care is related to questions of quality of life. The elderly and the chronically ill would prefer to remain in their independent living situations rather than be institutionalized in, for instance, a nursing home. Many families negatively value institutionalization and separation of the family members. Some cultural and ethnic groups are especially reluctant to treat the chronically ill and elderly in this manner. A desire for self-care as part of significant long-term changes in popular philosophy has also supported increases in home health care. Despite these significant trends in societal values, needed social and economic supports for the patients and family caregivers involved in long-term home care are rarely found.

Several emerging issues in home health care may also have an affect on the field in the next few years. Growth and extension of all the previous areas of influence can be expected. Some kind of reimbursement for long-term home care, either from private insurance or government support, may well develop in the next decade. The type and quality of support from health maintenance organizations whose influence on health care delivery is growing, is also a question. Will HMOs identify the strengths of home health care, or will their fiscal desire to restrict utilization patterns further limit home health care services?

Initiation and expansion of proprietary home care services will continue to change the features of the home health landscape. In some states, certificate of need still limits agency growth in numbers. Can adequate services be provided? In others, the profusion of agencies is complex and confusing to individuals seeking care and health care professionals alike. What kinds of standards of quality assurance will be necessary?

Community and Public Health Nursing

Two further factors will contribute to the determination of the types and kinds of patterns of home health care. Both the definition of the service field, in particular the understanding of community and public health nursing, and the prevailing definition of the concept of health will imply choices to be made by home health care nurses and providers.

Home health care is considered to be a part of community health nursing, which as been defined in different ways. Early in the development of the practice field, Lillian Wald innovated the term "public health nursing," referring to the "health nursing" concept of Florence Nightingale (who contrasted it to "sick nursing," the care of the ill). The use of the title spread with the National Organization for Public Health Nursing.

The term "visiting nursing" has also been used to refer to the provision of home health services, and has included both sick nursing and well nursing. Over the last few years, the term public health nursing has continued to co-exist with the newer term, community health nursing. These terms reflect both the similarities and differences in definition of home health care and related concepts based in the statements of the American Nurses' Association and the American Public Health Association.

Community health nursing is the term utilized by the American Nurses' Association (ANA). In their publication, *A Conceptual Model of Community Health Nursing*, the following definition is given:

> Community health nursing is a synthesis of nursing practice and public health practice applied to promoting and preserving the health of populations. The practice is general and comprehensive. It is not limited to a particular age group or diagnosis, and is continuing, not episodic. The dominant responsibility is to the population as a whole; nursing directed to individuals, families, or groups contributes to the health of the total population. Health promotion, health maintenance, health education, and management, coordination, and continuity of care are utilized in a holistic approach to the management of the health care of individuals, families, and groups in a community (American Nurses' Association 1973, 3).[*]

This statement of definitions and goals for the field proposed by the ANA should be contrasted with a similar definitional statement made by the American Public Health Association (APHA), as developed by its Public Health Nursing (PHN) Section. They state:

> "Public health nursing synthesizes the body of knowledge from the public health sciences and professional nursing theories for the purpose of improving the health of the entire community. This goal lies at the heart of primary prevention and health promotion and is the foundation for public health nursing practice.

---

[*] Reprinted with permission of the ANA.

To accomplish this goal, public health nurses work with groups, families, and individuals as well as in multidisciplinary teams and programs. Identifying subgroups (aggregates) within the population which are at high risk of illness, disability, or premature death, and directing resources toward these groups, is the most effective approach for accomplishing the goal of PHN. Success in reducing the risk and in improving the health of the community depend on the involvement of consumers, especially groups experiencing health risk, and others in the community, in health planning, and in self-help activities" (American Public Health Association 1982, 210).*

One similarity between the two definitions is their emphasis on the combination within community and public health nursing of public health and nursing concepts. Community and public health nursing utilizes the framework of the three levels of prevention: primary, secondary, and tertiary. In planning decisions, this field of nursing looks to problem-solving with groups based on epidemiologic concepts and tools.

One difference between the two definitions is the varying emphasis placed on primary care in the ANA definition, and on community level and aggregate goals of nursing in the APHA/PHN definition. While home health care is given in the community, one viewpoint is that this location does not alone constitute community health nursing practice. But it is important to clarify that the delivery of home health care services to individuals and their families does not automatically exclude the relevance of a population-based practice. The emphasis of the home health care nurse will reflect his interpretation of both definitions. Either a primary care-based practice or a population-based practice is possible in home health care nursing.

Concepts of Health

Health as the goal of nursing must be defined for home health care as the definition of health creates a further set of goals for the types of care and distribution of care provided under home health. Health, as a moral and political question, is informed moreover by other health provider groups, community values and standards, and the controls of the reimbursement system. The definition of health is part of the environment, part of the policy context for home health care.

Judith A. Smith (1981; 1983) has developed a framework, the ideas of health, to identify the fundamental concepts of health. These four distinctive types each have implications for the practice of home health care. All four models can be used to understand decisions about rehabilitation and prevention practices. It is not necessary to adopt one model, although the degree of emphasis on one compared to another may vary.

The clinical model is the basic model of health and is most represented in the practice of modern medicine. The health goal for this model is the absence of signs and symptoms of disease or disability. The next most inclusive idea of health is the

---

* Reprinted with permission of the American Public Health Association. 1982. The definition and role of public health nursing practice in the delivery of health care. *American Journal of Public Health* 72:210-212.

role-performance model, which adds the variable of the individual's ability to perform social roles with maximum expected output. Together, these two models represent what has most frequently been the goal of nursing services provided in home health care. The goal of the home health care nurse has been interventions toward decrease of symptoms and a return to the previous level of function.

The third idea of health, the adaptive model, adds the goal of effective interaction with the physical and social environment. Although free of disease, individuals' failure to demonstrate effective social functioning would constitute illness. Positive adaptation could be demonstrated in many ways, individually or not, and in relation to disease or not. One example, in relation to the APHA/PHN statement on the definition of public health nursing would be to include consumer representatives in the planning of health services. These consumers could provide, through their work on the planning, a means to interact effectively with their environment.

The fourth, and most inclusive idea of health, is the eudaemonistic model that health extends to general well-being and self-realization. This model is consistent with the definition of health contained in the Constitution of the World Health Organization (WHO) where health is: "A state of complete physical, mental, and social well-being and not merely the absence of disease or infirmity." Whatever utopian threads are present, this goal of health need not be seen as unachievable. For some, it is a goal represented in the contemporary consumer health movement. For the community as a whole, while probably not completely achievable due to a lack of resources, this concept is helpful because it directs practitioners toward what health could be.

Conclusion

The participation of nursing in the determination of home health care services to be delivered and in the style of organization will influence the actual care of the home health population in important ways. Nursing, in its partnership with home care patients and their families, can facilitate positive goals for health. Through political and advocacy efforts, nursing must work to fulfill its vision of health. Nursing, because of its experience in the role of home health provider, and because of its ability to work with patients and families toward health goals, must demonstrate a decisive and powerful role in the rapidly changing field of home health care.

References

American Nurses Association. 1973. *Standards.* Kansas City, MO: American Nurses Association.

American Nurses Association. 1980. *A conceptual model of community health nursing.* Kansas City, MO: American Nurses Association.

American Association of Retired Persons. 1985. *A profile of older Americans.* Washington, DC: American Association of Retired Persons.

American Public Health Association. 1982. The definition and role of public health nursing practice in the delivery of health care. *American Journal of Public Health* 72:210-212.

Buhler-Wilkerson, K. 1983. False dawn: The rise and decline of public health nursing in America, 1900-1930. In *Nursing history: New perspectives, new possibilities,* ed. E. G. Lagemann, 89-106. New York: Teachers College Press.

Dock, L. L., and A. M. Stewart. 1925. *A short history of nursing: From the earliest times to the present day,* 2nd ed. New York: G. P. Putnam's Sons.

McNamara, E. 1982. Home care: Hospitals rediscover comprehensive home care. *Hospitals* 56(21):60-66.

Roberts, D. E., and J. Heinrich. 1985. Public health nursing comes of age. *American Journal of Public Health* 75:1162-1172.

Rosen, G. 1958. *A history of public health.* New York: MD Publications, Inc.

Smith, J. A. 1981. The idea of health: A philosophical inquiry. *Advances in Nursing Science* 3(3):43-50.

Smith, J. A. 1983. *The idea of health: Implications for the nursing professional.* New York: Teachers College Press.

Chapter Two

Types of Agencies

The Home Health Agency
Judith Baigis Smith and Kathleen Williams

Historical Overview

The informal sympathetic care of the sick in their homes by relatives and friends has a very long history indeed. The delivery of systematic nursing care in the home, based on the best available knowledge of the natural history of disease, is a much more recent undertaking and is a result of Nightingale's program of secular scientific education for nurses (Smith 1983, 16). Admiring the skills of the "Nightingale" nurses, William Rathbone supported philanthropic projects aimed at the sick poor in Liverpool. The "Nightingale" nurses ran and staffed some of the projects (Woodham-Smith 1970, 346-347). This notion of delivering skilled nursing services to the sick poor was also developing in the United States.

Philanthropists in this country provided funds for the start-up of voluntary organizations, forerunners of our visiting nurse associations (VNA), with trained nurses hired to deliver home nursing services similar to their English counterparts. As local health departments developed and expanded in the early years of the twentieth century, health officers in charge of these so-called official agencies, also added nurses to their staffs. One of the nursing responsibilities was the delivery of services in the home. By the middle part of this century, a number of these voluntary and official agencies "combined" their resources to varying degrees in order to streamline their operations, and thus decrease overhead, costs, and service duplication. Such organizations are known, not surprisingly, as combination agencies.

In 1947, another innovative service model was instituted. E. M. Bluestone, a physician at Montefiore Hospital in the Bronx, introduced the notion of hospital-based home care. Patients discharged from that hospital were entitled to a wide range of nursing, social, and other related services all delivered in their own homes (Cherkasky 1949, 163-166). Such an arrangement, a health care institution operating a department of home care, is not limited to hospitals any longer. Rehabilitation centers and skilled nursing facilities also offer home health services. These departments of home care are referred to as institution-based agencies. In contrast, those agencies not part of an institution are referred to as freestanding.

Recent History

By the mid-1960s, there were approximately 1,200 of the aforementioned agencies delivering home health services (Mundinger 1983, 142), most of which were paid for by donations through structures like the local community chests and by the recipients of the care. The passage of Medicare, and to a lesser extent, Medicaid in the mid-1960s spurred the growth of the home health industry because these federal insurance programs ensure a stable source of income for the agencies eligible to participate in them. The growth of another type of agency for the delivery of home health services, the private agency, was further stimulated in 1982 when Congress and the Health Care Finance Administration (HCFA) opened up home health care to the for-profit sector for Medicare reimbursement. Table 2-1 shows the effect of the Medicare program on the growth in numbers of home health agencies during the past two decades. Since 1982, the growth of the proprietary agencies have been pronounced, over 75%. These proprietary agencies now comprise over 46% of the Medicare-certified home health agencies listed in the table. While the increase in the numbers of hospital-based home care agencies has been steady over time, the growth spurt between 1984 and 1986 has been due to the passage of the prospective payment system by Congress. Increasing numbers of acute care hospitals have been diversifying in order to broaden their revenue base and home health care has been one of the areas targeted for this diversification (Ginzberg 1984, 112). No one knows the number of noncertified agencies but the assumption made is that there are at least as many noncertified as there are certified agencies (Hoyer 1986). These noncertified agencies like homemaker-home health aide agencies, provide a variety of services under contract with the certified agencies.

This chapter provides an outline of the similarities and differences among these types of home health agencies (voluntary, official, private). They are similar in administrative structure and sources of funding. The major differences among the aforementioned types of agencies is one of positioning for tax purposes, and financial control or ownership.

Table 2-1 Medicare-Certified Health Agencies (1967-1986)*

Month	Year	Total	VNA	Combi-nation	Official	Hospital	Proprietary	Private Nonprofit
March	1967	1714	549	93	939	133	0	0
December	1977	2459	503	43	1242	281	81	309
July	1982	3346	520	55	1232	481	471	587
July	1984	4476	523	57	1231	691	1255	719
July 12	1986	5846	510	62	1192	1341	1915	826
Degree of change		4132	-39	-31	+253	+1208	+1915	+826

Source: Health Care Finance Administration via National Association for Home Care, Washington, DC, mimeographed, August 1986.

The numbers do not include categories of "rehab, SNF, and other" listed in the original table.

Financial Concerns

The phrase, not-for-profit is a designation that exempts organizations from taxation on profits or excess of income under Section 501 of the Internal Revenue Code of 1954. This excess is put back into the organization and no part of the net earnings can be used for the private benefit of owners, partners, or share holders. Thus, a voluntary organization like a VNA or a community-owned hospital would usually be not-for-profit. If a not-for-profit organization wants to engage in activities which are intended to make a profit or surplus which is shared or distributed, it would have to form holding companies or separate corporate entities to deal with those profit-making actions. Many VNAs and hospitals are doing this in today's competitive market.

The term for-profit or profit-making is also a designation for tax purposes. Agencies with this designation are called proprietary agencies and they are not eligible for tax exemption under Section 501 of the Internal Revenue Code. It must be remembered that such designations for tax purposes are not true differentiations of financial status. For example, all business organizations (voluntary and private) must make profits or at least have income equal to expenses in order to continue to exist.

Phrases like "governmental agency, nongovernmental, private, church-affiliated, etc." all refer to control or ownership, and not positioning for tax purposes. The health department is an example of an official governmental agency created to perform specified public functions, like drinking water purification and services, like public health nursing. It is maintained from revenues such as taxes, and fees collected from the people who are benefitting from its services or functions. Within this context then, a community-owned agency would usually be not-for-profit, but a privately owned organization like a home health agency could be either for-profit or not-for-profit.

Scope of Home Care

Home care is one of the many service components in the arena of long-term care, although it is not limited only to long-term care. Other service components of long-term care include for example, nursing homes, programs for substance abusers, the mentally retarded, the occupationally disabled, and the handicapped. In other words, many different age and population groups require continuing care.

Within this long-term care context however, the phrase home health care is used in two ways. On the one hand, it is used to refer to the range of in-home services provided to chronically ill people over a long period of time. On the other hand, it is also used to refer to the Medicare-reimbursed home-based services which are primarily for the acutely ill elderly and which are skilled, short-term, intermittent (Moyer 1986,7). Regardless of how home health is defined, however, nursing care is the foundation of the entire system.

Range of Home Health Agencies

The Medicare Conditions of Participation for Home Health Agencies define a home health agency as "a public agency or private organization... primarily engaged in providing skilled nursing services and other therapeutic services." (*Federal Register*

1968, 12901; 1973, 18978) Common to the certified home health agencies, since it is required for participation in the Medicare program is the Professional Advisory Committee. This group of professional persons establishes policies and governs the services provided by the home health agency. Appropriate professional discipline representation is required in addition to a minimum of one physician and one registered nurse. This committee must review the agency's policies on an annual basis and meet frequently to advise the agency on professional issues.

Governmental Agencies

Governmental ("Official") home health agencies are "created and given their power through statutes enacted by legislators." (Stewart 1979, 25) Home health services are frequently provided by the nursing divisions of state or local health departments. The organizational structure within the nursing divisions varies among agencies, with some agencies opting to have their public health nurses include their home health clients within their overall public health caseload. Other governmental agencies choose to form home health teams within their nursing departments whose primary function is to provide home health services. Combinations of these two approaches are seen even within a single health district. In the Commonwealth of Virginia, for example, each health district is certified as a separate home health agency, with several local health departments comprising that health district. These local health departments may have a combination of both public health nurses and home health team nurses providing home health services.

Governmental agencies usually provide home health services such as disease prevention, health promotion, communicable disease investigation, environmental health services, as well as maternal child health and family planning services.

Fiscal responsibility for the governmental home health agency rests with the city, county, or state governmental units or a combination of such organizations. The overall county-city-state budget restrictions can directly influence the provision of health services in a particular area. Home health caseloads of governmental agencies frequently include a disproportionate number of indigent patients since the agency cannot refuse services based on the client's ability to pay. There is a growing trend throughout the country for governmental agencies to decrease or eliminate the provision of home health services. This growing disinterest may be due to the indigent client issue as well as other politically motivated issues which influence the types of health services provided by a governmental agency. Many more governmental agencies are focusing on the more traditional public health services so we may in the future see a decline of government-sponsored, Medicare-certified home health agencies.

Voluntary Agencies

Home health agencies which do not depend on state and local tax revenues but are financed primarily with non-tax funds such as donations, endowments, United Way contributions, and third-party insurance providers (Medicare, Medicaid, Blue Cross) are referred to as voluntary agencies, such as the VNAs.

Voluntaries are governed by a Board of Directors of interested individuals, frequently, respected members of the surrounding community or service area. These agencies are considered to be "community-based" agencies since they provide services within a fairly well-defined geographic location or community. In recent years, however, traditional VNA boundaries have become less distinct due to increased competition for clients. In the past, voluntary agencies could depend on virtually all of the home health clients within their own catchment areas, but the growth of proprietary and institution-based home health agencies has now eroded their traditional referral base. The relationships between neighboring VNAs has turned in many instances from one of cooperation to one of competition.

Private Agencies

Private home health agencies can be for-profit or not-for-profit organizations. Some proprietary (for-profit) agencies participate in the Medicare home health program as part of national chains, administered through a corporate headquarters.

The entry of proprietary agencies into the home health care market has been marked with controversy, with some traditional providers claiming that their interest in providing services is primarily monetary (Stewart 1979, 36). Many proprietary agencies have countered this criticism with the statement that they have expanded service availability. This increased availability of home care services has led to the relaxation of rigid service policies held by some traditional agencies, such as VNAs and has increased the overall access to home health care (Stewart 1979).

Recently, there has been a merger of several proprietary chain providers which may forecast a consolidation of the proprietary home health industry into larger, national firms. These larger companies are able to generate sufficient revenues to cover overhead costs (Anderson 1986, 118).

While revenues are generated by some proprietary agencies through third-party payors such as Medicare and Blue Cross, other proprietaries rely on private-pay clients. These "private-pay" agencies offer services such as private-duty nursing to both acutely and chronically ill patients, a difference from most Medicare-certified providers, who provide most of their services to clients who have had a recent acute change in their medical condition. These private services are often on extended hours (2 to 24 hours) rather than on a per-visit basis (O'Malley 1986, 26). Many agencies also provide hospital staffing services.

Institution-Based Agencies

Home health agencies operating as departments in sponsoring health care organizations are certified under Medicare and hold a separate provider number but they are governed by the sponsoring organization's Board of Trustees or Directors.

In the past, home health services provided by institution-based providers consisted of "intensive level" services, intended for those clients requiring multiple discipline services and supplies. The client case mix of today's institution-based agencies reflects the change to a more balanced caseload, with clients requiring differing degrees of services. The principal source of referrals for these agencies is the inpatient population of the facility, with the discharge planner being the coordinator of services and case finder of potential home health clients.

The philosophy of the institution-based agency usually coincides with that of the sponsoring organization. Good continuity of care is frequently cited by these agencies as their primary advantage over other types of home health agencies (Stewart 1979, 39). This continuity can be "sold" to the medical staff of the institution by promoting the fact that the home care of the physicians' clients is being coordinated by persons familiar with the physicians and the institution.

A fiscal advantage of institution-based home health providers is the allowance by Medicare of the inclusion of a percentage of administrative and general overhead in the calculation of the visit costs. The Medicare home health reimbursement system also recognizes the higher costs of office space in hospitals and permits an "add-on" amount in the calculation of the visit costs. Another advantage enjoyed by the institution-based home health agency is the ability to draw from the resources of the other departments of the facility for service provision as well as formal and informal consultation services.

Hospice

An agency in which "services are provided by a medically supervised interdisciplinary team of professionals and volunteers" for terminally ill clients is defined as a hospice by the National Hospice Organization (1984). There are variations among home care hospice programs in their structure and staffing, but all profess to foster the provision of palliative and supportive services to the patient and family after the demise of the client. This service is unique to hospice agencies since other home health agencies cease services upon the death of the client.

The hospice concept was imported from Britain into the United States at New Haven in the mid-1970s and has grown to over 1,400 programs. Hospice services are reimbursed by many health insurance plans such as Blue Cross-Blue Shield as well as by the home hospice service Medicare benefit provided in the Tax Equity and Fiscal Responsibility Act of 1982 (Cunningham 1985, 124). Many hospice agencies have chosen *not* to obtain Medicare certification because of the current reimbursement schedule outlined by the regulations.

Structurally, hospices can be institution-based, owned by or affiliated with a certified home health agency, or be an independent agency.

Homemaker-Home Health Aide Agencies

Agencies providing homemaker-home health aide services are frequently private agencies in which clients pay for the home care services or the care is financed by private insurance policies (Stewart 1979, 36). These agencies can provide home health aides who are "Medicare-certified," that is, they have completed a Medicare-approved home health aide course of study (usually 40 hours in length). With these "certified" aides, homemaker-home health aide agencies are able to contract with Medicare-certified home health agencies who, in turn, are reimbursed by Medicare for the home health aide services. The Medicare-certified agency pays the homemaker-home health aide agency directly on an hourly basis. Such contracts are lucrative since they are guaranteed income for the homemaker-home health aide agency.

The distinction between homemakers and home health aides can at times be difficult to ascertain since both functions are often provided by a single employee. Homemakers function primarily as housecleaners while the principal duties of home health aides are in the area of personal care (such as bathing). Other more complex services such as range of motion exercises can be performed by the home health aide after proper instruction by a registered nurse.

Homemaker-home health aide agencies usually provide periodic continuing education sessions for their personnel. In addition, on-site performance evaluations are conducted by professionals such as registered nurses.

Other Home Health Care Providers

In addition to the types of home health agencies discussed in this chapter, there are home health services provided by durable medical equipment companies (DMEs), high-technology service companies (ventilators, total parenteral nutrition, etc.), home telephone reassurance programs, and companion services, to name a few. Many of these organizations refer to themselves, even in their titles, as "Home Care." With the increase in consumer awareness and demand for home care services, and as a result of the "aging" of the American population, all types of health care services provided in the home may blend with each other, thus creating even more confusion among consumers and professionals alike, about types of home health agencies.

Conclusion

The categorization of types of home health agencies has changed in the past two decades and the future may bring new organizational structures that are now beginning to evolve. These new alliances, formed mostly out of economic necessity, may continue to blur the distinctions between types of home health agencies, thus creating even more complexities with which a home health administrator must cope. Table 2-2 summarizes the preceding discussion of types of agencies, comparing each type of agency according to governing body, role of Professional Advisory Committee, client case mix and services provided, and revenue sources.

Table 2-2

	Governmental	Voluntary	Proprietary	Institution-Based	Hospice	Homemaker-Home Health Aide
Governing body	Local governmental units (Boards of Supervisors, Local Board of Health) by way of local health officer.	Board of Directors comprised of members of service area and local community.	Individual owner(s) or corporate headquarters (chain)	Sponsoring health organization's Board of Trustees	Board of Directors comprised of members of local community and service area (independent) or Board of Trustees of sponsoring health organization (institution-based)	Individual owner(s) or corporate headquarters (chain)
Role of professional advisory committee	Functions in advisory capacity as defined in Medicare regulations	Functions in advisory capacity as defined in Medicare regulations	Functions in advisory capacity as defined in Medicare regulations	Functions in advisory capacity as defined in Medicare regulations	Closely knit team of professionals and volunteers provide services as well as consultation	Usually no professional advisory committee; comply with appropriate Medicare personnel standards if contracted by a Medicare certified agency.

Table 2-2 continued.

	Governmental	Voluntary	Proprietary	Institution-Based	Hospice	Homemaker-Home Health Aide
Client case mix/services provided	Skilled home health clients; may have higher percent of indigents; also, provide public health services such as maternal-child health, family planning, environ-mental health.	Skilled home health clients of all ages; some screening activities such as health maintenance, other community health activities in senior centers, etc. services becoming more diverse.	Skilled home health clients of all ages: private duty services, hospital-staffing services.	Skilled home health clients of all ages; traditionally, clients have required more "intensive" services than community-based agency clients (this is changing).	Terminally ill clients (usually with less than a six-month life span prognosis), much involvement with significant others. Bereavement services also provided; volunteers used for services provided.	Skilled and un-skilled (custodial) home health clients of all ages; personal care and housekeeping services provided.
Revenue sources	Primarily from tax revenues, third party insurance payors (Medicare, Medical Assistance, Blue Cross-Blue Shield, etc.)	Donations (such as United Way), endowments, fundraising, third party insurance payors, private pay (usually on sliding fee basis)	Third party insurance payors, private pay	Third party insurance payors, private pay, donations, endowments, fund raising are usually in conjunction with sponsoring institution	Third party insurance payors (including Medicare hospice benefit), self-pay, donations, grants	Contract revenues from Medicare, certified home health agencies; private pay

A Case History: The New Proprietary Agency

E. Joyce Gould and Allan G. Ginsberg

The chief operating officer (COO)* of any organization is responsible for both its operational and financial survival. Successfully meeting this mandate is a prerequisite for fulfilling the agency's mission. Although for-profit and nonprofit organizations have similar services and similar missions (to fill a need in the community), the methods for measuring the performance of the COO and agency differ.

For the proprietary agency, profit can be viewed as a yardstick for measuring performance; profit is derived from successfully filling a need or void. For a nonprofit organization, benefit to the community is the criterion for determining success. For the former, profit is a concrete, easily identified and agreed upon measurement tool. For the nonprofit organization, the task of measuring success is more complex because there frequently are vague and divergent views on how to define "benefit to the community." The role of the COO is significantly influenced by these differences in defining success.

For the nonprofit agency, the COO must participate in an extensive round of board and committee meetings to gain input and support for all major decisions. This cumbersome process is necessary to ensure a reasonable amount of agreement and support so that any new course of action will be judged beneficial to the community it serves. With a clear mandate to produce a profit, the COO in a proprietary agency has a wider scope of authority which requires decisive action in dealing with the multitude of issues facing any home health agency.

The following description of developing and running a home health agency will illustrate the operational and funding differences which shape the role of the COO in a for-profit agency.

Planning Stage

United Medical Services, Inc. is a private corporation engaged in delivering a variety of quality medical and health services in a manner which enables community residents to easily obtain services and produces a profit for the company. Prior to 1981, United had two well-established businesses providing retail pharmacy services and medical and surgical supplies and equipment. As a dynamic organization, United views planning for the future as an essential ingredient for survival.

Planning is the critical factor in achieving organizational success. The planning cycle starts with the evaluation of all factors relevant to the particular venture or program under consideration. The first step is an assessment of the community (also called a market survey) to determine the types and amount of unmet needs. Once a need for service has been identified, there is another series of questions to answer. Does the service fit into the overall mission of the organization? Does the organization

---

* Chief operating officer (COO) will be used throughout this case history to identify the individual who is responsible for all day-to-day operations of a home health agency. Common titles for people in this position are: Administrator, Executive Director, President, Chief Executive Officer.

have the skills and abilities to meet the need? Is it financially feasible to deliver the service?

Changes in the Medicare regulations and the health care industry opened the door for United to begin planning to provide complete home care services. Since United's business was directed toward the aged, predictions of an increasing elderly population in the communities served by United clearly indicated a market for home care services. Evaluation of United's patient population revealed that they were not receiving these needed services. United's expansion into personal home care services was judged a natural extension consistent with the organization's mission.

Although the company possessed financial and managerial skills, it recognized the need to expand the management team to include experienced clinical managers. Investigation of the possibility of starting a home health agency required a year of research into the costs and benefits of providing the service. The financial decision to venture into this new area was based on the potential interrelationship among the three businesses: the inevitability of interdivisional referrals and the opportunity to offset fixed and variable expenses. The projected financial return on investment was analyzed and deemed acceptable.

Organizing Stage

Organizing the responsibilities, resources, and activities necessary to start and maintain a new service was the next phase toward achieving the goal of providing home health services. The governing body, three owners, had a vested and very personal interest in assuring the survival, growth, and marketability of the planned services. Therefore, the President, a health professional, was identified as the one responsible for organizing the necessary resources to bring this new venture to fruition. It required six months of intensive work to design and structure the home health agency. Start-up costs needed to be funded. Since it did not qualify for charitable donations or foundation grants, United capitalized this new venture by using financial reserves and bank loans.

A critical step in this stage of development was the hiring of a nurse consultant to assist in the creation of an organization which primarily delivers nursing care. The nurse consultant was responsible for drafting the administrative and clinical manuals to meet government requirements and United's expectations of efficient operation. The president of United reviewed and revised the manuals. After the nurse consultant and president agreed on the manuals, a multidisciplinary professional advisory board was appointed. Its first task was to review, revise, and accept the administrative and clinical manuals as the policies to guide agency operations.

In the course of designing the manuals, the role of the COO was defined as directing the agency. The president of United assumed the newly created position of Administrator. The next step was to seek Medicare certification. The administrator enlisted the help of the nurse consultant in preparing for the certification survey. Following successful completion of this hurdle, the administrator and nurse consultant began the search for a nurse to manage day-to-day clinical operations.

For any organization, hiring the right person for the job is one of the most important factors for success. Therefore, time was invested in selecting the appropriate person for the Director of Patient Services. With the advent of this new manager, the process of delineating tasks between the administrator and director began.

Operating Stage

Authority is very focused in the top management of a proprietary agency. The governing body delegates authority to the COO to act with a great deal of independence in a wide range of areas. Responsibility is viewed as twofold: to the community, on the one hand, for the services provided and to the investors, on the other hand, for a reasonable return on their financial investment. Authority in the nonprofit agency is diffused among the COO, the governing body, and the community. The agency is responsible to the community for both services and financial solvency. These differences are reflected in the decision-making processes used in daily operations of a for-profit agency.

At United, the governing body (owners) delegated authority to the administrator for all major and minor daily administrative and clinical decisions. Delegation of authority among the members of top management was a process of ongoing negotiation. This stage required a commitment to establishing communication and trust. Cooperation and confrontation were equally important in establishing a successful collaborative working relationship between the Administrator and Director of Patient Services.

This evolving relationship encompassed many changes in allocating responsibility for certain tasks. This process eventually resulted in the establishment of the new position, Assistant Administrator for Clinical Services, which was assumed by the director. With this change came a broadening of responsibility and a refocusing on positioning the agency to meet anticipated and unanticipated changes occurring in the home health industry.

Within this setting, the professionals on the Advisory Board functioned primarily as overseers and guides for clinical management. Their influence on day-to-day administrative operations was indirect.

Accepting the first patient launched the exciting and demanding juggling act of striking a balance between service delivery capabilities and community outreach efforts. Hiring and training staff required a significant investment of time and money. Predicting the need for staff to match the demand for service is, at best, an inexact science. At United, this necessitated that the Director of Patient Services establish a communication link with the professional representatives of the parent company. These representatives educated individuals and providers in the community about the company's services. A process of trial and error finally yielded a workable system to lessen the possibility of generating a demand for service that could not be met. Despite our best efforts, on several occasions, it became necessary to refuse referrals because we lacked sufficient staff to properly serve the patient.

An increased ability to match the fluctuations in demand evolved with experience and growth. The demand for home care services, however, continues to vary based on many external forces such as the advent of DRGs and the increase in the number of agencies providing home care. Management must be geared to expand and contract staff to meet these changing needs. For United, this meant establishing a core of full- and part-time salaried staff, utilizing contract staff to meet increased need.

Expansion necessitated reinstitution of the entire planning cycle to evaluate the need for additional layers of management. The agency has found that organizing management functions in cycles of decentralization and centralization is most effective in meeting the changing demands of a growing organization. The creation of a middle management layer for both clinical and administrative activities occurred over a two-year period.

For staff from middle management level down, there is no significant difference in their job functions in a for-profit or nonprofit agency. The adherence to professional standards of clinical practice are the same for all nurses and therapists regardless of where they practice. The daily tasks of office management are similar for both types of agencies.

Once the agency had all the daily routine clinical and administrative operations running smoothly, there was an opportunity to evaluate underutilized resources of the clinical and managerial staff. Again the planning and evaluation cycle was initiated to determine maximum use of their knowledge to benefit patients and enhance the agency's position in the home care industry.

The first project involved the development of standardized home health nursing care plans. This endeavor was spearheaded by the Director of Patient Services with extensive input from one of the staff nurses. As this quality assurance tool was being developed, it was shared with the professional community via presentations at local, state, and national educational programs, and via publications. The overall design of the care plans was geared to meet the twin objectives of improving patient care and reducing charting time.

The constant need for home care to address problems surrounding medication management for the homebound elderly revealed that a unique and unused resource was present in the agency. The administrator, a practicing registered pharmacist, was an untapped source of information who could assist the nursing staff in improving medication management for patients. Resources were allocated to develop a model for consultation with the pharmacist. Concurrently, a clinical rotation for pharmacy students was developed to foster interdisciplinary collaboration between nurses and pharmacists. This emerging role for pharmacists has generated interest when presented at state and national professional meetings.

Ongoing evaluation of market needs revealed a dearth of home care services for the psychiatric patient. The nursing supervisor at United had extensive education and experience in providing psychiatric nursing care in an inpatient setting. Utilizing her clinical expertise to meet specific patient problems led to the realization that this resource could be developed into a specialty program. Adapting clinical interventions to the home care setting required considerable clinical skill as well as managerial expertise to ascertain funding availability, required resources, and matching the two.

Reassessment of available resources and renegotiation of roles are integral parts of maintaining efficient agency operation and allows for development of new programs. The increased autonomy of the COO in the proprietary agency creates the flexibility to act quickly in moving through the planning and implementation phases.

Conclusion

Overall, both profit and nonprofit agencies have the same ideology: to fulfill a need in the community. There are operational and financial differences in the functioning of the two types of agencies. Managerial tasks are the same in any organization. Constancy of purpose tempered with flexibility to meet changing circumstances are keys to success. Starting and maintaining a proprietary home care agency illustrates the influences that shape the role of the COO.

Home Health Care in the Hospital Setting

Lori R. Sherman

When Medicare was first enacted in 1965, Congress added a limited home nursing coverage to its basic hospital benefit. Following hospital discharge, a beneficiary was allowed up to 100 home health visits a year under Part A; another 100 visits were available under Part B. The emphasis was on medical treatment of acute illness. To be eligible, a beneficiary had to be homebound and in need of skilled nursing. On the other hand, his need for care had to be "intermittent" rather than continuous, otherwise it was assumed he would be more appropriately placed in a nursing home.

Since that time, major demographic and technical changes have forced a reassessment of public policy. In the 1970s, even larger numbers of the elderly were sent to nursing homes, at great cost and dubious benefit. At the same time, hospitals were reducing their lengths of stay, causing patients to be discharged at earlier stages of recovery and advances in medical technology were making it possible to perform more complex procedures safely at home. Congress, in the 1980 Omnibus Reconciliation Act, responded to these changed circumstances by expanding the home care benefit and eliminating the prior hospitalization requirement and 100-visit limit, effective July 1981. At the same time, Congress removed restrictions on proprietary agencies' participation in the program. Home care was expected to take its place as an integral part of the health care continuum and a cost-effective substitute for institutionalization. Even so, the home care benefit, though still a miniscule fraction of the Medicare budget (approximately 3%) is its fastest growing component.

Hospital management of home health is by no means a new concept. Looking back to 1961, a United States Public Health Service survey reported that of the 46 home health programs then in existence, 40 were hospital-based (Littauer 1962). Today, care in the home is becoming even more accepted, primarily due to restricted reimbursement for inpatient care, and hospitals are therefore looking to home health as an attractive market to develop.

This is further supported by Health Care Financing Administration statistics, which demonstrate rapid growth in the number of hospital-based home health agencies in the United States (Table 2-3). Major reasons for increased hospital interest are the hospitals' unique position to address some of the basic impediments to home health utilization and the need to control this supplementary service which can significantly affect inpatient utilization. Length of stay is a particular concern nationally, as the country moves toward a "cost-per-case" method of reimbursement. Added to

Table 2-3 Medicare-certified home health agencies

Provider type	February 1984	February 1985	May 1986	Gain or loss (February 1985- May 1986)
Hospital-based	585	937	1,312	+375
Proprietary	1,018	1,626	1,924	+298
SNF-based	135	173	126	- 47
Rehab-based	19	22	19	- 3
Private not-for-profit	673	757	830	+ 73
Combination	58	60	62	+ 2
VNA	519	526	514	+ 12
Official (county agencies)	1,230	1,223	1,202	- 21
Other	32	19	4	- 15
Total	4,282	5,343	5,993	+650

Source: Health Care Financing Administration.

this are the economic incentives to broaden the institution's revenue base intrinsic to prospective payment.

Additional impetus for hospital-based home care can be cited:

- Such a program is consistent with the hospital's desire to assure the best possible service to its patients and medical staff. The patient will benefit from an enhanced quality and continuity of care, no longer being shifted from the hospital to another organization when home care is needed. To this end, a patient and his or her family and physician do not have to leave the umbrella of the health system to receive needed health care services. The hospital will be able to set quality standards, maintaining them in a consistent manner from the hospital to the home setting. When patients are referred to outside organizations, the quality cannot be controlled. For example, the hospital can orient its home care program to the needs of its own patients, assuring that those referred receive prompt attention following discharge. Patient outcome and satisfaction will not only keep the patient within the system, but it will also influence the patient's return to the system when needed. The physician's perspective on quality of care is also essential. In addition, the service standards and continuity of care established during the inpatient stay will not be interrupted.

- There will be a direct linkage between the home health staff and the physicians. Such a program can only serve to improve communications between all involved disciplines at the time of referral and during the ongoing management of the case. Further, the medical staff will have input to and monitor the professional policies and quality of home health services.

- A hospital-based program can serve as a means of diversifying and expanding revenue as well as assuming a significant portion of the hospital's overhead expense. Services provided generate revenues presently lost to the institution. These revenues will support the direct and indirect expenses of operating the program. If the hospital elects to make the program a department of the hospital, a significant portion of the hospital overhead will be allocated to home care and reimbursed there. With home health patients being predominately Medicare, these services are cost-reimbursed. A surplus may be generated from services to patients covered by commercial insurance and self-pay. This can offset losses which may be incurred on services which are not reimbursable, but are provided because the institution considers them important to the totality of its patient care program (i.e., free services for the indigent; sliding scale fee services).

- Hospital-based programs can effectively integrate discharge planning to further continuity of care. A home health intake nurse actively participates in ongoing discharge planning and follows potential home health candidates from the day of hospital admission. This key staff member also assures that referrals to home health are appropriate; arranges for various services that need to be in place when the patient returns home (i.e., scheduling of personnel, ordering and arranging delivery of durable medical equipment). Conversely, when the patient is referred to an outside agency, many of these services are not arranged for until the visiting nurse makes the first home visit.

- A hospital-based home health program enhances the image of the hospital in the community. Hospital-based home health departments are viable programs that can be well received by the patient and community, once the program is known. In this sense, the marketing gains outweigh themselves, with the hospital and medical staff receiving continual recognition.

- A home health program can be an integral component of the hospital's strategic plan and marketing plan. It may assist in improving or maintaining the hospital's competitive edge with other area hospitals (See Exhibit 2-1).

Organization as a Hospital Department or Freestanding Agency

A hospital has the option of establishing the home health program as a department of the hospital or as a freestanding agency. As a hospital department, the program is allocated indirect cost from the sponsoring facility. The amount is determined via the Medicare step-down and in some cases is higher than would be incurred if the organization were freestanding. In many instances, the step-down results in the provider-based organization being charged for some services from which the agency derives little or no benefit. With the consent of the intermediary, Medicare docs permit the use of alternate cost-finding methodologies which produce a more precise cost allocation to the home health program. While in theory this can resolve the indirect cost problem, the reality is that alternate methodologies often do not serve the best interest of the entire hospital entity.

Exhibit 2-1. Incentives/Objectives for Hospitals Entry into Home Health Care

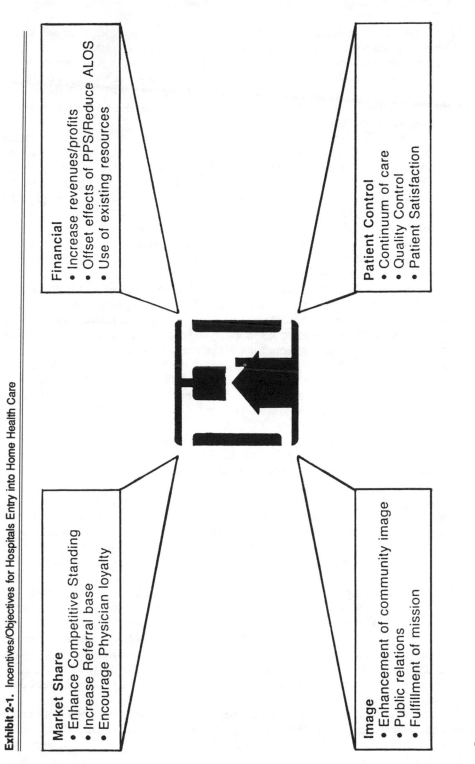

Financial
- Increase revenues/profits
- Offset effects of PPS/Reduce ALOS
- Use of existing resources

Patient Control
- Continuum of care
- Quality Control
- Patient Satisfaction

Market Share
- Enhance Competitive Standing
- Increase Referral base
- Encourage Physician loyalty

Image
- Enhancement of community image
- Public relations
- Fulfillment of mission

Source: Louden & Company

The Federal Government has recognized the higher indirect expense which provider-based home health programs experience as being an artifact of the cost-finding process. They allow provider-based agencies higher cost ceilings. Although freestanding providers have contested this (and demanded a single schedule of limits for provider-based and freestanding agencies), the Health Care Financing Administration has issued new limits. These limits provide an adjustment for hospital-based programs reflecting the additional overhead allocation.

There is a significant advantage to the home health program being a department of the hospital, particularly during the early phase of development. This relates to the ease with which the program can draw upon hospital support without having to account in detail for services used. There is no need to establish contracts covering the use of hospital staff or services on a regular or as-needed basis, such as physical therapy. (Staffing issues will be addressed later on in this chapter.) It also cushions the organization against cash flow problems until such time as a regular revenue stream can be established or home health department be qualified for participation in Periodic Interim Payment. Conceivably, an agency may not see its first Medicare dollar until six months after start-up.

The reimbursement mechanism differs among funding sources and is closely requested by Medicare to prevent fraud and abuse. Briefly, an agency may bill for services rendered once the intermediary has authorized eligibility for care. This ongoing process may take from one week to six months, depending on delays in billing, desk review by the intermediary for appropriateness, incomplete paperwork and so forth.

The concern is that the cost per visit not exceed the Medicare cost cap due to the allocation of indirect cost. For it to be advisable to establish the home health program as a freestanding provider, the amount of overhead reduction must be greater than the amount by which the cost caps would be reduced if the home health program were freestanding.

If, in a desire to reduce the cost per visit, the program is set up as a freestanding provider, the hospital should recognize that it will have to provide all of the legal, accounting, insurance, and managerial support associated with all independent business. The services drawn from the hospital would have to be costed and charged to the home health provider. While this option should be reviewed when the program has significantly grown, an independent organization may not be a significant advantage in the first (or second) year of operation. It is important to be aware that regardless of the fact that the independent provider may be owned by the hospital, once organized as a separate entity, it is subject to the lower cost caps which apply to freestanding providers.

With a freestanding agency structure, the hospital could elect to establish the program as either nonprofit of proprietary. A proprietary is permitted to include return on equity on its cost report as part of the allowable cost to be reimbursed by Medicare. Like hospitals, this report is excluded from nonprofit organizations. Due to the minor investment associated with the establishment of a home health provider, this is not a significant consideration. It only becomes pertinent where the home health program makes commitments in terms of ownership of office space, vehicles, and data processing equipment.

The decision, therefore, as to organizational form is made based upon state reimbursement policies as they impact on the parent organization, Certificate of Need rules when they differ for provider-based and freestanding, size of program, and the objectives of the sponsoring organization.

Finances

The start-up costs for the agency can be an expensive proposition and a substantial amount of capital is required. If the program is to be set up within the existing hospital, start-up costs can be significantly lowered by the sharing of facilities, office equipment and supplies. Whatever expenses are encountered during this time will be depreciated over five years.

The following expenditures are by no means all-inclusive, but list the likely start-up expenses:

- Desks
- Chairs
- Typewriters
- Calculator
- Computer hardware
- Office supplies
- Copier (or access to one)
- Telephone installation
- Bookshelf
- File cabinet

Once potential expenditures are identified, the hospital's financial advisor will need to develop a budget. Developing a budget will help the agency to plan for the growth required to cover all fixed and variable expenses. It is an essential tool that can be carefully scrutinized to determine an agency's viability.

A cash flow budget should be projected to identify monthly cash and total capital needs over a one-year period. Such projections should take into consideration cost report reconciliations. A new agency may have difficulty complying with the regulations because of a general lack of experience with home health care reimbursement mechanisms and requirements. To this end, the hospital may find the agency with a high percentage of visit denials and delayed payments.

After the decision is made to establish the program as a department of the hospital or as a freestanding agency, contact must be made to the appropriate state agency (usually State Health Department) to ascertain if there are any state licensure or certificate of need requirements. In addition, the home health program must receive separate Medicare certification and provider number than the hospital. (The same holds true if the hospital wishes to establish a Medicare-certified hospice program). Therefore, the hospital will need to request an application packet for Medicare home health certification from the State Health Department.

At this time, it is advisable to contact the state home health association to obtain any materials they have published on the home health requirements applicable in their state and often surrounding states. Most state associations are affiliated with the National Association for Home Care. The Pennsylvania Association of Home Health Agencies, Florida Association of Home Health Agencies, and California Association for Health Services at Home all have publications on quality assurance and standards, for example.

The hospital must further decide on the model of the agency. Among the most prevalent are the development of:

- A hospital-based home health agency which provides all of its own services.

- A hospital-based agency which provides some services directly and contracts for other services.

- A hospital-based home care department which affords the hospital control of patient care while contracting services with an existing home health agency.

- A joint venture with a home health agency.

- A contractual relationship with a home health agency.

Organizational Structure

The Medicare-certified home health department depicted throughout the remainder of this chapter is one that is hospital-based and considered a department within the structure of a medical center, with its staff hired as hospital employees. As part of the hospital, the program is accredited by JCAH and is reviewed for accreditation during the reviewer's visit to the hospital. The department, as well as the hospital, is certified by Medicare and Medicaid.

The initial inpetus for home care was based on the hospital's recognition of the need for continued care among patients who were being discharged from the hospital. Also recognized was the need for an appropriate and timely flow of information to be shared among providers as patients moved from one level of care to another.

The objective was to avoid fragmentation and to achieve the goal of fulfilling each patient's total health care needs by providing a complete package of integrated health care services in the patient's place of residence.

The department was integrated within the hospital's organization chart (Exhibit 2-2). An organizational structure was appropriately designed to implement the home care program and establish lines of responsibility and accountability, which is reviewed at least annually and revised as necessary.

To ensure the efficient operation of the program and the delivery of services which comply with quality standards, the responsibility for administration of the home care program was delegated by the hospital CEO to a member of the hospital administrative staff. The role of this administrative link is to assist the home care department director with interfacing agency policies and procedures and those of the hospital. For example, operation details such as parking, use of photocopy machines, cafeteria privileges, as well as basic patient-related procedures such as interviewing

Exhibit 2-2 Home Care Program Organizational Chart

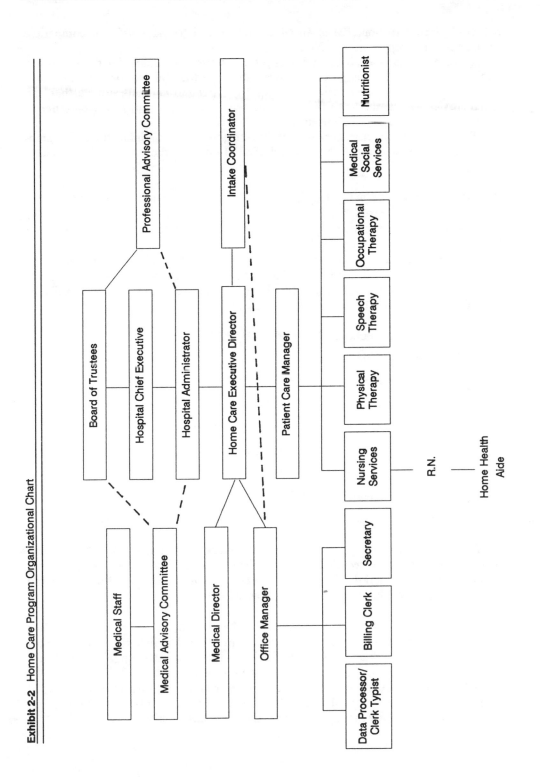

patients referred to home care, all which are crucial to maintaining a compatible working relationship.

The administrator designated in this setting is also responsible for the social service department. This supports cohesive interdepartmental working relationships while allowing for comprehensive administrative direction and support. Further, the social service and home care offices are located in close proximity of each other to foster optimum working relationships.

The executive director worked closely with the hospital administrator in establishing the following committees during the initial phase of the program implementation:

Professional Advisory Committee. Professional Advisory Committee (PAC) functions as an advisory and evaluative body to the program. The committee reviews and assesses the scope of services to determine the appropriateness, effectiveness, and adequacy of program services and objectives. During the initial period, the PAC was responsible for reviewing and approving the medical record system (including all forms and maintenance procedures), administrative policies, and professional practice manuals required for state licensure, Medicare certification, and to insure compliance with JCAH standards. The nine manuals include:

A. Administrative Policy and Procedure Manual

B. Nursing Procedure Manual

C. Physical Therapy Procedure Manual

D. Occupational Therapy Procedure Manual

E. Speech and Language Therapy Procedure Manual

F. Social Work Service Procedure Manual

G. Home Health Aide Procedure Manual

H. Operations Manual

I. Medical Relationship Policies and Emergency Procedures Manual

The committee meets quarterly, with its members appointed yearly by the governing body. Minutes are forwarded to the medical center's Medical Board, Joint Conferences Committee, and the Board of Trustees. Subcommittees were further created to deal with quality assurance review and program evaluation.

Medical Advisory Committee. The Medical Advisory Committee is responsible for advising the program in the area of professional practice. The five to seven physicians selected represent different medical specialties included on the hospital medical staff and submit minutes to the PAC and CEO of the hospital.

A key to the success of this program is the awareness, satisfaction and support of the medical staff. The hospital's success in developing that support will impact significantly on how quickly the home health activity reaches its potential.

A home health program that is part of the hospital is responsible to its medical staff. They are consulted regarding the program's professional policies and can monitor implementation of these policies. Medical staff and agency staff communication and collaboration are facilitated with an on-site agency. This direct collaboration leads to an improved quality of patient care and physician confidence in the program.

The Medical Advisory Committee plays a role in shaping the policy of the agency. It can be used as a vehicle for involving the medical staff in the planning process, educating them as to the direction planned for the program, and building support for this activity within the medical community. Initially, it was this committee that established the protocol and procedure granting those physicians not on staff at the center, the temporary home health privileges for management of their patients.

Clinical Records Review Committee. Clinical Records Review Committee conducts ongoing review of home care clinical records to insure that established policies and standards are observed in providing services to patients. The committee meets quarterly and submits statistics, summary findings, and follow-up actions to the PAC.

Prior to the initiation of services, the director established cooperative operational relationships with other hospital departments (i.e., accounting, admissions, central supply, business services, nursing services, social services, communications). For example, the department's hours of operation are Monday through Friday, 8:30 a.m. to 4:30 p.m., with services available on a 7-day-per-week, 24-hour-per-day basis. From 4:30 p.m. to 8:30 a.m. during weekdays and on weekends and holidays, the on-call system is channeled through the hospital switchboard operator, who contacts the on-call home health staff.

In order to communicate understanding and stimulate support of the home care program throughout the hospital and among community agencies, the director continually participates in staff education, orientation meetings, and serves on the hospital discharge planning committee. This has aided the hospital staff in maintaining a clear understanding regarding the administration and appropriate use of the home care program, along with outlining the role each staff member has in supporting this program.

Staffing

The services offered by this program include nursing, physical, occupational, and speech therapy, medical social work, nutritional guidance, and home health aide. In addition, laboratory services are provided by the nursing staff. (Under Medicare guidelines, this is considered to be a hospital outpatient service and is billed as such.) The department arranges with local vendors for all medical and surgical equipment and supplies necessary for the care of the patient in the home.

Initially, the department's full-time staff consisted of the director, intake coordinator, patient care manager, three visiting nurses, and secretary. The hospital opted to provide home health aide services through a linkage with a community-based agency. In addition, interdepartmental arrangements were established to "share" therapy and social work services. This allowed for a more cost-effective operation during the initial period when limited numbers of specialized personnel are required. The home health department presently has its own staff and relies on the hospital staff only to balance peaks in workload or employee vacancies.

Therapy services are generally provided through the use of contractual employees. Such contracts incorporate those provisions specified in JCAH standards and Medicare conditions for home health agency provider certification.

All contract personnel must meet the hospital home care program job qualifications. In addition to signing a contract, each individual utilized should be thoroughly familiarized with all home care program policies and procedures applicable to their role as a member of the health care team.

The intake coordinator is an active participant in the discharge planning process and takes part in formal and informal multidisciplinary discharge planning rounds on patient units. The coordinator facilitates case finding as well as serves as the focus for the close coordination between the hospital and home health. It is this coordination and the linkage it forms with other health care professionals that is one of the significant advantages of having the home health program hospital-based. The coordinator becomes an active part of the hospital's program in educating the staff to discharge planning and patient care needs. Once the coordinator receives a referral, he plans, develops, and coordinates needed home care services for only those patients who will receive care by the agency. Some of these duties include insurance verification, preparing a written treatment and care plan approved by the attending physician, and ordering of durable medical equipment, transportation, and medical-surgical supplies.

Discharge planning rounds also prove beneficial to the hospital staff as the home care representative is able to provide a report about the home care progress of a newly readmitted patient. The rounds are also an excellent vehicle to review each patient's care with a focus on the posthospital period of illness, while the interdisciplinary team develops individualized patient plans. The hospital is therefore able to identify patients having disposition problems at the earliest opportunity, allowing time for planning and implementation. This type of continuity of care between hospital care and home care is even more crucial as prospective reimbursement impacts the length of hospital stay.

Once the intake coordinator assesses the need for services, all coordination is documented on the patient's hospital chart, on a home health narrative. This serves as an informative tool regarding planned home health services. It becomes a permanent part of the hospital record, and later accompanies the written referral (and other pertinent documents) to the home care department.

The coordinator meets with the patient care manager on a daily basis to provide both a verbal report and the above documents on all completed referrals. Patient care assignments are then established by the manager according to designated geographic areas. The care must be under the order of a physician and the patient must be essentially homebound.

The patient care manager is further responsible for the supervision and direction of home health staff in the provision of direct care, and the evaluation, planning, and initial coordination of patient services. This includes scheduled weekly conferences and periodic home visits of each staff nurse to provide guidance in effective patient care, evaluation of job performance, quality of care, and record review for general program effectiveness. Other visiting staff are also supervised.

The community health nurses' focus of care is on disease prevention and health maintenance, with the provision of quality nursing services. He also functions as the case manager. Case management established a system of appraisal, care planning, and care evaluations in the home care department. To this end, the written plan of action became imperative to ensure that tasks are carried out, that established standards are complied with, and that there is continuous reassessment and evaluation.

Further, home care interdisciplinary team meetings were held initially biweekly. Attendance is required of the patient care manager, visiting staff, and home health aide representative. The medical director attends when able, while the director is present when so indicated. Other community and hospital representatives have also been invited at varying times to discuss specific patients.

These meetings help to integrate the services of each discipline into a harmonious style, in accordance with the department's policies and procedures. Discussions revolve around problematic cases, patients receiving services greater than 60 days, and those cases involving multiple disciplines. Documentation is then entered into the corresponding patient record. The home care department also established a designated time when the therapists, social service worker, and home health aide agency could contact the visiting nurses and patient care manager to discuss those case management issues that cannot wait until the team meeting.

The office manager, who has a clerical background in a health-related setting, became responsible for the clerical component of the program, including supervisory and coordination functions, once additional staff were hired. Initially, she functioned as the department's secretary.

The data processing system, kept in the department, includes hardware and specific software developed for the home health industry. Such a software package provides the department (and hospital administrators) with split payor billing, specific visit analyses, accounts receivables, worksheets, charge audits, all payor billing, employee productivity, tracking of recertification, assistance with the preparation of HCFA 485, 486, and 487 forms, census, admission and discharge material, and tracking of referrals by source, with manual charge entry override.

The responsibility for home care billing, including processing all charges and maintenance of all manual statistical reports, was one of the secretary's functions initially. With the addition of clerical staff to the department and the promotion of the secretary to office manager, this became a responsibility shared by the billing clerk and data entry staff member. This includes follow-up to billing problems and change of fee status. It should be mentioned that the physical preparation of bills has always been done by the hospital computer.

Conclusion

You may ask that with all the pressures of reimbursement and competition, and the demands for costly, comprehensive services, why should hospitals even bother with home care? Home care is one part of the entire continuum of care. Smart hospital strategy dictates a wide array of services along that continuum to keep the patient within the hospital orbit.

Moreover, the hospital home care program can serve as a base from which to diversify into such programs as hospice, private pay homemaker services, congregate care services, meals on wheels, and durable medical equipment. If hospitals are to evolve into centers for community health, a home care program can help lead the way.

The Wissahickon Hospice

Madalon O'Rawe Amenta and Priscilla D. Kissick

Planning, Feasibility, Needs Assessment

The Wissahickon Hospice, an administratively independent, community-based hospice program with an average daily census of 25 to 30, has been in operation since February 1982. Certified by Medicare as both a hospice and a home health agency, it is also accredited as a hospice by the Joint Commission on Accreditation of Hospitals (JCAH). The service area--covering a radius of 15 miles from the office, an average of 30 minutes driving time--incorporates the urban neighborhoods of Germantown, East and West Mount Airy, Roxborough, Wadsworth, and Chestnut Hill of northwest Philadelphia and the suburbs of Eastern Montgomery County. Socioeconomically heterogeneous with families ranging from the very poor to the very rich, there is a strong "Old Philadelphia" Quaker tradition of cooperation, voluntarism, and political activism.

Founding. The agency was founded in 1980 when a physician, a lawyer, and a clergyperson, realizing that hospices were burgeoning both nationally and locally, decided to explore the possibilities of establishing one in their community.

The physician, a widower who had taken care of his wife at home during her terminal illness, had a deep conviction that contemporary institutions have made too many inroads into people's private lives. Out of this conviction developed a strong commitment to the implications of hospice care both for the health care system and for society at large. It is notable that in the area in 1980 there was a climate of relative cooperation among the local health care institutions, especially the community agencies.

The original hospice planning group, expanded by the addition of nurse CEOs of three Visiting Nurse Associations, a representative of the Episcopal Diocese, the medical director of a life care community, and the CEO of a community hospital, submitted a proposal for start-up funding for a home care hospice to the Glenmede Trust and the funding began in November of 1981. By naming the proposed hospice for the Wissahickon Creek which runs through all the geographic sections of the service area, the founders linked it symbolically to its community mission.

The purpose was to expand, not duplicate the work of existing agencies. The hospice, therefore, contracted for nursing services with the participating VNAs (with nurses trained and supervised by the hospice director) and itself provided the hospice-specific services (e.g., total family support, volunteer care, spiritual support, round the clock coverage, bereavement care) not then available through any other reimbursement structure. The first hospice families were all patients of the three cooperating VNAs.

Needs Assessment. To determine service need, the planners used the formula based on the then nationally demonstrated demand of 25% of the annual number of deaths from cancer-related causes in the proposed service area. They factored in an additional 5% to allow for patients with progressively debilitating terminal conditions other than cancer such as end-stage renal disease, ALS, and COPD. Using a base figure of 210 (the cancer-related deaths in the service area in 1978, the latest year for which figures were available), the planners estimated that 30% or 65 to 70 patients and families a year would seek hospice care and that the program would average 20 patients and families at any one time.

Admissions to the program exceeded this estimate by the third year of operation. In the fourth year, there were 152 admissions. Ninety percent of all patients admitted have had a diagnosis of cancer with cancer of the lung, colon, and breast representing 75% of the cases.

Philosophy, Mission, and Long Range Plan

Philosophy. The philosophy of the Wissahickon Hospice is in keeping with the tenets of the modern hospice movement as it has evolved in the English-speaking world since the late 1960s. That is, a hospice program is a coordinated array of holistic services in which a dying patient is not required to accept cure as the therapeutic goal, but may instead choose treatment aimed at comfort--or palliation. Pain and symptom control are managed through a highly sophisticated technology and spiritual needs, whether or not related to a particular religious denomination, are identified and attended to. The family, which, if necessary, is followed with supportive care after the death occurs, merits the same concern as the patient. Since the work of the core hospice team is enhanced by the supportive services of nutrition, physio-, occupational, art and music therapies along with companionship provided by both professionals and volunteers, interdisciplinary team collaboration and special attention to team building are essential.

Within this holistic framework, the patient, even though dying, is considered a primary source for meeting his own needs through many still intact social, emotional, and spiritual strengths. As a consequence, the notion of the "appropriate" death assumes that the dying patient has warm, intimate relationships with family, friends, and caregivers. It assumes a "context of open awareness" in which forthright communication may take place.

Mission. The mission of the Wissahickon Hospice is threefold.

1. Service. To provide residential hospice care of high quality for terminally ill children and adults and their families in northwest Philadelphia and eastern Montgomery county.

2. Education. To provide education to the public regarding hospice principles, and to professionals in the application of these principles.

3. Research. To encourage and, where appropriate, initiate research about any aspect--professional, operational, or financial--of hospice services and programs.

Long-Range Plan. The long-range plans for this hospice program are to remain in as strong a financial position as possible and to increase the patient caseload incrementally. This will be done through more intensive and penetrating case finding in the service area, with special emphasis on the presently underserved. The hospice intends to begin to implement these goals by strengthening administrative capacity through the introduction of a management information system for more effective financial and programmatic planning purposes, and by establishing a planning committee at the board of directors level.

Governing Body

The governing body of the Wissahickon Hospice, responsible for the establishment of overall program policy and evaluation of the executive director, is the Board of Directors. This group, which according to the bylaws may consist of not less than 3 nor more than 21 members, now numbers 14. The intent is to keep it small, responsive, and highly active. In short, this is a working board. There are physicians, nurses, a lawyer, a funeral director, and a businessman. A teacher is the community representative. A specialist in organizational development, recently added to the board, chairs the long-range planning committee.

Executive Committee. The Executive Committee, appointed by the Board of Directors, exercises the powers and authority of the board (with the exception of changing bylaws and appointing new directors) between full meetings. It is a five-member group consisting of the President of the Board, a physician; the Vice President, a lawyer; the Secretary, another physician; the Treasurer, a businessman; and the Chair of the Professional Advisory Committee, a nurse.

Staff Organization, Job Descriptions

In 1983, when it applied for the Medicare Hospice Benefit, the Wissahickon Hospice hired its own clinical care-giving staff since the law requires that all core professionals--nurses, physicians, social workers, counselors--be direct employees. The staff currently engaged in total program implementation are arrayed on the Organization Chart. (See Exhibit 2-3.)

Executive Director. The Executive Director, a nurse with an MN degree, is a full-time administrator. In addition to supervising the entire operation--carrying responsibility for organization, administration, performance standards, and evaluation--she maintains liaison among the board of directors, the professional personnel, all contracting entities, and the staff. She also participates in community activities involving the hospice; e.g., seminars, workshops, meetings, research; and plans and conducts an orientation for board members, staff, students, as well as contracting agencies.

Director of Patient Care Services. The full-time Director of Patient Care Services is also a master's prepared nurse. Working very closely with the Executive Director, she

Exhibit 2-3 Wissahickon Hospice Organizational Chart

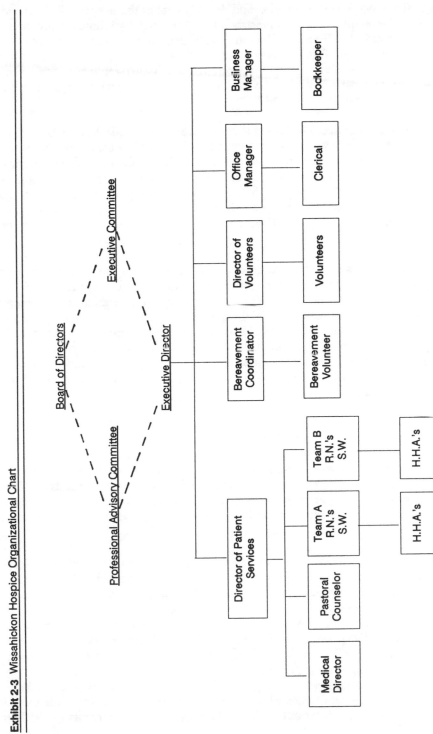

manages the day-to-day coordination and development of the hospice clinical services with particular emphasis on adminstration of the interdisciplinary team and the promotion of staff development. She participates with the team in determining those patients appropriate for admission, supervises the implementation of the interdisciplinary team care plan, and prepares the interdisciplinary team meeting agendas. She also participates in the educational, program evaluation, and research activities at the hospice.

Director of Social Service. The Director of Social Service, an MSW, is employed at .80 FTE and another social worker is employed at .40 FTE. They assess the psychosocial needs of patients and families; counsel patients and families, staff, and volunteers; and refer to appropriate community resources when the hospice's capacity for supportive care is insufficient. They manage bereavement follow-up by conducting support groups as needed for widows, other survivors, and children. They also participate in the educational, program evaluation, and research activities of the agency when appropriate.

Bereavement Coordinator. The Bereavement Coordinator, a retired librarian who is reimbursed for four hours a week, is responsible to the Director of Social Service. She organizes and maintains the tracking systems and documentation for monthly bereavement telephone, home visit, and correspondence contacts made by the social workers and the volunteers. She acts as liaison between staff and volunteers in relation to all pertinent information about the bereavement caseload and assists the social workers in planning bereavement support groups and volunteer educational activities. She also helps the Pastoral Counselor in the planning of memorial services for the hospice community.

Director of Volunteers. The Director of Volunteers, a .50 FTE employee, with a master's degree in social gerontology, supervises 65 active and 20 inactive volunteers in both the home care and the bereavement components of the program. She selects, assigns, and supervises volunteers and develops plans for all volunteer activities. She participates in the development of the volunteer training program, attends all classes, and coordinates ongoing in-house training and continuing education. In addition, she manages a regularly scheduled volunteer support group, and promotes the hospice volunteer program in the community.

Nurses. Professional nursing care for the patients enrolled in the Medicare Hospice Benefit is carried out by 3.8 FTE registered nurses each averaging 4.5 visits a day. Depending on the stage and severity of patient illness and the "problems" or symptoms of the family, one full-time nurse is generally able to manage seven to nine patients and families. When many patients have complex physical and psychosocial problems, four to five patients and families may be the limit of a reasonable caseload. Some patients not enrolled in the Medicare Hospice Benefit receive nursing services through a contracting Visiting Nurse Association.

The nurses, in addition to sharing on-call rotation in the provision of 24-hour-a-day, 7-day-a-week coverage, also plan and facilitate care and provide skilled nursing services on a part-time, intermittent basis. They do initial assessments in the home, counsel patients and families, participate in in-service education, and supervise and teach other nursing personnel such as home health aides whom they monitor every two weeks.

Home Health Aides. There is a .50 FTE home health aide on the staff and when more are needed, they are hired from home health aide agencies with which the hospice has contracts. The home health aides provide personal care services such as hygienc and comfort measures, assist with activities of daily living, and prepare meals. They promote easy communication between patient and family and report changes in patient and family status to the nurse in charge of the case. There is great emphasis placed on the hospice plan of care with these workers who document their activities in a manner appropriate to the clinical record.

Physiotherapist, Dietitian. The contracted services of the physiotherapist and dietitian, managed under nursing coordination, are the functions traditionally performed by these specialists.

Pastoral Counselor. The .25 FTE Pastoral Counselor, a clergyman reporting to the Director of Patient Care Services, coordinates spiritual care for patients and families and for survivors during the bereavement period. He shares observations of patients and families at team meetings and contributes to the development of the goals of the interdisciplinary plan of care. The chaplain also coordinates the work of the community clergy as it affects hospice families and staff, and provides education to the hospice team in all matters dealing with the spiritual aspects of care. He develops community education programs and participates in appropriate research projects.

Medical Director. The .25 FTE Medical Director reporting to the Director of Patient Care Services, shares 24-hour on-call rotation with other professional staff, provides hands-on medical care, and consults about palliative care to the rest of the hospice team. He recertifies patients enrolled in the Medicare Hospice Benefit. In addition, he provides direct medical care to patients when an attending physician cannot, and consults with attending physicians on matters of pain and symptom management and the hospice philosophy of care. He is responsible for decisions related to the admission and the discharge of hospice patients to and from inpatient services and also functions as the inpatient Chief of Service. Finally, he is responsible for establishing health policies for hospice employees.

Attending Physician. The attending physician and the hospice Medical Director cooperate in the medical management of patients at home. On the patient's admission to the hospice program both doctors evaluate the need for the attending to make house calls, designate which physician will sign the death certificate, determine the preferred hospital if an inpatient admission should be indicated, and discuss the appropriateness of the hospice Medical Director's writing medication and nursing orders if the attending is unavailable. A standing invitation is extended to the attending physician to participate in weekly team meetings via conference telephone.

Business Personnel. There is a .5 FTE business manager, a full-time office manager, as well as a part-time bookkeeper, transcriptionist, and file clerk all of whom function within the confines of their traditional occupational roles.

Volunteers. Volunteers have been central to the development of the hospice movement in the United States and in the Medicare Certified Hospice they are MANDATED as part of the interdisciplinary team. At the Wissahickon Hospice volunteers are recommended by two people (one of whom must be a physician) and are accepted for full service only after thorough evaluation. They must "fully participate" in the hospice volunteer training program of 24 classroom and six to eight observation hours with a hospice nurse. Volunteers make home visits to families on an appointment basis and assist in helping the family with household functions (washing dishes, child care, light meal preparation) and psychosocial and comfort care (reading, playing cards, listening to music). Through "active listening" they support the patient, the family, and the survivors during the bereavement period.

Staff Commitment. It should be noted that typical of hospices across the country all workers at the Wissahickon Hospice, paid and volunteer, give of themselves to a degree that goes beyond that of staff in traditional agencies. On-call nurses often make home visits in the middle of the night when they might easily have met the family's need by phone. Members of the business staff frequently work on their "own time" to catch up with the excess when the volume of paperwork gets out of hand. The pastoral counselor arranges for funeral services on very short notice when the patient and family have not been able to make appropriate arrangements in a more timely fashion. Some volunteers, in a crisis, drop their personal plans to go to a patient's home. All paid employees log more hours on the job than those for which they are reimbursed.

Development of Policies

As does any licensed, accredited, home health agency, the community-based independent hospice program must have policies providing for admission, continuation of and discharge from service, staff education, quality assurance and utilization review, program evaluation, and the maintenance of the medical record. In short, there must be a policy for every element of the program. For every service, there must be a job description spelling out how the function will be translated into actual care and how it will be evaluated. If a service is provided by someone who is not an employee of the program, for example, a physical therapist, there must be a contract delineating mutual responsibilities and communication requirements. In this discussion we focus on the policies that differentiate hospices from other types of home health agencies.

In developing the policies for guiding the day-to-day operations of the Wissahickon Hospice, the board of directors and the staff drew on four sources. In historical order they were: the National Hospice Organization Standards, the Conditions of Participation for Medicare-Certified Home Health Agencies, the Conditions of Participation of the Medicare Hospice Benefit, and the Hospice Standards of the Joint Commission on Accreditation of Hospitals (JCAH).

Admission Criteria. The eligibility criteria, reviewed annually, state that in order for a patient and family living within the service area to be admitted to the program there must be:

- A patient diagnosis of terminal disease with a six-month or less prognosis
- An understanding that cure-oriented treatment is no longer appropriate
- A desire for therapeutic efforts to be aimed at the provision of comfort and the enhancement of the quality of life for the patient and family
- A primary care person (PCP), or someone who will learn about and carry out the daily tasks of personal care in the patient's home
- A willingness on the part of the patient's doctor to agree with the hospice philosophy and procedures
- A willingness on the part of the patient's doctor to continue as the attending physician

Discharge Criteria. The discharge criteria state that families will be removed from the program rolls when:

- The patient and family request termination of the service
- The patient's life situation is unsafe or not conducive to the provision of hospice care or its supervision
- The patient and family are unable or unwilling to participate in attaining service goals
- More appropriate service can be offered by another agency (patient no longer needs hospice care)
- Attending physician fails to renew orders as required by hospice policy
- Patient has changed medical supervision

The Medical Director reviews all cases of potential discharge.

Patient and Family Rights Statement. The Patient and Family Rights Statement provides for information about the hospice's services and all related charges. It assures the patient the right to be informed by the physician and the right to participate in the plan of care. It assures the right to refuse treatment, the right of confidentiality, the right to be treated with respect and dignity, to be treated without discrimination, and to be treated by competent staff.

Informed Consent for Care. The informed consent for care includes the patient's request for service. It avers that the patient understands hospice care in relation to his terminal illness as palliative and not curative. It affirms that questions related to the terminal illness have been answered by the attending physician and that in the event of a cardiac or pulmonary arrest at home, the hospice does not have the capability of performing resuscitative measures. Patients are informed that pain-suppressing medications will be administered as needed and that all measures to assure physical and emotional comfort will be applied.

Continuation of Care. The policy outlining the criteria for the continuation of care states that service will be maintained when:

- Medical supervision is present or is to be obtained and a written plan of treatment has been or is being established by the supervising physician in collaboration with the hospice staff
- Hospice care is the on-going choice of patient and family
- Hospice care can meet the physical and psychological needs of the patient
- The plan of care is reviewed and revised as indicated by the hospice staff and attending physician at least as frequently as in compliance with Medicare regulations

Interdisciplinary Team Care Plan. The policy requiring an interdisciplinary team plan for each patient and family is central to a hospice program. The core professionals, and everyone else (patients and families, volunteers) involved with this highly individualized care has the opportunity to contribute to the goals of care and the assessment of treatment results.

In addition to certification by both the attending physician and the hospice program Medical Director that the patient has a life expectancy of six months or less, the interdisciplinary team plan includes a summary of patient and family physical, psychosocial, and spiritual needs based on the separate medical, nursing, and social service intake assessments and as determined at the initial interdisciplinary team meeting. The plan clearly indicates the interventions prescribed to meet the identified needs. The specific service to be provided is stated, the frequency and the personnel or type of service (e.g., chaplain, nurse, volunteer, etc.) are also indicated.

For example, if the patient has a lesion of the right breast and pain in the right upper quadrant, radiating to the right arm, the plan might read—Problem: Pain, right breast, ribs, arm; Service: Nursing, two times per week; Intervention: Monitor pain, medications, and compliance. Measure arm. Goals: Control pain, maximize comfort, teach primary care person (PCP) about the care of the arm. If the PCP is having difficulty coping, the plan might read—Problem: PCP anxiety. Service: HHA three times per week, Volunteer two times per week; Intervention: HHA bathe and provide other appropriate personal care, volunteer, sit, or provide companionship; Goal: Caregiver relief through respite.

Prescribed medications, dosage, frequency and method of administration must also appear on the plan. The hospice philosophy of pain management is to give enough of the correct medication to control the pain. Since levels and intensity of pain change often, measures are taken to allow the patient and family latitude in achieving relief. Orders may be written with a range of dosage, e.g., "Percocet 1 or 2 tablets, every 3 to 4 hours, as needed." If the patient when active experiences greater pain, two tablets of Percocet may be administered every three hours, but when the patient rests, the lesser dosage can be tried at a longer time interval. Medication orders are also written to cover the occasional possibility of pain breakthrough as well as to delineate alternative routes of administration, should swallowing become difficult.

The attending physician and the hospice Medical Director must each sign the plan of care as well as indicate all changes in writing. The plan must be reviewed and updated as often as necessary at interdisciplinary team meetings. A summary of the essence of the meeting and the goals for the coming week are recorded in the patient record and narratives dated and signed by each team member following each patient and family visit are also included.

Staff Support. Because hospice work can be intensive and the contributions of many professionals and volunteers are necessary to provide the round-the-clock care, a policy about staff support is necessary for hospice programs. The staff support policy of the Wissahickon Hospice states that an outside consultant will conduct a general support meeting monthly. Between these meetings, the staff members support each other informally through mutual counseling and day to day help with the technical problems of care.

Continuity of Care. Mechanisms for the smooth negotiation of continuity of care across treatment levels is another hallmark of hospice care. The process turns on effective communication. At the Wissahickon Hospice there are several policies designed to facilitate this process.

Levels of Care. One of these policies identifies the four major levels of care defined in the Medicare Hospice Benefit. Routine home care which is the primary service, consists of intermittent home nursing, home health aide, and social service as appropriate. Routine home care also assures the patient and family in their home all other needed hospice team services such as spiritual support, volunteer assistance, and physician consultation.

Continuous home care is the level of service provided for those patients whose needs go beyond those of routine home care. At times when, for example, pain control needs meticulous attention or ministration, or when there is intense family stress, nursing and home health aide services are provided in the home by the hospice program on a 24-hour basis.

Respite care is used when the family needs short periods of relief from the heavy demands of prolonged daily care of the dying patient in the home. At this level of care, a skilled nursing facility (SNF) accepts the patient for a few days during which it supplies all the services necessary to insure the patient's comfort.

Acute care in community hospitals is provided when the patient's symptoms are either too difficult to manage at home, special diagnostic procedures are required, or skilled nursing observation and intervention must be employed around the clock.

On-Call Policy. The On-Call Policy provides for the systematic rotation through 7-day-a-week, 24-hour-a-day coverage by professional staff. When the social worker or the physician are "on-call" there is always a back-up nurse assigned in case a nursing visit in addition to telephone support is required. The protocols for logging, documentation, and communication are all spelled out.

Contracts. Since the hospice program under the Medicare Hospice Benefit is clinically and fiscally responsible for the total span of services, all the institutions that have contracts with the Wissahickon Hospice must understand the hospice philosophy of care and the goals of the program. The staffs of contracting agencies must be oriented to the special needs of terminally ill patients and their families with special emphasis placed on interdisciplinary teamwork and the fundamentals of palliative care. An orientation outline containing the history of the agency, material about the service area and demographic information, service policies, job descriptions, and specific contractual elements is used by hospice staff in this educational activity.

Contracts itemize the services to be provided and the timeliness with which they must be delivered. Contracts also stipulate hospice policies applicable to the contracted employee, participation of subcontractors in the plan of treatment, daily reports and clinical documentation, lines of communication, reimbursement schedules, mileage allowances, and case conference participation.

As part of contractual arrangements with all participating agencies, there are transfer and discharge protocols. The protocol for admission to the emergency care unit (ECU) of the acute care hospital is significant. Services provided in the ECU are active treatment for the control of pain when home treatment has obviously failed, and symptom control with diagnosis and treatment for either a single symptom, i.e., nausea; or for multisystem deterioration. The procedures to be used are those compatible with palliative care that can reasonably be carried out in the emergency room setting, i.e., thoracentesis, paracentesis. There are special conditions--arrayed in a set of guidelines — under which blood transfusions or platelets and IV fluids or tube feedings may be administered. Any diagnostic tests must be part of the hospice plan of care. The policy for admission to the ECU stipulates that the "E.C.U. will provide required services to Wissahickon Hospice patients as requested by their attending physicians or the hospice Medical Director."

The contract with the acute care hospital is also significant. It states at the outset that "services will be rendered in accordance with the plan of care as developed and amended by the hospice team." This means that the hospice "retains authority and responsibility for the professional and medical management of patient care, discharge, and the documentation of hospice services in the hospital patient chart." It is agreed that when the patient's physician is a member of the hospital's medical staff, he or she will be the attending during the hospitalization. If the patient's physician is not on the hospital's staff, either the hospice Medical Director or his designee will fulfill the medical role. According to the terms of the contract, hospital visiting rules are altered to allow visiting of those close to the patient including small children. There is a clause assuring home-like decor, physical space for privacy, and arrangements for family to stay overnight if desired. Also, a facility for family privacy after the death is required.

When a patient is in the hospital, someone from the hospice team visits every day. Hospice professional staff, as expressly permitted in the contract, make entries into the hospital chart. These notes are then countersigned by the patient's attending physician. A note from the social worker might read "Please allow Mrs. Wilson's granddaughter to sleep overnight." When this is written as an order in the Physician's Order Sheet, the attending initials it. The only order, other than for medications or for diagnostic tests, that the non-physician members of the hospice team CANNOT write on the inpatient chart is a "Do Not Resuscitate (DNR)" order. If it is appropriate, this is done by either the attending or the hospice Medical Director at the time the patient is admitted.

DNR is NOT, in the Wissahickon Hospice, as it is in some, a blanket order. It is individually applied. For example, if a patient who is suffering, but not on the brink of death has been hospitalized to have a Hickman Catheter implanted so he can receive IV Morphine for pain, and is waiting to see his son who is flying in from Tokyo, the physician will not write a DNR order. Patients and families know on admission to the program that the hospice makes no provision for resuscitative procedures in the home (see discussion above re: policy for informed consent for care).

The Professional Advisory Committee

According to the bylaws of the Wissahickon Hospice, the Professional Advisory Committee (PAC), appointed by and responsible to the board of directors, must establish and annually review the hospice's policies related to scope of services, patient and family admissions, and medical supervision. The PAC also prepares comment on the emergency care plan, clinical records, and personnel qualifications. Finally, it reviews the program evaluation.

Under this rubric it reviews the procedures pertinent to each service (Nursing, PT, OT, ST, SSW, HA, Volunteers, Medicine and Pastoral Counseling). It examines the admission, continuation of care and discharge criteria, the standing orders for emergency care, the job descriptions, and the consumer evaluation. The PAC also reviews and advises on the yearly statistical reports and financial statements, staffing needs for new programs, staff development plans, contracts and all program changes.

Presently, the PAC consists of the President of the Board of Directors, the Medical Director, the Executive Director, and the Director of Patient Care. There are two nonemployee master's prepared nurses one of whom is also a board member. The other has extensive experience as a surveyor for the State Department of Health. In addition, there are two social workers. One, employed in an acute care hospital with a hospice program, has experience with cancer patients and their families and the other, a contract worker, does home health social service. There is a physiotherapist who holds an MBA and is in independent practice. A clergyman, engaged full-time in pastoral counseling, reviews the scope of services, job descriptions, and evaluations relevant to pastoral care on an as needed basis.

Financial Aspects

The Wissahickon Hospice, like any other contemporary community agency dependent on third-party reimbursement, experiences frequent cash flow problems. The normal period from time of service to the time of payment is approximately three months. With some payors, for a variety of reasons, there is a greater time lag than with others. When large payors, such as Medicare, fall behind in their payment schedules the hospice has to take out loans in order to continue in operation. It is important to note that the hospice has received very few denials of payment for Medicare services.

Sources of reimbursement by proportion of total income for the delivery of patient care services are Traditional Medicare (52%), Medicare Hospice Benefit

(18%), Blue Cross (10%), Medicaid (1%), HMO (3%), private insurance (6%), and contributions (10%). Free care for those patients with no source of insurance amounts to approximately 1% of the budget with uncovered services representing 15%. The total operational deficit is made up through foundation support, United Way, and community contributions. As the number of annual visits rises due to increased caseload and heightened nursing productivity--between 1985 and 1986 it increased 60%--the size of the budget increases as well. The 1986 budget of $375,000 was double that of 1985.

At the Wissahickon Hospice, items costing over $300 are capitalized. Approximately 6% of the annual budget is allotted for capital equipment. The next major expenses are expected to be a new photocopier and a computer system for billing and documentation of care.

Advantages and Disadvantages of the Independent Community-based Hospice

Disadvantages. The disadvantages for the community-based freestanding hospice are those of any small organization in an increasingly competitive health care economy. If third parties hold up their payments too long or too often, the financial base of the agency is threatened. If larger agencies that function with more resource reserves and larger overall budgets begin to fill community need for the service, the referral base may become eroded. The small agency cannot draw on the shared services such as accounting, public relations, and the clinical specialty departments that are available through large parent organizations. For instance, the Wissahickon Hospice is now developing its own management information system a task that would certainly be less costly, if not less difficult, if done in conjunction with a parent agency.

Advantages. The great advantage of the small community freestanding program, on the other hand is its administrative independence. When either program needs, or the service environment change, the response time of the governing body can be rapid. The staff of an agency like the Wissahickon Hospice can also function with great agility as the patient and family advocate in the wider health care system. Since the hospice program controls the patient and the plan of care, the hospice can run interference when the patient and family meet difficulties.

For example, the wife and caretaker of a hospice patient on the Medicare Hospice Benefit suffered an acute myocardial infarction. When she was taken to the cardiac care unit of the community hospital, the hospice program admitted the dying man to an SNF for respite care. The hospice social worker coordinated care with the hospital and arranged to have the wife (after her coronary condition had stabilized) admitted to the same SNF as her husband. Meanwhile, the hospice administration negotiated with the Medicare fiscal intermediary to allow the patient to receive reimbursement for routine hospice home care while remaining at the SNF after the allotted five days of respite care were exhausted. For this purpose, the fiscal intermediary agreed to consider the SNF the patient's residence. During their stay at the SNF, the patient and family received skilled nursing care, volunteer assistance, social service, and pastoral counseling. Their house was rearranged with the help of the hospice team to accommodate the two patients on their return and the husband eventually died peacefully, at home, surrounded by his wife and children.

The advantages to dying patients of a hospice program helping them negotiate various levels of care is demonstrated to the community through the education that has been provided to the traditional care facilities. Hospice patients, as previously noted, when admitted to inpatient facilities, in accordance with prior arrangements, do not have to stop for routine admission tests such as chest x-rays, extensive blood work and so forth. The admitting office is called and told that a hospice patient is coming in and what the physician wants done. If, for instance, the physician wants the patient to have a thoracentesis, the order is taken and the procedure done without the decision having to go through several layers of bureaucracy.

The Medicare Hospice Benefit is a great advantage in that patients undergoing medical crises at home receive around the clock nursing care, thus averting the trauma always associated with moving the fragile patient. Other advantages for Medicare hospice beneficiaries are that they are entitled to free use of durable medical equipment drugs (practically free) and hospitalization. As previously noted, the hospice program, not the inpatient facility, controls the conditions under which admission and transfer will take place and controls the patient's care while the patient is in the hospital.

Organizationally, it is easier for the small, independent, single purpose institution to affect the climate of the wider environment in favor of a greater understanding and acceptance of hospice care. The small, agile agency can do intensive education and networking. The Wissahickon Hospice has developed excellent relations with most of the attending physicians whose patients are participants in the program. There is a strong sense that in the four years of the life of the hospice, it has increased the understanding of palliation and enhanced good feeling for hospice care within the physician community.

The small independent hospice can attract dedicated, highly committed personnel who like the latitude of professional responsibility, teamwork, and the idealism of hospice care. The person who is one of 10 or 15 employees sitting around the table at a team meeting once a week is one who will more than likely develop a strong loyalty to the service, the team, and the patients. This member of a small group will also have the satisfaction of observing first hand his or her influence on care and organizational policy.

The independent hospice is free to move quickly in the establishment of not only clinical and social service arrangements with other agencies, but also financial ones. It can be a great advantage to be the first hospice in the community to get to the HMO with a contract proposal.

The Wissahickon Hospice as an independent community-based program has the sharp focus and elegant design that result from small size and a single mission. Policy, procedure, and organizational structure take forms that follow function. They are determined solely by the needs of the families served, and tempered only by the fiscal, legal, and accrediting accountabilities, themselves, created in the field. It is this kind of agency that provides a unique model of innovative care on the cutting edge of the health care system.

References

Anderson, H.J. Sept. 26, 1986. "Two recent home healthcare mergers may signal industry consolidation." *Modern Healthcare* 16: 118

Cherkasky, M. 1949. The Montefiore Hospital home care program. *American Journal of Public Health* 39: 163-166.

Cunningham, R.M., Jr. 1985. The evolution of hospice. *Hospitals* 59: 124

Federal Register. Subpart L. *Conditions of Participation.* Home Health Agencies. Vol. 33, No. 167, August 27, 1968, p. 12901; Vol., 38, No. 135, July 16, 1973, p. 18978.

Ginzberg, E., Balinskey W., and Ostow, M. 1984. *Home health care.* Totowa, NJ: Rowman & Allenheld

Hoyer, R. August 27, 1986. Research Director, National Association of Home Care, personal communication

Moyer, N. 1986. Public policy, politics, and home health care, *Home Healthcare Nurse* 4:7.

Littauer, D. 1962. *Bulletin of Academy of Medicine New Jersey* Volume 8.

Mundinger, M. O'N. 1983. *Home care controversy.* Rockville, MD: Aspen Systems Corp.

National Hospice Organization. 1984. *The basics of hospice.* Pamphlet.

O'Malley, S.T. 1986. Reimbursement issues, in S. Stuart-Siddal, ed. *Home health care nursing: Administrative and clinical perspectives.* Rockville, MD: Aspen Systems Corp.

Smith, J.A. 1983. *The idea of health.* New York: Teachers College Press.

Stewart, J.E. 1979. *Home health care.* St. Louis:The C.V. Mosby Co.

Woodham-Smith, C. 1970. *Florence Nightingale: 1820-1910* London & Glasgow: Fontana Books.

Part II

Standards for Home Health Agencies

Chapter Three

Agency Standards

Adherence to the Conditions of Participation

Peggie R. Webb

Trying to operate a home health agency without understanding the Conditions of Participation is analogous to building a house without a blueprint. It may be called a house and resemble a house from a distance, but a closer look reveals serious flaws and defects. Additionally, the people who reside in the house live with a nagging suspicion that one wrong move will reduce the structure to shambles. Needless to say, they do not remain in such a dwelling any longer than necessary.

The Conditions of Participation are the blueprint for the successful operation of the home health agency. However, reading the Conditions of Participation is not an enjoyable experience. It is no wonder that many home health managers prefer to have anyone who professes to be knowledgeable explain what must be done to comply with the conditions. Sometimes this method is effective; most times it is not.

The purpose of this chapter is to enable the reader to understand the Conditions of Participation as a working document, which delineates the requirements which must be met by every home health agency in order to become a certified provider eligible to receive Medicare and Medicaid funds. This chapter does not discuss the additional requirements imposed by some state laws and licensing regulations. These requirements would also have to be met in order for the agency to become a Medicare-certified provider.

For reference purposes, the Conditions of Participation are included in Appendix A. The discussion of each of the Conditions follows the presentation of the Conditions of Participation. Conditions of Participation 405.1201 General, 405.1202 Definitions, and 405.1230 Qualifying to Provide Outpatient Physical Therapy or Speech Pathology Services are self-explanatory and will not be discussed further. The appendix which includes the addenda for several states incorporating Conditions of Participation higher than those imposed by the Health Insurance for the Aged Program is not included.

It should be noted that the regulations have not been revised to include Amendment to Section 1861(o) made by the Medicare and Medicaid Amendments. The Amendments which are cited in the *Federal Register* (October 26, 1982) include the bonding and escrow requirements and enable proprietary agencies to participate in the Medicare program in states that do not have licensing requirements for home health agencies.

§405.1220 Condition of Participation: Compliance with Federal, State, and Local Laws

This condition requires that the home health agency comply with all applicable federal, state, and local laws and regulations at all times. Licenses, permits, and approvals of the agency must be readily available. It is recommended that the documents be prominently displayed within the agency.

While it is generally recognized that this condition refers to the agency's compliance with applicable laws and regulations, there is less recognition that this condition also requires the agency to have available a current license for all personnel who must meet license requirements in order to provide service. This includes personnel providing services on a contractual basis. A photocopy of the current license is acceptable. However, the agency should verify that the applicable state board does not forbid photocopying of the license. When a photocopy is acceptable, the photocopy should be clear and contain all of the information on the original. If not copied correctly, part of the expiration date may be omitted. Because the expiration dates vary, the agency should develop a system to identify when licenses expire and request proof that the license has been renewed.

Finally, to meet the intent of the condition, the agency should have available policies and procedures relating to the maintenance of records, reporting, communicable diseases, and drug control which meet the requirements of applicable state and local laws and regulations and concomitantly meet the specific needs of the agency.

§405.1221 Condition of Participation: Organization Services Administration

This condition requires the agency to have written materials which delineate the organizational structure, administrative procedures, and mechanisms for controlling all aspects of the agency's operation.

The organizational chart should depict the existence of the governing body, group of professional personnel, finance committee, and all current positions, as well as the relationships which exist among staff members, the governing body, and established committees. Some organizational charts depict all existing committees and subcommittees. When applicable, the chart should depict the personnel available at the branch office(s). Because subunits must be certified separately, organizational charts should be developed for the subunit. If a relationship exists between the agency and a parent agency, this relationship should also be represented. More than one organizational chart may be necessary in order to accurately depict relationships within the agency and with other entities. A legend should be included to explain how different relationships are represented. The organizational chart should always include the date it is approved by the governing body.

The agency should have written policies which delineate the operational practices and expectations of the agency as well as the mechanisms for maintaining accountability for the delegation of responsibilities down to the patient care level. A discussion of the content of these policies will be found in the remaining sections of this chapter. Usually the agency's written policies and procedures are available within an operations manual and are accurate at the time originally approved and incorporated in the manual. However, over time, one of three patterns frequently emerges which makes it difficult for the agency to establish that its operational practices and policies are in compliance with the Conditions of Participation. Variations in the patterns also occur depending on the degree of creativity exhibited by the management and supervisory staff.

The first pattern may be termed the "roundtoit" method of maintaining current written materials relative to the organization, administration, and services of the agency. In this instance, the agency changes internally; however, no one assumes responsibility for ensuring that the relevant written materials are updated to reflect the approved changes. These materials will be updated some time in the future when someone gets "around to it." Thus, the present operation of the agency becomes a secret which can be gleaned only by asking the right question of the "appropriate personnel" or reading minutes of governing body, committee, and staff meetings. Alas, the operation manual remains on the shelf collecting dust, becoming useful only as a historical reference.

The second pattern which emerges is the "new broom sweeps clean." This pattern is opposite of the pattern just described, and is more evident in agencies which experience frequent turnover in management and supervisory personnel. Each newly appointed administrator or supervising registered nurse changes the existing organizational chart, policies, and job descriptions to improve the agency's operation. These changes are made in the operations manual either by incorporating new materials or writing corrections and revisions directly on to the applicable existing materials. Materials deemed inappropriate are simply removed from the manual. Invariably, the revised material refers to a policy or position which has been deleted. Therefore, the manual should be read in the presence of the administrator or supervising nurse in order for one of them to fill in the missing pieces or to explain the inconsistencies noted. Additionally, with this pattern, the governing body, group of professional personnel, and other applicable committees are generally told of what has occurred some time after the changes have been implemented.

The third pattern is less often observed; however, it also creates problems documenting compliance. The pattern is called, "I'll put a stop to that right now!" Usually, but not always, this is a pattern demonstrated by administrators. It is exhibited whenever a problem arises in the agency. Although written policies exist to correct or address the problem identified, the administrator determines that a stronger course of action must be taken immediately. This action is specified in a memorandum which is distributed with the paychecks, posted on a bulletin board, or read at a staff meeting. The memorandum has the effect of policy and takes precedence over existing policies. Here again the governing body and appropriate committees are informed of that action taken long after it occurs. One cannot discern which policies are current without access to all the memoranda which have been written.

This condition includes nine standards which must be met. Compliance with these standards is evaluated in determining whether or not the agency meets the intent of the condition. Two of these standards may not be applicable if the agency does not use contracted personnel to provide therapeutic services.

a) *Standard: Services provided*

The agency bylaws, philosophy, mission statement, or similar documents should clearly specify the purpose of the agency. The agency must provide skilled nursing and at least one other service on a visiting basis, in a place of residence used as the patient's home. At least one of the qualifying services must be provided directly through agency employees; other services may be provided on a contractual basis.

b) *Standard: Governing body*

The governing body, usually called the Board of Directors, must keep updated minutes of meetings which are sufficiently detailed to verify that the body has not only fulfilled its mandated responsibilities, but also is operating in a manner consistent with its bylaws. The minutes should always include the list of members present.

The bylaws or an appropriate equivalent document should clearly specify the manner in which the governing body functions as well as its responsibilities. Bylaws which state that the Board of Directors will meet from time to time as necessary, within or outside the state, will be governed by applicable business laws and will engage only in lawful business practices including the purchase of real estate or property, are not appropriate for the home health agency. The agency's bylaws should include specific information regarding:

- Term of office, duties, and responsibilities of the members of the governing body.

- Frequency of meetings.

- Method of electing officers as well as the term of office and duties of each officer.

- Qualifications of members and officers.

- Committees of the governing body including method of appointment of members and committee responsibilities.

- To whom responsibility for direction and supervision of program and evaluation of practices is delegated.

The bylaws or acceptable equivalents should be received periodically to ensure that the document remains current.

c) *Standard: Administrator*

The agency must employ a qualified administrator. The job description should specify the required qualifications. At minimum, the administrator must meet the requirements specified in the definition cited in the Conditions of Participation 405.1202.

Written policies as well as job descriptions, the organizational chart, and other documents must establish that the administrator is responsible for directing the agency's operation. The job description should delineate the specific responsibilities assumed by the administrator to fulfill each of the duties cited in this standard. Agency policies, personnel files, meeting minutes, financial records, and public information materials should verify that the Administrator is appropriately directing the agency's affairs. A qualified person should be authorized in writing to act for the Administrator.

d) *Standard: Supervising physician or registered nurse*

Because a registered nurse usually fills this position, the term supervising nurse will be used throughout this discussion. The supervising nurse must be employed on a full-time basis. The incumbent or a qualified alternate should be available during operating hours. Written policies and procedures as well as the supervising nurse's job description should clearly delineate the course for directing, coordinating, and supervising all of the services provided. The supervising nurse also ensures that job descriptions are developed for personnel involved in the delivery of services and that these positions are filled by qualified personnel. The supervising nurse is involved in the recruitment and selection of patient care personnel and assures that these personnel complete an appropriate orientation program. The supervising nurse also participates in the development and implementation of staff development programs for direct service personnel.

The agency must establish criteria which enable the supervisor to maintain appropriate number and levels of staff and to plan and budget for sufficient staff to meet patient service needs. These criteria should be functional and appropriate to meet the specific needs of the agency.

e) *Personnel Policies*

The agency must have written policies which set forth the existing rules, regulations, benefits, and performance expectations for all personnel. The personnel policies should include information relative to wage scales and hours of work, fringe benefits, workman's compensation, orientation and staff development activities, employee performance evaluations, health examinations, and exit interviews. Job descriptions should be established for each category of personnel. The personnel records should verify that the personnel policies are followed.

Each employee should be oriented to the policies and objectives of the agency. Materials documenting completion of an orientation should be maintained for all personnel including those available on a contractual basis. The time and dates of the orientation program as well as the content and names of individuals who participated in the program should be documented.

Health examinations and employee performance evaluations should be completed on a timely basis. The health examination policy should specify the scope as well as the frequency of the examination. The performance evaluation should be an assessment of the employee's abilities to fulfill the duties established in the job description and provide information for planning staff development programs.

Position descriptions should clearly state functions and responsibilities as well as the specific qualifications necessary to perform the job. The job qualifications should clearly establish the license, certification, educational, experience, and training requirements which must be met. The Conditions of Participation definitions identify the required qualifications for direct service personnel. The agency must ensure that the job descriptions also include any additional state requirements.

All personnel are expected to participate in appropriate staff development activities. A record should be maintained to document the employee's participation in continuing education activities.

f) *Personnel under hourly or per visit contract*

The contract for the provision of therapeutic service should clearly designate the procedures followed to ensure that each of the six elements in this standard are met. The contract should specify the responsibilities of agency personnel as well as the obligations of the contractee. The contract should specify the titles of agency personnel who have responsibility for ensuring that certain activities are completed. If evaluation of the contractee's performance is conducted in part through the quarterly review of records by a designated committee, this information should be included in the contract. The contract should be reviewed and renewed on an annual basis.

The hourly or per visit contract is established between the agency and one individual. Another individual cannot be designated by the contractee to provide services instead of or in addition to the contractee. If more than one individual is utilized, the contract must specify the name of the group or organization providing services. When services are provided during normal working hours by a staff member employed by the same organization which is the parent for the home health agency, a written contract is not necessary; however, agency policies should establish the manner in which the service is available and supervised. It should be clear that services are available on a regular basis, not just when the employee is not busy working for the parent organization.

The personnel records should verify that the contractee meet applicable personnel policies including, but not limited to completion of an orientation program, educational and license requirements, physical examination, and performance evaluations. A record should be maintained of the contractee's participation in continuing education activities. The clinical record should document that the contractee meets performance expectations as specified in the job description and the contract and that services are provided as specified in existing policies and procedures.

g) *Coordination of patient services*

The agency should have a policy which establishes the purpose and procedures for conducting patient conferences. At minimum, the procedure should specify the frequency for conducting the conferences and the personnel who are expected to participate in the conference. Ideally, the case conference should be incorporated in the clinical record. The conference should document that all team members are coordinating and planning interventions as needed to meet the patients' needs. The clinical record should document the outcome of this plan of action developed during the case conference as well as any communication between team members relative to patient care.

The 60-day summary report should provide pertinent information about each therapeutic service that has been provided. The report should be sufficiently detailed to enable the physician to assess the patient's response to the treatment plan. Further, the summary should establish the need for continued service(s) to meet the goals established for the patients. If it is anticipated that the patient will be discharged soon, this should be indicated in the report as well as plans for follow-up care if appropriate.

h) *Services under arrangements*

Contracts between the agency and groups or organizations for the provision of therapeutic services must meet the same content provisions as contracts with individuals. The agency must have materials which document that each individual utilized completes an orientation program. It is not appropriate for the agency to allow a representative of the group or organization to conduct the agency's orientation program.

Some organizations have a physical examination policy which differs from the agency's policies. It is acceptable for the agency to have this policy on file as well as materials which verify that each employee adheres to the contracting organization's policy.

i) *Standard: Institutional planning*

The annual budget and capital expenditure plan, if required, must be prepared under the direction of the governing body by a committee consisting of representatives of the governing body, the administrative staff, and the group of professional personnel, and the medical staff, if any. One person may not act for more than one of the required representatives; however, this committee may include more than one representative. The governing body minutes should document the appointment of the committee members. Strange as it may sound, the governing body treasurer is often not a member of the committee which prepares the budget. The reasons for this omission have never been clearly explained.

The procedures followed to ensure that the annual budget is prepared on a timely basis should be available in writing. If the supervising nurse is not a member of the committee which prepares the budget, the procedure should indicate the manner by which the supervising nurse participates in planning and budgeting for the provision of therapeutic services, including supervisory and support personnel. This procedure or other policies which discuss the agency's fiscal practices should acknowledge that a capital expenditure plan will be prepared by the committee which prepares the budget, when appropriate.

The budget must be approved by the governing body. During the year the budget should be reviewed and revised as necessary under the direction of the committee responsible for its preparation. Minutes of committee and governing body meetings should document that the members are kept informed of the agency's fiscal affairs.

If the agency does not anticipate capital expenditures in excess of $100,000, a capital expenditure plan is not necessary. If a capital expenditure plan is required, it should be prepared in a manner which meets the requirements identified in this standard. Because of reimbursement issues for each capital expenditure, the plan must indicate whether it is likely to be required, or is required to conform to state and local comprehensive health planning standards, criteria, or plans, and whether the proposed expenditure has been submitted to a comprehensive health planning agency for approval in accordance with Section 1122 of the Social Security Act. If neither one of these requirements has to be met, the administrator should have information noting if the designated planning agency has approved or disapproved the proposed expenditure.

§405.1222 Condition of Participation: Group of Professional Personnel

This condition requires the agency to have a group of professional personnel who establish and annually review policies governing the delivery of services and personnel qualifications. The group also is responsible for ensuring that the annual program evaluation is completed, reviewed, approved, and subsequently submitted to the governing body. It is not necessary for the group to establish personnel qualifications or some types of policies when this responsibility is mandated for a higher authority. This frequently occurs in public health agencies operated by the state, county, or city health departments. In this instance, the group should review these materials and make such recommendations for revisions as the group believes is appropriate.

The agency bylaws and policy should specify the composition, purpose, and functions of the group. It is recommended that the responsibility for the group to have a representative on the committee which prepares the budget be included in the statement of functions. The group should include a broad representation of health care professionals as well as members of occupations who are knowledgeable about health-related issues and community affairs. Minutes of group meetings should document that the members are active participants. Members who regularly attend "in spirit" only should be promptly removed.

The bylaws and policy should also specify the mechanism for informing the governing body of the group's actions. The governing body, having assumed full legal authority and responsibility for the operation of the agency, must approve or disapprove all recommendations and newly developed or revised policies and personnel qualifications. Facility-based agencies may need to involve additional personnel in the chain of command or established committees which are authorized to act for the governing body on policy and related matters.

a) *Standard: Advisory and evaluation function*

The first action taken by many agencies upon learning that the group of professional personnel was no longer required by the Conditions of Participation to meet at least quarterly was to promptly change the meeting frequency to once each year. Unless the agency is operating in a vacuum, it is difficult for the group to fulfill its mandated responsibilities with this meeting schedule. When the group meets on an annual basis, the members do not attend a meeting, they attend a lecture. The minutes document that the group hears from one or more staff members about the myriad activities occurring and actions taken since the last meeting. Because the agenda is so full, dialogue among the group members is limited. However, the limited dialogue may occur because the group meets so infrequently, the members are not sure of what they should do. Indeed it appears the group's only purpose is to approve all actions that have already been taken.

Clearly, the group must meet frequently enough to fulfill its mandated responsibilities, and advise the agency on professional issues, participate in the evaluation of the agency's program. The members should be sufficiently knowledgeable to assist the agency to work cooperatively with other (noncompetitive) health care providers and inform the community of the services available.

§405.1223 Condition of Participation: Acceptance of Patients, Plan of Treatment, Medical Supervision

This condition requires the agency to demonstrate that patients are accepted for care only after a decision-making process determines that the resources available are sufficient to meet the patient's needs in a residential setting and that the patient is eligible for services. The agency must also demonstrate that the care provided is physician-directed.

Written policies must identify the scope of services offered, the manner by which the services will be provided, coordinated, and supervised, as well as the process for maintaining communications with the physician. The policies should set forth the criteria which are considered as part of the decision-making process to determine the patient's eligibility for care. Criteria which are considered should include at least the following:

- Adequacy and suitability of agenda

- Personnel and resources to provide the services required by the patient

- Assessment of medical, nursing, and social information, provided by the physician, institutional personnel, and agency staff

- Comparative benefit of home care for the patient as distinguished from care in a hospital, skilled nursing facility, or other institution or means of care

- A plan to meet medical emergencies

- Adequacy of physical facilities and equipment in the patient's residence for safe and effective care

- Availability of family or substitute family member who is able and willing to participate in the patient's care.

a) *Standard: Plan of treatment*

This standard specifies the information which must be contained in the plan of treatment. Agency policy must specify the necessity for each patient to have a plan of treatment established by a physician. If there are requirements the physician must meet in order to refer a patient for service(s), these requirements should be set forth in writing. Frequently, the patient has more than one physician providing medical supervision. Agency policy should specify how the provision of service is coordinated between physicians. In some instances, it is necessary to develop more than one plan of treatment to clearly establish the care ordered and source of medical supervision.

Frequently, the plan of treatment cannot be completed until after the initial evaluation visit. Agency policy should delineate the procedures followed to communicate to the physician findings and recommendations for additions or modifications to the plan. This is especially important for agencies that use contracted personnel who may not have completed the evaluation visit at the time the plan of treatment is submitted to the physician for certification.

b) *Standard: Periodic review of the plan of treatment*

Written policies must specify the necessity for the physician to review the plan of treatment at least every 60 days with the patient's progress reported to the physician. Written procedures should require the professionals who have provided care to participate in this review to assure that the plan accurately reflects the need and plans for continued care treatments and interventions provided. The plan must be submitted to the physician for review, modification as necessary, and recertification prior to the end of the 60-day period in order for services to continue uninterrupted. The agency should also have an established process to determine the accuracy of the plan when the patient is hospitalized for a short time (less than 7 days during any certification period). Finally, agency policies should specify the necessity for the professional to promptly inform the physician of any change in the patient's condition which suggests the need to alter the plan of care. The procedure for documenting verbal and written communication should be established in writing. The clinical records should include documentation reflecting staff adherence to these policies.

c) *Conformance with physician's orders*

Written policies must exist to assure that services are provided only as ordered by the physician. Verbal orders are accepted only by qualified personnel, promptly recorded, signed, and dated by the professional accepting the order(s) and submitted to the physician for countersignature. Verbal orders should be considered part of the plan of treatment; therefore, the orders must be sufficiently detailed to specify clearly what has been ordered.

Too often the physician's countersignature for verbal orders is not obtained on a timely basis. This omission is most frequently evident when the verbal order policy has been revised to delete a specific time period for obtaining the countersignature. It is reasoned that if a specific time period, e.g., 7, 10, or 14 days is not identified, the agency will avoid being cited for not ensuring adherence to establish policies when a recertification resurvey or a validation survey is conducted. Further, the reasoning continues, the verbal orders will be included when the plan of treatment is recertified and the fiscal intermediary for Medicare patients will be informed of the additional orders when the medical update and patient information is submitted.

Such reasoning throws the baby out with the bath water. First, the agency has attempted to abrogate the professional's responsibility to promptly obtain the physician's countersignature for verbal orders. Second, during the period treatments and interventions are provided without proper physician authorization, the care is not reimbursable. Third, and most importantly, the ability to document that care is provided only as ordered by the physician has been compromised in a manner which could have adverse legal consequences for the agency and the caregiver if patient care problems arise.

Written policies should specify the responsibility of the staff to review all medications that the patient is taking, including over the counter drugs. Mechanisms must exist to inform the physician of any problems with the medication regimen.

§405.1224 Condition of Participation: Skilled Nursing Service

This condition requires the agency to have written policies which clearly designate that skilled nursing services are provided by or under the supervision of a registered nurse, the manner by which supervision is exercised and the mechanisms for ensuring that care is provided in accordance with the plan of treatment and agency policies.

The policies should be consistent with the State Nurse Practice Acts and reflect current professional standards for care.

a) *Standard: Duties of the registered nurse*

Job descriptions, nursing service, and other appropriate policies should delineate the registered nurse's duties and performance expectations as a member of the health care team. When specialty nursing services, such as, rehabilitative, psychiatric, or pediatric nursing care are offered, a job description and policies relative to the provision of the specialty service should be established in collaboration with the group of professional personnel and approved by the governing body.

The clinical record should verify that the registered nurse consistently and appropriately completes each of the duties identified in the standard. The reader should refer to the specific chapters in this text in which some of these areas are discussed in detail.

The care plan is an important tool which enables the professional to identify problems and needs, approaches and interventions, and goals and outcomes. Standardized care plans for nursing care are available which are comprehensive and easy to use. However, to be useful, the care plan must be a working document which is tailored to meet the specific problems and needs of the patient and expanded or modified as needed during the period services are provided. In too many instances, the care plan is a format which is circled, initiated, and dated when service is initiated and never referred to again until the patient is discharged at which time the word "resolved" is written by every problem and need identified. A review of the clinical record would not confirm that resolution had, in fact, been achieved.

There appears to be a universal agreement that complete, concise, and accurate documentation in the clinical record is crucial from both a legal and financial standpoint. Unfortunately, it appears that many administrators believe that a warranty guaranteeing the ability to document properly in any health care setting is issued with the professionals with the nursing license. Therefore, if documentation problems are identified in the clinical record, it is because the nursing supervisor(s) "won't stay on top of those nurses." The course of action taken when this mentality exists is to assign the supervisor the responsibility to read every clinical note before it is incorporated into the patient's record. Woe be unto the supervisor who lets a poorly written note slip by. The supervisor's anxiety is communicated to the staff nurse as the stack of clinical notes get higher each day. This staff nurse, in turn, becomes anxious. Anxiety becomes fear and fear becomes the fuel on which the staff operates.

This penny-wise, but pound-foolish approach guarantees a high turnover among staff and supervisory personnel. Staff nurses are terminated or resign on a regular basis; supervisors are promoted and demoted so frequently that name pins say only "Nursing Supervisor," never the nurse's name. Equally distributing are the underlying implications in this approach. There is the manifest implication that the staff nurse's professional responsibility to document appropriately can be transferred to the supervisor. Moreover, there is a latent implication that the staff nurse can never learn to document properly; therefore, every note must be checked. This approach may also diminish the staff nurse's sense of professional responsibility to improve documentation practices since what is written will always be checked.

Earlier, this management approach was called penny-wise and pound-foolish. Rather than expend the resources necessary to prepare the staff to document appropriately in the clinical record, those in authority prefer to have the supervisor become a policeman of paper and continually face the expense of recruiting and orienting staff nurses while relying on contingency plans to provide service to the patients cared for by the departing nurses.

Although this discussion has been limited to nurses, it should be clear that this same approach is often employed for the therapists and social workers.

b) *Duties of the qualified licensed practical nurse*

The agency must have written policies which delineate the role and responsibilities of the qualified licensed nurse for providing care. These responsibilities must be consistent with the duties defined in the incumbent's job description. The policies must also identify the mechanisms which are utilized by the registered nurse to maintain coordination and supervision of the services provided by the qualified licensed practical nurse. Finally, the policies should clearly establish the role of the qualified practical nurse in performing the duties specified in this standard.

§405.1225 Condition of Participation: Therapy Services

This condition requires the agency to have written policies which clearly establish the scope of each therapy service offered and the manner in which these services will be coordinated and supervised. The written policies, job descriptions, and contracts, if applicable, should identify the mechanisms which exist to assure that the therapists fulfill the duties specified in this condition. These written materials, as well as the personnel records should verify that each therapy service will be provided only by a qualified therapist and that the therapist's responsibilities are consistent with the applicable state practice acts and professional standards.

The clinical records must verify that each therapist follows agency policies and performance expectations when care is provided, that the therapist maintains communication with the other members of the health care team, including the attending physician, and services are provided under the supervision of the qualified therapist when necessary. The personnel record or acceptable alternative should verify that each therapist meets the qualification requirements and participates in continuing education activities.

a) *Supervision of physical therapist assistant and occupational therapy assistant*

The agency's written policies must specify the manner by which therapy service will be supervised by the appropriate qualified therapist if assist therapists are utilized to provide care. The policies should specify the services which may be provided by the assist therapists. The job descriptions, written policies and contract, if applicable, verify that the therapist duties meet the intent of this standard.

b) *Supervision of speech therapy services*

The Condition of Participation (405.1202) definition specifies the qualifications for the speech therapist. If the agency uses personnel who are in the process of meeting the qualifications for the speech therapist, the agency's written policies must specify the manner in which supervision will be exercised by the qualified therapist. The speech therapist must also meet state license requirements. It must be noted that the definition of supervision specified in the same Condition of Participation requires the supervision of the speech therapist to be direct on-site supervision. The clinical record must document that this supervisory requirement is met.

§405.1226 Condition of Participation: Medical Social Services

This condition requires the agency to have written policies which clearly establish the scope of medical social work services offered and the manner in which the services will be coordinated and supervised. The written policies, job descriptions, and contracts, if applicable, should specify the mechanisms which exist to assure that the social work staff provides service in a manner which meets the requirements cited in this condition as well as applicable state practice acts and professional standards. When social work assistants are utilized, the written policies, job descriptions, and contracts, if applicable, should specify the plan for providing regular supervision by the qualified social worker.

The clinical record should verify that the social work staff adheres to agency policies when providing services and that the personnel meet the job performance expectations. Supervision of the social work assistant by the master's prepared social worker should be readily apparent. The personnel record or an acceptable equivalent documents that service is provided only by qualified personnel and that these personnel participate in continuing education activities.

405.1227 Condition of Participation: Home Health Aide Service

This condition specifies the content of the training program which must be completed to prepare the individual to function as a home health aide utilized by the agency. A certificate documenting completion of a home health aide training program may be accepted in lieu of the curriculum and list of instructors only when the individual completed a program conducted by a Medicare-certified home health agency. The agency must also meet any additional state requirements relative to home health aide training program. It should be apparent that the purpose and content of the training program is very different from the purpose and content of the home health aide orientation program.

The agency must have written policies which delineate the process for determining that home health aide services are needed and the manner in which the services will be provided and supervised. The job descriptions and service policies must specify the duties which may be performed by the home health aide when personal care services are necessary. The clinical records must verify that home health aide services are provided and supervised in accordance with established policies.

    a) *Assignment and duties of the home health aide*

        The agency's written policies should require the registered nurse to be responsible for assigning a home health aide to care for the patient for whom service has been ordered. The policies require the registered nurse or qualified therapist, when appropriate, to prepare written instructions for these services to be provided by the home health aide. These written instructions would identify the specific duties to be performed by the home health aide and would include, but not be limited to the duties identified in this standard for the home health aide. When the aide is expected to perform some duties as an extension of the therapy service(s), the therapist(s) must prepare written instructions for the home health aide. It is not sufficient to write on the home health aide assignment sheet, "Exercise program as instructed by the therapist." The agency policies must also specify the necessity for the home health aide assignment sheet and care plan to be updated as frequently as necessary to remain current.

        The assignment sheet should contain sufficient information to promote efficiency in meeting the patient's personal care needs. Too often pertinent information about the patient is not given to the home health aide. Only when care is initiated does the home health aide learn that the patient is hard of hearing, forgetful, speaks very little English, or prefers to ambulate unassisted even though this practice is not safe. Often the assignment sheet is not sufficiently detailed to complement the provision of other services. For example, the occupational therapist may be developing a program to enable the patient to become independent in bathing and dressing activities. Unless the information is shared with the home health aide, the aide may continue to assume much of the responsibility for these activities which could safely be performed by the patient.

The assignment sheet should always specify the change in the patient's condition which should promptly be reported to the professional nurse or the aide's supervisor.

b) *Supervisor*

The agency's written policies must clearly specify that the home health aide is regularly supervised by the registered nurse or therapist, when the therapist participates in the assignment of the care to be provided. At least every two weeks a supervisory visit is made to the patient's residence either when the aide is present to observe and assist, or when the aide is absent to determine if the aide has established relationships and consistently provided services in a manner which promotes achievement of the personal care goals established for the patient. The clinical record should verify that this supervision has occurred and that it is sufficient to ensure that the home health aide is completing all duties as assigned. The supervisory note in the patient's clinical record should establish if the aide was present or absent during the visit.

Agency policy may establish that the requirement for supervising the home health aide at least every two weeks is waived when the patient is receiving services of a custodial nature. However, the policy should specify the manner in which professional supervision is provided when the home health aide provides personal care and incidental household services in the circumstances.

The format completed by the home health aide identifying the services provided during each visit should also be reviewed to verify that the aide has completed the duties which were assigned. More often than one would expect, the format completed by the home health aide indicates that some duties are performed sporadically or not at all, or that the duties have been performed by the aide in the absence of written instructions to do so. The home health aide should be encouraged to write comments about the patient's condition. It is unfortunate when the home health aide's comments identify symptoms which could affect the patient's response to the treatment plan before these symptoms are identified by the appropriate professional.

Condition 405.1228 Condition of Participation: Clinical Records

This condition requires the agency to have written policies which specify the necessity for a clinical record to be maintained for every patient receiving home health services, the manner in which the records will be retained and protected, and the content of the clinical records. The review of clinical records should establish that the content of the records meets the requirements set forth in this condition as well as any additional requirements specified in the agency's policy.

The record is expected to contain specific detailed information which confirms that services and treatments and interventions were provided as ordered by the physician, documents the patient's course during the period the agency renders care, provides information on which to base immediate and long-term plans, supports communication between all members of the health care team, including the physician, and promotes continuity of care. For professional, financial, educational, and legal reasons, the importance of incorporating the appropriate information in the clinical record can not be overstressed.

The review of clinical records frequently indicates that the terms clinical note, progress note, and summary report have not been clearly defined in applicable agency policies. The clinical note is an updated written notation by a member of the health team of a contact with a patient containing a description of signs and symptoms, treatments and interventions provided. This most frequently occurs when a flow sheet type format is used and the caregiver documents that instruction, supervision, discussion, or evaluation of a specific parameter was completed. It also occurs when personnel use such phrases as, "treatments provided as ordered," or "exercise program completed as written" to document the care provided. Because the clinical record establishes the action of the caregiver in a permanent form, it is imperative that the specific actions of the caregiver, as well as the patient's condition and response to the action of the caregiver be accurately and completely described. The clinical note must always be written the day service is rendered and incorporated in the patient's clinical record at least weekly.

The progress note is a dated written notation by a member of the health care team containing specific information about the patient's response to the treatment and intervention which have been provided over a specific period of time. The progress note is written as frequently as necessary in order to evaluate the patient's need and responses to the treatment plan over a specific period of time. The frequency for preparing a progress note may vary; however, a progress note should be prepared for each therapeutic discipline at least every 60 days. The summary report is a compilation of the pertinent information from the clinical and progress notes which is submitted to the patient's physician. Summary reports must be submitted to the physician at least every 60 days and at the time the patient is discharged from service(s).

The agency should have procedures which establish the purpose for each of the formats utilized in the clinical record as well as instructions for accurately completing the forms. The review of clinical records should document that the formats are utilized appropriately. Personnel should not be able to use any other format instead of those approved for use by the agency.

The clinical record should be organized in a manner which facilitates use and promotes the incorporation of information in a systematic manner and the prompt retrieval of information.

    a)   *Retention of Records*

        The agency must have written policies relative to the retention and preservation of the clinical records. The policies must meet applicable state laws. In the absence of state laws, agency policy must specify that the clinical record will be retained for at least five years after the month the cost report to which the records apply is filed with the intermediary. The policies for retention and preservation of the records should establish the procedures for maintaining the clinical records in a systematic manner as well as the procedure disposing of the records appropriately.

The policies should clearly specify the manner in which the records will be retained if the agency discontinues its operation.

b) *Protection of the records*

The agency must have written policies which delineate how clinical records will be protected. The policies should also meet applicable laws relative to the release of information. The policies should establish under what circumstances information may be released from the clinical record, or the clinical record may be taken from the agency. The policy should identify those persons who may have access to the record as "authorized personnel." The system for storing and filing the records should ensure that although the records are readily available, there are safeguards to protect the record from damage, loss, or unauthorized use.

§405.1229 Condition of participation: Evaluation

This condition requires the agency to have written policies which specify that a written evaluation of the agency's operation will be completed at least annually, the manner in which this evaluation will be completed, and the process followed to ensure that the evaluation is promptly reviewed and acted on by the group of professionals and the governing body.

The agency should have a written plan for conducting the evaluation. The plan should specify the responsibilities of the individuals who participate in the review. The agency may retain the service's knowledgeable individuals and organizations to complete the annual program evaluation when it is determined that this process would provide a more objective and thorough assessment of the agency's operation.

a) *Policy and administrative review*

As part of the evaluation process, those responsible for conducting the evaluation should have access to patient service and personnel activity data to determine if the policies and administrative practices of the agency promote delivery of patient care that is appropriate, adequate, efficient, and effective. The agency must establish in writing the mechanisms for collecting and compiling the data necessary to assist in the evaluation process. At minimum, these data should include the information specified in this standard. The evaluation process should also include a review of board and committee activities as well as activities relevant to the management of the agency's fiscal affairs. The evaluation should identify the extent to which existing policies and procedures enable the agency to readily and appropriately respond to existing or potential problems.

b) *Clinical record review*

The agency has written policies which specify the necessity for the quarterly review of clinical records by a committee which includes at minimum a professional representative for each therapeutic service offered. The provision of home health services may be evaluated by the registered nurse or the qualified therapist when appropriate. Agency policies should specify the composition of the committee, the method of appointment, the frequency of meetings, and the process for selecting the open and closed records to be reviewed. This process should ensure that at least 10% of each service provided on a quarterly basis is reviewed. If a therapeutic service has been provided to less than 100 patients during the quarter, the committee should review at least ten records of documents in summary report that the service has been provided to less than 10 patients. If the agency provides service to more than 500 patients per month, the committee may review less than 10% of each service. The state survey agency should be contacted to determine the percentage of records which must be reviewed in this instance.

The committee findings should be summarized and reported to the group of professional personnel. The nursing supervisor should ensure that appropriate action is taken to correct any problems identified. Subsequent review of the clinical records should assess the extent to which the action taken has been effective.

In addition to the quarterly clinical review, the agency should have policies and procedures for conducting other quality assurance activities on a regular basis. These activities should also assist the agency to evaluate the quality, appropriateness, and effectiveness of care provided to patients; assess the utilization and coordination of services; identify gaps in service; obtain information relative to staff development, program, planning, and evaluation; and provide a mechanism for the resolution of problem cases.

Finally, the agency policies should establish the process for completing the 60-day review of records and specify the personnel expected to participate in this review. The clinical record should document that this review has been completed.

Accreditation: Quality Assurance for Shaping Nursing's Role in Health Care Delivery Systems

Stephen Paul Holzemer

Introduction

The National League for Nursing has been supporting the nursing profession in its quest for providing quality nursing care in home care and community health settings since the mid-1960s. This support has been channeled into an accreditation program to encourage professionals working outside institutional settings to provide the highest level of quality health care. This discussion of accreditation is intended to provide the reader with the clear understanding of the benefits of accreditation, with an overview of the process, and with a discussion of key concepts related to the process of accreditation.

Although this document will focus specifically on the potentials for nursing related to accreditation, it must be understood that the accreditation program sponsored by the National League for Nursing relates to services provided by all disciplines in home care and community health. The accreditation process is a peer review activity involving input from many health professions with particular focus on consumers as recipients of care. Accreditation fosters the belief that both the provider and recipient of care need to be directly involved in the creation and evaluation of services.

Purposes of Accreditation

Accreditation exists for a number of purposes. Home care and community health agencies (i.e., VNA's Home Care Departments, Public Health Units) become accredited for the purpose of stimulating the continuous improvement of services and also measuring an agency's progress in measuring up to nationally accepted standards. In addition, the process of accreditation promotes the coordination and integration of quality health care delivery by all disciplines providing care. Accreditation fosters the best possible use of available health personnel and fosters a climate for ongoing self-study and peer review. Accreditation distinguishes the excellent agency from its competition because peers from across the country have judged it as meeting high standards (Nassif 1985, 50). This process identifies for the consumer those agencies that have measurable structure, process, and outcome quality indicators.

Benefits

Accreditation must benefit the agency that wishes to complete the process--otherwise critical resources of the agency and staff are depleted. The agency should, as a whole, decide whether or not they wish to enter the process of accreditation and whether or not their resources can support the process to its completion. The process of accreditation can conserve agency and staff resources when the task is understood as having benefits for all participants. Accreditation becomes an organizing concept to foster staff and agency efficiency in care delivery. It is important for all participants to understand the benefits of accreditation; there are many.

The benefits of accreditation concentrate in two main areas: the first type of benefit is generic in nature and the second type of benefit is more specific to individuals served by the process. The second category separates into the areas of benefits for clients, personnel in the agency, and the agency itself.

To begin with, there are four major benefits of accreditation that are more generic to all individuals involved in the process. Accreditation:

1. Stimulates agency growth through the in-depth self-evaluation required by the process.

2. Determines an agency's quality in relation to nationally accepted standards.

3. Facilitates an agency's continuous improvement through implementation of peer body recommendations.

4. Demonstrates an agency's accountability to consumers, third-party payors, and other interested bodies.

Other benefits of accreditation relate specifically to providers and recipients of care.

Benefits to Clients: Developing an Interpersonal Relationship

The examination of benefits to clients using the agency's services should be considered before the agency enters the accreditation process. Involving key consumers in the process of accreditation helps them appreciate the complexity of agency functioning. Although standards for accreditation can be met without major client involvement, it is important to help clients appreciate the internal workings of the agency to gain their support for programs and services. Since all health disciplines essentially exist to meet the health and illness needs of clients, they (consumers) should be central, not peripheral, to all agency workings. Consumer involvement relates to the concept of their owning the services provided by an agency. If they feel comfortable with the services, they may well serve as public relations ambassadors for the agency.

Agencies can develop available and acceptable services for clients by involving selected consumers in decision-making about programs and services. The accreditation process clarifies to clients how services and programs are coordinated and how they relate to agency's resources. With the advent of various prospective payment systems, in acute and community-based settings, it is essential that the consumer of services and resources be clear about the strengths and potential of the process. It is not suggested that one sell the limiting aspects of prospective payment systems, but rather help the client understand the resources of the agency and how they are dispensed via services. An understanding of prospective payment system can foster a new and profitable working relationship with your clients. Involving consumers in accreditation is a major, yet inexpensive, risk management initiative. Clients are fully aware of the products and services of the agency and have established an interpersonal relationship with the staff and management team. The interpersonal relationship the agency strives to foster may well help identify risk situations which can be dealt with before a crisis occurs.

Benefits to Personnel: Developing a Team

There are also benefits of accreditation which relate specifically to the personnel who work for the agency in providing services. All types of agencies, from the most traditional to the most innovative, need to focus on securing a solid market for their services. All personnel represent the first line of marketing and selling for an agency. This newly emerging role may cause a role conflict for personnel: corporate goals versus professional expectations. Many professionals feel that corporate goals are in opposition to professional expectations. It becomes a critical benefit to personnel to help them work through these issues by the accreditation process. The agency can define and develop a market in consort with professional practice standards. Accreditation may be received as a process supportive of nursing's social contract with society (American Nurses' Association 1980). The accreditation process links the philosophy and expectations of the corporation with the strength of potentials of individual professionals.

Accreditation also provides a mechanism for personnel within a discipline and across disciplines to work collaboratively. The accreditation standards clarify roles and provide a mechanism by which all personnel can share in the process of setting priorities within and among the services and programs. Accreditation supports personnel in understanding the complexities of corporate goals and how they can best support the agency as well as provide the highest level of quality to their clients. It is a reality in today's economic environment (in health care) that budget cuts, shifts in programs and staff, and rapid development of new services to capture emerging markets are occurring daily. Accreditation can be instrumental in making these rapid changes more palatable to employees. Personnel develop an "agency wide" perspective of issues and can be less parochial in their vision of how the agency might evolve. The unintentional exploitation of professionals outside of their scope of practice is avoided when various disciplines work together to identify their own strengths and potentials, as well as in a collective mission that all personnel can support.

The accreditation process provides a matrix in which all personnel can be involved in decision making for the agency. Employees may become more involved in product and service development. The staff may also become more involved in the actual provisions of various services, or more involved in the administration of various programs and services. It is important, from the point of the administrator or management team, to know where every individual in the agency stands in their ability to support the corporation. The accreditation process provides a natural overlay for corporate goals and the performance appraisal mechanism used by the agency. Individual practitioners (professional and ancillary) become well aware of the expectations the agency sets for evaluation of their performance. Personnel are not only involved in having their clinical skills evaluated; they are evaluated in every aspect of supporting the corporation in meeting the needs of clients.

The accreditation process can be central to grooming "in-house" managers. It is important to develop a strong and committed cadre of managers to assist the agency in achieving care delivery goals that many times are seen as very costly. Through individual orientation plans for "budding" managers, and grooming these managers using principles of adult learning with the accreditation criteria and standards, the administrator can develop a blueprint for diagnosing areas in which managers need to strengthen their level of confidence and performance. Using accreditation criterion standards as the daily measures of management capability removes managers from a frequently experienced "crisis mode" and enables them to utilize their strengths and potentials to manage for the future viability of the agency.

Benefits to the Agency: An Investment in the Future

As previously mentioned, it is essential that accreditation become a major benefit for the agency itself--separate from the benefits to clients and the personnel that work for the agency. Accreditation must serve the agency. It must be a wise, acceptable investment: a wise and acceptable investment from the point of view of both the individual providers of care and the management team, from the board of directors to the first line managers. The process of accreditation will not miraculously benefit the agency; the agency must commit to use the process for continuous growth proactively. Some accredited agencies are probably disappointed when they find out that the process continuously demands their input for improved services in the agency. It's not a process that is completed every few years by completing forms and submitting documentation. It is a continuous investment in improvement of services and in the integrity of the agency. Benefits to the agency range from enabling the agency to develop a visionary strategic plan and marketing strategy, to developing continuing education programs to specifically meet risk management concerns. Other benefits relate to securing grants, obtaining contributions to the agency, and enabling agencies to enter joint ventures and diversify with the support of the community around them.

Of primary importance in today's health care sector is the concept of short-term funding. Accreditation may well give an agency the competitive edge when it is seeking local aid and state or federal funding for special projects. Accreditation may also serve to foster business relationships between various corporations within a community. Agencies, whether acute care or community-oriented, are continuously examining the potential for joint ventures and diversification of services within a community. Meeting national standards and developing a blueprint for quality services through the accreditation process may well put an agency ahead of the competition when joint ventures and diversification of services are developed. The accreditation process can magnify its strengths in both public relations and a financially creative posture.

Another benefit to agencies in relationship to accreditation relates to the recruitment and retention of personnel. The enormous cost of attracting and retaining qualified personnel plagues many agencies. The mobility of personnel and changing general economic conditions may rapidly change any stability an agency may have within its staff mix. The components of accreditation serve to orient, promote, remove, and retain personnel working for an agency. The agency can be presented to health providers as an agency that promotes professional standards while emerging as a secure business in service to the community. The agency takes a position of offense, not defense, in securing an appropriate staff mix for the agency. This benefit of accreditation relates directly to the use of students in the health care delivery environment.

In the rapidly changing health care delivery system, we need new practitioners that have sharp skills, both mechanical and theoretical in providing their usefulness to society by providing health services. The staffs of agencies have an opportunity (and some feel an obligation) to serve as role models for the next generation of health providers. An agency using accreditation criteria and standards can complement the educational process by offering a quality clinical experience that is deeply rooted in the current realities of health care delivery. A frequent concern related to providing clinical experiences for students relates to the cost to the agency for providing this experience. Using the criterion standards for accreditation, an agency can quickly andefficiently identify where student placement could be useful. In this framework, students are not used simply for provision of clinical care to clients, but in a number of roles within the process of strategic planning for the agency. If an agency wants students skilled at a basic level at graduation, it should aggressively seek out schools of nursing, medicine, and health professions that can provide it with technical support from their faculty, as well as from their students.

The most important concept related to the education of students relates to their roles when they graduate as gatekeeper of a health care delivery system. It is important for agencies to extend beyond nursing education, but also look at providing experiences for student physicians, and student social workers, for example, that are in many situations the nation's gatekeepers in community health. Many agencies spend financial and time resources attracting professionals that arc already out of the educational system. It is important to help students of health professions learn why an agency is different, and why it has a documented ability to provide quality services. They will more readily use the agency's services when they become the gatekeepers of tomorrow, if that agency has courted them while they were students.

In summary, the benefits of accreditation are both generic and specific. It is imperative for agencies to decide which benefits they wish to receive from the process of accreditation. The accreditation process, however, is one that will demand continuous commitment to services and programs by staff within the agency. Benefits of accreditation developed by the agency, assume an ongoing commitment of time and energy to improve agency functioning. The benefits of accreditation for the future productivity and fiscal solvency of the agency cannot be underplayed.

For some agencies, the accreditation process of continual involvement of staff in improving services does not cost the agency money, but actually makes money for the agency. When the types of cost savings that an agency would accrue by decreasing turnover of staff, increasing referrals, and increasing staff productivity are examined, accreditation no longer "costs" money. The accreditation process actually becomes a revenue-generating source for the corporation.

Overview of the Accreditation Process

The accreditation process is not one that is completed late at night solely by the administrator. The process of accreditation is the collective vision in work of nurses, social workers, dietitians, and consumers. The process of accreditation moves from the structure of excellence that is required by the various criteria and standards to an outcome-oriented quality assurance system. Accreditation, as a marker of excellence, reflects the agency success in coordinating a system of services which are rooted in the theory and practice of various health management and care providers. Various therapists, religious and volunteer support personnel, and physicians as well as board members all become part of the growing movement of excellence for the individual agency.

The most succinct components of the accreditation process are the concepts of peer review and voluntary self-study. The question, "Where is the agency in its movement toward reaching its mission?" becomes the focus of a voluntary self-examination by the agency (self-study) according to the guidance of peers also providing services to the community (sitc visit and board of review). The self-study process includes a detailed examination of all personnel and material resources which provide care delivery to the community. These resources are explicated when the agency addresses each of the criteria and standards that have been established by a national group of experts in home care and community health. The peer review component of accreditation relates to the meeting of the board of review, made up of administrators, consultants, and consumers from across the nation.

Accreditation is viewed as an act of good faith with consumers who use the home care and community health services provided by the agency. Consumers use the resources of an accredited agency knowing that institution has "done its part" in their contractual agreement between provider and recipient of health care. Knowing that the agency has met nationally recognized standards becomes quite instrumental in allowing clients to participate more freely in their health choices. Accreditation stands for proven excellence in the quality of care provided to consumers. The self-study report, written by the agency, identifies the areas of excellence in five major categories. The organizing concepts which cluster the criteria and standards for accreditation relate to the following areas: strategic planning and marketing, organization and administration of the agency, the programs provided, the staff involved in providing care to the public, and the overall plan for evaluation of the agency.

Submission of the self-study report represents the interest of the agency in beginning the accreditation process. When the document is received at the National League for Nursing, it is examined briefly for its completeness. Site visitors are then assigned to visit the agency to verify, clarify, and amplify the self-study document. Site visitors, oriented to evaluate the agency according to accreditation requirements, may be program administrators, consultants, or staff from the National League for Nursing. The site visitors examine documents retained at the agency (i.e., confidential information), interview personnel, and discuss overall agency concerns with individuals from the agency-governing body as well as clients that are using services at the agency. The site visitors write a report that complements the agency's self-study report. Both documents are used by the accreditation board of review in making an accreditation decision.

Members of the board of review are elected by accredited agencies. They represent individuals which have expertise in home care and community health and have demonstrated competence in working with the criteria and standards for accreditation. The board of review examines the self-study document and the site visitor's report in making their accreditation decision. During the board of review, site visitors and the agency administrator may be contacted in case there are questions about either report. Actions of the board of review include granting an initial accreditation, granting continuing accreditation, or deferring, denying, or withdrawing accreditation from an agency. These decisions are made after the agency is discussed at length by the board of review members. Changes in the agency's accreditation status do not occur without a lengthy period of consultation in support from the accreditation program.

Agencies that are reviewed by the board of review receive a detailed description of their strength and potentials. The board of review identifies specific recommendations for improvement and commendations for excellence every time a self-study report is submitted to the board. Between the time full self-study reports are submitted and site visits occur, the agency submits an interim report. The interim report relates to changes that have occurred in the agency as well as specific requests for information by the board of review. Special reports and progress reports may be required at any time by the board of review to help the agency continue providing services at a level of excellence. Agencies are requested to provide documentation of changes in their structure and mission whenever they occur so that the board of review can assume a position of support for agencies as they diversify their services. Once an agency is accredited, it may submit names of individuals working in the agencies for the role of site visitor and board of review member. Agencies are strongly encouraged to participate at every level in the accreditation process.

The Accreditation Program for Home Care and Community Health seeks to assist both accredited and nonaccredited agencies in their development. Consultation is provided for agencies that are accredited as well as agencies that are simply interested in the process. New agencies find the criterion standards excellent tools for developing their services to clients. Whether they enter the accreditation process formally or not, they find the accreditation program sponsored by the National League for Nursing to be a great asset in their development. Many agencies have used the criteria and standards initially to establish programs or changes in programs. They then enter the process when they have the personnel and material resources to commit themselves to a continued growth and development experience through accreditation.

The accreditation program continuously undergoes change as agencies change in both form and function. As the field changes, the accreditation program also changes to be of assistance to agencies meeting the demands of the marketplace. Agencies involved in the accreditation process are moving toward a "critical mass" which will give them a collective, political, and professional clout in changing health care systems. The criteria and standards serve to support the agency in becoming a prime mover in changing the health care system. Nonaccredited agencies are encouraged to review and critique the criteria and standards of accreditation for how they feel the process would be useful or not useful for them. The accreditation program includes the suggestions of nonaccredited agencies in its program development.

Key Concepts in Accreditation: The Criteria and Standards

It is important for agencies entering the accreditation process to understand the significance of both the criteria and standards for accreditation. A criterion describes the variables that are to be measured in the accreditation process. Standards, on the other hand, specify the level of achievement the agency must abide by in order to become accredited. It's important to understand the process of meeting both the criteria and standards in a specific area of accreditation. The criteria are examined here to provide a flavor of the expectations of accreditation. The criteria are grouped under the five major categories discussed previously. The criteria which follow and the information presented in the paragraph immediately preceding, reflect the accreditation requirements at their last revision (National League for Nursing 1985a).

Strategic planning and marketing is central to the survivability of any agency currently providing services to the community. The overall expectation for agencies seeking accreditation in the area of strategic planning and marketing relates to the following statement.

> The agency utilizes information gathered from the community to establish and alter programs and services as well as developing a strategic (multi-year) plan for future community/provider needs. (There are two criteria that relate to the area of strategic planning and marketing. They are:)

Criterion 1

The provider accesses the community served and develops a mission statement which reflect attention to current and anticipated community needs.

Criterion 2

A multi-year strategic plan for example (a long range or business plan) incorporates actual and potential community needs, in provider resources.

The standards that relate to these criteria involve the agency community assessment and identification of what needs can be realistically met by the agency. The agency identifies who created the strategic plan as well as how it is supported by the governing body. The agency is provided an opportunity to relate critical management data such as number of clients seen, visits made, productivity of discipline, to the development of a realistic strategic plan.

The next major area of accreditation concerns organization and administration of the agency. The following represents a synopsis of what is expected in the organization and the administration of accreditation.

Health services are provided in a community wide basis. Services may be provided by one agency or maybe a component one or more providers possibly of different types. The provider has legal authorization to operate, in the area of the governing body accountable for the management of the agency. The provider in its subunit/branch offices is organized effectively and efficiently to deliver home care and community health services.

Accreditation criteria 3 to 10 identify the expectations in organization and administration for completing the requirements for accreditation. These criteria are listed below.

Criterion 3. The provider has a legally constituted body that is responsible for the effective governing of the agency. It involves consumers in broad agency affairs when possible.

Criterion 4. Administrative responsibilities and relationships are established and clearly defined.

Criterion 5. The governing body delegates to the qualified individual the authority and responsibility for overall agency administration.

Criterion 6. If the provider has a person (or persons) other than the administrator responsible for the administration and direction of the provider's program, this individual (or individuals) is delegated the authority and responsibility for program adminstration.

Criterion 7. If the provider has a person other than the administrator responsible for the fiscal and business affairs of the provider, this individual is delegated the authority and responsibility for fiscal and business practices.

Criterion 8. Fiscal policies and practices assure effective and efficient implementation of the program(s) of the provider.

Criterion 9. The provider has agreements with organizations, agencies, and/or individuals for securing or providing services.

Criterion 10. The provider evaluates its organizational structure and administrative policies and practices.

Resolving concerns in the organization and administration of the agency would be helpful in an attempt to coordinate resources to provide the most supportive environment for quality care delivery. Typically, agency administration is seen as far removed from care of clients. The accreditation process attempts to clearly articulate the relationship between a well managed agency and a supportive environment for excellence in care delivery.

Agency programs are examined in the next section of criteria. The natural evolution of programs occurs out of the strategic planning process and the organization and administration superstructure of the agency. The overview of expectations in this section are provided below.

Programs are planned and provided in accordance with the provider's purpose, in relation to community health needs and the total community health program. When appropriate, the provider's resources are available for preparation of health practitioners.

Criterion 11. The management information system (MIS) promotes effective planning and implementation of programs within the provider.

Criterion 12. The provider has established programs which reflect the multi-year strategic plan for the provider. Objectives are established to monitor client progress with services.

Criterion 13. For each program and service, the provider has priorities that are responsive to provider purpose and community need. All services are coordinated.

Criterion 14. The provider has policies and procedures governing programs, services, and professional practices.

Criterion 15. Service records are maintained for each client.

Criterion 16. The provider has the responsibility for participation, if feasible, in the education of student health personnel.

Criterion 17. The provider evaluates its program(s).

Programs represent the visible commitment of an agency to the clients for whom they care. It is in this context that the accreditation concerns of utilization review (of services) and peer review (of care delivery) are most closely examined.

Staff concerns are examined next in the process and these concerns dovetail with the agencies programmatic needs. The introductory statement and criteria in this area are developed with a special emphasis on appropriate use of personnel resources.

The purpose of the provider is reflected in staffing patterns, policies and practices. Administrative, supervisory, direct service, and supportive personnel are essential for effective delivery of health services. Professional staff have the responsibility for planning providing, and supervisory services to patients and families and for coordination of the activities of multidisciplinary personnel.

Criterion 18. The staff composition is commensurate with the needs of the provider's programs. There are written job descriptions for all classifications of personnel.

Criterion 19. The provider has written personnel policies and personnel records for all personnel.

Criterion 20. The provider provides ongoing professional and/or technical supervision and/or consultation for all personnel.

Criterion 21. The agency provides for staff development.

Criterion 22. The provider evaluates its staffing patterns, policies, and practices.

The last component of the accreditation process, which brings the agency full cycle in meeting client needs relates to overall agency evaluation. Although evaluation has been addressed in the previous sections, overall evaluation is expected to provide a comprehensive view of the agency with special emphasis on evaluation as a critical component of strategic planning and marketing.

The provider is accountable to the community for the quality of its care. Accountability is insured by an effective evaluation process. Evaluation is the essence of a strategic plan and of marketing activities.

Criterion 23. The provider has a structure and plan for evaluation.

Criterion 24. The provider establishes goals as a result of its overall evaluation which become central to continued strategic planning and marketing. It communicates its status to the public.

Summary

Accreditation provides a mechanism whereby cost containment and quality of care can coexist. The very difficult balance between these two "implacable imperatives" (Donabedian 1984, 142), can be addressed by the examination of accreditation criteria and standards.

The benefits of accreditation are many; they can be clustered into more generic benefits for all participants (i.e., recognition of meeting national standards) and specific benefits to clients, agency personnel, and the agency itself. Benefits to clients center on issues of their increased functioning in health care decision making. Key consumers are also encouraged to participate in developing a clearer understanding of agency strengths and potentials of programs and services. Developing a strong supportive relationship with the community served cannot be undervalued. Accreditation provides the tools to foster that relationship.

The agency's personnel also receive benefits of accreditation primarily by clarifying their role in relation to the agency's future development. Accreditation assists employees in accepting responsibility for better staff coordination in care delivery and program planning. The accreditation process may also foster bridging the gap between clinical expertise and management essentials. As managers in an agency are groomed, accreditation criteria and standards can be used to structure the new manager's transition. The criteria and standards can represent a blueprint where new managers need to demonstrate important business skills related to strategic planning and evaluation, for example.

Agencies invest in their future by entering the accreditation process. It is an investment in establishing a sound base on which to build for upcoming changes in care provision and program development. Agencies set themselves above their competition when they meet the nationally developed standards of accreditation.

The accreditation process makes the criteria and standards more than abstract comments. The process, from application by the agency to the decision of the board of review, is one of continuous growth. The agency interprets its status in a self-study--professional visitors verify, clarify, and amplify the report on site--peers in home care and community health identify strengths and limitations in the agency for their continuous self-improvement.

The accreditation process provides a challenge to agencies to accept responsibility for their growth and development in the areas of strategic planning and marketing, organization and administration, programs, staff, and overall agency evaluation. When examined as a total process, accreditation examines structure, process, and outcome components of quality assurance. The criteria and standards are continuously evaluated and revised for their appropriateness in the contemporary care delivery scene.

Accredited agencies also reshape how care is provided by their thoughtful critique of the program and their work toward improving the process by suggesting change. The challenge to become a part of a measurable quality assurance process, making it more care outcome-sensitive, faces agencies and professionals involved in accreditation.

Editor's Note: The Deficit Reduction Act of 1984 authorized the Secretary of Health and Human Services to deem national accrediting bodies, thereby, recognizing the decisions of those bodies in determining whether a provider meets requirements for Medicare participation. The National League for Nursing's application for deemed status has been satisfactorily reviewed by staff of the Health Standards and Quality Bureau and the Bureau of Eligibility, Reimbursement and Coverage of the Health Care Financing Administration. It is anticipated that deemed status will become effective in 1987. The review will change from a five to a three-year cycle with an annual written report.

Certificate of Need and Licensure

E. Michael Flanagan

Introduction

At first glance, a health care entrepreneur's interest in home health as a business is understandable. The product to be furnished is readily identifiable and labor- rather than material-intensive. This means that the anticipated capital outlay for start-up costs should be minimal.

It is only when the entrepreneur confronts the complex and often confusing array of federal and state regulations concerning home health agencies (hereafter referred to as "HHAs") that the hidden costs of establishing a home care program are realized.

This chapter discusses two aspects of this regulatory scheme: Certificate of Need (hereafter referred to as "CON") and licensure. As you will discover in reading the following pages, the impact of CON and licensure requirements on HHAs will vary dramatically depending on the state in which the HHA operates.[1] It is important, however, from the standpoint of marketing feasibility, to understand the specific requirements of the jurisdiction in which you plan to establish a home health program.

Finally, because many states have merged their state licensure function with their responsibilities concerning certification of new Medicare providers, some discussion of Medicare certification will be inevitable in this chapter, even though that topic will be covered in more detail elsewhere in the book.

HHA CON Requirements

Background. When Congress passed the National Health Planning and Resources Development Act of 1974,[2] it sought to rationalize the distribution of health services throughout the United States and give individual states a legal mechanism to make prospective determinations of need for new health care services. These laudable objectives proved more problematic in practice than originally envisioned and the 12 years since enactment of the law have seen the once energetically federal initiative become almost exclusively a creature of state law. Federal funding for health planning has declined considerably in recent years and some states, such as California, have repealed their CON laws and substituted more stringent licensure requirements for health care facilities.

The establishment of a home health agency historically has required a limited capital expenditure. Moreover, the existence of CON requirements for HHAs in certain states has thus far failed to demonstrate a positive correlation between restricted market entry and lower costs per unit of service.[3] Consequently, states are beginning to reconsider the need to include HHAs in their CON laws and at least four states (Texas, Tennessee, California, and Virginia) have eliminated HHAs from CON review.[4] The continuing trend toward less regulation and greater free market competition for health care services generally will likely convince more states in the future to eliminate HHAs from CON review.

Impact on Feasibility Study. When someone decides to explore the possibility of entering the home health care market as a provider of services, essentially two options are available. The first is acquisition of part or all of an existing home health care business. The second is the creation of a new HHA that will compete for a share of the existing market. The presence of a CON law for HHAs in the state of intended operation is often the single most important determinant in deciding whether to go forward with the project in that state and under which option.

Some form of feasibility study is desirable for any prospective entrant into the home care business. The first consideration identified in a creditable feasibility study will be barriers to entry into the market. For example, some states (including Florida, Georgia, Alabama, Kentucky, and Mississippi) have at one time or another imposed moratoriums on the issuance of new HHA CONs. This would mean that the only opportunity for entry in these states would be acquisition or the establishment of a private-pay HHA (i.e., an agency that provides no services to Medicare or Medicaid beneficiaries), if that is not a reviewable event under state law.[5]

If the state of operation in the new entrant's business plan is not predetermined, the existence of CON requirements could lead to the selection of a different state. Such a move is not without its risks.

Selecting a Non-CON state. The selection of a non-CON state will have the immediate beneficial effect of eliminating the need for significant start-up costs for consulting, legal, and accounting expenses related to obtaining CON approval. On the other hand, absence of CON means that any other competitors (including local hospitals) can invade the market at any time and steal away referral sources and valued employees.

Survival in such a competitive environment is difficult. Hospitals more than likely will have their own facility-based HHAs to capture their own home health referrals. At the same time, these hospitals will put pressure on their staff physicians to refer to the hospital-based agency. In addition, national chain home health providers are generally more active in these markets because their size allows them to endure the financial strains of longer start-up periods.

Thus, the decision to pursue a non-CON state is not a panacea. In fact, certain state home health associations (Florida and Georgia, for example) have fought to preserve their state CON programs for HHAs motivated in large measure by its belief that CON is the only way to preserve the free standing community-based HHA.

Acquiring an HHA in a CON State. Recognizing the difficulties of surviving in a non-CON state, it may be advisable to explore acquisition opportunities in the CON state.[6] In most CON states, the acquisition of an HHA's stock or a transfer of assets is considered a change of ownership. As such, unless the change of ownership is accompanied by a change in the scope of services or service area, it will be determined to be a nonreviewable event.[7]

It is often the case, however, that the state health planning agency will require notice of the change of ownership at some time in advance of the event.[8] Thus, the recommended manner of proceeding is to identify the intended acquisition, negotiate the purchase offer, and then send a formal letter of intent to acquire the HHA to the state health planning agency. The letter should also request a written confirmation that the acquisition is a nonreviewable event under the state CON law. Once the confirmation letter is received, the need to focus on CON issues is at an end unless a later modification of service or service area necessitates review.

If the acquisition entails simply a transfer of part or all of the existing agency's stock, the transaction might not even fall under the CON law's change of ownership rules. Thus, as in all potential CON matters, a careful review of the law and regulations could avoid unnecessary headaches.[9]

Obtaining a CON. This discussion is not for the faint of heart. Under the best of circumstances, obtaining a CON in a conscientiously regulated state can be a brutal affair involving intense political influence wielding and courtroom battles with established HHAs in the affected service area.

Based on experience, it can be anticipated that obtaining a CON will add $50,000 to $100,000 to agency start-up costs. This figure can rise significantly if an adversely affected HHA files suit to enjoin issuance of the CON. In one of the more famous CON wars, Johnson & Johnson waged a major campaign to obtain HHA CONs in Florida. The widely publicized assault on the state CON program ultimately brought the Florida Association of Home Health Agencies into the fray on the side of the state health planning agency. After having the regulatory basis upon which need determinations had been made in Florida since 1975 declared invalid,[10] Johnson & Johnson abandoned the effort, having spent approximately $3 million in a losing cause.

If you are still undaunted by the bleak prospects of obtaining a CON, then the first step to take would be to examine the CON law and regulations to see if there is any way validly to claim entitlement to an exemption from the review requirement.

Exemptions may be available for a number of reasons based on your particular circumstances. We have already discussed the exemption based on change of ownership (see p. 47, above). Some states also exempt from review new HHAs whose operating expenses will not exceed a certain amount in the first year of operation.[11] Obviously, this exemption would not help an agency that expects to be very busy in the first year of operation. It should be remembered, however, that it is the applicant that makes the estimate of first year operating expenses. Thus, you have control over your figures and even if you succeed beyond your expectations in the first year, it is never easy for a state health planning agency to pull a CON on an HHA already in operation. Further, state planning agencies lack the resources presently to police CONs after they have been issued.

Finally, some states have so-called "grandfather" provisions in the CON laws that exempt from review existing HHAs that have been providing home health services continuously in the state since a time prior to the effective date of the CON law. The "grandfather" provision in the Florida licensure law[12] furnishes an excellent illustration of this type of exemption:

> Any home health agency operating and providing services in the state and having a provider number issued by the U.S. Department of Health, Education and Welfare on or before April 30, 1976 shall not be denied a license on the basis of not having received a Certificate of Need.[13]

Historically, Florida has administered its CON program on a county-by-county basis. Because of this, HHAs that were Medicare-certified and operational in the state prior to April 30, 1976 have successfully used the "grandfather" provision to expand their service areas. By simply demonstrating to the state health planning office that it had seen one or more patients in the expansion county prior to the effective date, the HHA is able to obtain a determination that it is exempt from review and able to serve that entire county as fully as any other preexisting HHA already serving the county.

Another exemption category that may become the subject matter of litigation in the future applies to Health Maintenance Organizations (HMOs) that seek to furnish home health services directly. Most states generally exempt HMOs from the coverage of their CON laws.[14] It is unclear, however, if the exemption would apply to all services the HMO furnishes directly.[15]

Even though Florida has an exemption provision for HMOs, the state health planning office maintains that any HMO that seeks to furnish home health services directly must obtain a CON. The federal government, on the other hand, through the Health Care Financing Administration's Bureau of Eligibility, Reimbursement, and Coverage, has taken the position that HMOs seeking to furnish home health services directly are exempt from state CON review, presumably as a matter of federal preemption of state law. To my knowledge, this issue has not yet been brought to a head in the filing of a lawsuit, but the potential for conflict is there.

Obviously, exemptions are exceptions to the rule that new HHAs must submit to CON review. If no exemption is available and acquisition is not feasible, it is important to have some understanding of the typical CON review process so that a strategy can be developed to ensure the best chance of a favorable outcome.

A Typical CON Review Process. All state CON laws differ in certain respects concerning the formalities of the review process, but I will attempt to outline a typical review sequence based on Maryland law.

The first step in the filing of a CON application is the submission of a letter of intent to the health planning agency.[16] If you are unfamiliar with the process generally, a telephone call to the agency would be advisable. Our experience indicates that health planning staff persons can be extremely helpful in guiding applicants through the maze of red tape that invariably accompanies CON actions.

The letter of intent is designed to alert the agency of an impending CON application. It usually includes the following information: (1) a description of the proposed project; (2) the nature and scope of new health services to be offered; (3) the location of the project; and (4) the estimated total project cost.[17] The letter of intent normally sets in motion a time period within which to file the CON application. Under Maryland law, the CON application must be submitted at least 60 days after the submission of the letter of intent, but the application must be received before the expiration of 180 days from the date of submission of the letter of intent.[18] If the application is received too early, it can be held over until the next review period after the expiration of the 60 days. If no application has been received by the expiration of the 180 days, the letter of intent is null and void and the applicant must start over.[19] The time requirements vary from state to state, so it is essential to know your particular state's rules.

It is also important to realize that a CON application takes a good deal of time and effort to complete and the burden of proving entitlement to a CON rests squarely on the applicant. If you are serious about obtaining a CON, it is advisable at this point to hire a consultant who specializes in completing and justifying CON applications. It is also a good idea at this time to start lining up whatever political assistance is available to you to begin the necessary lobbying effort to convince the agency of the need for a new HHA.

Once the application is submitted, the planning agency reviews it for completeness and assigns a docket number.[20] The agency will then notify the applicant in writing of the docketing and will also publish notice of the docketing in a newspaper of general circulation in the area of the proposed project.[21]

Some state planning programs (such as Florida's) have routine review cycles into which similar applications are "batched" for the purpose of comparative review. In other words, if three new HHA CON applications are submitted in the same month, they will be assigned together to the same batching cycle and their individual merits will be assessed in comparison to one another. Thus, if only one new HHA is justified in the area, the best applicant of the three will be selected.

Parties that will be affected by the project (referred to in CON laws as "interested persons" or "interested parties")[22] are entitled to request an evidentiary hearing to be conducted by the planning agency.[23] As a general rule, the hearing must be requested within a certain time period after the notice of docketing is published. The evidentiary hearing is conducted in a fashion similar to a courtroom trial, with counsel representing the parties, oral testimony including examination and cross-examination of witnesses, and a written report by the presiding officer with findings of fact and conclusions of law.[24] The final action of the evidentiary hearing is the issuance by the presiding officer of a Proposed Order that will become final after the parties to the hearing have had an opportunity to file written objections and give oral testimony before final action on the application.[25] The final order in most instances is a grant or denial of the application.

Another type of forum available to affected persons to comment on a proposed project is the public informational hearing.[26] Unlike the adversarial evidentiary hearing, the public informational hearing is more or less an open forum to provide the public with an opportunity to express their views on the project.

Regardless of whether the application is submitted to an evidentiary hearing, or comparative or individual review, its merits will be judged against certain parameters of need established by the state health planning program. These considerations will generally include: (a) the identification of a need for such a service in the State Health Plan;[27] (b) the need of the population served or to be served (a supplemental analysis to the general need determinations included in the State Health Plan); (c) the availability of less costly or more effective alternatives for addressing the unmet needs identified by the applicant; (d) the immediate and long-term financial viability of the project, and (e) the adequacy of staffing, community, and professional support for the project.[28]

The decision of the planning agency on the application must be issued within a certain time period of docketing.[29] The planning agency can decide either to grant the application, deny it, or grant it subject to specific conditions.[30] The decision must be in writing setting forth the reasons for the action.

Assuming that the project has been approved either completely or with acceptable conditions, you might be lulled into thinking that your new HHA is home free. This, however, may be only the beginning of the ordeal. The final decision has created a new class of participants in the CON process called "aggrieved parties." An aggrieved party is essentially an affected person (see page 51 above) who has been adversely affected by the final decision.[31] An aggrieved party (which obviously includes the applicant if the decision was a denial) has the right to request, upon a showing of good cause, a hearing for the purpose of reconsidering the final decision.[32] This reconsideration hearing must be requested within a short period of time after the date of the final decision (normally within 15 days), and a reconsideration decision is considered a new final decision for purposes of appeal (and renewed requests for reconsideration hearings, etc. . . .).

Finally, an aggrieved party that has not been able to show good cause for a reconsideration hearing, or has not been satisfied by a reconsideration decision, has the right to take a direct judicial appeal within a specified time frame of the date of the final decision.[33] The judicial appeal is normally made to the trial court level of the state court system, but the review of the case is normally limited to the record that has been developed in the administrative process. Further, any decision at the trial court level may be appealed to the highest appellate level of the state courts, and ultimately (carrying the process to its most sublimely ridiculous extent) to the United States Supreme Court if a sufficiently national issue can be demonstrated.

Summary. It should be clear from the tenor of the above presentation that it is the opinion of this author that the CON process is an ineffective tool to insure the appropriate distribution of health care resources. It is tedious, expensive, and ultimately incapable of preventing the granting of unnecessary projects to those with the will and financial and political backing to outlast the process. It is, however, a mandatory precondition to the establishment of a new HHA in 34 states and the District of Columbia. Thus, if there is no alternative to submission to the CON process, then the above information should prove useful.

HHA Licensure

Background. Because in states that have HHA licensure laws the license requirement is not used as a barrier to entry into the marketplace, there is no need to go into elaborate detail about the nuances of the licensure process. The political, practical, and economic realities of licensure are unambiguous: if the HHA meets certain conditions established by the state, it will be issued a license; if not, the HHA will not be permitted to operate until the conditions are met.

In some states, such as California, the licensure laws are so stringent and enforced so vigorously that, from the standpoint of economic feasibility, they may constitute a barrier to the establishment of a new HHA. The California experience, however, is clearly the exception.

Of the 35 state licensure laws (including the District of Columbia) for HHAs, virtually all have requirements that track closely with the Medicare program's conditions of participation.[34] In fact, most states have unified their state licensure and Medicare certification functions into one office which coordinates survey activities for both.

Prior to the Omnibus Budget Reconciliation Act of 1980, if an HHA was established in a state that had no HHA licensure law, the HHA was prohibited from participating in the Medicare program unless it had obtained status as a charitable organization under Section 501(c)(3) of the Internal Revenue Code. This restriction was apparently based on the assumption that for-profit HHAs are inherently suspect without a state regulatory body in existence to police their operations. The 1980 legislation abolished such distinctions as a matter of federal law, but at least one state (New York) had retained the restriction as a matter of state law until two years ago.

State HHA Licensure laws have generally been administered without much controversy, but it is important to understand your state's law (if any) so that potential problem areas can be anticipated.

Typical Licensure Law. Most states that have HHA licensure laws make it a criminal offense for anyone to operate an HHA without a license. In many instances, however, the licensure requirement applies only to those HHAs that intend to participate in the Medicare or Medicaid programs. An HHA that is treating only private insurance or private-pay patients will not be required to be licensed. Thus, in these days of separate Medicare and private HHAs, it is important to know the coverage of your state's licensure law.

The licensure law sets out minimum operational standards for HHAs operating in the state that must be met at all times. An applicant for initial licensure must furnish the following information to the licensing office: (a) formal assurance that the applicant complies with all requirements of the state CON law, if applicable; and (b) disclosure of the names and addresses of each officer and director of the HHA.[35]

Upon receipt of the application, the licensing office will schedule a survey to insure that the HHA meets all requirements. The timing of the licensure survey in relation to the operational start-up of the HHA varies from state to state. It is important to make contact with the licensure office in advance of the survey to ascertain the level of activity the survey team is expecting to see by the date of the survey. Most states will not permit the HHA to see a patient before the license is issued. Others will expect to review a patient chart or two and thus require some minimal visit activity prior to the licensure survey.

Essentially, the survey team will be seeking to determine that: (1) the key personnel of the HHA have the requisite skill level; (2) the required scope of services will be provided either directly or through contractual arrangements; (3) the HHA complies with all applicable state and federal laws; (4) the HHA has appropriate liability insurance to cover all employees and contractual indemnity to cover services provided under arrangement; and (5) the HHA has the requisite recordkeeping capability.[36]

If the HHA passes the survey, the state will issue a license for a one-year period. Most states require that the annual application for relicensure be submitted well in advance of the expiration date (generally 60 days) so that any reinspection can be done and a new license issued prior to the expiration date. In at least one state (Florida), an administrative fine of $100 per day is levied against any HHA submitting its relicensure application less than 60 days before the expiration date.

If the HHA fails to meet licensure requirements, it will be denied a license. This decision is subject to appeal under the state's Administrative Procedures Act.

Finally, under certain circumstances, the state can issue a provisional license (of normally 90 days in duration) to an HHA that is not in substantial compliance if the HHA has submitted an acceptable plan of correction to resolve the areas of noncompliance.[37]

Once the license is issued, it must be displayed in a place viewable by the general public.[38] If the HHA decides to voluntarily relinquish the license, or if it is denied, revoked, or suspended under administrative action, the HHA must provide requisite notice to the patients, their authorized representatives, attending physicians, and third party payors.[39]

The licensing agency has the right to investigate complaints and to insure that the HHA is maintaining compliance with all licensure requirements, including: (a) the governing authority of the HHA;[40] (b) proper personnel;[41] (c) staff supervision and training;[42] and (d) the maintenance and safeguarding of clinical records.[43]

Some Legal and Practical Considerations about Licensure. Although licensure issues do not often arise as legal problems, some points about licensure in the context of CON and Medicare certification should be kept in mind.

As has already been mentioned, in CON states for HHAs, a CON or a formal exemption determination is a precondition to the issuance of a license. It is also true in many states, however, that the continuing viability of the CON is dependent on uninterrupted licensure. Thus, if for some reason the HHA License is suspended or revoked, or the agency ceases to operate for any period of time, the state or, more likely, a competing HHA, could assert that the CON has lapsed. It is important, therefore, that any licensure defects be rectified as soon as possible to avoid threatening the CON.

Licensure problems also seem to arise almost magically when an HHA is forced to fire one of its key employees. An unannounced inspection always seems to follow shortly on the heels of a terminated administrator. Accordingly, if it becomes necessary to fire a key employee, it is often wise to alert the licensure office that the action is pending and that you have taken appropriate steps to hire a qualified replacement. A preventive phone call could save you the aggravation of being visited by licensing inspectors carrying an order to show cause as to why the HHA should not be closed down for being improperly staffed.

Another problem with the license as it affects CON is the fact that health planning authorities look to the license to ascertain the HHA's service area. In states in which the service area is not clearly articulated in the CON, the counties or subdivisions listed on the HHA's license are looked upon as the best evidence of the HHA's service area. Thus, whenever a licensure form needs to be completed that asks for any identification of service area (for example, "single county" or "multicounty"), to the extent that your answer is not clearly inconsistent with your CON approval, always select the most expansive definition.

Finally, it should be kept in mind that licensure is a precondition to Medicare certification, and although the two offices generally work closely together, they do not always coordinate their efforts carefully enough. If a new HHA obtains Medicare certification before licensure is effective, or if licensure is lost for any period of time, the HHA will be forced to forfeit all payment for Medicare services furnished during the period without licensure.

Conclusion

If you are interested in becoming involved in the ownership and operation of an HHA, and you are still convinced after reading this chapter, press on. As the chapter indicates, there are often ways to circumvent the costly and time-consuming burdens of confronting the CON process head-on. Licensure, on the other hand, must be faced, but it is not nearly so cumbersome or threatening a process. The important principle to keep in mind in dealing with CON and licensure issues is that anticipation and prevention of problems can save enormous headaches and expenses that come as a result of reacting to crises. Before you go flailing headlong into the regulatory process that encompasses home health care, establish a business plan, do a marketing feasibility study, retain competent advisors who are knowledgeable in the area, and develop a good working relationship with the government agencies that will determine your entitlement to CON and licensure. The game plan is to accomplish your objectives with the least possible expenditure of your resources. In the present home health care marketplace, there is no substitute for cost consciousness.

Endnotes

1. At the present time, only 34 states and the District of Columbia have CON and/or licensure requirements for HHAs. It should be noted that not all 34 states with HHA CON requirements have HHA licensure laws. In other words, some states (Arizona and California, for example) have licensure but not CON Laws, and others (like Alabama and Alaska) have CON but no licensure requirements.

2. Pub. L. No. 93-641, 88 STAT. 2225 (January 4, 1975).

3. See generally, Anderson, K. B., and D. S. Kass. *Certificate Of Need Regulation Of Entry Into Home Health Care.* (Bureau of Economics Staff Report to the Federal Trade Commission, January 1986).

4. Texas and Tennessee have recently reinstated their CON requirements for HHAs after a rapid expansion of new HHAs in those states threatened to destabilize the entire industry. California, as noted previously, has dropped its CON program in its entirety.

5. Most of the 34 CON states only require review if the HHA intends to seek reimbursement from the Medicare or Medicaid programs. Some jurisdictions, notably Kentucky and the District of Columbia, require CON review for all in-home services without regard to payment source.

6. Acquisitions of existing HHAs in non-CON states do occur when the purchaser is seeking to acquire an established patient base and/or goodwill.

7. See, for example, Annotated Code of Maryland ("Md. Ann. Code") section 19-115 (k)(5)(ii); Code of Maryland Regulations ("COMAR") section 10.24.01.03A(1).

8. *Id.*

9. We are aware of one instance in which a new entrant fought a long, costly, and ultimately successful battle to obtain a new HHA CON, only to realize later that it would have been entitled automatically to a CON under the CON law's "grandfathering" provision.

10. Florida had been using the so-called "Rule of 300" to make need determinations for new HHAs. The Rule of 300 would prevent a new HHA from obtaining a CON unless it could demonstrate that all of the existing agencies in the relevant market area had an average daily census of 300 patients. The Rule was ultimately struck down by the Florida state courts as having been adopted without proper reliance on any empirical data justifying such a criterion.

11. Ohio and Nevada both have provisions exempting from review new HHAs whose operating expenses will not exceed $305,750 in the first year.

12. Because in states having CON laws governing HHAs CON approval is a precondition to licensure, it is not uncommon that certain provisions in the licensure law will have a bearing on CON requirements. This is a point to bear in mind when determining whether to pursue CON.

13. Fla. Stat. Ann. Section 400.504 (1980).

14. See, for example, Md. Stat. Ann. section 19-116 (1985 Cumulative Supplement); Fla. Stat. Ann. section 381.495(4)(a).

15. The Florida exemption provision lists three reviewable events that would be exempted under certain circumstances: (1) the offering of an inpatient institutional health service; (2) the acquisition of major medical equipment; and (3) the obligation of a capital expenditure. It can be argued as a matter of the legal interpretation of statutes that the inclusion of these three exempt categories in no way implies that the HMO would be exempt from all possible categories of review.

16. See COMAR section 10.24.01.06C.

17. COMAR section 10.24.01.06C(2).

18. COMAR section 10.24.01.06C(3) and (5).

19. *Id.*

20. COMAR section 10.24.01.07A.

21. *Id.*

22. Under Maryland law, an "interested person" is defined as "an affected person who has made a written request to the Commission to receive copies of relevant notices concerning an application." COMAR section 10.24.01.01.B(16). An "affected person" includes, among others, the applicant, local health planning authorities, consumers of health care services in the area of the project, existing health care facilities, insurers, and any competing applicants. COMAR 10.24.01.01.B(1).

23. COMAR section 10.24.01.07C.

24. COMAR section 10.24.01.07E.

25. COMAR section 10.24.01.07F.

26. COMAR section 10.24.01.10.

27. The State Health Plan is a document that sets present and projected need for the distribution of certain health care services and equipment throughout the state. Need is normally projected for a five-year period.

28. See COMAR section 10.24.01.07H.

29. See COMAR section 10.24.01.07K. In Maryland, the time period is 150 days if an evidentiary hearing is held, 120 days if not.

30. *Id.*

31. COMAR section 10.24.01.01B(2).

32. COMAR section 10.24.01.17.

33. COMAR section 10.24.01.18.

34. For a comparative illustration of the various state HHA licensure laws and key elements of Medicare conditions of participation, see *The "Black Box" of Home Care Quality,* a Report Presented by the Chairman Of The Select Committee On Aging, House Of Representatives, Ninety-Ninth Congress, Second Session, Prepared By The American Bar Association (August 1986).

35. See COMAR section 10.07.10.02B.

36. See COMAR sections 11.07.01 and 10.07.03. Most licensure laws require HHAs to provide skilled nursing services and at least one of the following: a, physical therapy; b, occupational therapy; c, speech therapy; d, medical social services; or e, home health aide.

37. COMAR section 10.07.10.04.

38. COMAR section 10.07.10.06.

39. COMAR section 10.07.01.05.

40. See COMAR section 10.07.01.07.

41. See COMAR section 10.07.01.08.

42. See COMAR section 10.07.01.09.

43. See COMAR section 10.07.01.10.

The Accreditation Program for Hospice Care
Barbara A. McCann

The Joint Commission on Accreditation of Hospitals

The Joint Commission offers the only national voluntary accreditation process for hospice services. The standards and accreditation process emphasize the delivery of quality interdisciplinary team care to terminal patients and their families in the in-patient and home care settings. The standards encompass the principles of hospice care and palliative care as first stated by the International Work Group on Death, Dying, and Bereavement, the National Hospice Organization, and the American Nurses Association.

The standards were developed between 1981 and 1983 by the Joint Commission through a grant by the W. K. Kellogg Foundation. The Commission worked with national organizations representing the various hospice providers and others to develop the current hospice standards. These standards represent a field consensus of quality hospice care. The process and results of the development project are presented in detail in *The Hospice Project Report* (McCann 1985).

Eligibility Criteria. Accreditation is available to independent hospices and to hospice programs that are a service of a home health agency, a hospital, a long-term care facility, a psychiatric facility, or other health care provider.

Eligibility for survey includes the following criteria:

- The hospice serves individuals who have a diagnosed terminal illness and a projected limited lifespan, and it must emphasize the management of pain and other physical symptoms as well as psychosocial problems of the patient and the patient's family;

- The hospice provides interdisciplinary team services both at home and in an inpatient setting, including bereavement care as appropriate following the death of a patient;

- The hospice provides a continuum of care in the home care and inpatient settings either directly or through an agreement;

- The program has the permission of the agency or individuals who provide hospice services through an agreement to be surveyed to be in compliance with the standards as stated in the *Hospice Standards Manual*;

- The hospice program has been in operation and actively caring for patients and families for at least six months before survey so a record of performance is available;

- The hospice program is in compliance with applicable federal, state, and local laws and regulations, including any requirements for licensure;

- The hospice program operates without restriction by reason of sex, race, creed, or national origin.

The Hospice Standards. The accreditation award and the survey process are based on the standards as stated in the *Hospice Standards Manual*. The standards are presented in an outline format to organize and clarify their content. The format consists of a statement of a general standard and, under that statement, specific required characteristics against which a hospice program's compliance with the standard will be measured.

Although the standards are comprehensive and apply equally to all hospice programs that seek accreditation, the Joint Commission recognizes that the methods used to comply with these standards may vary with the type and size of the hospice program. Acknowledging the variety of organizational types of hospice programs, alternative procedures may be acceptable provided that the hospice program can demonstrate that the desired results have been attained.

Independent hospices and hospice programs which are a service of a home health agency are surveyed for compliance with all applicable standards in the *Manual*. When JCAH surveys a hospice program in a facility which is currently JCAH-accredited, the survey of the hospice program is limited to assessing compliance with standards in the *Manual* which are pertinent to hospice care. For example, governing body standards are not surveyed once for hospice and again for hospital accreditation. In this way, organizations are not surveyed twice for compliance with comparable standards in both standards manuals. Survey burden and cost is therefore also reduced.

Although all of the standards stated in the *Hospice Standards Manual* are considered to be important in the process of assuring quality patient and family care, there are standards against which an organization must demonstrate compliance to become accredited. These standards are stated below:

Sufficient Staffing. The program must demonstrate that there is sufficient staffing in the inpatient and home care settings for the following services:

- Nursing

- Psychosocial

- Spiritual

- Bereavement

- Homemaker and home health aide and

- 24-hour, 7-day-a-week availability of a registered nurse

Whether or not a hospice has a sufficient number of staff is determined by the individual program's own acuity system and observed needs of patients or families during the course of the survey which were or were not met. Specific patient to staff ratios are not dictated by the Joint Commission.

Staff Qualifications. All staff in the inpatient and home care settings which are directly responsible for providing care to the patient and family must have demonstrated competency in their particular area of service.

- There are stated minimum education and training requirements for all services, and current staff meet these requirements.

- The training and education required is appropriate to the scope of services offered and the needs of the patients and families served.

- There is evidence that all staff participate in appropriate training and in-service education to maintain their skills.

- There is appropriate training for those providing bereavement services.

- There is orientation of all employees to the hospice program and concept of care.

- There is a periodic evaluation of every employee's performance.

Direction and Licensure. There is appropriate clinical and administrative supervision of all care providers. Also, there is evidence of current licensure or certification as required by the state for each caregiver.

- There is an appropriately qualified registered nurse who provides clinical supervision of nursing care. There is a designee appointed to act in his or her absence.

- There is an appropriately qualified clinical supervisor(s) for psychosocial and bereavement services.

- There is appropriate supervision of volunteer services.

- There is evidence of appropriate supervision of homemakers and home health aides by a registered nurse.

- There is registered nurse supervision on all inpatient shifts.

- There is delineated supervision and responsibility throughout the hospice program.

Assessment and Review. Assessment and ongoing review is a key patient care process in both the inpatient and homecare settings.

- There is evidence that appropriate written admission criteria are followed.

- There is evidence of signed informed consent of the patient to receive hospice services.

- There is a clear process for initial assessment of patients' needs in regard to all services provided.

- There are regular and documented team conferences for all services involved in patient and family care.

Care Planning. Care planning is the key to the successful process of patient and family care in a service such as hospice which involves more than one discipline often in more than one setting.

- There is evidence of the involvement of the patient and family in care planning.

- There is evidence of the approval of the care plan by the attending physician.

- There is an interdisciplinary team care plan for every patient and family. The care plan reflects problems, goals of intervention, and services involved.

- There are appropriate written agreements when not all services are provided directly by the hospice.

- There is an appropriate resuscitation policy for patients at home and in the inpatient setting that is effectively implemented.

- There are delineated procedures for death in the home.

Patient and Family Services. A key element in hospice care is the appropriate provision of interdisciplinary services to meet identified needs of patients and families.

Physician Care.

- Each patient has a designated attending physician.

- The attending physician is fully licensed.

- There is evidence of ongoing communication between the team and physician.

Nursing Care.

- There are appropriate initial and ongoing assessments conducted by a qualified registered nurse.

- There is evidence of appropriate nursing care process which includes, but is not limited to:

- Periodic physical assessments addressing pain and other symptoms;

- Notation of treatment and outcome, changes in the patient's physical condition, and patient family instruction and compliance.

- There is evidence of following appropriate policies and procedures for treatment modalities such as IV therapy, chemotherapy, etc.

- There is documentation of medications administered, of indication errors, and of adverse reactions.

- Nursing documentation reflects standards of current practice and indicates appropriate assessment, action in response to identified needs, and plans for ongoing care.

Psychosocial Service. Psychosocial services can be provided by any member of the team who is qualified by appropriate education, training, and experience.

- There is a psychosocial assessment of each patient and family which is conducted by a qualified individual.

- Psychosocial documentation reflects current standards of practice and it includes an appropriate assessment of the needs of patient and family, actions in response to these needs, and realistic plans for follow-up and intervention, if any.

- There are periodic assessments noting the psychosocial status of the patient and family, any intervention provided, outcome, and change in psychosocial status.

Spiritual Services. The spiritual needs of the patient and family can be met by appropriately trained members of the team, a chaplain or other trained clergy, or through an ongoing relationship with the patient's community clergy or spiritual counselor.

- Spiritual services are available in the home care and inpatient setting.

- If services are provided through community clergy, there is documentation of ongoing communication.

- The provision of spiritual services by a team member reflects an assessment of spiritual needs, and the plan for follow-up, if any.

Bereavement Services. The provision of care to survivors is another critical element in hospice care. The survey process looks at how the hospice determines the needs of the survivors in their community and what is an acceptable mode of follow-up in regard to cultural, social, or religious factors, as well as survivor need.

- There is regular survivor contact for at least one year after the death of the patient.

- The process of bereavement care reflects current standards of practice. It includes an assessment of need, action based on the need, and plans for follow-up.

Quality Assurance. Central to the Joint Commission's accreditation process is the demonstrated ability of the hospice to monitor the quality and appropriateness of their care against accepted clinical standards of practice.

- There is appropriate assignment of responsibility within the program to implement quality assurance activities which encompass both home care and inpatient care.

- There is a written quality assurance plan which delineates how the process will occur; who is responsible for implementation; how results will be shared with appropriate management, care providers, and the governing body; and how contracted services will be involved.

- There is evidence that action has been taken when problems are identified, and that the action is evaluated.

- The process to monitor and evaluate care encompasses all interdisciplinary team services and care provided in the inpatient and home care settings.

- The criteria used to evaluate care is clinically sound.

Medical Records. Although providers emphasize the importance of the actual delivery of care, standards also recognize the importance of documentation of that care. This is especially important in a care process which now primarily involves home care services which are often provided in the absence of easy access to supervision and often demand great skill and flexibility on the part of the caregiver

- There is timely submission of documentation by all services providing care, including volunteers.

- Medical records must be complete and include a record of bereavement services provided, if any.

- Noting that hospice care is provided in a number of settings and by different individuals, the standards do not mandate one hospice record. However, information must be easily assembled when needed by either the inpatient or home care team members.

Inpatient Services. Hospice involves two settings, home care and inpatient. All of the above standards apply equally to hospice care provided in either setting; however, the following standards are unique to the provision of care in an institution. They are applicable to freestanding hospice facilities, leased hospice units, or services provided in unaccredited inpatient settings. If the inpatient setting the program works with is JCAH-accredited, the survey of these items is waived.

- There are pharmacy services consistent with the medication needs of the patients.

- There are appropriate policies and procedures for prescribing, dispensing, administering, controlling, storing, and disposing of all drugs and biologicals, as well as supervising pharmacy services.

- There is an organized medical staff.

- There is a facility-wide infection control program which includes an appropriate plan for prevention and control of infection.

- The building is in compliance with the National Life Safety Code and there is implementation of appropriate safety practices.

The Survey Process

All of the hospice surveys are conducted by a hospice surveyor who has at least three years of clinical and administrative experience in a hospice program. The survey is therefore conducted by peers who use their experience as practitioners and administrators and their national experience as surveyors to advise programs on better ways of achieving desired results. The surveyor assumes the role of evaluator, consultant, and educator.

The Survey Duration. The duration and cost of the survey varies by the type of program. The average survey of a community-based hospice is 1.5 days. The survey is conducted by a single hospice surveyor. An exception to this process is when the program is working primarily with an inpatient facility which is not JCAH-accredited. In this instance, the survey involves three days, and an engineer is added to the team to conduct the life safety survey of the building and safety practices. In this instance, the second half day of the hospice surveyor's agenda involves assessing the inpatient nurse staffing pharmacy, infection control, and arrangements for radiology and laboratory services etc.

The survey of a hospice which is a service of a JCAH-accredited organization involves one day, and is always conducted by a hospice surveyor. The reduced time is due to the duplication of survey items as discussed in Section II, "the Hospice Standards."

Cost. The base 1986 charge for a hospice survey is $940/day, plus a $250 application fee for a three-year accreditation. These charges may vary according to the type of survey as outlined below. Independent hospice programs or those programs which are a service of a community-based agency are charged for 1.5 days plus a $250 application fee or a total of $1,665.00 for three years.

Exception. The total cost of an initial survey of a program whose average unduplicated monthly census is 45 or less, and who work primarily with a JCAH-accredited inpatient facility, through December, 1987 is $940.00. No additional application fee is added, and the survey duration remains 1.5 days. The resurvey of all programs is charged at the usual 1.5-day fee of $1,665.00.

Hospices which are a service of a JCAH-accredited organization are charged $940 for a one-day survey. No additional application fee is charged for the hospice survey.

The Survey Agenda. The following is a brief outline of a typical survey of an independent or community-based hospice program for 1.5 days. The emphasis of the survey process is contact with the patients and families served, and the team members who provided the day-to-day care. While documentation and policy review is involved, emphasis of the survey is on the implementation of the policies and procedures and the patient and family care process. Throughout the day the surveyor advises individual team members of strengths and weaknesses, and the recommendations that will be made. The surveyor also shares with staff knowledge and experience which is individualized to the program's problem. At the end of the day, the surveyor summarizes the findings of the survey. Board members, staff, and other interested individuals are encouraged to attend and enter into a dialogue with the surveyor.

Day One. The first day provides time for an opening conference, review of documentation, and individualized interviews with team members providing care. The surveyor also visits one of the inpatient sites and reviews continuity of care in the inpatient setting.

Day Two. The second day is often devoted to visiting a patient and family to observe care, as well as completing the review of home care program. The summation conference is scheduled for the last hour of the survey.

The Accreditation Process. The hospice surveyor submits his or her findings to the staff at JCAH headquarters. The results are analyzed by staff members with hospice experience to assure that the intent of standards was met by the hospice and the surveyor, that the documentation supports any recommendations, and that the decision made is consistent with others made for programs with similar results.

Following this review and approval by the staff, the results are presented to the JCAH Accreditation Committee of the Board of Commissioners. The Commissioners can render one of three types of accreditation decisions:

- Accreditation without contingencies
- Accreditation with contingencies
- Nonaccreditation.

A contingency is a proviso that the hospice is accredited pending evidence that a particular problem(s) in the patient and family care process is corrected within a specified time. The evidence may be requested in the form of a written progress report or a return visit of a surveyor may be required. Which type of follow-up is requested depends on the type of problem. If the hospice does not demonstrate adequate progress in addressing the problem(s) in the specified time period, the Accreditation Committee can initiate nonaccreditation.

If a hospice program fails an initial survey, the program has the option to request the Accreditation Committee to deem this a consultative and educational visit. In this instance, the nonaccreditation decision would not remain on the record. This option is not available for the initial survey of a hospice based in an already JCAH-accredited organization.

All information as to whether or not a hospice has or does not have a contingency is confidential, and is not revealed by the Joint Commission.

The Ongoing Accreditation Process

Of great importance to the voluntary accreditation process is the ongoing development and revision of standards by which the services provided by a hospice can be evaluated. A standard is developed because there is an identifiable need to measure or enhance the quality of a particular aspect of hospice care or interdisciplinary team service. Innovations in techniques, advancements in knowledge, or issues identified by consumers can bring about the need to revise or develop new hospice standards. Cost considerations are also an integral part of the standards development and revision process. (Please see Appendix on home care standards being developed by JCAH.)

Input in this process from actual providers of hospice care is very important. In this regard, there is a national Hospice Professional and Technical Advisory Committee (PTAC) who meet on a regular basis to monitor the compliance of hospices with the standards, the effectiveness of the survey process, and the need for changes in the existing standards or development of new standards. The members of the PTAC include representatives who are actively involved in hospice care appointed by the following organizations: American Hospital Association, American Medical Association, American Nurses Association, American Psychiatric Association, American Psychological Association, Association of Community Cancer Centers, The College of Chaplains, National Association for Home Care, National Association of Social Workers, National Hospice Organization, and the National League for Nursing.

Through the ongoing development and revision of standards to be used in the hospice voluntary accreditation process, the Joint Commission helps hospice providers improve and maintain the quality of the care they provide. Our goal is to continue to respond to the needs of hospice providers and consumers to maintain quality care in the United States.

The Benefits of Accreditation

In today's competitive health environment, the most valuable asset a program has is the quality of the care provided to patients and families. The JCAH hospice accreditation process is one of the best ways to demonstrate the provider's commitment to quality. Accreditation provides a means to let the public, the consumer, know that the staff provides high quality care.

Some of the benefits of accreditation include the following:

- Assistance in program efforts to improve the quality of patient and family care and provide a procedure to organize and improve management systems.

- Provision of an on-site evaluation based on realistic, nationally recognized standards for hospice care.

- Provision of individualized consultation and education to caregivers to help them in their self-improvement efforts.

- Assistance in qualifying for grants and donations.

- Facilitate reimbursement from insurance companies and other organizations and agencies.

- May favorably influence liability insurance premiums.

- Give physicians and organizations you work with a recognized measure of assurance that you are striving to provide quality health care.

- Encourage referrals.

- Enhance team morale and pride in a job well done.

The central premise of voluntary accreditation is that health care providers, such as hospices, can and should take responsibility for evaluating and assessing the quality of care they provide. The Accreditation Program for Hospice Care signifies the professional commitment of hospice caregivers to provide quality care to terminal patients and their families.

Standard Setting & Accreditation by the National HomeCaring Council*

Nancy Day Robinson

The National HomeCaring Council sets standards and conducts an Accreditation Program for homemaking-home health aide services. Accreditation by the National HomeCaring Council assures people who receive home care that the service conforms to national standards for safe and reliable care. Accreditation assures those who pay for the service--taxpayers, individuals and their families, insurance companies--that their dollars are being used efficiently. Finally, it assures home care workers that they work for a reputable agency.

The National HomeCaring Council's standards and accreditation process provide an agency with guidelines for setting up a good in-home service, and a means of self-evaluation and stimulus for improvement. At the same time, the standards are broad enough to allow the agency flexibility to adapt to local conditions.

Accreditation--An American Phenomenon

Voluntary accreditation is peculiar to the American scene. In other countries the government generally sets regulations for services and educational programs and polices conformity to the regulations. In this country, standard-setting by industry and monitoring by peers is widely accepted. However, there is still an interaction between the public and private sectors. Growing numbers of public agencies recognize and support standard-setting and monitoring by nongovernmental bodies, thereby strengthening the system.

Dr. William K. Selden, former Executive Director of the National Commission on Accrediting, is perhaps the nation's foremost authority on accreditation. Selden tells us that as far back as 1787, the New York State Board of Regents was required to visit every college in the state and report annually to the legislature, and that this was probably the first step in the evolution of voluntary accreditation (*Accreditation: Its Purpose and Uses,* Washington, DC: The Council on Postsecondary Accreditation, 1977).

Most historians mark the start of accreditation in the early 1900s . At this time medical schools became accredited by the American Medical Association, spurred on by a gadfly, Abraham Flexner. Still in the early 1900s, accreditation of hospitals was instituted. This pattern is significant, for, to this day, accreditation of education is more universally demanded by the public than accreditation of services. In many professions graduation from an accredited school is necessary to attain a certificate to practice.

---

* The National HomeCaring Council is now a division of the Foundation for Hospice and Homecare.

Generally the public waits to demand accreditation of services until a widely publicized scandal or series of abuses underscores the need for it. With a wider understanding of and use of home care, attention to the need for standards in the field is increasing. In December 1985, the *Wall Street Journal* published a feature, "As Health Care at Home Rises, So Do Problems." Now is the time for greater emphasis on standards and self-policing by the field.

History of Standard-Setting and Accreditation

Standards for homemaker-home health aide service have a long history. In 1937 a national conference on the service was called, in part "to think through . . . satisfactory standards of service." As a result a National Committee for Homemaker Services was formed and met over the years. In 1961 the Committee requested the National Social Welfare Assembly and the National Health Council to "bring into being a new, independent national organization with a board broadly representative of health and welfare interests . . . (to promote) homemaker services of high quality . . . such promotion to include standard-setting consultation and research." As a result the Council was incorporated in 1962 as the National Council for Homemaker Services and almost immediately a Code of Standards was written. One of the most important standards concerned the proper training of homemaker-home health aides. Solid job skills, which form the basis for safe, reliable care, depend on adequate training. In 1967 the Council published a training manual for instructors of homemaker-home health aides.

In 1969 and again in 1970 the Council was designated in the *Federal Register* as a standard-setting body for the service. The 1970 citation stated that homemaker services were to "be in accord with the recommended standards of related national standard-setting organizations such as the National Council for Homemaker Services." This recognition and requests from agencies in the field led to the development of an Accreditation Program in 1971. Initially it was called an "approval" program because the review was based on a self-study and other written materials, without a mandated site visit. However, five years later full accreditation with a site visit was instituted. Agencies now have the option to apply for accreditation or approval of their homemaker-home health aide services (the history of the national HomeCaring Council's Accreditation Program is adapted from "The Approval Program — How It Came To Be," 1972, an unpublished paper by Florence Moore, former Executive Director of the Council.)

Recognition by the Federal Government and the States

Since those first citations in the *Federal Register,* recognition and use of the National Council's standards and accreditation have grown.

Maine's Department of Human Services was the first to tie funding for contracts for homemaker-home health aide services to accreditation or approval by the Council. It did so after Sabra Burdick, an Administrator in the Department, analyzed the cost of setting up a state monitoring program versus the Council's fee for accreditation and concluded accreditation was clearly more cost-effective.

The late Dr. Ellen Winston, an early president of the National Council, and the first US Commissioner of Welfare, Department of Health, Education and Welfare, under Presidents Kennedy and Johnson, was deeply involved in the Accreditation Program for many years. She worked tirelessly to link federal funding of services to accreditation. Although unsuccessful on the federal level, she was able to get her home state of North Carolina, through the Division of Aging, to provide start-up funds for homemaker-home health aide services to agencies, provided they applied to the National Council for accreditation or approval.

Dr. Winston's influence reached into the neighboring state of Tennessee. There, the Chattanooga Area Regional Council of Governments enacted the requirement that recipients of Older Americans Act funding for homemaker-home health aide services apply for accreditation or approval by the National HomeCaring Council.

This stipulation was particularly notable because in many states contracts under the Older Americans Act are awarded to the lowest bidder, without regard to the quality of care.

The State of Alaska has a long and interesting history with respect to in-home services. Because of its climate, its expansive distances, and its multi-ethnic population which speaks diverse native languages, the services have problems and characteristics unlike those found in any other state. In spite of operational difficulties, three of the first programs approved by the National HomeCaring Council in 1974 were in Anchorage, Fairbanks, and Juneau. These agencies had the State Title XX contracts for homemaker services. In an effort to save the state money and at the same time spread services over the entire state, the state funding body developed a plan for maximum use of an individual provider system. However, the fiscal agent for the individual providers spent all the money allocated for service midway through the fiscal year, and a crisis ensued. Meantime the three approved agencies had closed their doors.

After several unsuccessful stopgap measures, Alaska finally awarded its statewide contract to an agency accredited by the Council. Alaska's Department of Health and Social Services, like all wise consumers, realized that conformity to standards would safeguard their investment. It now requires its contractors to seek accreditation from the National HomeCaring Council.

The latest formal recognition of Council accreditation is by the New Jersey Department of Human Services. In November 1985 an agreement between the Division of Medical Assistance and Health Services and the Council was signed, based on new state regulations. These require agencies receiving funding for the New Jersey Medicaid Personal Care Assistant Program or the Community Care Program for the Elderly (Medicaid waiver) to apply for Council accreditation or accreditation available through the HomeCare Council of New Jersey.

The chief reason for New Jersey's action was its desire to expand the availability of home care service through heretofore unauthorized state use of proprietary agencies. The first New Jersey proprietary, Alan Health Care Services, to apply for review of its homemaker-home health aide service under the new regulations, has now been accredited by the National HomeCaring Council.

One major advantage to states that work with the National HomeCaring Council toward a monitoring system for quality care is that the Council will tailor its accreditation process to fit the state's needs. One tool developed by the National Council for use by state administrators is a model request for proposal. It can be used by any third-party funder in any state.

At least a dozen other states have incorporated all or part of the national Council's standards into their requirements for in-home services. Criteria for content and length of training taken from the Council's training standard have become the nationally recognized basis for training of homemaker-home health aides.

In several instances the federal government has awarded "deemed status" to accrediting bodies; that is, the government will accept accreditation by the deemed national voluntary organization as evidence that federal conditions for receiving funds have been met. For example, hospitals accredited by the Joint Commission on Accreditation of Hospitals are deemed to have met the *Conditions of Participation* in Medicare. In 1985 the National HomeCaring Council responded to a request by the Administrator of the Health Care Financing Administration (HCFA) for renewal of the National Council's earlier request for such recognition of its Accreditation Program. As of the date of this writing, the decision by HCFA is still pending.

Accreditation by the National HomeCaring Council

Every accreditation program is a plank set on two sawhorses: the standards-setting function and the standards-monitoring function. In the National HomeCaring Council, the standards are adopted as policy by the Board; however, they are developed by the Standards committee, made up of agency administrators, federal administrators, and representatives of other voluntary health/social service-based national organizations. The 11 standards cover the essential aspects of homemaker-home health aide programs (see Exhibit 3-1). Several years ago the committee significantly revised the standards based in part on comments from council agency members. So the standards are truly set by the field.

The other sawhorse, standards-monitoring, is the responsibility of the National HomeCaring Council's Accreditation Commission. It meets quarterly for a two-day period to review and act upon applications for accreditation. This Commission is comprised of a dozen agency administrators and volunteers and there is always a consumer representative.

The Standards Committee would like to set ideal standards of practice. However, it is aware of the realities of agency funding problems and the need for strict conservation of resources. Therefore, it sets the minimum standards consistent with protection of the consumer and the buyer. Safety and accountability are the watchwords of the National Council's Accreditation Program.

Three basic documents are used in the Accreditation Program: the Standards, the *Interpretation of Standards* and the Self-Study:

- The *Interpretation of Standards* contains the criteria, or operational definitions of the Standards, the "spelling out of the Standards."

- The Self-Study documents conformity to the Standards.

Information required for documentation is broken down into simple discrete items, so that only short answers, not essay responses, are required.

Exhibit 3-1. Basic National Standards for Homemaker-Home Health Aide Services

STRUCTURE

Standard   I.   There shall be legal authorization to operate the agency.

Standard   II.   There shall be a duly constituted authority and a governance structure for assuring responsibility and for requiring accountability for performance.

Standard   III.   There shall be compliance with all legislation relating to prohibition of discriminatory practices.

Standard   IV.   There shall be responsible fiscal management.

STAFFING

Standard   V.   There shall be responsible personnel management including:
     A. Appropriate processes used in the recruitment, selection, retention, and termination of homemaker-home health aides;
     B. Written personnel policies, job descriptions, and a wage scale established for each job category.

Standard   VI.   There shall be training provided to every homemaker-home health aide for all service to be performed.

SERVICE

Standard   VII.   There shall be written eligibility criteria for service and procedures for referral to other resources.

Standard   VIII.   There shall be two essential components of the service provided to every individual and/or family served:
     A. Service of a supervised homemaker-home health aide;
     B. Service of professional persons responsible for case management functions.

COMMUNITY

Standard   IX.   There shall be an active role assumed by the service in an ongoing assessment of community health and welfare needs and in planning to meet these needs.

Standard   X.   There shall be ongoing interpretation of the service to the community.

Standard   XI.   There shall be evaluation of all aspects of the service.

Agencies already accredited by another body, such as the National League for Nursing or the Council on Accreditation of Services for Families and Children, need complete only a short form of the Self-Study.

The Review Process

The Council's accreditation procedures parallel those of other accrediting bodies. Exhibit 3-2 summarizes the Council's process.

The Focus of the Accreditation Program

The Council's Accreditation Program, which focuses primarily on the paraprofessional, the homemaker-home health aide, serves a vital public service. Generally, other home care workers such as nurses or therapists are certified by their professional associations and may be licensed by the state as well. As a rule, homemaker-home health aides are not subject to any certification or licensure, therefore, there is a critical need for standards for homemaker-home health aide service.

In the early days of the Council a major issue was whether to certify the aide or to accredit the service. After a great deal of deliberation the Council opted for accreditation on the rationale that a homemaker-home health aide was one member of a care team, and that the employing agency must carry accountability for the service. Furthermore, until aide training became more extensive, the sanctioning of private practice by a homemaker-home health aide through national certification would possibly undermine the Council's intent of ensuring safe, reliable care.

Another issue that arose was whether an agency that provided homemaker-home health aide-type services through several programs (e.g., homemaker-home health aide, chore worker), usually funded through different sources, could apply for accreditation of just one of its programs. The Board ruled and has consistently held that the safety and efficiency of service should not depend on the funding source. Under this policy, for example, an agency which meets the Council's standards for training and supervision in its home health aide services but uses untrained homemakers for private pay services cannot become accredited until all its services are in conformity with the Standards.

The Major Standards

A standard is a statement based on a principle. The training standard, for example, is based on the simple principle that a homemaker-home health aide should be trained for the tasks assigned.

Standard-setting bodies rarely set specific figures; they allow too little flexibility to adapt to local situations and changing demands of the service. Figures are also subject to controversy and change. The training standard is a case in point. The National HomeCaring Council's present standard requires a very specific 60 hours of basic classroom training and 8 hours a year of in-service training.

When the National Council began setting standards, the general belief in the field was, as one executive director put it, that the "aide was sanctified and prepared to go

Exhibit 3-2. The Accreditation Process

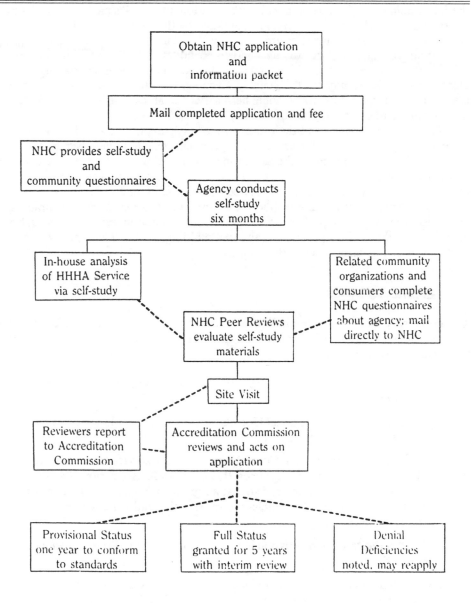

to work by walking through the door of a nursing agency" (or social work agency). On-the-job training was the accepted mode. The National Council's early standard was 40 hours of generic classroom training. Acceptance by the industry of this standard was slow. As the numbers of agencies grew and uses for homemaker-home health aide service expanded, the standard was changed to 60 hours of training within the first six months of employment. A 1985 Council study found that this 60-hour training requirement is now used throughout the country. Even so, the United States lags far behind many European countries where home help service is an established vocation requiring several months or even years of training.

Recruitment of aides and their appropriate assignment are also important components of quality care. Unfortunately some agencies hire a homemaker-home health aide over the telephone and at the same time assign the aide to a case. The Council's Standards require selection and employment to include an initial personal interview, checking for references and a pre-service health examination. Personnel practices must be in strict accord with allapplicable federal and state laws. For example, agencies must comply with regulations covering nondiscrimination, minimum wage, Social Security, Worker's Compensation, and withholding taxes. The agency may not delegate these responsibilities to the client.

Checks and Balances

The greatest asset of an accreditation program is its integrity. The National Home-Caring Council's program has many built-in checks and balances to maintain the integrity of the accreditation.

- Separate committees maintain responsibility for Standard-setting and accreditation.

- Accreditation by the National HomeCaring Council is independent of membership in any organization.

- The National HomeCaring Council represents the service rather than the self-interests of individual agencies. It is not a trade association. The Board and committees are structured so that a significant number of members are not employees of home care agencies but rather other individuals with a commitment to the field.

- The Accreditation Commission is autonomous from the Board in ruling on applications.

- Confidentiality is strictly maintained. The Commission reviews applicants under code numbers, not agency names. The only information about an application made public by the Council is that the service has been accredited or approved.

- A Council-developed "Index of Compliance" safeguards applicants against subjective decisions by the Commission. This validation tool is a first in the field of accreditation.

- All requirements and processes, including an appeals procedure, are matters of public record.

Why Seek Accreditation?*

The awarding of accreditation is the outcome of successful peer review based on the agency's own self-study. The self-study alone, regardless of outcome, is valuable in that it guides the agency through a careful review of its structure, policies, and procedures. The recommendations of the Accreditation Commission can assist an agency in identifying its strengths and weaknesses, and overall, in improving its program.

Once accredited, a homemaker-home health aide service presents an image of safety and accountability that agencies can use to market their services to the community at large. Clients are reassured; third-party payers have a basis for favoring the services of the accredited agency over others; the board and staff can take pride in its service. The National HomeCaring Council stands behind the agency, attesting to the quality of its services, proud to have it use the Council's logo. The service is listed in the Council's Directory of Accredited/Approved Services, thereby attaining national visibility. The agency can take part in the Council's central purchasing plan, and is given priority in participating in projects conducted by the Council. The agency which demonstrates conformity to basic national standards through the self-study and peer review process and becomes accredited shows that it takes responsibility for its services and merits public trust.

References

American Nurses' Association. 1980. *Nursing: A social policy statement.* Kansas City, MO: American Nurses' Association.

Department of Health and Human Services. 1985. *Code of Federal Regulations* (Title 42):298-301. Washington, DC: Government Printing Office.

Donabedian, A. 1984. Quality, cost, and cost containment. *Nursing Outlook* 32:142-145.

Health Care Financing Administration (HCFA). 1980. State Operations Manual, Provider certification; Interpretive guidelines—Home health agencies.

Joint Commission on Accreditation of Hospitals. 1983. *Hospice standards manual.* Chicago, IL: Joint Commission on Accreditation of Hospitals.

McCann, B. 1985. *The hospice project report.* Chicago, IL: Joint Commission on Accreditation of Hospitals.

Nassif, J. Z. 1985. *The home health care solution.* New York: Harper & Row.

National League for Nursing. 1985. *Accreditation for home care and community health: Accreditation criteria, standards, and substantiating evidences.* New York: National League for Nursing.

National League for Nursing. 1985. *Policies and procedures for the NLN accreditation program for home care and community health.* New York: National League for Nursing.

---

* Reprinted by permission of the National Association for Home Care, from *Caring* magazine, April 1986, pp. 34-39.

Appendix A

Medicare Conditions of Participation

CHAPTER IV*
HEALTH CARE FINANCING ADMINISTRATION § 405.1202

Subpart L—Conditions of
Participation; Home Health Agencies

§ 405.1201 General.

(a) In order to participate as a home health agency in the health insurance program for the aged, an institution must be a "home health agency" within the meaning of section 1861(o) of the Social Security Act. This section of the law states a number of specific requirements which must be met by participating home health agencies and authorizes the Secretary of Health and Human Services to prescribe other requirements considered necessary in the interest of health and safety of beneficiaries. Section 1861 (o) of the Act provides:

(o) The term "home health agency" means a public agency or private organization, or a subdivision of such an agency or organization, which—

(1) Is primarily engaged in providing skilled nursing services and other therapeutic services;

(2) Has policies, established by a group of professional personnel (associated with the agency or organization), including one or more physicians and one or more registered professional nurses, to govern the services (referred to in paragraph (1)) which it provides, and provides for supervision of such services by a physician or registered professional nurse;

(3) Maintains clinical records on all patients;

(4) In the case of an agency or organization in any State in which State or applicable local law provides for the licensing of agencies or organizations of this nature, (A) is licensed pursuant to such law, or (B) is approved, by the agency of such State or locality responsible for licensing agencies or organizations of this nature, as meeting the standards established for such licensing;

(5) Has in effect an overall plan and budget that meets the requirements of subsection (z); and

(6) Meets such other conditions of participation as the Secretary may find necessary in the interest of the health and safety of individuals who are furnished services by such agency or organization; except that such term shall not include a private organization which is not a nonprofit organization exempt from Federal income taxation under section 501 of the Internal Revenue Code of 1954 (or a subdivision of such organization) unless it is licensed pursuant to State law and it meets such additional standards and requirements as may be prescribed in regulations; and except that for

---

*AUTHORITY: Secs. 1102, 1842, 1861, 1862, 1870 and 1871 of the Social Security Act; 42 U.S.C. 1302, 1395u, 1395x, 1395x, 1395y, 195gg, and 1395hh, unless otherwise noted.

SOURCE: 38 FR 18978, July 16, 1973, unless otherwise noted. Redesignated at 42 FR 52826, Sept. 30, 1977.

purposes of Part A such term shall not include any agency or organization which is primarily for the care and treatment of mental diseases.

(b) The requirements included in the statute and the additional health and safety requirements prescribed by the Secretary are set forth in the conditions of participation for home health agencies.

§ 405.1202 Definitions.

As used in this subpart, the following definitions apply:

(a) *Administrator, home health agency.* A person who:

(1) Is a licensed physician; or

(2) Is a registered nurse; or

(3) Has training and experience in health service administration and at least 1 year of supervisory or administrative experience in home health care or related health programs.

(b) *Bylaws or equivalent.* A set of rules adopted by a home health agency for governing the agency's operation.

(c) *Branch office.* A location or site from which a home health agency provides services within a portion of the total geographic area served by the parent agency. The branch office is part of the home health agency and is located sufficiently close to share administration, supervision, and services in a manner that renders it unnecessary for the branch independently to meet the conditions of participation as a home health agency.

(d) *Clinical note.* A dated written notation by a member of the health team of a contact with a patient containing a description of signs and symptoms, treatment and/or drug given, the patient's reaction, and any changes in physical or emotional condition.

(e) *Nonprofit agency.* An agency exempt from Federal income taxation under section 501 of the Internal Revenue Code of 1954.

(f) *Occupational therapist.* A person who:

(1) Is a graduate of an occupational therapy curriculum accredited jointly by the Council on Medical Education of the American Medical Association and the American Occupational Therapy Association; or

(2) Is eligible for the National Registration Examination of the American Occupational Therapy Association; or

(3) Has 2 years of appropriate experience as an occupational therapist, and has achieved a satisfactory grade on a proficiency examination conducted, approved, or sponsored by the U.S. Public Health Service, except that such determinations of proficiency do not apply with respect to persons initially licensed by a State or seeking initial qualification as an occupational therapist after December 31, 1977.

(g) *Occupational therapy assistant.* A person who:

(1) Meets the requirements for certification as an occupational therapy assistant established by the American Occupational Therapy Association; or

(2) Has 2 years of appropriate experience as an occupational therapy assistant, and has achieved a satisfactory grade on a proficiency examination conducted, approved, or sponsored by the U.S. Public Health Service, except that such determinations of proficiency do not apply with respect to persons initially licensed by a State or

seeking initial qualifications as an occupational therapy assistant after December 31, 1977.

(h) *Parent home health agency.* The agency that develops and maintains administrative controls of subunits and/or branch offices.

(i) *Physical therapist.* A person who is licensed as a physical therapist by the State in which practicing, and

(1) Has graduated from a physical therapy curriculum approved by:

(i) The American Physical Therapy Association, or

(ii) The Council on Medical Education and Hospitals of the American Medical Association, or

(iii) The Council on Medical Education of the American Medical Association and the American Physical Therapy Association; or

(2) Prior to January 1, 1966,

(i) Was admitted to membership by the American Physical Therapy Association, or

(ii) Was admitted to registration by the American Registry of Physical Therapists, or

(iii) Has graduated from a physical therapy curriculum in a 4-year college or university approved by a State department of education; or

(3) Has 2 years of appropriate experience as a physical therapist, and has achieved a satisfactory grade on a proficiency examination conducted, approved, or sponsored by the U.S. Public Health Service except that such determinations of proficiency do not apply with respect to persons initially licensed by a State or seeking qualification as a physical therapist after December 31, 1977; or

(4) Was licensed or registered prior to January 1, 1966, and prior to January 1, 1970, and 15 years of full-time experience in the treatment of illness or injury through the practice of physical therapy in which services were rendered under the order and direction of attending and referring physicians; or

(5) If trained outside the United States,

(i) Was graduated since 1928 from a physical therapy curriculum approved in the country in which the curriculum was located and in which there is a member organization of the World Confederation for Physical Therapy.

(ii) Meets the requirements for membership in a member organization of the World Confederation for Physical Therapy,

(iii) Has 1 year of experience under the supervision of an active member of the American Physical Therapy Association, and

(iv) Has successfully completed a qualifying examination as prescribed by the American Physical Therapy Association.

(j) *Physical therapist assistant.* A person who is licensed as a physical therapist assistant, if applicable, by the State in which practicing, and

(1) Has graduated from a 2-year college-level program approved by the American Physical Therapy Association; or

(2) Has 2 years of appropriate experience as a physical therapist assistant, and has achieved a satisfactory grade on a proficiency examination conducted, approved, or sponsored by the U.S. Public Health Service, except that such determinations of proficiency do not apply with respect to persons initially licensed by a State or seeking initial qualification as a physical therapist assistant after December 31, 1977.

(k) *Physician.* A doctor of medicine or osteopathy legally authorized to practice medicine and surgery by the State in which such function or action is performed.

(l) *Practical (vocational) nurse.* A person who is licensed as a practical (vocational) nurse by the State in which practicing.

(m) *Primary home health agency.* The agency that is responsible for the service rendered to patients and for implementation of the plan of treatment.

(n) *Progress note.* A dated, written notation by a member of the health team summarizing facts about care and the patient's response during a given period of time.

(o) *Proprietary agency.* A private profit-making agency licensed by the State.

(p) *Public agency.* An agency operated by a State or local government.

(q) *Public health nurse.* A registered nurse who has completed a baccalaureate degree program approved by the National League for Nursing for public health nursing preparation of postregistered nurse study which includes content approved by the National League for Nursing for public health nursing preparation.

(r) *Registered nurse.* A graduate of an approved school of professional nursing, who is licensed as a registered nurse by the State in which practicing.

(s) *Social work assistant.* A person who:

(1) Has a baccalaureate degree in social work, psychology, sociology, or other field related to social work, and has had at least 1 year of social work experience in a health care setting; or

(2) Has 2 years of appropriate experience as a social work assistant, and has achieved a satisfactory grade on a proficiency examination conducted, approved, or sponsored by the U.S. Public Health Service, except that such determinations of proficiency do not apply with respect to persons initially licensed by a State or seeking initial qualification as a social work assistant after December 31, 1977.

(t) *Social worker.* A person who has a master's degree from a school of social work accredited by the Council on Social Work Education, and has 1 year of social work experience in a health care setting.

(u) *Speech pathologist or audiologist.* A person who:

(1) Meets the education and experience requirements for a Certificate of Clinical Competence in the appropriate area (speech pathology or audiology) granted by the American Speech and Hearing Association; or

(2) Meets the educational requirements for certification and is in the process of accumulating the supervised experience required for certification.

(v) *Subdivision.* A component of a multi-function health agency, such as the home care department of a hospital or the nursing division of a health department, which independently meets the conditions of participation for home health agencies. A subdivision which has subunits and/or branches is regarded as a parent agency.

(w) *Subunit.* A semi-autonomous organization, which serves patients in a geographic area different from that of the parent agency. The subunit by virtue of the distance between it and the parent agency is judged incapable of sharing administration, supervision, and services on a daily basis with the parent agency and must, therefore, independently meet the conditions of participation for home health agencies.

(x) *Summary report.* A compilation of the pertinent factors from the clinical notes and progress notes regarding a patient, which is submitted as a summary report to the patient's physician.

(y) *Supervision.* Authoritative procedural guidance by a qualified person for the accomplishment of a function of activity with initial direction and periodic inspection of the actual act of accomplishing the function or activity. Unless otherwise provided in this subpart, the supervisor must be on the premises if the person does not meet qualifications for assistants specified in the definitions in this section.

§ 405.1220 Condition of participation: Compliance with Federal, State and local laws.

The home health agency and its staff are in compliance with all applicable Federal, State, and local laws and regulations. If State or applicable local law provides for the licensure of home health agencies, an agency not subject to licensure must be approved by the licensing authority as meeting the standards established for such licensure.

[47 FR 47391, Oct. 26, 1982]

§ 405.1221 Condition of participation: Organization, services, administration.

Organization, services provided, administrative control, and lines of authority for the delegation of responsibility down to the patient care level are clearly set forth in writing and are readily identifiable. Administrative and supervisory functions are not delegated to another agency or organization and all services not provided directly are monitored and controlled by the primary agency, including services provided through subunits of the parent agency. If an agency has subunits, appropriate administrative records are maintained for each subunit.

(a) *Standard: Services provided.* Part-time or intermittent skilled nursing services and at least one other therapeutic service (physical, speech, or occupational therapy; medical social services; or home health aide services) must be made available on a visiting basis, in a place of residence used as patient's home. A home health agency must provide at least one of the qualifying services directly through agency employees, but may provide the second qualifying service and additional services under arrangements with an agency or organization.

(b) *Standard: Governing body.* A governing body (or designated persons so functioning) assumes full legal authority and responsibility for the operation of the agency. The governing body appoints a qualified administrator, arranges for professional advice (see § 405.1222), adopts and periodically reviews written bylaws or an acceptable equivalent, and oversees the management and fiscal affairs of the agency. The name and address of each officer, director, and owner are disclosed. If the agency is a corporation, all ownership interests of 10 percent or more (direct or indirect) are also disclosed.

(c) *Standard: Administrator.* The administrator, who may also be the supervising physician or registered nurse (see paragraph (d) of this section), organizes and directs the agency's ongoing functions; maintains ongoing liaison among the governing body, the group of professional personnel, and the staff; employs qualified personnel and ensures adequate staff education and evaluations; ensures the accuracy of public information materials and activities; and implements an effective budgeting and accounting system. A qualified person is authorized in writing to act in the absence of the administrator.

(d) *Standard: Supervising physician or registered nurse.* The skilled nursing and other therapeutic services provided are under the supervision and direction of a physician or a registered nurse (who preferably has at least 1 year of nursing experience and is a public health nurse). This person, or similarly qualified alternate, is available at all times during operating hours and participates in all activities relevant to the professional services provided, including the developing of qualifications and assignments of personnel.

(See Connecticut, Massachusetts, New Jersey, and Rhode Island Addenda in the Appendix.)

(e) *Standard: Personnel Policies.* Personnel practices and patient care are support by appropriate, written personnel policies. Personnel records include job descriptions, qualifications, licensure, performance evaluations, and health examinations, and are kept current.

(f) *Standard: Personnel under hourly or per visit contracts.* (1) If personnel under hourly or per visit contracts are utilized by the home health agency, there is a written contract between such personnel and the agency clearly designating:

(i) That patients are accepted for care only by the primary home health agency.

(ii) The services to be provided.

(iii) The necessity to conform to all applicable agency policies including personnel qualifications.

(iv) The responsibility for participating in developing plans of treatment,

(v) The manner in which services will be controlled, coordinated, and evaluated by the primary agency,

(vi) The procedures for submitting clinical and progress notes, scheduling of visits, periodic patient evaluation, and

(vii) The procedures for determining charges and reimbursement.

(g) *Standard: Coordination of patient services.* All personnel providing services maintain liaison to assure that their efforts effectively complement one another and support the objectives outlined in the plan of treatment. The clinical record or minutes of case conferences establish that effective interchange, reporting, and coordinated patient evaluation does occur. A written summary report for each patient is sent to the attending physician at least every 60 days.

(h) *Standard: Services under arrangements.* Services (see paragraph (a) of this section) provided under arrangements must be subject to a written contract conforming with the requirements specified in paragraph (f) of this section and with the requirements of section 1861(w) of the Act (42 U.S.C. 1395x(w)).

(i) *Standard: Institutional planning.* The home health agency, under the direction of the governing body, prepares an overall plan and budgeting budget and a capital expenditure plan.

(1) *Annual operating budget.* There is an annual operating budget which includes all anticipated income and expenses related to items which would, under generally accepted accounting principles, be considered income and expense items (except that it is not required that there be prepared, in connection with any budget, an item by item identification of the components of each type of anticipated income or expense).

(2) *Capital expenditure plan.* (i) There is a capital expenditure plan for at least a 3-year period (including the year to which the operating budget described in paragraph (i)(1) of this section is applicable), which includes and identifies in detail the anticipated sources of financing for, and the objectives of, each anticipated expenditure

in excess of $100,000 for items which would, under generally accepted accounting principles, be considered capital items. In determining if a single capital expenditure exceeds $100,000, the cost of studies, surveys, designs, plans, working drawings, specifications, and other activities essential to the acquisition, improvement, modernization, expansion, or replacement of land, plant, building, and equipment are included. Expenditures directly or indirectly related to capital expenditures, such as grading paving, broker commissions, taxes assessed during the construction period, and costs involved in demolishing or razing structures on land are also included. Transactions which are separated in time but are components of an overall plan or patient care objective are viewed in their entirety without regard to their timing. Other costs related to capital expenditures include title fees, permit and license fees, broker commissions, architect, legal, accounting, and appraisal fees; interest, finance, or carrying charges on bonds, notes and other costs incurred for borrowing funds.

(ii) If the anticipated source of such financing is, in any part, the anticipated reimbursement from title V (Maternal and Child Health and Crippled Children's Services) or title XVIII (Health Insurance for the Aged and Disabled) or title XIX (Grants to States for Medical Assistance Programs) of the Social Security Act, the plan states:

(a) Whether the proposed capital expenditure is required to conform, or is likely to be required to conform, to current standards, criteria, or plans developed pursuant to the Public Health Service Act or the Mental Retardation Facilities and Community Mental Health Centers Construction Act of 1963, to meet the need for adequate health care facilities in the area covered by the plan or plans so developed;

(b) Whether a capital expenditure proposal has been submitted to the designated planning agency for approval pursuant to section 1122 of the Social Security Act (42 U.S.C. 1320a-1) and implementing regulations; and

(c) Whether the designated planning agency has approved or disapproved the proposal capital expenditure if it has been so presented.

(3) *Preparation of plan and budget.* The overall plan and budget is prepared under the direction of the governing body of the home health agency by a committee consisting of representatives of the governing body, the administrative staff, and the medical staff (if any) of the home health agency.

(4) *Annual review of plan and budget.* The overall plan and budget is reviewed and updated at least annually by the committee referred to in paragraph (i)(3) of this section under the direction of the governing body of the home health agency.

[38 FR 18978, July 16, 1973, as amended at 40 FR 24325, June 5, 1975; 40 FR 56661, Dec. 4, 1975. Redesignated at 42 FR 52826, Sept. 30, 1977; 47 FR 47391, Oct. 26, 1982]

§ 405.1222 Condition of participation: Group of professional personnel.

A group of professional personnel, which includes at least one physician and one registered nurse (preferably a public health nurse), and with appropriate representation from other professional disciplines, establishes and annually reviews the agency's policics governing scope of services offered, admission and discharge policies, medical supervision and plans of treatment, emergency care, clinical records, personnel qualifications, and program evaluation. At least one member of the group is neither an owner (185 405.1221(b)) nor an employee of the agency.

(a) *Standard: Advisory and evaluation function.* The group of professional personnel meets frequently to advise the agency on professional issues, to participate in the evaluation of the agency's program, and to assist the agency in maintaining liaison with other health care providers in the community and in its community information program. Its meetings are documented by dated minutes.

(See New Jersey Addendum in the Appendix.)

§ 405.1223 Condition of participation: Acceptance of patients, plan of treatment, medical supervision.

Patients are accepted for treatment on the basis of a reasonable expectation that the patient's medical, nursing, and social needs can be met adequately by the agency in the patient's place of residence. Care follows a written plan of treatment established and periodically reviewed by a physician, and care continues under the supervision of a physician.

(a) *Standard: Plan of treatment.* The plan of treatment developed in consultation with the agency staff covers all pertinent diagnoses, including mental status, types of services and equipment required, frequency of visits, prognosis, rehabilitation potential, functional limitations, activities permitted, nutritional requirements, medications and treatments, any safety measures to protect against injury, instructions for timely discharge or referral, and any other appropriate items. If a physician refers a patient under a plan of treatment which cannot be completed until after an evaluation visit, the physician is consulted to approved additions or modifications to the original plan. Orders for therapy services include the specific procedures and modalities to be used and the amount, frequency, and duration. The therapist and other agency personnel participate in developing the plan of treatment.

(b) *Standard: Periodic review of plan of treatment.* The total plan of treatment is reviewed by the attending physician and home health agency personnel as often as the severity of the patient's condition requires, but at least once every 60 days. Agency professional staff promptly alert the physician to any changes that suggest a need to alter the plan of treatment.

(c) *Standard: Conformance with physician's orders.* Drugs and treatments are administered by agency staff only as ordered by the physician. The nurse or therapist immediately records and signs oral orders and obtains the physician's countersignature. Agency staff check all medicines a patient may be taking to identify possibly ineffective drug therapy or adverse reactions, significant side effects, drug allergies, and contraindicated medication, and promptly report any problems to the physician.

§ 405.1224 Condition of participation: Skilled nursing service.

The home health agency provides skilled nursing service by or under the supervision of a registered nurse and in accordance with the plan of treatment.

(See Connecticut, Massachusetts, and Rhode Island Addenda in the Appendix.)

(a) *Standard: Duties of the registered nurse.* The registered nurse makes the initial evaluation visit, regularly reevaluates the patient's nursing needs, initiates the plan of treatment and necessary revisions, provides those services requiring substantial and specialized nursing skill, initiates appropriate preventive and rehabilitative nursing procedures, prepares clinical and progress notes, coordinates services, informs the physician and other personnel of changes in the patient's condition and needs, counsels the patient and family in meeting nursing and related needs, participates in inservice programs, and supervises and teaches other nursing personnel.

(b) *Standard: Duties of the licensed practical nurse.* The licensed practical nurse provides services in accordance with agency policies, prepares clinical and progress notes, assists the physician and/or registered nurse in performing specializes procedures, prepares equipment and materials for treatments observing aseptic technique as required, and assists the patient in learning appropriate self-care techniques.

§ 405.1225 Condition of participation: Therapy services.

Any therapy services offered by the home health agency directly or under arrangement are given by a qualified therapist or by a qualified therapist assistant under the supervision of a qualified therapist in accordance with the plan of treatment. The qualified therapist assists the physician in evaluating level of function, helps develop the plan of treatment (revising as necessary), prepares clinical and progress notes, advises and consults with the family and other agency personnel, and participates in inservice programs.

(a) *Standard: Supervision of physical therapist assistant and occupational therapy assistant.* Services provided by a qualified physical therapist assistant or qualified occupational therapy assistant may be furnished under the supervision of a qualified physical or occupational therapist. A physical therapist assistant or occupational therapy assistant performs services planned, delegated, and supervised by the therapist, assists in preparing clinical notes and progress reports, and participates in educating the patient and family, and in inservice programs.

(b) *Standard: Supervision of speech therapy services.* Speech therapy services are provided only by or under supervision of a qualified speech pathologist or audiologist.

§ 405.1226 Condition of participation: Medical social services.

Medical social services, when provided, are given by a qualified social worker or by a qualified social work assistant under the supervision of a qualified social worker, and in accordance with the plan of treatment. The social worker assists the physician and other team members in understanding the significant social and emotional factor related to the health problems, participates in the development of the plan of treatment, prepares clinical and progress notes, works with the family, utilizes appropriate community resources, participates in discharge planning and inservice programs, and acts as a consultant to other agency personnel.

§ 405.1227 Condition of participation: Home health aide services.

Home health aides are selected on the basis of such factors as a sympathetic attitude toward the care of the sick, ability to read, write, and carry out directions, and maturity and ability to deal effectively with the demands of the job. Aides are carefully trained in methods of assisting patients to achieve maximum self-reliance, principles of nutrition and meal preparation, the aging process and emotional problems of illness, procedures for maintaining a clean, healthful, and pleasant environment, changes in patient's condition that should be reported, work of the agency and the health team, ethics, confidentiality, and recordkeeping. They are closely supervised to assure their competence in providing care.

(See Connecticut and Oregon Addenda in the Appendix.)

(a) *Standard: Assignment and duties of the home health aide.* The home health aide is assigned to a particular patient by a registered nurse. Written instructions for patient care are prepared by a registered nurse or therapist as appropriate. Duties include the performance of simple procedures as an extension of therapy services, personal care, ambulation and exercise, household services, essential to health care at home, assistance with medications that are ordinarily self-administered, reporting changes in the patient's conditions and needs, and completing appropriate records.

(b) *Standard: Supervision.* The registered nurse, or appropriate professional staff member, if other services are provided, makes a supervisory visit to the patient's residence at least every 2 weeks, either when the aide is present to observe and assist, or when the aide is absent, to assess relationships and determine whether goals are being met.

(See Massachusetts Addendum in the Appendix.)

§ 405.1228 Condition of participation: Clinical records.

A clinical record containing pertinent past and current findings in accordance with accepted professional standards is maintained for every patient receiving home health services. In addition to the plan of treatment (see § 405.1223(a)), the record contains appropriate identifying information; name of physician; drug, dietary, treatment, and activity orders; signed and dated clinical and progress notes (clinical notes are written the day service is rendered and incorporated no less often than weekly); copies of summary reports sent to the physician; and a discharge summary.

(a) *Standards: Retention of records.* Clinical records are retained for 5 years after the month the cost report to which the records apply is filed with the intermediary, unless State law stipulates a longer period of time. Policies provide for retention even if the home health agency discontinues operations. If a patient is transferred to another health facility, a copy of the record or abstract accompanies the patient.

(b) *Standards: Protection of records.* Clinical record information is safeguarded against loss or unauthorized use. Written procedures govern use and removal of records and conditions for release of information. Patient's written consent is required for release of information not authorized by law.

§ 405.1229 Condition of participation: Evaluation

The home health agency has written policies requiring an overall evaluation of the agency's total program at least once a year by the group of professional personnel (or a committee of this group), home health agency staff, and consumers, or by professional people outside the agency working in conjunction with consumers. The evaluation consists of an overall policy and administrative review and a clinical record review. The evaluation assesses the extent to which the agency's program is appropriate, adequate, effective, and efficient. Results of the evaluation are reported to and acted upon by those responsible for the operation of the agency and are maintained separately as administrative records.

(a) *Standard: Policy and administrative review.* As a part of the evaluation process the policies and administrative practices of the agency are reviewed to determine the extent to which they promote patient care that is appropriate, adequate, effective, and efficient. Mechanisms are established in writing for the collection of pertinent data to assist in evaluation. The data to be considered may include but are not limited to: number of patients receiving each service offered, number of patient visits, reasons for discharge, breakdown by diagnosis, sources of referral, number of patients not accepted with reasons, and total staff days for each service offered.

(b) *Standard: Clinical record review.* At least quarterly, appropriate health professionals, representing at least the scope of the program, review a sample of both active and closed clinical records to assure that established policies are followed in providing services (direct services as well as services under arrangement). There is a continuing review of clinical records for each 60-day period that a patient receives home health services to determine adequacy of the plan of treatment and appropriateness of continuation of care.

§ 405.1230 Condition of participation: Qualifying to provide outpatient physical therapy or speech pathology services.

(a) Section 1861(p) of the Social Security Act provides in pertinent part as follows:

(p) The term "outpatient physician therapy services" means physical therapy services furnished by a provider of services, a clinic, a rehabilitation agency, or a public health agency, or by others under an arrangement with, and under the supervision of, such provider, clinic, rehabilitation agency, or public health agency to an individual as an outpatient — ***
The term "outpatient physical therapy services" also includes speech pathology services furnished by a provider of services, a clinic, rehabilitation agency, or by a public health agency, or by others under an arrangement with, and under the supervision of, such provider, clinic, rehabilitation agency, or public health agency to an individual as an outpatient, subject to the conditions prescribed in this subsection.

(b) As a provider of services, a home health agency may qualify to provide outpatient physical therapy or speech pathology services if such agency meets the statutory requirements of section 1861(o) of the Act and complies with other health and safety requirements prescribed by the Secretary for home health agencies, and, additionally, is in compliance with applicable health and safety requirements pertaining to rendition of outpatient physical therapy or speech pathology services. The applicable health and safety requirements pertaining to outpatient physical therapy or speech pathology services are included in the conditions of participation in Subpart Q of this part. (See §§ 405.1717, 405.1718, 405.1719, 405.1721, 405.1723, and 405.1725.)

[41 FR 20871, May 21, 1976, Redesignated at 42 FR 52826, Sept. 30, 1977]

Appendix B

The Home Care Project
Barbara A. McCann

The Joint Commission initiated a two-year project in January, 1986, to develop standards for the delivery of home care services by both facility-based and community-based organizations.

Background. The Joint Commission currently accredits approximately 1,000 hospital-based and -affiliated home care organizations. The survey process is based on the standards as stated in the "Home Care Services" chapter of the 1986 edition of the *Accreditation Manual for Hospitals*. The survey is conducted by the nurse surveyor during the accreditation of the parent hospital. There is currently no additional charge for the survey of the home care service.

The existing home care standards primarily address the provision of skilled intermittent care in the home, most often associated with the traditional Medicare-certified home health agency. In addition, the standards require the involvement of the hospital medical staff in ongoing review of the quality and appropriateness of patient care provided. This function, however, is just one element of the agency-wide monitoring of patient care. The Joint Commission requires that there is a planned and systematic process established to review the quality and appropriateness of all major clinical functions in the home care setting utilizing objective clinical criteria.

Scope of the Home Care Project. The goal of the Home Care Project is to review the existing JCAH home care standards and as appropriate, revise and expand them to address the variety of services now provided in the home. The proposed scope of the standards will address the following services:

- Acute intervention provided on a short-term or long-term basis,

- High technology services such as IV therapy and chemotherapy,

- Hourly services provided by nurses, homemakers, and home health aides, and

- Durable medical equipment provided in conjunction with patient care.

The standards will emphasize meeting the needs of the patient and consumer. They will include elements which are common to all home care providers such as appropriate governance and management, as well as elements which are particular to the service provided, such as 24-hour accessibility to qualified staff for patients receiving home IV therapy services.

Provider Participation. Provider input in the development of the standards is critical to their relevance and value to the field and the consumer. To facilitate provider participation, several modes of review of the proposed standards are proposed. First, the Joint Commission has invited national associations representing consumers and the variety of organizations and disciplines providing home care, to participate as members of a national Home Care Advisory Committee. The members include the American Association for Retired Persons; American Federation of Home Health Agencies; American Hospital Association; American Medical Association; American Nurses Association; American Occupational Therapy Association; American Physical Therapy Association; American Speech Language, and Hearing Association; Blue Cross and Blue Shield Association of America; Health Insurance Association of America; Health Care Financing Administration; Home Health Services and Staffing Association; National Association for Home Care; National Association for Social Workers; National HomeCaring Council; and the Visiting Nurses Association of America. This Committee works directly with project staff to develop, review, revise, and approve each draft of the standards. In addition, there is also a Home Care Consultant Panel which is composed of organizations and individuals who have particular expertise to offer in regard to specific areas of home care such as IV therapy, pediatric home care, etc.

Home care providers across the nation will also be able to review and comment on the standards either in writing through the normal field review process, or through participation at one of the six regional conferences where providers can meet with staff and committee members to discuss the standards. In addition, representative agencies will be selected across the country to act as sites for pilot surveys in the Spring of 1987 utilizing the draft standards. The feedback from the survey process will be critical in developing an accreditation process that is of value to the home care provider.

It is expected that the accreditation process will be completed and available by 1988. Accreditation will be available to community- or hospital-based organizations, as well as to home care services which offer only one service or a continuum of home care. The home care standards used in the survey will represent a consensus of home care providers nationwide.

Chapter Four

Benefits of Organizations

The Relationship of the HHA to the State Trade Association

Mary Kay Pera

Introduction

An individual can satisfy basic needs for food and shelter, but he must have contact with other human beings in order to be complete. People joining together for a common purpose is the basis of institutions, trade, and professional associations. Group participation fulfills human needs; it stimulates economic activity and provides a way for people to work together for mutual benefit.

Modern associations have their roots in trade associations that existed thousands of years ago. Throughout the ages, people banded together for mutual protection and advancement. In ancient Chinese, Japanese, and Indian civilizations, evidence exists of class trade groups which operated for the betterment of members. Trade groups in the Roman Empire served regulatory protective functions and applied the concept of apprentice training. Seagoing Phoenician merchants protected their vessels from pirates by sailing together, and the Aramaeans formed large caravans to protect themselves from bandits while they transported goods over land.

Craft guilds and merchant guilds grew rapidly to serve an important function in society in general during the transition from ancient to medieval times. In England, the "guilds-craft" were formed to safeguard the rights of craftsmen and artisans and set quality standards for their work. "Guilds-merchant," associations of traders and merchants, protected members and increased profits. Early guilds served important functions by encouraging new industries, improving processes, and promoting individual skill and training.

During early US history, merchantilism was the dominant economic force. Carryovers from guilds existed particularly among craftsmen, and a degree of cooperation was found with colonial political authorities.

A parallel exists between the period of transition from medieval guilds to modern associations and the progress of civilization, as education and prosperity became more widespread. Governments improved, inventions were ingenious, and communication and transportation became available to the masses rather than only to a privileged few.

Several associations existed in the United States before 1800, some of which are functioning today. Most associations of home health agencies, however, are comparatively young. As the home health industry has grown, individual agencies have experienced a need to join together to accomplish through the group what they could not alone.

Association Structure

The democratic process is epitomized in the organizational structure of most home health agency associations. Associations represent, protect, promote, and are a reflection of their members. The members are the foundation of any association. Ultimate decision making regarding rights and duties occurs at the membership level. The function of the association is to carry out the policies and programs that reflect the views of the majority of the membership. Members choose their leadership which, in turn, sets the policies of the association.

The leadership of the association is most often called the board of directors or board of trustees. The board is essentially the association's most important committee. These members are expected to be knowledgeable about the needs of the association, and use this knowledge to transact the business and supervise the affairs of the association so that its purpose may be achieved.

Officers are elected from the members of the board of directors either by the members of the board or by the membership, according to the policies of the association. The elected officers usually comprise the executive committee which acts as a liaison and functions for the board between meetings.

Committees, which are usually appointed by the chief elected officer, represent the membership by providing input into the decision-making process and ensuring that all diverse interests of the membership are made known. The number, size, and type of committees vary according to the objectives of the association.

Staff members implement the policies and programs of the association. The chief staff person is hired by and reports to the board of directors through the executive committee.

The organizational structure of an association must allow for continued flexibility and responsiveness to member needs. Priorities change according to member needs. A strong, vital organization anticipates and accepts change.

What Associations Do

The reasons for the existence of home health agency associations are as numerous as the agencies themselves. Typically, however, there are some broad activities that an agency might expect from its association, depending on the availability of resources to support that organization.

The overwhelming majority of home health associations report some involvement in educational activities through sponsorship of seminars, workshops, and other programs. Many provide continuing education credits, awards, or certificates for completion of educational programs.

The majority also are involved with government relations programs. Action at the state and federal levels in both the legislative and regulatory branches can affect the operation of the agency and the care that agency provides to patients. For example, a decision by Congress on Medicare, which is the Medicare agency's biggest payor, could alter significantly the provision of care by that agency.

The association opens the lines of communication, education, and persuasion between the association membership and the legislators and regulators. It becomes a two-way street. The association keeps members up-to-date on governmental action and the legislators and regulators informed about home health industry issues and concerns. At times, news from "Capitol Hill" is fast-breaking. The association monitors events as they develop and disseminates information at once, placing the member agency at an advantage over the nonmember agency. Some associations have also formed political action committees through which the membership can support political candidates and incumbents who share their views.

One of the most valuable resources in association membership is the opportunity to meet colleagues in an informal setting and to exchange experiences. It is comforting to know "you are not alone" and helpful to learn what has worked and not worked for others. Many new ideas for resolutions to problems are spinoffs from ideas of others.

Communication is a key function of most home health agency associations. Through the newsletter, membership directory, annual report, position papers or other bulletins, and audiovisual productions, associations disseminate information to the membership or the general public. Publicity and public relations activities are a part of the associations communications program, which members can often use as promotional material in their local areas.

Another program which is part of many home health associations is setting professional standards for home health agencies. The membership has a stake in each agency providing quality home health care. Through standardization of professional home health care, a direct short- and long-term benefit occurs to the members as well as the consumers they serve.

Some associations are also involved in collecting data about the home health industry, researching trends and reporting outcomes.

The ultimate test of an association's effectiveness, however, is not how many or what types of programs it offers; rather, it is whether the association is meeting the needs and purposes of the membership.

Getting the Most out of Membership

The home health agency which is actively involved in its trade association is the agency that is likely to benefit most from membership. Involvement can take place at many different levels. Each agency must determine its reasons for belonging to the association and choose the appropriate level of involvement to meet those identified needs.

Participation at the board level requires the greatest level of involvement in and commitment to the association. The board of directors is involved in policy-making, program-planning, initiating change, and getting things done. A successful director is knowledgeable about home health; sensitive to the diverse needs of the membership; flexible; courageous; and following deliberation, decisive on the issues. By virtue of election to the board, the member is recognized as a leader in the association, is on the cutting edge of the industry and has the opportunity to effect the direction that the association and industry take.

Committees afford another major opportunity for involvement in the association. Committees are the backbone of the association and the means by which it functions. Service on a committee, which is generally for a year at a time, provides the member with a framework to bring issues before the association for consideration and action. The member with expertise in a given area is often welcomed on a committee that has a responsibility in that area. For example, the member with a strong background and interest in finance would be valuable to the association on the finance committee; a member with legislative or regulatory expertise could contribute to the association on a legislative committee, etc.

An agency may choose not to participate on the board or a committee and remain involved in the association, deriving maximum benefits from membership. An involved association member has a number of important responsibilities. The member should:

1. Stay informed on the issues by reading all the information disseminated by the association.

2. Learn to know the association's leadership and communicate individual issues and concerns to those people.

3. Share experiences, what has worked and what hasn't worked, and solicit experiences from others.

4. Respond to requests for data on agency operations. Every member's input is vital when the association is assessing industrywide trends.

5. Ask questions. All questions are worth asking, no matter how insignificant they may seem.

6. Initiate requests for information. Make the association accountable for responding to individual agency needs.

7. Attend educational programs. Provide suggestions for additional, meaningful programs.

8. Respond to requests from the leadership for calls and letters to legislators. Elected officials pay more attention when they hear from large numbers of constituents on a given issue.

The association can also be an invaluable resource in times of difficulty. An agency administrator may think the agency is alone in facing a particular dilemma only to learn upon calling the association, that many others are experiencing a similar difficulty. Even if the solution is not immediately found, it is comforting to know you are not alone.

In approaching the association for assistance there are certain steps that should be taken: 1) identify the problem; 2) be specific about what you are requesting of the association; 3) supply supporting information, such as copies of correspondence, pertinent records, or details of what has transpired while attempting to resolve the situation on your own. It is helpful to follow up any discussion of the sequence of events with a letter.

Conclusion

Membership in an association can yield substantial benefits to a home health agency. The collective wisdom of individual agencies is absolutely essential to compete in the complex health care environment. Individual agencies working alone can progress. However, it is the association with others of similar interest, the sharing of ideas and resources, and the discussion, modification, and filtration that can result in the greatest accomplishments. This, of course, is the essence of belonging to an association.

The National Association for Home Care

Val J. Halamandaris

The National Association for Home Care (NAHC) is the nation's largest and most broadly based organization representing home care professionals and is an aggressive advocate in Washington, D.C. Committed to principles and activities designed to foster an environment where home care can thrive, the association works to support the dedicated efforts of home care providers who are helping Americans live dignified, independent lives regardless of age or physical ability. Its membership represents the full spectrum of the home care industry. Members benefit from comprehensive direct services designed to meet their specific needs.

Perhaps the most dramatic evidence of NAHC's successful representation of home care is the growth of the association itself. From the initial 500 home care agency members in 1982 (after a merger of National Association for Home Health Agencies and the National League for Nursing's Council of Home Health Agencies/Community Health Services), NAHC has grown to include more than 5,000 members in every area of home care. This includes more than two thirds of all Medicare certified home care agencies.

How NAHC Works

As the nation's voice for home care, the association presents a united front promoting trend-setting ideas, programs, and legislation on behalf of all those involved in home care from the nurse, therapist, and homemaker-home health aide, to the patient and his or her family. The components of home care include: skilled nursing, homemaker-home health aide services, social work, therapy, physician services, adult day care, respite care, Meals on Wheels, transportation services, and many others. Because there are so many components of home care, NAHC retains a professional team of lobbyists, lawyers, policy specialists, and researchers, all of whom combine their efforts becoming "watchdogs" of this old-turned-new again area of health care.

Expressed more broadly, the purposes of the Associations are as follows:

1. to represent the interests of those Americans described as being on the "fringes of life"--the elderly facing compound problems of illness and advanced age in the twilight of life, millions of fragile children facing major health problems in the dawn of life, and the disabled, too often relegated to the shadows of life;

2. to heighten the political visibility of home care services;

3. to affect legislative and regulatory processes impinging on home care services;

4. to gather and disseminate data on the home care industry;

5. to promote home care as a viable component of the health care delivery system;

6. to foster, develop, and promote high standards of patient care in home care services;

7. to provide an organized and unified voice of home care provider organizations;

8. to disseminate information and provide for the exchange of information with those interested in home care services and total health care;

9. to interpret home care services to governmental and private sector bodies affecting the delivery and financing of home care services;

10. to collaborate with state organizations representing home care interests and other organizations at the state, national, and local levels;

11. to initiate, sponsor, and promote educational programs for and with providers and consumers of home care, health care, social service, governmental bodies, and other professional individuals and associations interested in home care;

12. to initiate, sponsor, and promote research related to home care services directly through its own programs or through grants, contracts or other arrangements with individuals and organizations;

13. to engage in any and all other activities permitted by law for the promotion of or related to any of the above purposes; and

14. to foster a mutually beneficial relationship with other organizations interested in the well-being of the population of infirm, disabled, or medically fragile of all ages.

Furthermore, NAHC remains in close contact with the White House, the United States Congress, the Health Care Financing Administration (HCFA), Veterans Administration (VA), and other government agencies, the courts, the state capitals, private enterprise like insurance companies, corporate executives, benefits managers, as well as the rest of the established American health care system. Lastly, NAHC nurtures a close, friendly relationship with the media, both local and national.

Legislative and Regulatory Advocacy

In 1986 for example, NAHC's diligent lobbying efforts resulted in substantial legislative relief for home care providers. Included in the Omninbus Reconciliation Act of 1986 (OBRA: P.L. 99-509) were these provisions:

- Extending the Medicare presumption of waiver of liability to include hospice services, and establishing a separate 2.5 percent waiver for technical denials.

- Upholding the rights of providers to assist beneficiaries in appealing denied claims. (NAHC had already won a major court victory on this issue, but HCFA planned to appeal it).

- Requiring prompt payment of all clean Medicare claims (95 percent of clean claims to be paid in 30 days in fiscal year 1987, with more prompt limits in the years thereafter).

- Requiring hospitals to provide discharge planning.

- Requiring HHS to develop an instrument for uniform patients needs assessment.

- Permitting states to provide optional coverage of respiratory care services at home to Medicaid ventilator-dependent individuals without regard to whether the state extends similar benefits to other Medicaid patients.

In addition to these provisions, Congress also enacted National Home Care Week to promote home care and to honor those who provide care for people in need.

NAHC's efforts are not just limited to working with our nation's elected leaders. The following are some of the issues which were hammered out between NAHC and the regulatory agencies:

1. worked with HCFA on revisions to the Medicare forms 485-8 and obtained significant concessions for providers;

2. commented on many proposed HCFA regulations for issues like bonding and escrow, calculation of lesser costs or charges, and return on equity; and

3. monitored HCFA actions in such matters as the transition to 10 fiscal intermediaries, coverage and interpretation, medical review issues, audit issues, PIP, discrete costing, and sampling.

Judicial Intervention

When legislative and regulatory avenues are not enough, NAHC sometimes finds it necessary to apply judicial pressure to protect home care providers and beneficiaries. In this manner, NAHC has been instrumental in obtaining legal actions that intervene on behalf of home care providers. Recent judicial interventions include a lawsuit to stop governmental agencies from using illegal statistical projections of claims to increase an agency's rate of claims denials. Another lawsuit upheld the right of Medicare beneficiaries to select a home health agency as their representative when appealing a Medicare claims denial.

An Information Source

The Association offers its' members access to vital market research, and computerized information with up-to-the-minute statistics on home care.

Public relations is another resource area for those interested in finding out about home care. Press kits are always available to members prior to the yearly celebration to National Home Care Week, the last week in November. Other promotional items such as brochures, posters, films, and video cassettes for television spots are sold at a discount to members.

Publications receive a lot of national attention and the NAHC Report, which is sent to members on a weekly basis, is a "hot sheet" of information about the home care industry and community. This newsletter includes important national legislative, regulatory and major policy issues, and reports on state and local home care issues of national importance. *Caring* is a highly-acclaimed monthly magazine that offers in-depth analyses of legislative, regulatory, business/financial, and education issues that impact the home care industry. Feature stories focus on new treatment methods and the latest high-tech developments in the field. *Homecare 87* is a monthly newspaper of the who's and what's of home care. Coverage includes what is happening in the home care industry today. This publication also facilitates networking among home care professionals. There are also a number of special reports that focus on new research, market studies, and statistical data on issues in the field.

Education is another top priority for NAHC. There are so many new and constant discoveries in the home care field that it is essential to keep members up-to-date. This is accomplished through an annual meeting given each autumn in different parts of the country. This meeting features prominent speakers and home care advocates, hundreds of educational workshops and exhibits of services, supplies, and the latest in high-tech equipment.

Each spring there is also a legislative and regulatory conference. This meeting brings the providers to Washington, D.C. so they may visit their Senators, Congressmen, and legislative staffers to discuss issues of concern to the home care industry. The conference also features presentations from key regulatory staff, fiscal intermediaries, and other policymakers. Other meetings include regional meetings that go on throughout the year.

The Future

Through NAHC and its three affiliates, The Foundation for Hospice and Homecare, The Hospice Association of America (HAA), and the National Association for Physicians in Home Care (NAPHC), there exists quite an ambitious agenda for the future. This agenda, which is printed each year in January, is called The Blueprint for Action. In this blueprint, NAHC lists all improvements that need to be made on the national, regional, and local level.

As a general outline, this agenda includes the framework for homecare, recommending improvements to the private and public sectors dealing with homecare, recommending legislative changes, and presenting cost-effective home care services in order to expand rather than limit the delivery of such care.

As always, NAHC attempts to protect the field of home care while helping to establish quality control issues, serving the areas of the population that do not receive sufficient health care, thereby expanding the home care benefit.

The Visiting Nurse Associations of America
Robert F. Leduc and Rebecca Wolf

The Visiting Nurse Association of America (VNAA) was formed as the American Affiliation of Visiting Nurse Associations and Services (AAVNA/S) in 1982 for the purpose of fostering communication and cooperation among individual visiting nurse associations, promoting a national image, and pooling resources for marketing, advertising, and other operational needs. VNAA is the first formal linkage of VNAs in the history of the VNA movement. The linkage was necessary and desirable because of an increase in competition in the home care provision market, a decrease in reimbursements from sources of significant funding to VNAs, and because of demographic changes that ultimately lead to increased demand for the type of services that VNAs desire to provide to American citizens. The national coalition of VNAs was established because the VNA movement concluded there would be strength in numbers. Individual VNAs made a choice that their individual needs and internal competition must be subordinated for the greater good of the movement. As a result, the Visiting Nurse Association of America was founded and is now becoming a dominant organization in the home care marketplace.

VNAA has developed a member services program with five major objectives:

- Decreasing costs through central purchasing and negotiating

- Increasing revenues through national fundraising and contracting

- Improving local and national imaging

- Advocating for the voluntary, community-based model of home health delivery

- Maximizing the operational capacity of member agencies.

The first area of concern to VNAA is to decrease the cost of home health services to patients. VNAA is coordinating a central purchasing program to lessen the cost of buying products frequently used by VNAs. Items to be centrally purchased include: medical and surgical supplies, durable medical equipment (DME), pharmaceutical products, office furniture, equipment and supplies, as well as employee benefit insurance (health, life, dental, etc.).

Furthermore, VNAA will facilitate cost reductions through a national audit service contract with a Big Eight accounting firm, and through the services of a captured travel agency and a print shop.

VNAA is also involved in efforts to increase revenue for affiliate members. VNAA meets with potential partners, including: insurance firms, HMOs, PPOs, and such other entities as the American Association of Retired Persons (AARP). Joint ventures with these groups will lead to programs whereby VNAs shall serve as preferred providers to home health services, thereby increasing their base and share of the marketplace.

VNAA is also involved in the promotion of a national image which will help educate and inform the country of the high quality services provided by VNAs. To promote a national image, VNAA will help to: place ads in key periodicals, establish a Preferred Patient Card program, design a national uniform, and otherwise spotlight the work of its members. VNAs have been providing high quality home care for over a century, and a national imaging program will help to tell this story.

VNAA is also providing advocacy for its affiliates. Generally, this effort is designed to insure that the voluntary, community-based option of delivering home health services is represented to the legislative and executive branches of government and to such other entities as necessary to the fairest expression of this model of service delivery.

Finally, to strengthen each individual affiliate, VNAA provides training sessions and video and audio tapes on management and other issues that concern the VNA movement. The national office also provides on-site consulting, turnaround management services, and other types of management support as requested by individual members.

Members and Markets

VNAA has 90 affiliates in 27 states across the country. (See Exhibit 4-1.) In order to be eligible to join VNAA, agencies must meet each of the following criteria:

1. Agencies must meet the requirements of Sections 501 (c) (3) and 590 (a) (1) or (2) of the Internal Revenue Code of 1954.

2. Agencies should operate under the legal name of or do business as a Visiting Nurse Association, a Visiting Nurse Service, a VNA, or a VNS.

3. Agencies must be freestanding.

4. Agencies must have majority control by an independent voluntary board of directors.

To get an application, agencies should write to the national office at:

> 518 Seventeenth Street
> Suite 388
> Denver, CO 80202

VNAA helps affiliates and recognizes market differences across the country. In addition to common problems faced nationally, each region also has special needs. For instance, florida, the state with the largest population over age 65, is a state where VNAs rely heavily on Medicare reimbursements. New England, on the other hand, deals in greater numbers with private insurance companies that reimburse for home health care costs. In order for the national office to help increase the operational capacity of its member agencies, it must address Medicare reimbursement and deter-

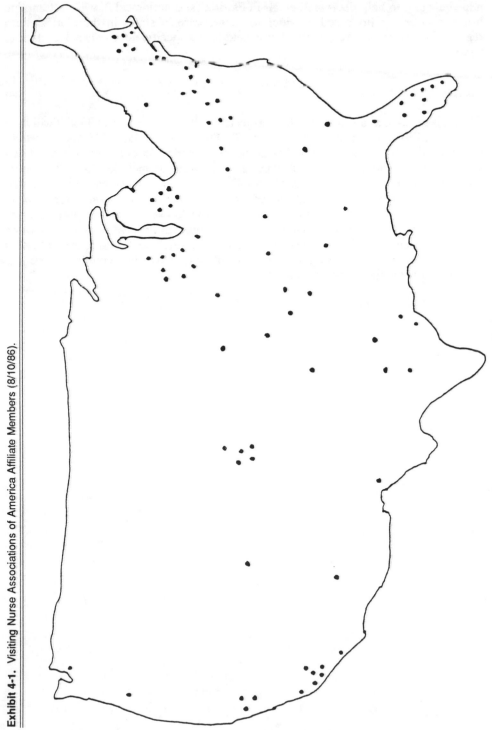

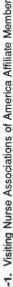

Exhibit 4-1. Visiting Nurse Associations of America Affiliate Members (8/10/86).

mine how best to help decrease denials in Florida (and nationwide), while attempting to contract as the preferred provider for home care in states in the Northeastern region of the country. Similar attention is paid to the specific needs of each section of the country.

Future

VNAA is growing at a rapid rate. It is projected that by December of 1986 it will have over 100 affiliates throughout the country. By December of 1987, VNAA expects to have virtually all of the largest VNAs across the country. In order to best assist this growing membership, VNAA will expand its services to include: "SWAT" teams, professionals in the VNAA network that will go in and help agencies in crisis, mediation, negotiation, and amalgamation services to assist agencies as an alternative to their absorption by other home care programs; and to expand central purchasing to include: employee insurance, some legal aid, and joint venures with other groups who deal with the elderly. VNAA is a strong, viable force which continues to expand and is dedicated to helping Visiting Nurse Associations across the country to be the dominant force in the home care industry.

Chapter Five

Professional Standards

Standards and Certification Options for Personnel in Home Health Care

Ann H. Cary

Agency administrators are constantly challenged to place well-qualified individuals in agency positions. While the supply and demand for well-qualified individuals never seems to be stable, the aspect of distribution of personnel in urban and rural areas poses an additional strain on an agency's efforts. Rural agencies report unique problems in attracting and retaining top notch personnel.

There are several sources of guidelines that exist from federal, state, and local jurisdictions, as well as from organizations that promote agency accreditation. These guidelines will be reviewed in an attempt to discuss the minimum standards proposed for agency personnel. A discussion of the various certification and licensure options for the home care administrator will be presented subsequently with a focus on the unique opportunities to develop a measure of distinction for the home health care administrator.

Current guidelines and standards for the administrators in home care can be found in the Conditions of Participation (COP) issued by the Department of Health and Human Services (DHHS 1985, 298-301). For agencies that operate under COP guidelines, the definitions provided in Section 405.1202 provide that the administrator is a licensed physician, a registered nurse, or a person with training and experience in health service administration. The administrator should also have at least one year of administrative and supervisory experience in either home health care or other health-related programs.

A second level person in the agency who may have administrative responsibility for supervising the skilled nursing and therapies is referred to as the supervising physician or registered nurse. COP guidelines suggest that this individual should have at least one year of experience and is a public health nurse. This specialty is defined as a registered nurse who has graduated from a National League for Nursing (NLN) baccalaureate program or who has completed a post-registered nurse study program which included public health nursing content approved by the NLN.

While these federal regulations guide the directors, administrators, and supervisors in Medicare-certified agencies, other state and local requirements for agency licensure may present different guidelines. For example, a few states (Massachusetts, New Jersey) require or prefer (Connecticut, Rhode Island) that the administrator possess a master's degree in community or public health, health care administration, or public administration (DHHS 1985, 306). Whether this will become a trend in licensure and certification requirements for the agencies can only be determined by monitoring adaptations in the state licensure laws for home health care agencies.

In addition to the public regulations available to guide the standards of preparation and experience for the administrator, there are standards generated by the professional organizations who may represent personnel or that accredit home health agencies.

The National League for Nursing (NLN) has an accreditation program for Home Care and Community Health Agencies (National League for Nursing 1985, 11-12). Their standards for administrators include preparation at the master's level in a health field and a minimum of two years of health administrative experience, or a bachelor's degree and five years of administrative experience in the health field. Equivalent groupings of experience, training, and education can be used to determine if the administrator meets this standard. As with the COP clause, the NLN also provides standards for individuals who may be delegated by the administrator to direct the agency's programs. This individual must possess qualifications respective of the professional organization of which they are a member as well as statutory and regulatory mandates. The individual should be a qualified health professional with community health experience. The standards for NLN accreditation were revised in 1985.

Standards of Nursing for Home Health Care Practice is a publication of standards developed and in the process of being field-tested by the American Nurses Association. The draft of Standard I states that in the Organization of Home Health Services, the "services will be planned, organized and directed by a master's prepared professional nurse with experience in community health nursing and administration" (American Nurses Association 1986a, 8). The draft *Standards* include comprehensive process and outcome criteria for nurses in home health care and will be finalized upon field comment to provide guidance to all registered nurses in home health settings in achieving excellence in the provision of health care.

The Joint Commission on the Accreditation of Hospitals (JCAH) accredits the home care departments of hospitals (JCAH 1986, 49). Characteristics required for the administrative director are that the individual be a physician, a registered nurse, or a person with training and experience in public health or health services administration. The individual should also possess at least one year of supervisory experience in home health or related health care programs. These characteristics are noted as key factors in the accreditation decision process by JCAH. In May of 1986, the JCAH announced that it was developing the first national accreditation standards for both hospital home care departments and community-based home care agencies. The timetable for these new standards included a field comment period in late 1986 with publication of the standards in 1988 (American Hospital Association 1986). The differences in accreditation standards for home health agencies and the impact on administrators' credentials will become increasingly clear as the evolution of the JCAH process progresses.

While the National Association for Home Care (NAHC) docs not establish standards for the administrators of their member home health agencies, the *Code of Ethics* adopted by the NAHC board in 1982 addresses the ethical responsibility of an agency to hire qualified employees who are utilized at their level of competency (National Association for Home Care 1982).

Standards for the qualifications of home care administrators can be found through public regulations and professional organizations. These standards change as the context of leadership needs in home care evolve. Additional standards for other professionals delivering care in the home health agency are also found in public regulations and professional standard criterion.

Current Guidelines for Non Administrators

A comprehensive guide to the qualifications of personnel who deliver skilled nursing, therapies, or support to the therapists can be found in the October 1, 1985, edition of the 42 CFR (Chp. IV.) issued by Health Care Financing Administration (DHHS 1985, 299,300,304). Definitions of what constitutes the qualifying standards for each are extensive. Although the COP guidelines will be generally discussed, the reader is referred to the document referenced above, specifically Section 405.1202 for an in-depth description of personnel criteria.

Skilled nursing is provided by or through the direction of a registered nurse. The RN must have graduated from an approved professional school of nursing and be licensed as a registered nurse in the state of practice.

Licensed Practical Nurse standards entail that the person is a licensed practical (vocational) nurse in her state of practice.

Home health aides (HHA) have general descriptive standards of literacy, compassion, maturity, and training in the maintenance of the client as well as the reporting of detected changes in the client's condition. Some states require that the HHA have a state approved training certificate in addition to the guidelines in the COP.

Physician standards include holding a Doctor of Medicine or Osteopathy degree and licensure to practice medicine and surgery in the current state of practice.

Physical therapists need to maintain current licensure as physical therapists in their state of practice. The educational preparation, training opportunities, and qualifying exam criteria for those trained within and outside of the United States are clearly described (405.1202,i) (DHHS 1985, 299).

Physical therapy assistant standards include state licensure to practice where applicable, experience, and proficiency examination demonstration. For exceptions see (405.1202-j2) (DHHS 1985, 299).

Occupational therapist standards include any combination of being a graduate from an approved accredited school, eligibility for the National Register Examination of the American Occupational Therapy Association, or the combination of experience and satisfactory grade performance on a proficiency exam. For exceptions see (405.1212-f) (DHHS 1985, 298).

Occupational therapy assistants must be certified as an assistant by the American Occupational Therapy Association or have two years experience as an OT Assistant and demonstrate a satisfactory proficiency score on exams conducted, approved, or sponsored by the USPHS. For exceptions see (405.1202-g2) (DHHS 1985, 298-299).

Social worker standards include a master's degree from a school of social work accredited by the Council on Social Work Education and one year of experience in a health care setting.

Social work assistants must have a baccalaureate degree in social work or a related field and have had at least one year of social work in a health-related setting or a combination of two years of experience as a social work assistant and achievement of a satisfactory grade on a government-sponsored exam. For exceptions see (405.1202-52) (DHHS 1985, 300).

Speech pathologist or audiologist requirements include the necessary education and experience to obtain a Certificate of Clinical Competence granted by the American Speech and Hearing Association, or having met the educational requirements is currently accumulating the supervised experience necessary for certification.

The regulatory standards for nonadministrative personnel are diverse within titles and between professional and semiprofessional categories. Mechanisms for determining qualifications include licensure, certification, work and educational experiences, and proficiency exam grades. As new therapies are included in reimbursement packages, standards for these specialists will need to be developed.

Concurrent monitoring and support for the maintenance and improvement in personnel capabilities are discussed in COP items relating to the participation in in-service programs, orientation programs, and reviews of the currency of personnel employment requirements. Contract personnel are obligated by the agency to be held to the same qualifications as the noncontract personnel (DHHS 1985, 301).

The NLN standards for nonadministrative personnel are broad in nature. Employment qualifications and responsibilities are congruent with education and experience, provider needs, professional standards, and regulatory guidelines (National League for Nursing 1985, 24).

JCAH standards demand that the home care personnel must have qualifications and abilities equivalent to the personnel providing comparable services in the hospital (JCAH 1986, 50).

Both organizations promote standards for staff development in keeping with professional currency, licensure, or certification criteria.

Credential Options Utilized by Home Care Administrators

At present, there are multiple options available to the home care administrator in obtaining an additional validation of professional administrative competency. Although none of the mechanisms have been specifically designed to measure home care administrative competency, these methods serve as peripheral measures of distinction.

Nursing Administration Certification

The American Nurses Association (ANA) sponsors a two-level certification process for nurses in administrative (midmanagement and executive level) positions (American Nurses Association 1986b). This voluntary professional organization sponsors a voluntary certification process for nurses. Applicants do not need to be ANA members but must be currently licensed as a registered nurse.

The first level certification requires that the applicant hold a baccalaureate or higher degree in nursing, have held a position equitable to the composite tasks listed for the first level certification for at least 24 months during the last five years, and a passing score on a written exam.

The advanced level certification recognizes the executive level nurse's administrative tasks and functions. Requirements include a master's degree (if it is a non-nursing master's degree the baccalaureate must be in nursing), have held the executive level position for 36 months within the last five years (congruent with published tasks listed for the advanced level), and a passing score on a written exam.

Consultants and educators can apply for certification by meeting specific guidelines in the certification manual.

Recertification is obtained every five years either by evidence of continuing education or by obtaining a passing score on the exam. The credential designations are either CNA (certified nurse administrator) or CNAA (certified nurse administrator, advanced). In the 10-year period since its inception in 1975 more than 30,000 nurses have received all types of specialty certification through this process.

Admission to the "College": American College of Health Care Executives (ACHE 1985).

ACHE is a voluntary professional society composed of members who have demonstrated career paths in health services administration. Affiliates of ACHE receive recognition through the sequential advancement in status: Nominee, Member, and Fellow. Each level has certain requirements for acceptance and there are special categories of affiliation available: student associate, honorary fellowship, and faculty associate.

Nominee status is characterized by an initial commitment to health services administration. Eligibility requirements include a baccalaureate degree and three years of administration experience; or, a graduate degree outside of health services administration and at least one year of administrative experience; or, a graduate degree in health services administration and in a current administration position. In the absence of a baccalaureate degree, the affiliate must have 10 years of administrative experience. Nominees must submit references and position descriptions and can remain a nominee for five years with a one-year extension. They must attend at least one educational program a year and may petition to advance to membership after two years in this status.

Membership confers permanent status indicative of knowledge, participation, and capacity for competence in health services administration. The applicant must have been a nominee, be a chief administrative officer or assistant administrator, pass a written exam and pass an oral exam on the concepts of health services management. Attendance at one educational program per year is required and advancement to the Fellowship level can be petitioned after five years.

The Fellowship status recognizes the individual's growth beyond typical expectations. The applicant must have been a member and occupy a Chief Administrative Officer position. Requirements include the favorable review by the Committee on Credentials of either a written thesis project or four written case reports. The continuing education requirement is the same as described for other levels and the Fellowship credential designations are FACHE.

As of 1986 there were more than 20,000 health care affiliates in varying status in the "College."

Licensure Model: Nursing Home Administrators

(National Association of Boards of Examiners (NAB) for Nursing Home Administrators, Inc.) (NAB 1985).

The licensure of nursing home administrators is a legal process instituted by each state. The criteria for eligibility for the license of administrators is state-sponsored. Each state regulates its own minimum age, educational level, presence of an administrator-in-training program, passing score requirements on an examination, continuing education, and reciprocity rules. A standardized national exam is required by 49 states and the District of Columbia while Texas constructs its own exam. Since the licensure requirements of nursing home administrators are mandated but diverse among states, this model of professional distinction may not achieve the comparable equity portrayed in the first two models. There are approximately 37,000 licensed nursing home administrators.

In a purposeful survey of home care administrators, the author found that of those administrators who had administrative credentials, all of these methods were represented in this group (Cary 1986).

New Certification Strategies for Home Health Care Administrators

Rationale. There are no current mechanisms available to specifically validate the qualifications and knowledge unique to home care administrators. With home care services being provided in diverse and remote sites from the institutional setting there are unique challenges to financial management, quality control, risk management, supervision methods, policy implementation, and organizational development. Reimbursement mechanisms place special demands on home care systems and their operations. The skills of providers are distinct, and are much more complex than simply moving the personnel from a hospital to a home care delivery mode where independence and resourcefulness are critical to success. Jim Kingsbury, president of the VNA of Greater St. Louis, cites differences in the administrative perspective in home health care systems. Having served as both a hospital and home care administrator, he relates that home care administrators must have a broader perspective on the community's services, programs, needs, and networks. Home care has a broader focus in "treating a problem, . . . (and) educating and assisting the patient and patient's family in ongoing care. If I go back into a hospital position some day, it will be with a much broader and improved perspective" (Kingsbury 1985, 32).

The rationale for the creation of a certification process for administrators of home health agencies goes beyond the assumption that the challenges to these administrators reflect a diverse knowledge level.

1. States are beginning to mandate certain credentials for administrators in home health agencies in order for the agency to be licensed.

2. Most other recognized delivery models, hospitals, nursing homes, public health agencies, have some type of credential process in place to recognize the unique qualifications and knowledge of professionals in these respective systems. Certification is a profession's endorsement of that individual. Home

health care administrators as an aggregate do not have that professional endorsement and unique opportunity.

3. Home health administrators represent a diversity of educational backgrounds, and professional and nonprofessional experiences. There are no parameters in place to offer boards, consumers, corporate headquarters, certifying agencies, and organizational personnel a measure of comparable worth in the credentials of administrators.

4. There is a new professional breed of health care manager emerging from the competition, conflict, and decreased autonomy of the health care system in general. This is the same manager who is the gatekeeper guru of health care, the physician administrator.

Note the recent trends for physicians (Flory 1986): smaller incomes; less influence; diminished perceptions of satisfaction from practice; oversupply of specialists and practitioners; strong competition among MDs as they woo the cost-conscious, well-informed purchaser; migration of MDs to salaried positions with hospitals, HMOs, PPO, community-based care centers; and consolidation of physician practices to develop broader referral bases.

As a result, there may be more physician involvement in the management of health care delivery systems in general. As physicians assume the power in management they will control the organizational agenda. There have been proposals to develop physician trade organizations and develop specialists in executive medicine so physicians can be properly trained in management roles (Johnson 1986).

This last activity clarifies the perspectives of other professionals in the management of a health care organization such as home health agencies: *Directors need preparation, education, and training in order to effectively apply their management roles in a complex, dynamic marketplace.*

Although the executive medicine, physician manager model is not currently in vogue for free standing home health agencies, the experiences of the sister HMO agencies and hospital-based agencies show us that the competition for administrator positions in health care is incorporating a newly prepared breed of manager.

As hospitals and multihealth chains move toward more fully integrated corporations, many income-producing ventures will emerge. In taking advantage of these opportunities health care organizations will involve members of the medical staff in equity and management participation.

One of the characteristics of a profession is its ability to regulate itself and to set its standards of practice. A certification process is a dimension that can assist in the perception of home care administrators as professionals. This has distinct advantages in being recognized as professional peers by others who are distinguished in the health industry.

A unique certification process for administrators of home health agencies can enhance professional distinction. In the formulation of the certification process, many questions clarifying the philosophy, sponsorship, eligibility, and ramifications can be posed. These questions reflect the issues inherent in designing, implementing, and evaluating a certification process.

Issues for Consideration in a Certification Process for Home Health Administrators.

Who?

- Who might be appropriate sponsors of a certification process?
- Should the sponsorship be placed in an organization committed to high standards in home health care or in an organization with no affiliation with the home care industry?
- Who might be the personnel in an organization who could be eligible for the process?
- Who, external to the agency, might be the individuals most interested in the certification process (consumers, insurers, and boards).

What?

- What is the goal of a certification process for HHC Administration?
- What currently exists to certify individuals in home health care agencies?
- What is the focus of the content to be measured in the process (i.e., administration, geriatrics, technology, legal issues?)
- What structures for administering the measuring tools exist in a certification process?
- What can individual certification do for my professional growth, the organization, consumers, and insurers?

When?

- When should the issues of certification be brought to the attention of providers and consumers?
- When in the careers of home care administrators should the process be available?
- When will the process of certification become mandatory for licensure and accreditation by regulating bodies?

How?

- How timely is the process in today's marketplace?
- How does the certification process compare to the standards of other professional processes?
- How can a certification process distinguish among professional administrators?
- How can the certification process be used as an advantage among my peers?
- How will the certification process be designed, implemented, and evaluated?

● How can I contribute to the creation of the process?

Why?

● Why consider standardizing certification for home health administrators?

● Why do consumers and reimbursers consider it important or unimportant?

In considering the forementioned standards existing among other professional administrators and the changes occurring in the administrator marketplace, the time is ripe to propose a certification process as a measure of distinction, a reflection of initiatives toward excellence, and the home care profession's endorsement of credentials in its administrators. Agency administrators can contribute to the creation of the process by verbalizing suggestions and concerns; volunteering to serve on organizational committees exploring the process; validating with other professionals the successes and pitfalls of their own certification process; participating in feasibility studies as well as job analyses studies that can form the foundation for the process; and by challenging one's creativity to generate ideas to measure professional distinction. While this idea may not be a popular one with all home care administrators, it offers the opportunity for self-regulation and a demonstration of skills and achievements not currently attributed in a standard way to home care administration. This avenue of change can create unparalleled opportunities for professional enhancement and recognition.

References

American Hospital Association. 1986. *Hospitals Weekly* 29(19).

American Nurses Association. 1986a. *Standards of Nursing Practice for Home Health Care* (draft). Kansas City: American Nurses Association.

American Nurses Association. 1986b. *Certification Catalogue.* Kansas City: American Nurses Association.

Cary, A. 1986. Unpublished survey: Administrators attending the *New Directions in Home Health Care Conference,* Clearwater, FL, March 6, 1986.

Department of Health and Human Services. 1985. *Code of Federal Regulations* (Title 42):298-307. Washington, DC: Government Printing Office.

Flory, J. 1986. Editor's Notes. *Healthcare Executive* 1(2):7.

Johnson, W., Jr. 1986. Upfront. *Healthcare Executive* 1(2):9.

Joint Commission on Accreditation of Hospitals.

1986. *Accreditation Manual for Hospitals.* Chicago: Joint Commission on Accreditation of Hospitals.

Kingsbury, J. A. 1985. *Transitions Changing Careers in Healthcare Management.* American College of Healthcare Executives 1984 1985 Annual Report. Chicago, IL: American College of Healthcare Executives.

National Association for Home Care. 1982, adopted. *Code of Ethics.* Washington, DC: National Association for Home Care.

National League for Nursing. 1985. *Accreditation Program for Home Care and Community Health.* New York: National League for Nursing.

1985 State Roster of Licensure Boards. 1985. Washington, DC: National Association of Board of Examiners.

Regulations Governing Admissions Advancements. 1986. Chicago, IL: American College of Healthcare Executives.

Part III

Management Issues in Home Health Agencies

Chapter Six

Discharge Planning

Joann Kelly Erb

Discharge planning is defined as "the process of activities that involve the patient and a team of individuals from various disciplines working together to facilitate the transition of that patient from one environment to another." (McKeehan 1981, 66).

Successful discharge planning requires thorough understanding of the concepts described in this definition and attention to all these elements as a plan is developed.

As a process, discharge planning consists of a series of well-defined steps to achieve an outcome. Volland (1982) discusses discharge planning as a decision-making, problem-solving process. Use of the decision-making model in the discharge planning process encourages consideration of the multidimensional nature of the problem, and the impact of a plan on all aspects of the patient-family-provider system. It also encourages involvement of the patient and family in the development of the plan and assists in formulating reasonable goals and identifying appropriate outcomes. This process promotes the movement of the patient along the health care system's continuum of care.

The involvement of the patient and the family in all aspects of plan development is essential to success. Since discharge planning occurs at a point in a patient's life when he is vulnerable, health care professionals must be sensitive to the patient's fears and supportive of his needs. Including patient and family in the planning process demonstrates concern for the patient and family and affirms the patient's rights and responsibilities for his own health. By presenting alternatives and helping the patient and family to choose the best option for their unique situations, discharge planning affirms the dignity of the individual and helps assure the success of the plan.

Another essential element of the discharge planning process involves multidisciplinary cooperation and collaboration. Because of the complexity of patient's needs, input from various disciplines such as physical therapy, occupational therapy, speech therapy, and dietary, as well as nursing and social service may be necessary to establish a comprehensive discharge plan. In this era of cost containment it is imperative that turf issues do not hinder the discharge planning process. Coordination, collaboration, and communication among health care professionals are imperative for successful discharge planning. Edwards (1978, 71) proposes "alliance of health care professionals to optimize effectiveness." He stresses flexibility, communication, and the ability to compromise as key points in being more responsive to patients' needs.

Historical Development

Heightened interest by hospitals in discharge planning has resulted from the implementation of the prospective payment system by HCFA in 1984. As in previous

157

eras, change in society and in the health care delivery system has influenced the development of discharge planning.

Prior to World War II, the sick were traditionally treated at home by the physician and cared for by their family. As medical technology advanced, the hospital became the center of physicians' practice and the ill were increasingly treated in hospitals.

The entrance of large numbers of women into the work force during World War II and a decline in the role of the extended family resulted in decreased availability of the family to care for sick members after hospital discharge.

Interest in discharge planning as a method to reduce costs, lower hospital readmissions, and provide the patient with options spurred the development of discharge planning after World War II.

Other societal changes that impact on discharge planning include increased life expectancy, and increase in chronic illness. More individuals now require some sort of posthospital care and rely on their elderly spouses and often elderly children to provide assistance.

One early example of the interest in discharge planning was the Montefiore Hospital Home Care Program, the first hospital-based program, established in 1947. This program coupled physician home visits with visiting nurse services to produce a therapeutic environment for patients in their own home. This program highlighted the need for health care professionals to consider the patients' posthospital situation and develop a plan to extend the benefits of hospitalization after discharge.

The inception of Medicare in 1966 added legislative clout to the development of discharge planning as an essential component of patient care. Hospitals were required to provide discharge planning functions as a condition of participation.

The Joint Commission on Accreditation of Hospitals also has emphasized the importance of discharge planning in its *Accreditation Manual for Hospitals* (1974).

JCAH standards emphasize continuity of care and require a discharge plan that coordinates medical and nursing plans of care and discharge planning services that are integrated into the health care delivery system. Documentation of discharge planning in the medical record is required and institutions must have a formal Discharge Planning Program. Coordination and cooperation with community agencies and an interdisciplinary approach to institutional discharge planning are also essential components for success.

Legislation enacted in 1972 established the Professional Standards Review Organization Program to review the quality and appropriateness of medical services to Medicare beneficiaries. PSRO required regular documentation of the development of the discharge plan.

Professional Review Organizations replaced PSRO in 1984 and are charged with monitoring patient care under prospective payment. The focus of PRO review is quality assurance, including the appropriateness of hospital admissions and discharges. Appropriate discharge can only be confirmed by documented discharge planning activities.

The American Nurses Association's *Standards of Nursing Practice* (1973) emphasize the importance of discharge planning as an essential component of the nursing process. McKeehan (1981, 66) notes "consideration of each of the eight standards illustrates how application to practice builds in discharge planning as an inescapable component of nursing care for every patient."

Goals and Objectives of Discharge Planning

The goals of discharge planning are: 1, to assist patients to return to or improve the level of functioning experienced prior to hospitalization; 2, to insure continuity of care in the transition from hospital to posthospital environment; 3, to promote cost-effectiveness and appropriate use of institutional and community resources.

The discharge planning process impacts not only on the patient, but also on the hospital and community. As acute care hospitals are now viewed as only one point on the continuum of care, the discharge planning process has been recognized as an essential element in patient care that contributes to the patient's progress along that continuum.

Because discharge planning impacts on three systems, patient, hospital, and community, each system will have its own expectations.

Patient Expectations

1. Discharge planning must recognize the individuality of the patient and family and promote the development of a plan of care that recognizes and utilizes the resources of the patient and family.

2. Discharge planning must accurately identify patients' needs and develop a plan to ensure continuity of care in the transition from hospital to posthospital environment.

3. Discharge planning must educate patients and families to the options available and encourage their participation in the decision-making process.

4. The discharge plan must promote attainment of a patient's maximal potential and personal dignity.

5. Discharge planning must assist patients and families in resuming control of their welfare and educate them of the resources available to assist in that process.

Institutional Expectations

1. Discharge planning will promote quality patient care by providing a mechanism to identify patients' needs and develop a plan to meet them.

2. Discharge planning will provide for cost effectiveness by promoting early identification of high risk patients, timely discharge, and by reducing inappropriate readmissions.

3. The discharge planning process will educate health care professionals on the structure and function of the discharge planning process, how that process promotes compliance to regulations, and utilizes community resources available to meet patients' needs.

4. Discharge planning will promote holistic patient care by focusing attention of the impact of illness on patient and family.

5. Discharge planning will promote good public relations by demonstrating the institution's responsiveness to the needs of patients.

Community Expectations

1. Discharge planning will provide for needed services to individuals, vulnerable from illness, returning to the community.

2. Discharge planning will promote utilization of health resources at the proper level and promote cost effectiveness.

3. Discharge planning will promote identification and utilization of community resources and will identify gaps in services and community needs.

4. Discharge planning will promote linkages between health care institutions and community agencies.

Conceptual Framework for Discharge Planning

Discharge planning is based on the philosophy that patients are individuals with unique health concerns and have the right to coordinated discharge planning and that hospitals have the responsibility to provide discharge planning as an essential component of patient care.

The discharge planning process demonstrates a holistic approach that considers the patient's and family's physical, psychosocial, and financial needs and assets in the development of a plan of care. Discharge planning is an essential element of continuity of care and must be integrated into the health care delivery system.

Successful implementation of an effective discharge planning program requires the involvement and support of hospital administration to assure access to necessary hospital resources. The philosophy and objectives of the discharge planning program must be clearly stated and must compliment the philosophy and objectives of the institutions.

For a discharge planning program to be comprehensive requires the support and involvement of a multidisciplinary team that includes the physician. This requires education of hospital staff and an opportunity for physicians and representatives from involved disciplines, such as physical therapy, occupational therapy, and dietary to join with nursing and social work in the development of a discharge planning program.

McKeehan (1981) describes the scope of discharge planning as consisting of four interacting elements, patient and family, available resources, regulations, and primary providers.

The involvement of the patient and family is essential to successful discharge planning and has been discussed in detail previously.

Evaluation of the resources available to patients will influence the development of the discharge plan. If community resources are inadequate to support a patient in their own home, other options such as the patient going to the home of a family member, or disposition to a boarding home, nursing home, or extended care facility must be considered.

One important community resource for patients returning home after hospitalization is the home health agency. There has been a dramatic increase in the number of agencies since 1980, improving access to skilled home care services, including 24-hour on-call availability and capabilities to care for patients with high-tech needs, such as home IV therapy or ventilators.

Unfortunately, access to unskilled services has not kept pace. Medicare does not cover custodial care, and therefore, chronically ill patients with long-term needs cannot receive homemaker services under Medicare. These are the types of services that many chronically ill, elderly individuals require to remain in their own homes. Availability of low cost supportive services varies by locality, but is generally agreed to be insufficient (Mundinger, 1983).

The Philadelphia Inquirer, June 16, 1986 edition, reported some alarming figures concerning the access to homemaker services in Philadelphia. Philadelphia Corporation for Aging, the Philadelphia agency that supplies supportive services to the elderly, reports a six-month waiting list for services and a total of 1500 clients awaiting assistance.

The lack of homemaker services impacts heavily on patients' ability to remain independent and families' ability to maintain patients at home. Mundinger (1983) notes that between 25-50% of nursing home patients could be maintained at home with supportive services. Lack of adequate homemaker services may require a discharge plan that is contrary to patient and family desires--a change in living situation.

The availability of senior transportation service, adult day care, Meals on Wheels, hospice and respite care, all influence the discharge plan. Transportation services provide free or low cost transportation for eligible individuals. Elderly patients who require frequent follow-up visits with physicians or frequent outpatient treatment may not be able to manage if a transportation service is not available in their area.

Adult day care is another service that influences patients' discharge disposition. These programs provide structured, supervised activities for individuals who are unable to be left alone for long periods of time. These programs offer families an option to institutionalization by providing care during the time when families are unable to care for these individuals. They may provide enough of a respite to caregivers to enable them to continue caring for the patient at home.

Another supportive service that benefits many elderly individuals is the Meals on Wheels program. This provides two meals a day, one hot and one cold, five days a week, at a nominal charge and makes available nutritious, balanced meals to those unable or reluctant to do their own cooking.

The ability of families to care for a terminally ill individual often hinges on the availability of a hospice or palliative care program. These programs offer skilled, Medicare-covered care and supportive services, including volunteers, chaplains, and multidisciplinary team approach to the care of the dying. Focus is on symptom control and support to the patient and family members.

Respite care is a concept of providing temporary relief to the caregivers of the chronically ill. Some facilities provide short-term inpatient care for patients to allow families to temporarily relieve themselves of the burden of caring for a chronically ill individual.

Availability of all of the supportive services affects the discharge planning process. Patients who might otherwise be destined for nursing home placement may be able to be maintained at home with the community services described previously. However, cost is an important consideration as many elderly on fixed incomes are unable to afford the regular supportive services they require to remain independent. Since unskilled services are not covered by Medicare, but are usually funded through state programs access varies considerably from area to area. Urban areas are more likely to provide a wider range of services than are available in rural areas. It is imperative that discharge planning professionals remain aware of community resources and educate patients, families, and health care professionals of their existence.

Thus far, discussion of resources has focused on services available to patients returning home. Other factors that impact heavily on the discharge planning process include availability of rehabilitation centers, skilled nursing facilities, nursing homes, drug and alcohol treatment centers, and vocational training centers. Since acute care institutions are just one point of care on the health care continuum, access to other specialty facilities promotes optimal patient care. Access can be hindered by availability or cost considerations. Discharge planning professions must be cognizant of not only the existence of such programs, but also of their financial and medical requirements. This requires interagency cooperation and communication.

The third element described by McKeehan (1981) as influencing the discharge planning process is the regulations affecting the delivery of health care in general and discharge planning in particular. As discussed earlier, the Medicare legislation has had a tremendous impact on health care delivery. This influence has not always been positive, however, as Medicare has encouraged the use of a medical-based model in the care of the elderly when most of the elderly's needs are social or nursing-related. To qualify for unskilled services under Medicare, the elderly must be eligible for skilled services. It is important that individuals involved in discharge planning be active in influencing the development of future legislation and in educating society of the impact of proposed legislation.

The final element affecting the discharge planning process is the integration of discharge planning activities into all aspects of health care delivery by primary providers. This requires awareness of the impact of illness on patients and of the need to plan for postillness care. Physicians, in particular, as gatekeepers of the health care system, must recognize that the health care delivery system is a continuum and that progress along that continuum requires planning and multidisciplinary cooperation.

Steps in the Discharge Planning Process

Since the goal of discharge planning is continuity of care, the same concept that is the foundation of nursing, it is not surprising to note that the steps in the discharge planning process mirror the steps of the nursing process: assessment, planning, implementation, and evaluation.

Assessment

This process involves identification of patients who will require assistance in planning for postdischarge disposition and evaluation of the patient's medical and nursing needs, psychosocial and financial characteristics

Because of DRGs and resultant decrease in length of stay, this phase of the discharge planning process has grown in importance. Prompt identification of patients requiring intervention by discharge planners promotes development of a suitable plan and timely discharge.

In order to effectively accomplish this step, discharge planning professionals must have open access to all patients. They must be able to screen patients and begin to develop a plan without a physician's order. Screening activities include the use of high-risk criteria and patient care rounds to identify patients needing assistance.

Some high-risk criteria commonly used are:

1. Age; over 65-70.

2. Living situation: lives alone or with poor support systems.

3. Life-threatening illness: cancer, AIDS.

4. Conditions requiring a change in lifestyle: CVA, fractures, amputation.

5. Disease conditions requiring instructions or supervision after discharge: insulin-dependent diabetics, colostomy, open wound, catheter or other body tube, cardiac or respiratory patients.

6. Suspected abuse or neglect.

7. Admitted from nursing home.

8. Patients with multiple readmissions or those with a history of disposition problems.

In an effort to further refine screening of patients for discharge planning needs, unit-specific criteria are now being developed. *The Discharge Planning Advisor* (Fall, 1985) published criteria developed at Burkham Hospital, Champaign, IL for neurological, surgical, pediatric, and orthopedic units.

The purpose of using high-risk screening criteria is to identify patients quickly and reduce the possibility of patients "falling through the cracks." However, even though high-risk criteria are becoming more sophisticated and sensitive, there is still the chance that patients will not be identified. All professional personnel, and nurses in particular, must be alert to identify patients who require discharge planning activities and refer them to the appropriate person.

Tools have also been developed to assist in the identification of patients. Rasmusen (1984) developed a screening tool to assist primary nurses in identifying patients who should be referred to the discharge planner.

Another tool developed by Quaschnick (1985) is an assessment form that identifies patients' areas of need and resources. A questionnaire developed by Hardy (1985) is aimed at assisting patients to identify potential problems they may experience after discharge. This tool focuses on ADL function prior to admission and allows patients to voice concerns about postdischarge problems.

An innovative approach to early discharge planning was recently described by Smeltzer and Flores (1986). This program involves expanding preadmission testing to include assessment of discharge planning needs. Information obtained during the preadmission assessment is utilized immediately on the nursing units and aids early identification of high-risk patients.

Once a patient has been identified as requiring discharge planning, a multidisciplinary assessment must be done. Areas to be assessed are the patient's medical and nursing needs, ADL ability, mental status and understanding of and adjustment to illness. Other factors to be evaluated include the patient's and family's strengths and coping skills, support systems, and financial resources.

The second part of the assessment involves the evaluation of community resources available to meet the patient's needs on discharge. Availability of skilled nursing facilities, rehabilitation centers, nursing homes, and home care services, as well as the patient's eligibility for them, must be identified.

The most important area to be evaluated is the desires of the family concerning discharge disposition. The family must have a realistic expectation of the patient's abilities and prognosis. This requires that the health care professionals involved in the patient's care communicate with the patient and the family on a regular basis.

Planning

Once a thorough assessment has been completed, planning can be initiated. The goal should be to return the patient to the least restrictive environment possible to promote the most independent level of functioning. The plan should include short-term and long-term goals and reflect a mechanism to adapt the plan to changes in the patient's condition.

Family involvement in the planning stage helps identify any areas of confusion or conflict and allows for resolution of any problems prior to discharge. Families need to understand what resources (such as home care or rehabilitation centers) offer and what their role in the patient's care will be.

Input from physicians and other health care professionals is necessary to formulate a successful plan. Some methods of promoting multidisciplinary communication and collaboration include regularly scheduled patient care conferences and discharge planning rounds and the use of a discharge planning communication form on patients' charts. The discharge planner must ensure the involvement of appropriate disciplines, collaborate with the physician, and communicate with the patient and family as the plan develops. Once there is agreement between health care professionals and the patient and family, the plan can be implemented.

Implementation

Implementation of the discharge plan involves making the referral for follow-up care and coordinating continuity of care in the transition. If a patient is to be transferred to another institution, such as a rehabilitation center or nursing home, the initial communication concerning the patient's condition and care can be transmitted verbally, but a written referral with pertinent information and a copy of the patient's chart should accompany the patient at the time of transfer. It is imperative that details of the nursing care plan, such as wound care, bowel and bladder regime, and educational needs be communicated to the receiving institution. Likewise, information about the patient's progress in physical and occupational therapy and the therapy goals must be communicated. It is also important to include pertinent social history and family dynamics in the referral.

For patients who will be receiving home care services, a referral should also be made prior to the patient's discharge to assure a smooth transition from hospital to home. The referral should include information about the hospital course, medical and nursing diagnosis and plans of care, discharge instructions, medication, and plans for medical follow-up. Since the home care personnel do not have access to the patient's medical record and patients are often unclear about aspects of hospital treatment, the referral should include as much information as possible about the patient's history and treatment. Only by thorough and timely communication can continuity of care be assured.

Arrangements for other community services such as Meals on Wheels, adult day care, transportation, and homemaker service should be initiated prior to discharge to ascertain that the plan is workable prior to the patient's discharge.

Evaluation

The final phase in the discharge planning process is the evaluation of the plan. This phase may be more difficult than it appears, as it is easy to "forget" patients once they leave an acute care hospital and move on to the numerous other patients that need discharge planning services.

In order to evaluate the discharge plan, adequate documentation must have taken place. Documentation should be ongoing and include the elements of the discharge plan as it develops. Documentation should also be concise and outline the options available to the patient and the patient's and family's response. At the time of discharge, a summation note should include disposition, community services to be provided, and agencies to be involved.

If a patient is returning home, families should be given information about the agencies that will be involved in the patient's care. This includes the agencies' telephone numbers, the date services are to begin, and a description of the services to be provided.

It is important to have a procedure for evaluating the discharge plan. The two most important aspects of the plan to be considered are the quality of the plan and its suitability. Pertinent points to consider in the evaluation of the plan are:

1. Was the plan appropriate?

2. Was there adequate coordination with posthospital providers?

3. Did the patient and family have input into the plan and were they satisfied with the final plan?

4. Did the plan ensure continuity of care in the transitional period?

In order to answer these questions, data must be collected. Some techniques that can be used in data collection are direct contact with the patient after discharge by means of telephone surveys or written questionnaires, feedback from the posthospital environment, and ongoing communication with patients and agencies. The degree of sophistication utilized depends on the resources available to the discharge planning department. Even departments with limited resources can accomplish the evaluation procedure by utilizing trained volunteers or clerical staff to collect data. In addition, not every patient needs to be contacted as long as the selection is random and the sample size is adequate.

Discharge Planning and the Nursing Process

The relationship between the discharge planning process and the nursing process was mentioned briefly in an earlier discussion. The steps of both processes are the same as is the goal--continuity of care.

Because no other discipline is as closely involved with the patient as is nursing, it is essential that nurses recognize their vital role in the discharge planning process and participate in all aspects of the plan development. So much of the data necessary to plan for the patient's discharge is routinely collected in the nursing assessment, for example living situation, support systems, ADL ability, and teaching needs. Provision of quality care requires that nurses utilize and communicate this information in the delivery of care, including the development of the discharge plan.

Professional nurses are guided in their practice by the American Nurses Association Standards of Nursing Practice. These eight standards provide guidelines for the practice of nursing to ensure quality nursing care. Field (1981) examines each standard and demonstrates how adherence to the nursing standards incorporate discharge planning as an essential element of nursing care.

Models

Numerous organizational models exist for discharge planning programs. There is no "perfect" model and the best model for a particular institution depends a great deal on the institution itself. Hospitals are all unique with different structures and power bases and this must be considered in deciding where a discharge planning program should fit within the organization. The program should be placed where it will be most successful.

Three of the most common sites for discharge planning departments are in the social work department, nursing department, or in a separate department under administration. Wherever the placement, it is essential that the process be a multidisciplinary effort, primarily by nursing and social work, but involving all appropriate disciplines.

Social work was traditionally responsible for discharge planning in acute care institutions. Recently, however, changes in health care delivery have necessitated increased understanding of sophisticated medical treatment and the "skilled" needs of patients to develop an effective discharge plan. This requires increased involvement by nursing.

Discharge Planning Update, a quarterly publication of the American Hospital Association, published various models submitted by hospitals throughout the country over a three-year period. Some programs were based in the social work department with nurses working in the department, and some were freestanding departments that include social workers and nurses. The placement of the program was not considered as important as the type of collaboration and communication that took place.

One interesting model described in the *Discharge Planning Advisor* (1986) involves consolidating utilization review and discharge planning functions. Since the UR department is the only department that reviews the chart of every hospitalized patient, it is extremely efficient to combine the two roles and utilize data already being collected by UR to facilitate discharge planning. This allows for prompt identification of patients requiring discharge planning intervention and facilitates the planning process. Because the same nurses are responsible for both UR and discharge planning functions, they are aware, not only of the patient's medical condition, but also the psychosocial factors that affect discharge. As in any model, communication and collaboration with all other departments, especially social work, is essential for success.

The fall, 1983 issue of the *Discharge Planning Update* highlighted what are considered the key points to any discharge planning model. They are:

1. Philosophy statement that reflects administrative support for the program and the patient's right to continuity of care and his right to be involved in a plan to insure it.

2. Goals and objectives that describe the responsibilities of each discipline and the methods to involve the patient and family.

3. Need to have an identifiable coordinator of the discharge planning process and a plan for interdisciplinary communication and collaboration.

4. System of early identification of patients needing discharge planning.

5. Development of a discharge plan that reflects comprehensive assessment and patient and family involvement.

6. Documentation that includes the progress of the discharge plan and summaries by all involved disciplines.

7. Evaluation process that defines the type and frequency of audits and program evaluation.

Quality Assurance in Discharge Planning

Quality assurance can be defined as a process in which standards of care are identified, observed, and measured to insure the achievement of proper standards; the goal of quality assurance is to make certain that care practices will produce satisfactory patient outcomes.

Quality assurance activities can be viewed as an extension of the evaluation phase of the discharge planning process, because quality assurance activities also focus on the quality and suitability of the discharge plan. These "outcome criteria" include: (1) patient and family satisfaction with and compliance to the plan; (2) appropriateness of the plan and the adequacy of information provided by the hospital discharge planner; (3) quality of the services delivered to the patient by the posthospital provider.

There are other outcomes of interest to the institution that should also be evaluated, such as: (1) length of stay and decrease in discharge delays; (2) decrease in number of readmissions due to inadequate discharge plans; (3) improved coordination and efficiency in service delivery and decrease in duplication of efforts.

In addition, quality assurance also addresses the "process" of discharge planning. Examples of criteria that evaluate the discharge planning process include:

1. The procedures for timely identification of patients requiring discharge planning activities.

2. The timeliness of response to referrals for discharge planning.

3. Evidence of patient and family involvement in the plan development.

4. Documentation of physician involvement in discharge planning activities.

5. Documentation of interdisciplinary communication and collaboration.

6. Integration of discharge planning activities into all health care delivery by all disciplines.

The objective of a quality assurance program is to identify areas of deficiencies and make data available to aid in developing solutions to problems and improve the quality of patient care.

Ethical Issues in Discharge Planning

Prospective payment for hospitals and diminished community resources have caused changes in health care delivery that can result in ethical dilemmas for discharge planning professionals. As hospitals are pressured to reduce length of stay to maintain financial solvency, the frail elderly are increasingly being discharged "quicker and sicker."

At the same time, more stringent interpretation of the Medicare home care benefit has resulted in reduction in eligibility for home care services. Tightening restrictions have also decreased availability of nursing home care under Medicare. The vise is closing and the victim is the patient.

Concepts such as the inherent dignity of man, his right to self-determination and access to optimal health care may be in conflict with an environment created by prospective payment and inadequate community resources. Discharge planning professionals, whose practice has been guided by those concepts that protect the rights of individuals at a vulnerable period in their lives, are being required to facilitate discharge of patients without having adequate community resources available for postdischarge care.

This is a major stressor for discharge planners as they realize the plans they have developed are inadequate or only temporary solutions to patients' problems. One common situation is that a frail, chronically ill elderly individual will be admitted with an exacerbation of a chronic condition or an acute episode of illness superimposed on a chronic illness. Because the patient has been acutely ill, he often will qualify for short-term home care services. However, since Medicare does not cover custodial care, once the patient has become stable, he must be discharged from home care service. Discharge planners may make referrals for home care services realizing that these services are very short-term and that there is inadequate long-term care for the majority of patients who need it.

Another example of an ethical dilemma that discharge planners face is a patient being discharged with complex care needs such as, pump-regulated enteral feedings, a biliary tube requiring irrigation or a Hickman catheter. These patients no longer require hospital level care and want to return home, but in some communities home care agencies may not have the sophistication or the 24-hour availability to be an adequate resource for the family.

Because these problems are complex, multifaceted solutions must be sought. Community agencies may need to expand services and receive education to care for patients with more complex needs. Hospitals may need to be made aware of limitations in community resources and the need to develop solutions to these problems. Families may need to receive more intensive education in the care of patients prior to discharge.

Most importantly, discharge planning professionals must join forces and lobby for programs to ensure the availability of care to those who need it.

Discharge Planning and the Home Health Agency

Discharge planning directly affects the delivery of service by home health agencies. In order to provide efficient, cost-effective care, home health agencies must have accurate information about the patient's living situation, caregivers, insurance data, diagnosis, and prescribed plan of care. Equipment and supplies must be available, patients must have received discharge instructions and prescriptions at the time of discharge. If any of these items is missing or inaccurate, agency personnel must spend valuable time tracking down correct information. If the medical information that has been given is inaccurate and the visiting nurse finds that the patient has no skilled needs as defined by Medicare, that visit cannot be billed and represents a loss to the agency.

Lack of coordination of services can result in omission or duplication of needed care. An incomplete referral results in agency personnel attempting to provide quality care without adequate data. Because the patient's well-being depends on the care delivered by the home health agency, it is imperative that discharge planners provide thorough, accurate information about the patient at the time of the initial referral.

Discharge planners need feedback on the quality of the plans they have developed and areas that need improvement. Home health agencies should maintain close contact with discharge planners to alert them to problem areas and also to changes in the condition of patients referred to them. This information is necessary for refining discharge plans if the patient is readmitted.

Summary

Discharge planning is a multifaceted process that seeks to promote optimal care for patients in the transition from the hospital to the posthospital environment. Prospective payment for hospitals has resulted in increased attention to discharge planning as a means to reduce length of stay while promoting optimal patient care. Multidisciplinary cooperation, communication, and collaboration, and the involvement of the patient and family in the plan development are key elements in the discharge planning process. This process consists of four stages: assessment, planning, implementation, and evaluation. Discharge planning programs must have an established evaluation procedure to identify areas of weakness and develop strategies to improve delivery of service. Discharge planners must educate health care professionals, patients and families, and communities of the services available and the limitations and gaps in service.

References

American Nurses Association. 1973. Standards of Nursing Practice. *Kansas City, MO: American Nurses' Association.*

Discharge Planning Advisor. September 1985. Hospital Peer Review *10(9).*

Discharge Planning Update: An Interdisciplinary Prospective for Health Care Professionals. *(Serial published quarterly by the American Hospital Association.)*

Edwards, R. C. 1978. Professionals in "Alliance" achieve more effective discharge planning. Hospitals, J.A.H.A. *52:71-72.*

Field, L. 1981. Discharge planning: A staff nurse's perspective. In Continuing care a multidisciplinary approach to discharge planning. *Ed. by K. McKeehan. St. Louis: C. V. Mosby.*

Hardy, G. 1985. A simple tool for early patient involvement. Coordinator *4(8).*

Joint Commission on Accreditation of Hospitals. 1974. Accreditation Manual for Hospitals. *Chicago: The Association.*

McKeehan, M., ed. 1981. Continuing care: A multidisciplinary approach to discharge planning. St. Louis: C. V. Mosby.

Medicare regulation. 1972. Chicago: Commerce Clearing House.

Mundinger, M. O. 1983. *Home care controversy.* Rockville, MD: Aspen Systems Corp.

Philadelphia Inquirer. 1986. 314(16) Philadelphia Newspapers Inc.

Quaschnick, M. S. 1985. Discharge planning in a small hospital. *Coordinator* 4(4).

Rasmusen, L. A. 1984. A screening tool promotes early discharge planning. *Nursing Management* 15(5).

Smeltzer, C. H., and S. M. Flores. 1986. Preadmission discharge planning--Organization of a concept. *Journal of Nursing Administration* 16(5).

Volland, P. J. 1982. Practice in action: Decision making in discharge planning. *Brook lodge symposium: Discharge planning to home care.* Upjohn Health Care Services.

Chapter Seven

Referral Sources

Michele Lucas and Lynne D. Pancoast

Definition

The referral is at the very core of the home health care industry. Without it, the business would certainly not survive. The referral is a critical component of the discharge planning process, a process which is crucial in every health care setting. Discharge planning, as defined by the American Nurses' Association (1975, 3) is "the part of the continuity of care process which is designed to prepare the patient or client for the next phase of care and to assist in making any necessary arrangements for that phase of care, whether it be self-care, care by family members, or care by an organized health care provider."

Discharge planning includes three components: (1) the assessment and identification of the actual and potential physical and psychosocial needs of the client; (2) the planning for care which is needed when a change in or cessation of services by the present health care provider is indicated; and (3) the preparation of the client for self-care when organized care is terminated, or the preparation and referral of the client for transfer to another health care organization (American Nurses' Association 1975).

In light of the above, a referral may then be defined as the compilation of pertinent client-related information which is communicated to an organization for the purpose of obtaining the needed health care services. In home health care, this information would include demographic as well as health-related facts about the client. The referral information may be given to or by the home health agency and may vary depending on the needed phase of care as determined by the discharge planning process.

Referral Sources

The sources of referrals to home health agencies can be described simply and in one word, limitless. In other words, an agency can receive a referral from almost any source. The types of sources for any given agency would depend on factors such as its size, structure (freestanding, hospital-related, public, nonprofit, voluntary, or proprietary), location, services offered, surrounding competition, and so on. For example, a hospital-affiliated agency would probably receive most of its referrals from the hospital. Other examples of referral sources would include skilled nursing facilities, intermediate care facilities, personal care boarding homes, rehabilitation facilities, outpatient facilities, community centers, physicians, families, neighbors, clients themselves, and almost any other imaginable source.

Each of the above-mentioned referral sources would probably differ in its reasons for making the referral and in its expectations of the needed services. For example, a health care facility should be able to provide the agency with more complete referral information and should be more realistic in its service expectations. On the other hand, lay referral sources would probably require more intense screening and are probably very limited in their understanding of the agency's role. Physician referrals generally vary in their reasons, quality of information, and service expectations depending on the individual.

The collection and maintenance of referral source data is a wise idea for all home health agencies. Analysis of these data can be very useful for internal agency evaluation, as well as agency marketing practices. Agencies are, in fact, recommended by Medicare (Department of Health, Education and Welfare 1973) to use referral source data as a tool for the required policy and administrative review part of the overall agency evaluation (Section 405.1229a).

Referral Information

As stated earlier in the chapter, home health referrals generally include both demographic and health-related information about the client. The quantity and quality of this information may vary and depend on factors such as the referral source, the needed level of care, the amount of information available, and the purpose of the referral (intake versus interagency referral). Even though this is true, the agency can exert some control over the information that is received or provided by its staff via the design of its forms. Agency referral forms serve as guides for the staff in receiving or relaying pertinent information. Their content is therefore crucial. Two types of referral forms, intake and interagency, will now be discussed and examples provided.

Intake Referral Form

This referral form is designed for initial intake purposes and can be thought of as a preadmission screening tool. The staff use this form for collecting or receiving information from an outside source about a prospective client. The form itself is usually developed by agency staff and will vary depending on the agency's needs. If the agency is Medicare-certified, it is subject to federal requirements on clinical records. In addition to other information, the record must contain " . . . appropriate identifying information; name of physician; drug, dietary, treatment, and activity orders . . . " (Medicare 1973, Section 405.1228). It is therefore advisable for the agency to obtain at least these facts when taking the preliminary information during the intake process. It is even more beneficial for the agency to obtain as much information as possible when receiving a referral.

If the referral source is unable to provide all of the desired information, the staff should be encouraged to pursue other possible sources. For example, if the original referral source is a family member, the staff person would be wise to confer with the appropriate physician for the desired medical information. Or if a physician refers a case and offers only scant information, the staff person would be wise to confer with the prospective client and family for additional facts if needed.

Please refer to Exhibit 7-1 for a sample of an intake referral form. It is important to consider that this agency is a hospital-affiliated, Medicare-certified agency which provides the six most common home health services and can arrange for in-home laboratory studies and delivery of medical supplies. Most of its referrals come from its affiliated hospital and skilled nursing facility companies, and include a significant amount of health-related information. It is also important to note that the agency utilizes a full-time nurse liaison to gather the referral data in these facilities once a referral is received. This same form, however, is also utilized by the agency's supervisory staff when referrals are made directly to the office. They utilize the back of the form to document telephone calls made to all parties for the purpose of obtaining additional information.

Interagency Referral Form

This referral form is designed for interim referral purposes and can be thought of as a transfer summary. The staff use this form to convey pertinent demographic and health-related facts about a client who has been under their service and will be followed by another agency. The most common reason for an interagency referral is a move to another geographical area. Sometimes such a move involves a great distance and the staff can find it difficult to locate an agency in the new area. The *National Home Care Directory,* published by the National Association for Home Care, is an excellent reference for locating an agency in an unfamiliar area.

Like the intake form, the interagency referral is usually developed by agency staff and will vary depending on the agency's philosophy. And although there are no specific content requirements for Medicare-certified agencies, there is a general requirement that "if a patient is transferred to another health facility, a copy of the record or abstract accompanies the patient" (Medicare 1973, Section 405.1228a). Thus, it is wise to develop and use a form which provides a sufficient amount of information about the care rendered, client's status, and needed services.

Please refer to Exhibit 7-2 for a sample of an interagency referral form. Any additional information is placed by agency staff on the back of the form and a copy of each side is maintained in the client's record.

Criteria for Service

The development and utilization of service criteria is a wise practice for all home health agencies. Agency policies can be of immense benefit to the staff when making a decision about whether any referred client is appropriate. Of particular benefit is the agency's policy on criteria for acceptance to service. These criteria provide parameters for the staff in determining whether the agency can safely and adequately provide the needed services. This is especially important in light of the increased demand for high technology therapies to be provided in the home. Many agencies have developed additional policies for these requested special procedures which in-

Exhibit 7-1. Jeanes Home Health Referral Form

<u>JEANES HOME HEALTH REFERRAL FORM</u>   Date of Referral _____
Patient seen by Liaison: YES NO

Patient Name		#		D.O.B.		Age	M.S.	Race	Sex

Address   T/P

Resp. Person/Relationship   Address   T/P

Referral Source   Hosp. Adm./Disch.   ECF Adm./Disch.

H.I.C. #   Other Ins.   Worker's Comp./No Fault
                                               Yes ___ No ___
DX   Pt./Fam. Informed
                                               Yes ___ No ___
P.M.H.

Hosp. Attending/Phone   FMD/Phone   Consultants/Phone

Surg. Procedure/Date

Diet   Mental Status   Funct. Limits

Hx this admit:

Meds: Allergies: Labs./Additional Information:

Home Services (circle or ?)   PT:
RN:

                                 ST:

                                 OT:

    D/C Rx -
    D/C VS. -
    M.D. Appt. -
                                 DME/Supplies:
HHA:
                                 Referral Called:
MSW:
Date	To		Date	To

JHH18 (8/85)

Exhibit 7-2. Jeanes Home Health

INTERAGENCY REFERRAL

Client Name: _____   Agency Referred To: _____

Address: _____   Address: _____

_____   _____

Telephone: _____   Telephone: _____

DOB: _____ Age: _____   Contact Person: _____

Fee Source: _____

HI #: _____   Emergency Contact: _____

Other Insurance: _____   Contact Address: _____

Hosp./Dates:_____   _____

ECF/Dates: _____   Contact Telephone: _____

Diagnosis: _____

_____ Pt. Informed yes no/Fam. Informed yes no

Surgical Procedure/Date: _____

Prognosis: _____ Pt. Informed yes no/Fam. Informed yes no

Allergies: _____ Diet: _____

Medications: _____

_____

_____

Mental Status: _____   Activities: _____

Status/Significant Info: _____

_____

_____

Services Requested: _____

Referring Physician: _____   Accepting Physician: _____
                                          (if known)
Address: _____   Address: _____

_____   _____

Telephone: _____   Telephone: _____

                                          Referred By: _____

JHH (8/84)   Date: _____

clude admission criteria specific to each. Here, the staff would utilize both the general criteria and the special procedure criteria to see if the client is appropriate.

If any referred client is determined to be inappropriate and is therefore rejected for service, the reasons should be clearly documented on the referral form and the form maintained in a separate file. Agency staff may need to access these data later, should a question arise about why service wasn't provided. Medicare (1973) also recommends that agencies analyze " . . . the number of patients not accepted with reasons . . . " as part of their evaluation process (Section 405.1229a).

The admission or acceptance criteria may vary among home health agencies. These differences may result from such factors as the agency's size, structure, location, services offered, philosophy, goals, and so on. In some agencies, the staff may develop the criteria. If the agency is Medicare-certified, however, it is required to have a Group of Professional Personnel, which is responsible for advising and evaluating the agency, as well as establishing and annually reviewing agency policies, including admission and discharge policies (DHHS 1973, Section 405.1222). Medicare also provides a general guideline on admission policies when stating, "Patients are accepted for treatment on the basis of a reasonable expectation that the patient's medical, nursing, and social needs can be met adequately by the agency in the patient's place of residence" (Section 405.1223). The agency therefore needs to include at least this concept when developing its admission criteria. In addition, the criteria for continuation of service (if used) and termination of service should logically flow from those for acceptance in order to remain consistent.

Please refer to Exhibit 7-3 for a sample of acceptance criteria. Some general admission policies then follow.

Rejection of Referrals

An agency that rejects referrals runs the risk of alienating the referral source, even if the patient is totally inappropriate for the services a particular agency provides. The dilemma lies in whether an agency should (1) simply accept all referrals for evaluation and be responsible for the disposition; or (2) explain to the referral source why the patient does not qualify for their services and leave the disposition to the referral source. One advantage of the former is the sense of ease a referral source will have in expediting patients to any agency. In the harried world of discharge planners, physicians, or any others trying to arrange follow-up home care services, the referral process must be facilitated in the most efficient manner possible.

On the other hand, if all referrals are taken for evaluation, it is reasonable to expect that some will be inappropriate for acceptance. The agency then has the responsibility to advise the patient or family member of other local community resources from which specific needed services could be obtained. A decision must then be made whether to inform the referral source of the disposition.

The other approach offers the advantage of having an opportunity to clarify to the referral source the agency eligibility requirements and admission criteria. Because of the frequently changing interpretation of eligibility for services under third party payers (in particular Medicare), it is not possible for referral sources to keep abreast of all home care regulations. Agencies are in a position to provide the most current information to those sources as inquiries are made about referrals. It is important that

Exhibit 7-3. Jeanes Home Health Policy and Procedure Manual Criteria for Services

I. Acceptance for Service

  A. Criteria

    1. The request for service is based upon a health need, not primarily a social or environmental need. There is a need for skilled professional service.

    2. A physician will assume responsibility for medical direction. If the source of medical care cannot be identified, a home visit may be made at the discretion of the Agency supervisory staff.

    3. The patient is essentially homebound.

    4. Someone is available to the patient to provide care between Agency visits if necessary.

    5. The Agency has the capacity to provide the kind and amount of service required and/or requested.

    6. The home setting is safe for the patient. There is provision for shelter, food, clothing, and protection of the individual.

    7. The patient and/or significant other is capable and willing to participate in the patient's care as necessary.

    8. The situation does not endanger Agency Staff.

    9. The environment is one in which service can be provided effectively.

  B. Policies

    1. Acceptance of a request for service does not insure continuation of further service beyond the initial visit. The decision to accept a patient for service is made after the initial visit when it is determined that the Criteria for Acceptance have been met.

    2. The patient or significant other will be contacted within 72 hours of receipt or referral, or sooner/later as indicated by the situation of the referral; at that time the plan for initial home visit (if appropriate) will be established.

    3. If an individual meets these requirements, he or she will be accepted for home health services regardless of age, race, creed, color, religion, sex, sexual preference, handicap, national origin and socioeconomic status.

---

an agency which refuses to evaluate a patient for admission to service consider giving the referral source a reason why. Reasons may include: (1) no skilled services are required; (2) the patient is not homebound; (3) the agency does not provide service in that patient's home area; (4) services required are not available through that particular agency (e.g., high technology therapies, pediatric care), and so on.

The disadvantage of giving feedback to the referral source about the inability to provide requested services can, however, result in "agency shopping" by the referral source. In the event this "shopping" is successful, a rapport with another agency may be initiated that will continue. That particular referral source may be lost to the agency for all future patients.

In light of the above choices, it is incumbent upon agency management to clearly define how an inappropriate referral is to be handled. Confusion on the part of intake personnel will impact negatively on the agency. Therefore, intake policies should be established and communicated clearly to the staff.

Intake Person

The intake person is one of the more important agency persons in terms of public image. He is the agency's link to the "outside," and can make the difference between whether or not a referral source utilizes the agency again. An agency is wise to choose the intake person with care.

Ideally, the intake person should be a registered nurse since the majority of referrals require home nursing services. While it is possible for a clerical person to take the demographic data, health-related information will be more accurately interpreted and transcribed by a health care professional. A referral involving only therapy services could be taken by a rehabilitation specialist such as a physical or occupational therapist, if available.

Other qualifications that should be considered for the intake person include: (1) a pleasant and dynamic voice; (2) the ability to get along well with people; (3) good communication skills; (4) good working knowledge of the agency's policies regarding patient eligibility for service; (5) an ability to seek out and obtain appropriate patient information; (6) knowledge of other community resources; (7) a nonjudgmental and caring attitude; (8) an organized approach to information collection; (9) knowledge of community health principles and practices; (10) a sense of humor; (11) good listening skills; and (12) the ability to maintain a positive professional attitude.

As much as possible, the agency should have an intake person readily available to receive information or referrals as soon as the call comes in. The easier the referral process is made, the more likely the referral source is to utilize the same agency again. The following can have a negative impact on a referral source: (1) a constant busy signal on the telephone; (2) being put on hold (for more than a minute or two); (3) constant interruptions to the intake person; (4) inefficient taking of information by the intake person (writes too slowly, constantly requesting the referral source to spell words or repeat, etc.); (5) inability of the intake person to hear information being conveyed; (6) indecision about whether the referral is appropriate or not; (7) asking too many questions; (8) sarcasm; and (9) inappropriate, nonprofessional behavior.

Some agencies provide the services of a liaison person to major referral sources such as hospitals and skilled nursing facilities. The liaison is an employee of the agency, usually a registered nurse, who collects information on patients referred to the agency from that institution. He can also act as a resource for questions regarding home care services and appropriateness of referrals. The liaison can facilitate the transition from institution to home by meeting with referred patients and families and discussing and arranging the following: (1) available, appropriate home services; (2) the roles of the home care staff; (3) scheduling of the first visit; and (4) necessary medical supplies and equipment that can be arranged for prior to discharge. Services from the agency can be processed and initiated more promptly since the liaison is in a position to personally evaluate the patient's needs prior to discharge from the institution. The liaison can ascertain directly from the institutional nurses how the patient is learning and performing specific techniques such as insulin administration, emptying of drainage bags, changing dressings, etc.

Two of the major responsibilities of the liaison are to review the medical records of all patients referred and to complete the referral form noting relevant demographic data, past medical history, history of the current problem, a brief description of pertinent facts regarding this admission, rehabilitation notes, discharge medications, psychosocial information, and pertinent laboratory and x-ray findings. Special instructions for the home care staff such as specific dressing techniques, monitoring of weight, and requests for laboratory studies at home can be obtained by the liaison as well.

The liaison position must not be confused with the role of a discharge planner who is an employee of the institution. This distinction is particularly important in terms of separating the job responsibilities and the costs attributed to these positions. The differences in these positions are further clarified in the *Medicare Provider Reimbursement Manual* which discusses the coordination of home health referrals.

The discharge planner is responsible for the discharge needs of the institution's patients. This may include such planning as nursing home placement, evaluation for a rehabilitation center, arrangement for private-pay homemaker service, or home-delivered meal services. The discharge planner can also initiate the referral to the home health agency through the liaison or other intake person. The liaison may not solicit patients in the institution. A referral process between the discharge planner and the liaison should be established and adhered to by all parties. Good communication between them will ensure more efficiency and smoother transition for the patient from institution to home.

Seasonal Trends

Agency management needs to be acutely aware of any trends in the referral pattern which will impact on staffing. For example, the agency who employs sufficient staff to handle 50 referrals a week, will experience a significant amount of downtime for their staff and resultant financial difficulties if the referral rate suddenly drops to 25 per week. One way of tracking trends is to plot agency activity such as numbers of referrals and total visits on graphs. These data can be analyzed to identify any trends related to seasons of the year, holidays, new legislation, etc., that will impact on the census. The ability to predict and anticipate referral patterns will allow an agency to better handle the overflow and to staff appropriately for the leaner times.

The agency administration can utilize trend data from the previous year to develop a realistic budget for the upcoming fiscal year. Projections for staffing can also be made based on these data. Because the home health industry is labor-intensive, salaries and wages account for a major portion of the expenses. The fluctuation in caseload can be managed in a more fiscally prudent fashion through the use of part-time staff and contractors. The referral profile can assist in overall agency planning and budgeting.

Marketing

The 1980s has seen a change in the health care field from interest in the public relations area to an absolute necessity for marketing and selling services. The increasing number of home health agencies requires an active sales campaign for many agencies in order to capture a share of the market. Word-of-mouth advertising is not enough in today's atmosphere of competition, particularly for those agencies that do not have joint ventures or other arrangements with health care institutions to guarantee a minimal flow of patients.

Marketing simply means selling your agency's services. This can be accomplished in many ways, but the process involves increasing the agency's visibility. The process begins with choosing an appropriate agency name that is easy to remember and relates to the services offered. Brochures and pamphlets describing the agency and its purpose should be developed and distributed in as many locations as possible, preferably where referrals are initiated. Examples would include physician's offices and waiting rooms, hospital waiting areas in various departments, senior citizens' centers, community social service agencies, school nurse offices, church bulletin boards, rehabilitation centers, nursing homes, retirement communities, and so on. Brochures can be included in admission packets given to patients in hospitals and the health care institutions where appropriate arrangements exist.

Each member of the staff can market the agency on a daily basis. Name pins bearing the title of the agency, as well as the individual's name, should always be worn. Staff should always introduce themselves by name and give the agency name as well ("I am Ms. Smith from the Jeanes Home Health Agency," rather than "I am Ms. Smith from the home health--or visiting nurse--agency"). The latter is too generic and does not give the agency recognition. Equipment bags carried by the staff should have the agency emblem and name predominately displayed. Vehicles owned by the agency should be lettered with the agency name and phone number. For staff using their own vehicles, identification cards can be placed in the window.

Public appearances such as speaking to different community groups on a variety of health-related subjects can also allow more visibility for the agency and its staff. Health fairs, school fairs, and shopping mall displays provide additional opportunities to achieve this. Giveaways of items with the agency's name such as pens, pencils, refrigerator magnets, telephone stickers with emergency numbers, memo pads, key chains, etc., all help to keep the agency's name in the public eye. Public service announcements on radio and television are also appropriate.

An agency designee should periodically visit their referral sources to discuss problems or issues of mutual concern. Requests should be made for feedback from these sources, and suggestions solicited on ways to improve service or add to services already being provided. Personal contact with a referral source will make a more lasting impact than a letter or evaluation card. Referral sources should be encouraged to be involved in the agency, if possible, as consultants, as members of an advisory committee, or as part of the record review process. Those who have more frequent and personal contacts with the agency will tend to use it more.

In conclusion, the best way to market an agency is through satisfied clients and referral sources. Appropriate, timely, good quality services will speak for themselves.

Legal Issues

Various providers in the health care system, such as acute care facilities, have become increasingly more cognizant of liability issues in the past few decades and have actively taken steps to avoid legal problems. A more recent example of this is the development of ethics committees in hospitals.

Home health agencies have, especially in the last few years, joined their provider colleagues in becoming more aware of potential liability concerns. Increased numbers of home health agencies and more creative business arrangements have resulted in greater competition and increased likelihood of liability and legal problems. One of the major areas in which agencies need to exercise caution is in their referral practices. Some of the issues surrounding these practices will now be addressed.

Collection of Referral Information

It is crucial that the agency's intake staff collect as much information as possible when taking a referral. This serves two very useful purposes. First, it provides agency personnel with the facts necessary to make a decision about whether the client's needs can be met adequately by the agency. Fletcher (1985) discusses this when she relates information from a presentation given by Patricia A. Peters, director of hospital services for Parkside Home Health Services in Park Ridge, IL. Ms. Peters, who spoke at the 1985 annual meeting of the American Society for Hospital Risk Management, reports that the assignment of a client to an inappropriate level of care could result in a liability claim for a home health agency. She uses an example of an agency providing part-time nursing care when full-time or private duty nursing was actually needed. Ms. Peters advises that "clearly worded admission and discharge standards and a clear description of services available" (Fletcher 1985,10) would help to circumvent such a problem. In addition, a more thorough screening during the referral process may have resulted in a more appropriate assignment of services.

The second purpose served by the collection of more complete referral information is a reduction in the amount of staff time spent in home visits. It could especially impact on the initial visit when much time is typically spent in obtaining information needed to complete documentation requirements and plan for appropriate service. As a result, the client, who is often frustrated with the many questions asked, may feel more relaxed and may perceive the agency as being more organized and knowledgeable about his situation.

Maintenance of Referral Information

Having gathered as much referral information as possible, a decision is then made about what types of service, if any, are indicated. If the agency plans to evaluate or admit a client, the referral should then become a part of the legal record. If, however, the client is deemed inappropriate and will not be seen, the reasons should be documented and the referral maintained in a special file. With this practice, the agency can later access the information should a question arise about why service was not provided or should the client be referred to the agency again in the future.

Agency Policies

In determining whether a client is appropriate for agency services, the intake staff would benefit from having parameters by which to be guided. One way in which to provide such guidelines is through clearly stated agency administrative and clinical policies. A home health agency, like any other health care provider, is compared to the standard practice when any legal situation arises. The agency should therefore model its policies after those of the agencies in the surrounding area. The more highly regarded agencies should be used as role models if possible.

Agency policies will probably vary depending upon the location of the agency, as well as other factors. Examples of administrative policies which can be used by the intake staff for referral-taking purposes may therefore include, but are not limited to, statements of philosophy, goals, services provided, geographical area served, service hours, and nondiscrimination practices. Clinical policies on topics such as admission criteria and medical supervision may also be helpful. The individual policies need not be lengthy or elaborate to be of value to the staff; rather, they need to clearly state the agency's perspective so that the staff can refer to and be guided by them in making referral decisions.

Antitrust Issues

As stated earlier, the significant changes in the home health care industry have resulted in increased competition. In particular, hospitals have sharply increased their participation in the business by either developing their own agencies or establishing arrangements with already existing agencies. These trends have begun to raise concerns about potential antitrust issues. Some of these concerns are addressed by Fletcher (1985) in her article on home care liability. She reports that, according to Patricia A. Peters, antitrust issues may arise when there is an unusually close relationship between a home health agency and a hospital or physician. Ms. Peters advises that "a home health care agency should have a clear understanding of legal implications related to contractual arrangements" (Fletcher 1985, 12).

Philp (1985), an attorney with a Washington, DC firm, discusses that as a result of increased competition, hospitals may attempt to ensure that their clients utilize their own affiliated agency by "steering" them to it. Ms. Philp reports that this action may take any of several forms, including hospital discharge planners recommending the affiliated agency or disparaging other agencies' services. Another method is the withholding of information about other available agencies by hospital staff. A third "steering" tactic is that of the hospital allowing staff from the affiliated agency to participate in its discharge planning activities, while preventing the same by competitor agencies.

The above tactics may be challenged through antitrust actions, particularly if the hospital represents a significant source of referrals and other agencies are prevented from obtaining or competing for the business.

Antitrust concerns may also arise when a hospital either becomes an equipment supplier or establishes a referral arrangement with a supplier. In conclusion then, antitrust concerns may be raised in any situation where a hospital participates in a business which depends substantially on referrals of hospital clients and the hospital tries to steer the clients to its own business (Philp 1985).

Referral Process

In consideration of the above information, the following case studies represent two examples of the entire referral process. The first includes the steps in the referral process from a liaison nurse. The second is an example of a referral from a physician.

Case Study 1

Referral From Liaison Nurse

Scenario

Mr. S., an 80-year-old male, is being discharged from an acute care facility after a 10-day stay for deep vein thrombosis. Mr. S. also experienced bladder outlet obstruction during this hospitalization, requiring an indwelling Foley catheter for an indefinite period of time. Mr. S. was placed on anticoagulant therapy and is being discharged on Crystalline Warfarin Sodium (Coumadin). Periodic Prothrombin Times will be required. His past medical history includes congestive heart failure and a myocardial infarction two years ago.

Mr. S. lives with his elderly wife in a two-story home. Because of generalized deconditioning, he is unable to negotiate stairs and will be set up on the first floor. A hospital bed and commode will be required. Mr. S.'s wife has recently recovered from a total hip replacement and ambulates with a quad cane. The extent to which she can assist Mr. S. is not clearly established. No other family members live close by; however, a neighbor has been assisting with shopping and transportation.

The teaching process for catheter care has been initiated by the hospital nursing staff one day prior to discharge. However, because of the high anxiety level of both the patient and his wife, further teaching and reinforcement will be required.

Steps in Referral Process

1. The hospital discharge planner and attending physician identify Mr. S. as a home care candidate. The patient is asked if he has ever had home health services.

2. Mr. S. is referred to the affiliated home health agency if appropriate. The liaison nurse is notified and given the above information.

3. The liaison nurse performs an initial review of the hospital record of the client, collecting pertinent demographic data, past medical history, history of

current problem, surgical procedures, allergies, diet, attending physician, mental status, and a brief synopsis of the hospital stay.

4. If possible, the liaison interviews the client and family to evaluate for and explain home health services. The liaison deems the case appropriate. Skilled nursing and physical therapy services are ordered immediately. The community health nurse will evaluate the need for a home health aide to assist with personal care, and for a medical social worker to assist with long-term planning. The liaison discusses how and when the home visits will be initiated. A brochure that describes the agency services is given to the client at this time with instructions to call the agency if any questions arise. Fees for service and insurance coverage of home health services are also clarified by the liaison.

5. Durable medical equipment and supply needs are identified and ordered for delivery prior to the client's arrival home. In this case, a hospital bed, commode, and catheter supplies are ordered by the liaison.

6. Specific discharge information is then collected by the liaison such as medications (dosage, frequency, and route of administration), catheter instructions (irrigations, frequency of changing, etc.), activity level, and needed in-home laboratory tests.

7. All pertinent information is documented on the intake referral form and submitted to the home health agency.

Case Study 2

Referral From Physician

Scenario

A physician calls the home health agency requesting home skilled nursing services for a patient he has just seen in the office. The patient is evidencing signs of congestive heart failure and wants to avoid hospitalization.

Medications have been changed and the physician wants the nurse to monitor their effectiveness and note any increase in symptoms. Because he is in the middle of office hours and is already behind schedule, minimal information is forthcoming from the physician except for the new changes in medications, the patient's name, and a brief description of past medical history. He then refers the agency intake person back to his office receptionist to obtain more information.

Steps in Referral Process

1. The intake person obtains as much information as possible from the physician.

2. The intake person then confers with the physician's clerical (and nursing) staff to obtain any additional information. If speaking with the clerical staff, mostly

demographic information would be obtained. The nursing staff, on the other hand, should be able to provide more health-related data.

3. The intake person then calls the patient and significant others to obtain any other information that would be useful to have. Eligibility requirements, services, and insurance coverage are also discussed. The agency's name and number are given and an initial visit plan is established.

4. All pertinent information is then documented on the intake referral form including dates and times of all phone calls and to whom they were made.

References

American Nurses' Association. 1975. *Continuity of care and discharge planning programs in institutions and community agencies.* Kansas City: American Nurses' Association.

Fletcher, M. 1985. Trend toward home care poses new liability worries. *Business Insurance* 19:10, 12.

Department of Health, Education and Welfare. 1973. Conditions of participation for home health agencies. *Federal Register.* 42:405.1201-405.1230.

Philp, M. S. 1985. Home-health referrals: some legal guidelines. *Hospitals* 59:72-75.

Chapter Eight

Self-Care Systems in Community Health Nursing

Joan Reynolds Yuan

As practice in a profession is based on theory, this chapter will address systems of care based on Dorothea Orem's Nursing Theory, the clinical applicability to community health nursing, and the implications for the nursing administration in a community health agency. In the American Nurses' Association's (ANA 1980, 2) publication, *A Conceptual Model of Community Health Nursing,* community health nursing is defined as follows:

> Community health nursing is a synthesis of nursing practice and public health practice applied to promoting and preserving the health of populations. . . .
> Health promotion, health maintenance, health education, and management, coordination, and continuity of care are utilized in a holistic approach to the management of the health care of individuals, families, and groups in a community.

In the current cost-conscious environment, there are many changes occurring in health care and in community health nursing. The role of the nurse as client advocate is crucial in the delivery of community health nursing services. Of growing concern is the ability of the client to pay for care, the provision of adequate care, access to health services, and the developing tiers of care based on affluence and the reimbursement system (ANA 1985). Community health nurses are in a position to develop systems of care for people in the community, based on health maintenance and promotion as well as ill care in the home.

In *A Guide for Community-Based Nursing Services,* it states, "Consumers are moving from nearly total reliance on hospitals and other institutions to community-based services. This shift has been prompted by rising costs and diminishing resources, changing demographic patterns, and a rediscovery of the benefits, and perhaps the necessity, of self help . . ." (ANA 1985, 4.)

Community health nurses have long practiced the concept of self-care. Since Lillian Wald conceptualized public health nursing (currently synonymous with community health nursing) at the turn of the century, self-care has been incorporated into the practice of this specialty. Consumer involvement is important in the development of the plan of care in community health nursing because the goals and desired outcomes ultimately will be the responsibility of individuals for self-care (ANA 1985).

Portions of this chapter have been reprinted with permission of the McGraw-Hill Book Co. from *Nursing: Concepts of Practice,* Second Edition by Dorothea Orem, McGraw-Hill, 1980.

Orem's theory of self-care has significance for community health nurses. According to Dorothea Orem, Nursing's special concern is: "Man's need for self-care action and the provision and management of it on a continuous basis in order to sustain life and health, recover from disease or injury and cope with their effects." (Orem 1980, 6). Self-care is purposeful. It is the practice of activities that are initiated and performed for oneself or for one's dependents to maintain life, health, and well-being. Self-care requisites are descriptive of the kinds of purposive self-care that are required. Universal self-care requisites are common to all human beings adjusted for such factors as age, developmental state, and environment. For example, the maintenance of sufficient intake of air, water, and food. Developmental self-care requisites are associated with developmental processes and conditions or events that affect development. This includes the provision of care to prevent the occurrence of deleterious effects of conditions that can affect human development. Health deviation self-care requisites are associated with genetic and constitutional defects, structural and functional deviations, and with their diagnosis and treatment (Orem 1980).

The assessment phase of Orem's nursing process relates to diagnosis and prescription (Orem 1980). It includes data collection, determining why the patient needs nursing care such as the requirements for therapeutic self-care, and the ability of the patient to engage in self-care. In community health nursing the nurse must also look at family and community needs. The planning phase of this nursing process is defined as

> The designing of a system . . . that will effectively contribute to the patient's achievement of health goals through therapeutic self-care . . . Planning for the delivery of nursing according to the designed system includes specifications for roles, resources, coordinating activities, and time, place, and frequency of performance of activities by nurse, patient, or others (Orem 1980, 202).

Implementation and evaluation are included in the third phase:

> The initiation, conduction, and control of assisting actions to (1) compensate for the patient's self-care limitations to ensure that self-care is given and is therapeutic and to enable the patient to adapt his or her behavior to existing limitations, (2) overcome when possible self-care limitations of the patient (or care limitations of the family) so that the patient's future short-term or long-term therapeutic self-care requisites can be met effectively, and (3) foster and protect the patient's self care abilities and prevent the development of new self-care limitations (Orem 1980, 202).

Self-care agency is the human ability to engage in self-care. The content of self-care agency derives from meeting self-care requisites (Orem 1980). In order for nursing to take place, the nurse must have the ability to view patients as self-care and dependent-care agents and to diagnose patients' abilities for engagement in continuous and effective care. "Unless self-care agency is accurately diagnosed, nurses have no rational basis for (1) making judgements about existing or projected self-care deficits and the reasons for their existence, (2) selecting valid and reliable methods of helping, or (3) prescribing and designing nursing systems" (Orem 1980, 84).

The self-care that the patient can or cannot manage and the reasons why, guide the nurse in the selection of the appropriate methods of helping. These methods include: acting for or doing for another, guiding another, supporting another, providing an environment that promotes personal development in relation to becoming able to meet present or future demands for action, and teaching another (Orem 1980).

Considering the concept that either the nurse or patient or the nurse and patient can act to meet patients' self-care requisites, three nursing systems have been identified: (1) wholly compensatory; (2) partly compensatory; and (3) supportive-educative (developmental) (Orem 1980). The need for a wholly compensatory nursing system is identified when the patient is unable to engage in those self-care actions requiring self-directed and controlled ambulation and manipulative movement or the prescription to refrain from such activity. Three subtypes have been identified: (1) persons unable to engage in any form of deliberate action; (2) persons who are aware and may be able to make decisions about self-care, but cannot or should not perform actions requiring ambulation and manipulative movements; (3) persons who are unable to make rational judgements and decisions about self-care, but are ambulatory and may be able to perform some measures of self-care with continuous guidance and supervision (Orem 1980). Frequently the helping method utilized by the nurse in this system is that of acting and doing for another. The nurse must be able to design and manage effective care systems. This includes providing guidelines and supervising others who can contribute to the wholly compensatory care system (Orem 1980).

In the partly compensatory system, both nurse and patient perform care measures or other actions involving manipulative tasks or ambulation. The distribution of responsibility varies with the patient's limitations for ambulation or manipulative activities, knowledge and skill required, and the patient's psychological state. In this system, all five helping methods may be utilized (Orem 1980).

The third system, supportive-educative, is used when the patient is able to perform or can and should learn to perform therapeutic self-care measures, but cannot do so without assistance. Helping methods include: support, guidance, provision of a developmental environment, and teaching (Orem 1980).

Historically, the community health nurse has cared for patients with many functional limitations that would be considered wholly compensatory. Systems of care have been designed to include care provided by family, friends, and neighbors, as well as professional and ancillary staff. The numbers in this group are growing at a time when society is unprepared to care for them. Due to changes in reimbursement, a frequently seen phenomenon is that patients are discharged home from the hospital quicker and sicker. This occurs at a time when many of the traditional supports are unavailable due to the increased numbers of women in the work force outside the home, the migration of family members to other parts of the country, and the limited physical and financial resources of many of the young-old who are attempting to care for the old-old.

Some of the patients in the wholly compensatory level have chronic problems and third-party payors will not reimburse for services provided. This is an area that must be addressed by the nursing administration. Is there an agency servicing that community that can provide home health aide, homemaker, and companion services that is affordable to the people in the community?

Many of the people currently being discharged home from the hospital have needs that must be addressed by highly skilled professionals. With advances in technology, patients are now at home with equipment such as ventilators. In many instances, family members will assume responsibility for the provision of care that was designed by the nurse in the wholly compensatory system. The community health nurse is responsible for the coordination of services. Not only is this good nursing practice, it is also mandated in Section 405.1224 in the Conditions of Participation for Medicare reimbursement: "The registered nurse . . . coordinates services . . . " (Department of Health, Education, and Welfare 1973, 18981) Services provided by the agency such as physical therapy, occupational therapy, speech therapy, social service, and home health aide must be coordinated. Services outside the agency such as respiratory therapy and the provision of specialized equipment must also be coordinated.

The nursing administrator should consider the special needs of the population in the community served by the agency. For example, some communities adjacent to a children's hospital may require private duty nurses for children home on ventilators. Although the structure of a nonprofit organization would not support this activity, a reorganization into various corporations could. Some patients in the wholly compensatory system are terminally ill and could benefit from hospice care. During the course of a terminal illness a patient may shift from one system to another. This is impacted by the reimbursement system. Although a patient is terminally ill, and could benefit from nursing in a supportive-educative system, it is possible that these services would not be third-party reimbursable due to the strict interpretation of regulations such as homebound status. In these instances, other sources of reimbursement should be investigated.

Many of the patients seen at home by the community health nurse are in a partly compensatory nursing system. Frequently, this skilled hands-on care is reimbursed by third-party payors. Patients that are receiving services in the home such as intravenous therapy, are often able to participate in their care, and can become independent in such activities as the administration of intravenous antibiotics. It continues to be the responsibility of the nurse to carry out such activities as monitoring the IV site for infection or infiltration and changing the IV catheter. Patients in this system may require multiple services. For example, a patient recovering from a cerebrovascular accident may be able to perform some self-care activities, but to become rehabilitated may require extensive services including all the therapies.

Other patients admitted to service in a community health agency are in a supportive-educative system. In this system, the patient's requirements for assistance relate to decision-making, behavior control, and acquiring knowledge and skills (Orem 1980). Changes in the patient's knowledge, understanding, or behavior should be documented. In this system, the nurse's role is frequently consultative. Many experts such as adult nurse practitioners and pediatric nurse practitioners are used in this role within an agency. Some patients may be performing continuous ambulatory peritoneal dialysis or hyperalimentation in the home and may only require the support and guidance of the nurse.

Preventive health care is an important area for community health nurses. Three levels of prevention are recognized: primary, secondary, and tertiary. Primary prevention is required before the onset of disease and is directed to the promotion of health and prevention of disease (Orem 1980). Every person requiring nursing care has requirements at the primary level of prevention. Universal self-care and have developmental self-care when therapeutic constitute prevention at the primary level (Orem 1980). Community health nurses select or assist the patient in selecting methods for meeting self-care requisites that promote and maintain health and development and prevent specific disease (Orem 1980).

Secondary prevention is required after the onset of disease and is directed to the prevention of complications and prolonged disability. Tertiary prevention is appropriate when there is disability and limited functioning. It is directed toward bringing about effective functioning in accord with existing abilities. Health deviation self-care when therapeutic is health care at the secondary or tertiary level of prevention (Orem 1980). Self-care measures are utilized to regulate and prevent effects of the disease, complications, prolonged disability, or adapt functioning to compensate for the adverse effects of permanent dysfunction (Orem 1980).

It is essential that the nursing administration of a community health agency be knowledgeable of the benefits of self-care and have the personnel necessary to promote self-care in this high-tech era. The theory of self-care can be utilized in the provision of care to those in the community who require health promotion, health maintenance, and health education and management.

References

American Nurses' Association. 1980. *A conceptual model of community health nursing.* Kansas City, MO: American Nurses Association.

Department of Health, Education, and Welfare. 1973. Conditions of participation for home health agencies. *Federal Register* 38:18978-18983. Washington, DC: Government Printing Office.

Orem, D. 1980. *Nursing: Concepts of practice* second edition. New York: McGraw-Hill Book Company.

Chapter Nine

Staffing Issues

Staff Recruitment and Retention

Elizabeth Z. Cathcart

A few years back the hotel chain, Holiday Inn, advertised as part of its services a "no surprises" policy. The idea was to let travelers know exactly what to expect prior to check in.

Although this may seem a bit revolutionary and even risky, two home health care executives have had much success using a similar technique. Whether it's volunteer services they're seeking or the expertise of paid professionals, they found that the "no surprises" policy is the secret to securing good people that are compatible to their organization. Here's how they go about it.

". . . Recruitment and retention of qualified personnel really begins with the development of an Agency's mission, its philosophy of service delivery, its programs and its policies. Priority must be given to the end product--the quality of care delivered and the level of services necessary to meet the patient's needs. If the focus remains on the results, an Agency can more effectively retain employees rather than constantly recruit.

Information does reach the professional community that an Agency has a reputation for the delivery of quality care. As a result, nurses come to the Agency seeking employment. In other words, the market has expanded beyond the advertisement of positions. It is still necessary to advertise in order that all Equal Opportunities and Affirmative Action criteria are met, even though the "ideal" candidate for a vacancy may have been identified.

We interview many of those who fill out an application, even though a position might not be immediately available. This prevents "desperate" hiring and dilution of quality care goals. Desperate hiring--and who hasn't been in that situation--creates or multiplies staff problems when the individual does not meet the professional standards expected by the other members of the team.

A key to successful recruitment is through the initial interview. During the interview, an assessment of a prospective employee is done. We look at what they have to offer, their potential for growth, and most important, their philosophy of health care. While it is not necessary that the Agency's philosophy and the employee's are duplicates--there should be some similarities. For example, we feel community health nursing practice involves more than the delivery of acute care to the patient. It involves the family, too. Other health problems in the family and their coping mechanisms are as important to the full recovery of the client as the hands-on care given by the health professional. In addition, the community itself should be involved in health care--support groups, and prevention of illness are likely areas for involvement. How do we ascertain whether the person being interviewed can assist us in meeting these needs? We look for previous involvement in the community, or a concern expressed about discharged hospital patients--i.e., "I often wondered how they managed when he/she went home." This awareness that assistance may be needed beyond the acute care environment is important where an employee may have to utilize several alternatives to find the best solution for someone being cared for at home.

At the same time we are learning about a prospective employee, we promote home health care in a positive way--both as an alternative to institutional care and as an exciting opportunity to practice independent and professional nursing. During this initial interview job responsibilities, skills needed to function effectively and personnel policies are reviewed with the applicant. We discuss job functions, time off, impact of the job on other family responsibilities and so forth, in order to avoid future misunderstandings.

The second part of successful recruitment is a result of staff interaction with the prospective employee. We encourage new field staff to spend a morning seeing patients with one of our employees. Because we recruit for three offices, it is important that the prospective employee and her "future" supervisor be able to relate to each other in a positive way. Thus, we provide an opportunity for this initial interaction to take place in a relaxed non-threatening situation.

In the field I'm sure the staff are verbal in discussing not only what the job entails, but also the Agency--what's good and what could be better. Since our employment is in the home setting--away from familiar support systems and where patients have much more control over their care--it helps for individuals to see the situation under which they will be expected to provide quality nursing care. Not everyone is comfortable working in this type of environment. It also makes obvious that our caseload is primarily senior citizens, or young adults with chronic or terminal illness. The nurse who hopes to see some maternity or pediatric cases must now face the reality that this is not really where most of our service occurs.

Retention and job satisfaction are based on the prevention of unrealistic expectations. We feel the extra time spent on this area benefits us both.

Assuming that after this process there are several likely prospects for a vacancy, a decision must be made. Again, working towards a goal of staff retention we verify references and look critically at skills. Does the prospective employee strengthen weak areas or add a new skill or dimension to services provided? What is the employee's plan in terms of career goals? Will the job help the nurse move ahead toward a career expectation of clinical or supervisory advancement, or is it a job that permits more regular hours to care for a family? These personal goals also impact on our expectation of an employee's work and the employee's expectation of the job.

With a national turnover rate for nursing personnel running between 32 and 40 percent, it is no wonder our emphasis is on the prospective retention of personnel within the Agency.

Recruiting a good employee is one thing, but there is always the added responsibility of promoting job satisfaction for both new and long-term employees.

To assure a smooth transition from new employee to valued staff member, an orientation which builds on existing skills while integrating home health care concepts is of paramount importance. We found that our orientation, while it adequately covered the delivery of care, was not consistent with day-to-day details. We asked the staff what they wished they had been told about our Agency, the position, the training, etc., but hadn't. From this an orientation guide was developed by the staff. It allows new employees to indicate their experience with regard to specific job requirements. Using a key, new employees can rate their nursing abilities from IV therapy to problem oriented recording. Another section deals totally with information on how the Agency works (i.e., requesting time off; using the answering service, etc.) Many items are covered prior to employment, but have little significance until an actual situation arises. Because this list was developed by the staff it contains those items which could easily be overlooked during an orientation yet, if not dealt with, may create unnecessary problems for a new employee. The orientation tool is referred to regularly during the probationary period in an effort to fill in the gaps while providing for a distinctly individualized beginning.

By the end of the probationary period we begin emphasizing productivity and increase our expectations. Added to these administrative expectations are days when, due to illness or vacations, staffing is less than ideal. Then, as staff perceives that it is not possible to provide the level of care they feel is acceptable, they can become unhappy with the work environment.

The staff at our Agency--knowing that chaotic times are cyclic due to referral patterns, vacations and holidays--suggested that supplemental staff be hired on a per diem basis. Our administration decided this idea had merit and established guidelines for per diem help. The program has literally been a life saver. Clients are scheduled based on their needs, regardless of the availability of full time staff. Knowing that this help is available when we are really busy, we believe alleviates some of the pressure on our staff, and also goes a long way in promoting quality care.

The feeling of professional self worth and job satisfaction is more evident among our staff since control over the work environment is encouraged. Opportunities for employees to make schedules and help develop patient care policies allows our staff to understand the constraints on their practice, as well as the rationale to continue striving for the optimum in service delivery.

We believe this promotes quality patient care--our end product, while at the same time providing a satisfying job for our employees. Satisfied customers give positive feedback to the staff and to the community, who will then be the best advertisement for new employees as well as for the retention of present staff."

Contract Versus Direct Staffing

Michele Lucas and Lynne D. Pancoast

Scenario

The idea for this particular home health agency was conceived during the restructuring of a hospital. Those involved in the planning phase decided that the agency would be structured as a division of one of five sister companies in the newly developed corporate health system. The agency was categorized as a hospital-affiliated (rather than hospital-based) home health agency because of its indirect relationship with the system's hospital (one of the five companies).

The planners further decided to contract for home health services with two already well-established agencies. The nursing supervisor and the rehabilitation supervisor, who were directly employed by the agency, were given the responsibilities of taking all referrals and case managing all agency clients. The nursing supervisor and director rotated administrative on-call duties. Both the supervisors and the director decided that the agency would coordinate all the care, including communication with physicians, completion of physician order forms, receiving of all client calls, and arranging for laboratory studies and supplies. The clinical services themselves were coordinated via conference calls. The contract agency staff were responsible for making the home visits, completing all visit-related paperwork, and calling the appropriate agency supervisor for a conference after the initial visit. In addition, they were required to call during interim service as needed and upon discharge. The agency supervisors assumed responsibility for documenting all conference information. Interdisciplinary referrals were generally handled by the agency supervisors as well.

The agency caseload grew very rapidly and another nursing supervisor had to be hired within the first five months of operation to assist in the case management process. The agency director and supervisors met regularly with appropriate representatives from each of the contract agencies for problem resolution. The major problem encountered by the agency was a lack of control over the service provided. Contract agency staff were accustomed to the style of their own agencies and often had difficulty in adapting to the requirements of the agency. Most importantly, the agency found that significant client-related information was not always communicated as needed. In addition, documentation requirements of the agency, which differed from those of the two contract agencies, were not consistently followed. Agency management became frustrated and considered hiring its own staff directly.

Therapists were the first to be added. They were brought on as independent contractors (rather than as employed staff) by their own preference. Medical social workers were the next group and they, like the therapists, were hired as independent contractors. Agency management was somewhat reassured by these changes and felt an increased control over services provided. However, they still perceived a major need for direct nursing staff. Seeing this through to fruition would also require a move to a larger location, as well as arranging for home health aides. This entire package had to be approved by the company's board of directors and took several months. Meanwhile, the agency's caseload continued to grow and the nursing supervisors were keeping long hours in an effort to keep up and maintain as much control over service as possible. The agency did manage to hire a full-time nurse liaison to receive referrals from the hospital social service workers and gather needed information from the hospital record.

Finally, approximately 16 months into operation, the agency hired its first component of staff nurses. Arrangements were also made to contract with one home health aide agency until direct home health aide staff could be hired. The agency also moved to a larger facility in order to accommodate the larger number of employees. During this time, the nursing supervisors faced a great challenge; they had to continue with case management of the contract agency clients, and simultaneously assume responsibility for the orientation and supervision of new nursing staff. Therefore, they put in even longer hours for the first several months of this transition period. Finally, the agency reached the point where it was able to provide direct nursing staff to all clients who required it. The agency also managed to bring on a full-time staff physical therapist; the remaining therapy clients were serviced by the therapy contractors. Another nursing supervisor was hired to create and oversee a home health aide program. Contracts with the same social workers were maintained with plans to later hire a part-time staff social worker.

Advantages of Contract Staffing

1. Initiation of services is easier--services are already in place within the contract agency.

2. Personnel management needs are less--advertising for, interviewing, hiring, and orienting visiting staff is accomplished by the contract agency.

3. A new and undetermined or fluctuating caseload is easier to manage.

4. Clinical versatility of the professional staff is greater in a larger, established agency; e.g., handling high technology therapies in the home.

5. Policies and procedures are already developed and available.

Disadvantages of Contract Staffing

1. Loss of control over service delivery occurs, but there is still ultimate responsibility by the agency.

2. Referral source dissatisfaction results from utilizing the agency as a third party--referrals can be made directly to the contract agency.

3. Clinical responsibility ultimately rests with agency supervisors who have had no direct contact with the clients.

4. Contact with contract agency staff is conducted entirely on the telephone.

5. Confusion exists on the part of clients regarding which agency is following them.

6. Problems in recordkeeping are caused by delays in obtaining original forms from contract agencies.

7. Compliance with documentation requirements is more difficult to monitor.

8. The process of transition to direct staff is more difficult once the agency is operational.

Flextime Scheduling

Diane Chaloux, Sharon Dezzani Martin, and Carol Brocker

The experience of a large private, nonprofit home health agency in developing a flextime policy is described. A task force was formed to examine current models utilized in business and their suitable application to home health. The task force developed definitions, measurable goals and objectives, a policy statement, and implemented a three-month, multisite, multidiscipline pilot study with 16 employees flexing. The pilot was evaluated from multiple perspectives. Pre- and post-testing of all agency employees revealed that flextime is seen as a major benefit to employees by allowing them to better meet personal and family commitments. Evaluation also demonstrated that flextime did not positively or negatively affect productivity or sick time utilization, and that the majority of participating employees opted for flexing to earlier work hours.

Introduction

One strategy cited in the literature for recruiting and retaining valued staff and increasing morale is the use of flexible patterns for scheduling and staffing (French 1982; Werther 1983). Flextime, also known as flexi-time, is a work schedule that allows employees some choice of when to start and stop their workday. It provides an opportunity for the person working outside the home to mesh job, family, and personal responsibilities more easily. It can assist with meeting patient needs for variations in regular caregiving hours. Best of all, in this age of clinical and corporate complexity, it is a refreshingly simple concept to implement. The following article is a description of the processes used to develop, implement, and evaluate flextime at our home health agency.

Background

The 40-hour workweek has been the prevalent schedule of employment for approximately four decades. The Fair Labor Standards Act of 1938, which mandated overtime pay for work over 40 hours, seemed to influence the development of the five-day, eight-hour workweek norm. It was the most obvious schedule to fit the 40-hour mandate and it has prevailed ever since. Sometime during the 1970s, options to that norm began to be explored (Werther 1983). At the same time Poor's book, *4 Days, 40 Hours, and Other Forms of Rearranged Workweek* published in 1970, spread the idea that the traditional workweek was not the only option (Poor 1970) (Exhibit 9-1).

As with any change there are forces occurring in society encouraging that change. One of the major social forces encouraging the initiation of flextime is the rise of the dual career family in which both husband and wife work. This results in a rise in income with a resultant desire for more leisure time. Also, if children are involved, it becomes inconvenient for parents to work the traditional hours as family obligations may be difficult to satisfy with both parents unavailable during the same hours. Single parent families find satisfying family demands even more difficult and need even greater flexibility in the work place to survive (Skeler 1981; Werther 1983).

A second force for change lies in the labor market. Firms have been forced to find innovative ways to attract and retain the staff that they need while attempting to keep labor costs down. Flextime stands out as an excellent new benefit that in most cases costs the organization very little. In many cases, such as understaffed hospitals, flextime offers a solution to attracting staff besides costly salary increases. Very often staff

Exhibit 9-1. Different Forms of Flextime

The different forms of flextime, from the least to the most flexible, include:

Staggered Hours—Employees are assigned a variation of regular established work hours.

Flextime—Employees choose a starting and quitting time, stick with that schedule for a period, and work eight hours a day.

Gliding Time—Employees may vary their starting and quitting time daily, but they must still work eight hours, or another company-set length, every day.

Variable Day—As long as employees work the number of hours required by the end of the week or month, they can vary the number of hours they work each day.

Maxiflex—Employees may vary their daily hours and do not have to be present for a "core" time on all days.

Compiled from: J. M. Roscow and R. Zager, 1983. Punch out the time clocks. *HBR* March/April, 12 - 29; and State of Maine, Department of Personnel, Memorandum 4-83, Alternative Work Schedules, p. 3.

who would otherwise have been unable to work at all have returned to the work force because of creative flextime schedules (Skeler 1981; Werther 1983).

A third force for change is demographics. The baby boom years have passed. The future probably will hold a decreased work force with decreased unemployment. Competition for the available employees will be greater. Innovative techniques such as flextime may be necessary to attract and retain sufficient staff (Skeler 1981; Werther 1983).

Task Force on Flextime

The request for flextime, originating from staff, resulted in the formation of a task force composed of administrative and first-line managers. The task force was formed to examine the models currently utilized in other business settings, determine their suitable application to the agency, and develop a flextime policy. The task force developed definitions, measurable goals and objectives, a policy statement, and implemented a three-month multisite, multidiscipline pilot study with 16 employees. The pilot was evaluated according to criteria established initially by the task force group that included the perspective of the patient, the employee, the supervisor, the team, the payroll department, and administration.

The work of the task force took place through several meetings over a period of seven months. The task force consisted of one administrator and four first line managers representing the central and branch offices of the agency. It was believed that the burden of implementation would be at the first line manager level, therefore they should have a major role in policy formulation. The task force gathered and disseminated information to staff at team meetings so that there was ongoing planning utilizing staff input.

The task force utilized the problem-solving approach in the development of the flextime policy. The first step was the identification of problems and generation of goals. Problems identified were as follows:

- Management time is spent on special requests made by staff.

- Staff desire greater freedom in managing their own time.

- Rigid hours interfere with patient needs and desires.

- Having no RN available after 4:30 p.m., except the on-call nurse, interferes with physician communication.

- Management reorganization has left "downtime" in the late afternoon for some home health aides.

- With rapid growth and resulting increases in staff, there are problems accessing free telephone lines and sharing office space.

Goals established by the task force provided the direction for developing policy. Goals identified were:

- There will always be coverage from 8:00 a.m. to 4:30 p.m. Flextime shall not disrupt the established levels and hours of coverage.

- Productivity will meet or exceed budgeted levels.

- Patient needs and desires will be met.

- There will be decreased management time spent on special requests made by staff.

- Staff satisfaction and morale will increase.

- There will be no lateness and less absenteeism.

- There will be increased capacity to "cover cases" in other than 8:00 to 4:30 time slot.

- There may be increased opportunity for physician and nurse conferencing to occur.

The next step of the task force was to develop definitions of flextime and core hours (Exhibit 9-2) and develop a policy statement (Exhibit 9-3).

Exhibit 9-2. Definition—Flextime

A work schedule that leaves the standard number of working hours unchanged but allows employees some choice of when to start and stop working within the limitations set by management. There is usually a flexible window at the beginning and end of each day which surrounds a core set of hours when all employees must be present.

Exhibit 9-3.

Policy

The manager arrives at decision to approve individual requests for flextime. The day-to-day decisions of a short-term nature such as alteration of staff schedule to accommodate physician appointments, etc., also falls within the jurisdiction of the manager. However, this policy is intended to address longer term alternative work schedules.

Under all circumstances, patient and team's needs will be met. Arrangements for supervision of flextime staff is the responsibility of the manager.

Core hours will be 9:30 a.m. to 2:00 p.m., Monday through Friday. The range of visit hours will be 6:00 a.m. to 6:00 p.m.

Starting time governs quitting time each day. Once hours are chosen they may not be changed without due notice. Anything outside scope of this policy requires administrative approval.

Eligibility Criteria

1. All full-time and part-time regular staff can be considered.
2. Staff must have demonstrated themselves to be responsible and independent by meeting expected agency behaviors via the performance evaluations.
3. Paperwork must be up to date.
4. Productivity stats must meet or exceed agency expectations.
5. Staff must have worked at AHHS for at least six months.
6. The number of individuals participating per team is at the discretion of the manager.
7. Award of the flextime benefit is for a period of six months.
8. Management reserves the right, based on performance and productivity, to require flextime participants to return to traditional schedule after suitable notification. A two-week time frame whenever possible is the maximum notice time.

The Pilot Project

Planning. Initial planning involved a literature search and survey of state and out-of-state community health agencies. Information was obtained via a literature search regarding experience with flextime in the health care setting and a procedure for considering implementing a flextime program (Rosenberg 1983). One agency surveyed had a formal policy regarding flextime.

Specific objectives for a flextime program were developed. As a result of the flextime program, there would be: (1) increased ability to meet patient needs; (2) productivity would be maintained at current budgeted figures; (3) increased staff morale; and (4) decreased or no increased supervisory involvement in managing patient care, or program issues as a result of flextime. These objectives were to be utilized in planning and evaluating the pilot as well.

The next step was to determine the feasibility of a flextime program in each of the offices and departments. Each of the managers was responsible for assessing whether a flextime program was feasible in that office or department. The feasibility was based upon the function of the office or department, as well as the needs of the staff and community. The flextime program was determined to be feasible by each of the managers.

Eligibility criteria for the employees were determined for the flextime program and were to be utilized for the pilot project. These eligibility criteria considered eight specific elements and were based on those developed by the Cambridge, MA VNA: (1) all full-time and part-time regular staff could be considered; (2) staff must have demonstrated themselves to be responsible and independent by meeting expected agency behaviors via the performance evaluation; (3) paperwork must be up-to-date; (4) productivity stats must be met or exceed agency expectation; and (5) staff will have worked at AHHS for at least six months. In addition, the following considerations were made: (1) The number of individuals participating per team is at the discretion of the manager; (2) award flextime benefit for period of six months; and (3) management reserves the right, based on performance and productivity, to require flextime participants to return to traditional schedule after suitable notification.

The last step of planning for the pilot project involved developing the evaluation criteria and the methods by which the pilot would be evaluated. The criteria developed were based upon the objectives and included the perspective of the patient, the manager, the employee, team, payroll, and administration.

Implementation. The flextime task force recommended that a three-month pilot study be done utilizing employees who had indicated an interest in flextime and who met the eligibility criteria. Managers in all offices and departments selected the individuals to participate in the flextime pilot.

Five nurses, five home health aides, three outreach workers, two payroll and billing clerks, and one occupational therapist representing all four locations participated in the pilot. Supervision was accomplished during flexed hours via telephone availability of manager and the on-call nurse (Exhibit 9-4).

Evaluation. At the end of the third month, an evaluation of the pilot was conducted by the task force. Evaluation efforts focused on input from the following areas: the patient, manager, employee, team, payroll, and administration. Employees kept a log

Exhibit 9-4 Employees Adjusted Work Hours--Regular Workday 8 a.m. - 4:30 p.m.

No. of staff	Flextime Hours
12	7:00 - 3:30
1	6:30 - 3:00
2	7:30 - 4:00
1	8:30 - 5:00

of patients and clients whose visits had been scheduled outside the 8:00 a.m. to 4:30 p.m. workday and submitted a brief narrative statement discussing their experience participating in the pilot. A telephone survey was done by managers to assess patient satisfaction. Individual and team visit stats were compared to budgeted projections. Increases and decreases in lateness and absenteeism among team members were assessed. Advantages and disadvantages of flextime were elicited from the managers and administration. A pre- and postsurvey was administered to team members. Increased time spent processing payroll was measured. The task force compiled the above data and analyzed the results based upon each of the established objectives.

Results

Increased ability to meet patient needs. The results of the log of patient visits outside the 8:00 a.m. to 4:30 p.m. workday were that many of the staff used the early hours to do their charting rather than to make patient visits. The telephone survey of patients indicated only three negative responses of 29 surveyed. A flextime program would formalize what is already occurring. Still to be addressed by other means would be the increased opportunity for physician and nurse conferencing to occur. Many staff comments reflected the availability of physicians for consultation in late afternoon; however, the majority of interest to participants was to flex to earlier hours.

Results of the pre- and post-testing did not focus on improved ability to meet patient needs. However, it is felt that the results were skewed because we currently adjust work schedules to meet patients needs.

Productivity would be maintained at current budgeted figures. Productivity and sick time did not seem to be affected positively or negatively with flextime. Employees with health problems continued to use sick time; employees with known productivity problems did not improve their performance due to flextime. In general, if there were problems before the pilot study with individuals, they remained. If there were no problems, flextime scheduling did not create any additional ones.

Increased staff morale. The results reflected that staff morale increased. Flextime was valued as a real benefit to participants in the pilot.

Decreased or no increase in supervisory involvement in managing patient care issues or program issues. The managers indicated difficulties in scheduling team meetings to accommodate varying schedules as a disadvantage. Advantages were increased staff morale and increased flexibility to meet patient needs.

The results of the pilot study revealed that the major benefit of flextime was an improved ability for staff to meet family and personal needs, with subsequent increase in staff morale. The majority of employees were satisfied with the current 8:00 a.m. to 4:30 p.m. Of those flexing, most chose to flex to earlier hours.

Overall, the flextime pilot was successful. It was the recommendation of the flextime task force to approve the flextime policy. The flextime policy was approved by the Board of Directors.

Limitations of Study

Identifying objectives of the program, as well as the means for determining success or failure of the project, should be established before a flextime study is even attempted, according to Rosenberg (1983). Clearly identifying these objectives prior to implementation allows comparison and a means to determine if what was planned initially was actually accomplished.

Evaluation criteria established prior to the study rested heavily upon a pre- and postpilot questionnaire which was intended to gauge staff satisfaction and morale. One of the project goals was to increase these two factors in staff. It is important to note that it was never determined by objective measurements, if satisfaction was to be increased in all staff, whether on flextime or not, or just staff utilizing flextime. However, the pre- and post-test was administered to all staff. Some problems can be identified with this procedure. First, by administering the pre- and post-test to everyone it may have measured general satisfaction with work rather than response to flextime. Many of the questions reflected factors besides flextime. This was borne out when staff discussed the test. When answering the questions, frequently, they were considering events of the office at the time which did not relate to flextime. In addition, Rosenberg suggests the pre- and post-tests should be administered no sooner than six months apart, giving staff enough time to feel as if flextime is the usual state of affairs. Our post-test was administered at the two-month interval in order to meet the deadline of a three-month report of pilot. This was probably too soon to test any real changes. In fact, if the test is examined, we find that there is little or no difference between the pre- and postanswers. Because of the broadness of the questions, the fact that the test was given to all employees, and the short time between administration of the test, the validity of the results as a means to gauge morale in relation to flextime is questionable.

Another goal of the project was that patients' needs would be better met. From patient response, via the telephone or in person, it would appear that patients enjoyed the flextime visits. Those who did not were rescheduled for visits later in the day. The third goal of the project, that there would be decreased management time spent on special staff requests, was not evaluated by objective criteria. No pre- and postcriteria had been developed. Subjective reports were sole means of the evaluation of this goal. A fourth objective, that there would be no tardiness and less absenteeism, was only partially measurable. Due to the fact that starting and stopping times were not measured by time clock it was difficult to gauge tardiness. Absenteeism, however, was measurable and there was no change found in comparing pre- and postflextime. The fifth goal, increased capacity to cover cases outside the 8 a.m. to 4:30 p.m. time slot, was measured only by subjective report of staff, patients, and supervisors, all of which were positive. The sixth goal, increased opportunity for MD and RN conferencing, was not met due to the majority of staff flexing earlier.

An important factor for consideration is the use of a control group to compare with the experimental group of flextime staff. It would have given us valuable comparative information.

Conclusions

Overall, the flextime pilot was successful and has been incorporated as a permanent personnel policy. According to the literature, attempts at flextime fail only about 5% of the time, generally because management has not included supervisors and staff in the planning (French 1982). For this reason, widespread participation was used. Also, flextime, as the first step to alternatives to time management, has formed the basis for future consideration of compressed work weeks, variable day and job-sharing. As one flexing staff member puts it, "Its nice to come and go when it fits the rest of your life."

Evaluating Productivity*

Lazelle E. Benefield

This section will discuss the definition of productivity and how productivity is analyzed in home health services. Environmental and staff factors that affect productivity are analyzed and a procedure to follow in determining the current productivity of staff is suggested. This discussion centers onlyon how to determine current productivity of staff that provide direct service; i.e., make visits (although useful for all caregivers, this information was originally written for use with professional staff). Determining current productivity is only one part of a program that measures and improves productivity. Information on how to determine the standard necessary for agency viability (and positive bottom line) and how to institute a productivity improvement program in an agency can be found in other sources (Benefield, In press; Levy 1979; Olson 1983; Rozelle 1977).

What is Productivity?

Several assumptions are listed below and form the basis for how productivity is viewed in this chapter.

1. Productivity *is* an issue in every agency. It's the current buzz word and many even think of productivity improvement as the sole method of improving the generation of income. (This is, by the way, incorrect.) In the past, productivity issues took a back seat in health care management. The curriculum in most clinical professions focused on improving skills in the care of individual clients and families, giving little attention to any systematic review of the relationship between efficiency and quality of services delivered. Now, the growing concern over rising health care costs and the need to better evaluate and control factors that improve efficiency has prompted a surge of interest in the productivity issue.

---

* Reprinted with permission from *Home Health Care Management* by Lazelle E. Benefield, The Brady Co., 1987.

2. Productivity evaluation is a greater issue for some agencies more than others, specifically agencies that use full-time (FT) and part-time (PT) staff. In the past, agency managers with contract staff usually were not concerned with increasing contract staff visitations per unit of time. (Contract staff is defined as a worker who is paid a flat fee per visit.) Historically, managers focused on FT/PT staff who were paid a salary for the hours worked (and not the visits made). This may be changing as many agencies are investigating payment of FT/PT staff on the basis of the number of visits completed (Griffin 1986).

3. The word productivity is usually viewed with some discomfort by most staff. Expect a negative response, either verbally or behaviorally, when the issue is first discussed. Staff often fear an assembly line approach, staff cutbacks, or unrealistic increases in workload, which means (to them) that they must work faster and give less quality (again, not necessarily true). [Are there research data to indicate that a two-hour visit is more effective than a one-hour home visit?]

4. Productivity is a management issue and not exclusively an employee issue. First line managers and above should be involved in the process of determining, monitoring, and if necessary, improving productivity. An excellent resource for further reading is White Collar Waste: Gain the Productivity Edge (Olson 1983) which covers this issue in depth.

5. Quality can improve at the same time that productivity increases (Rozelle 1977), even though many professional staff and managers would initially disagree. The most pressing need in this area involves accurately determining when quality exists: when has the client outcome been achieved? If we have a clear and measurable method of determining when quality exists, then it's easier to determine the type of services needed to achieve the outcome.

Productivity is defined as any or all of the following:

- "The efficiency with which resources are consumed in the effective delivery of service" (Rozelle 1977)

- ". . . output per given input" (Federa and Bilodeau 1984)

- "The relationship between the use of resources and the results of that use" (Olsen 1983)

The definitions fit when measuring productivity in industry (e.g., assembly line work). It's easy to measure the amount of items or products produced in a given period of time. It's difficult to do this in a health service industry. The Olson definition, "the relationship between the use of resources and the results of that use," was developed to include those in white collar positions, and for the purpose of this chapter it does fit for those in professional positions in a service industry such as home health care.

For example, in home care the "use of resources" may include everything necessary to complete the home visit (the product). This can include the caregiver's time, supplies, agency management time, and other indirect expenses. The "results of the use" (of resources) historically has been defined as the "number of visits per discipline per time period." The time period may be one day, one week, or one month. Visits may be separated by type (maternal child, pediatrics, hospice) or by discipline (registered nurse (RN), therapist, social worker). Examples include: Six reimbursable visits per RN each day; 25 pediatric visits per therapist per week; 120 reimbursable RN visits per week (Monday through Friday) four RNs at 30 visits each week; each RN averaging six visits per day.

As an aside, it's little wonder that when staff hear the word productivity they think of only increasing the number of visits, since the measurement for productivity is the number of visits done. Staff never assume that work can be simplified, reorganized, or delegated. Because of the "negative press" surrounding productivity, all agency personnel need a great deal of information and reeducation to understand exactly what productivity is and what it means to the agency.

This is an appropriate time, after defining productivity and before we analyze how it is determined, to clarify why there is concern over productivity. First, a cost-efficient operation is a primary goal. No agency will survive without being at least self-sustaining, and to do that personnel must be efficient: a productivity analysis program can assist in monitoring efficiency. Second, a quality operation is also a primary goal, and monitoring productivity can enhance the likelihood of providing quality services. A quality service is expected and wanted by clients (this means not just safe care, but quality care). Providing quality services involves allowing staff (the most valuable resource) to work toward their potential; e.g., to use the skills they were trained to use. The premise here is that monitoring and analyzing productivity assists staff because it frees them to use their skills efficiently.

What We Know About Productivity

What is known about productivity in home health care can be summarized below:

1. Productivity is difficult to measure in a health service industry (Linn and Karsten 1982).

2. Improving only one area or component of an agency will not affect overall production; assessment includes all areas.

3. When evaluating productivity, look at the 20% of the budget that amounts to 80% of the dollars and work on these areas (this is usually the labor costs) (Orefice and Jennings 1983).

4. "White collar productivity does not depend on how fast an employee works, it hinges, rather, on the efficient use of time." (Olson 1983)

Productivity is difficult to measure in a health service industry. It is difficult to measure because of our limited knowledge of what we're measuring; the quantity (number) of home visits can be measured, but we're less able to measure and evaluate the quality of the visit. Thus, the product (the provision of a service, namely a home visit) is so variable. The components of a home visit (the tasks, the staff behaviors) are very complex and difficult to quantify. In addition, the recipient of the service or action (the client) is so variable (Linn and Karsten 1982). The client will demonstrate changing characteristics, and no two clients with the same diagnosis will ever demonstrate the exact same needs. Physical, psychosocial, and environmental needs (e.g., lack of financial resources, limited support system) make each client and each visit unique and therefore difficult, at best, to quantify and evaluate.

Linn suggests that we have an "uncertain product definition," meaning that it's unclear what the agency is trying to produce--visits? --or health? To take it a step further the "problem sets the stage for a related health production issue --'How much of whatever health is do we wish to produce?" (Linn and Karsten 1982). The agency's philosophy statement (service to anyone regardless of ability to pay; service to those with the ability to pay) and management style begin to define what the mission of the agency is and what exactly the agency is producing (health, visits, or both?). In addition to using agency philosophy as a guide, managers at the service delivery level are helped to define "health production" by insurance companies who define the services to be reimbursed, and consumer demand for certain states of health (Linn and Karsten 1982). (In other words, agencies provide services that are reimbursable and that consumers are willing to pay for.) With little agreement over what range or depth of services that should be provided, it's understandable that it has been difficult to measure productivity in the health services industry. This sums it up: "Economic approaches to productivity definition and measurement tend to be mathematically oriented, and the complexity of services rendered. . . does not lend itself to easy formulation" (DHEW 1975).

Improving only one component of an agency will not affect overall productivity. Productivity improvement involves a systematic assessment of the entire organization, rather than just a staffing review. As an example, a physical therapist's job (and the tasks performed) may be tied to secretaries (who answer the phones and screen calls) and to data processing (records may not be transcribed and back to the therapist for the scheduled visit), and to other disciplines (the therapist may have to wait for the home health aide (HHA) to arrive to supervise the visit or meet with an RN regarding the client). Don't assume that any one discipline can improve or change productivity unless other components of the system are evaluated (e.g., don't expect the RN staff to increase productivity unless you also look at other components of the system that RNs work with).

Start by looking at the 20% of things that cost 80% of the dollars, and initially work on these areas. Look at a budget sheet for a home health agency; the majority of costs are attributed to staff or personnel (Orefice and Jennings 1983). This includes staff who deliver the service (the product = home visit) and other personnel whose job it is to support the caregivers. First, evaluate this area, then expand to the larger organization. Remember, productivity is a people issue (Olson 1983).

"White collar productivity does not depend on how fast an employee works; it hinges, rather, on the efficient use of time!"(Olson 1983). This is the key to beginning an analysis of productivity and probably the most important statement in this section. Staff are not encouraged to "work faster" (to rush through visits, to do more with less time); rather, they are encouraged to use time efficiently (spend time doing those skills they were trained to use).

To do this, managers assist staff to (1) identify their own professional skills; (2) refer the services best done by others to other professionals; and (3) continually focus on whether the task or action being performed is relevant to achievement of client outcomes. This is simply stated, but it does make the point that productivity is clearly a management issue and not solely an employee issue. "Management personnel create the climate and set the pace for effective productivity" (Riddell 1981). This process of improving productivity through effective management is beyond the scope of this section; further resources are listed at the end of this chapter.

An agency that embarks on a productivity analysis would assess the entire organization for (1) unnecessary activities; (2) simplification of work; and (3) the definition of the product (home visit) (Bermas 1984). The goal is not to improve one subset or the organization (personnel), but to maximize the entire organization's productivity.

Research data to help understand and measure the efficient use of time (how efficient and how well a job is done) are scarce. In the past, the focus was on hospital services, and only recent attention has been paid to home health care service delivery. Previously, there was a lack of sophistication in how to measure what staff did, how staff use and analyze outcomes when providing care, and perhaps a lack of knowledge in determining what client outcomes to look for to indicate health.

Analyze Service Delivery: Efficiency, Effectiveness, Equity

Analysis of productivity involves looking at variables that are unique to each agency. It includes both an agencywide and personnel review. Before review of personnel productivity, determine the efficiency, effectiveness, and equity (Linn and Karsten 1982) of services provided by the agency (or program) as a whole. Look at what each of these mean in the agency, use them as background information, and then embark on a productivity review of personnel.

Efficiency may include a goal to increase the amount of output produced by a given input, or to decrease the amount of input (skilled services) required to produce a given output (home visits) (Linn and Karsten 1982). Consider more than just the volume of service; also include information on service intensity (complexity level of client) and the case mix (types of clients: severity of illness, the service admitted under) of the population served. At this stage, the degree of agency efficiency is hard to identify, so list the methods and strategies the agency has used in the past to maintain efficiency. Identify which worked and why (incentive pay for visits over a certain number, fear of job loss if visit numbers were not increased, streamlined organization of paperflow?).

Effectiveness of the service, a second variable to consider in productivity analysis, or the "degree to which a production process has accomplished what it was intended to do" (Linn and Karsten 1982), should evaluate whether "the correct job got done." This relates to the quality of service provided. Determine (through staff and management input) what the expectations are for the outcomes of the services (what "correct things" should occur in a home visit). This will establish or clarify guidelines (standards) by which you can measure the care given and received. During this initial planning process use historical data and clinical judgment to evaluate effectiveness (while beginning a more systematic review later). In other words, what things should occur during a home visit for a diabetic client, what things should the staff do and say (the process of doing the home visit), and what are the client responses (outcomes). These data may be retrievable through the agency's quality review program.

The equity of services is defined as "the distributional effects of a given productivity scheme" (Linn and Karsten 1982). In other words, which population receives the service and is it "fairly" distributed (how one defines "fairly distributed" is based on agency philosophy and policy). Horizontal equity is "how the effects of production are distributed across the population as a whole" (e.g., identify all the types of clients that are seen by the agency from the geographic areas served). Vertical equity is "how a given production function affects a specific target population" (Linn and Karsten 1982) (e.g., identify all the clients who need intravenous therapy (IV); have they received the service, does the agency wish to provide service to all, or to only a segment of the population). Determine what the agency philosophy is regarding equity (service to clients with the ability to pay, quality care to all) and use that as a framework when analyzing productivity.

Don't expect a greater level of productivity than is possible. For example, if the agency services a large rural area, the staff productivity standard will be different from an agency who provides only hospice services to a population in a circumscribed city area, and different from a maternal child health program that services essentially a healthy population.

Evaluate Current Productivity

To develop productivity standards in an agency use the following sequence of steps:

1. Analyze environmental factors that affect productivity.
2. Analyze staff factors that affect productivity.
3. Determine current productivity of staff.
4. Develop "standard" through management blueprint.

Table 9-1 is an overview of the process that is detailed here. The process, simply stated, is to (1) identify and review the specific characteristics of the agency's service delivery (including office and field); (2) identify the current productivity (looking at efficiency, effectiveness, and equity); (3) determine what productivity standard is needed to break even; and finally, (4) determine whether a productivity improvement program is needed to meet the productivity standard. This section will analyze environmental and staff factors and determine and evaluate current productivity.

In determining and analyzing direct caregiver productivity, analyze the work (meaning the environment and the direct client care). Look at environmental and staff factors that contribute to the efficient (good use of time) use of staff expertise (staff are challenged). Look at areas that hinder and help staff to complete their work.

Environmental Factors. Include all nondirect care factors that impact on the staff member's delivery of the direct client care (meaning the visits done per time period).

Table 9-1. How to develop productivity standards

Analyze environmental factors that affect productivity.

    Geographic area
    Paperwork
    Type of program
    Amount and quality of group work
    Staff scheduling
    Percent of unnecessary activities
    Other

Analyze staff factors that affect productivity.

    Experience
    Length of service with agency
    Morale, motivation
    Other

Determine current productivity of staff.

    Baseline data on staff
    Collect visit data
        Type, diagnosis, complexity
        Reimbursement
        Completed visits
        Travel between visits (time, distance)
        Time spent in direct service, preparation
        Documentation, other
    Determine productivity (product number divided by hours of labor)

Assess and analyze productivity data.

Determine standard.

Geographic Area

- Determine, if not already known, the geographic area served by the caregiver: is it a densely populated urban area, a sparsely populated rural area?

- Is travel time great? What is the distance between clients (in time and in miles)?

- Do staff physically report in each morning or afternoon from the field? (what is the time allotted for travel?)

Paperwork

- Which programs generate the most paperwork; the least paperwork?

- Determine how long it takes to admit a client. For which type clients (older, complex diagnosis) does it take less or more time?

- Are charts available for charting when needed? Are computer terminals available and used, are dictaphones used, and are progress notes called in for transcription?

- Are secretaries used for completing all insurance forms or does staff do this?

- If staff does paperwork by hand, ask them where changes can be made to reduce redundancy (do they write the client's name on four different sheets when admitting the client? Are addresses copied on more than one form. . .1,?).

Type of Program

- List the programs the caregivers are involved in (hospice, pediatrics, high-tech, maternal child health, adult care).

- Is the average visit length different for each type of program? Are there different lengths within a program (based on severity of client)? Which programs consume longer visit time (look at your own agency and its setup to determine why particular programs have a longer visit time)?

- Which programs "wear staff out" emotionally (productivity and motivation may be decreased due to the type of clients cared for; e.g., pediatric oncology clients, stroke clients)?

- Which programs do staff shy away from, and why? Is it because it's emotionally draining, the clients are noncompliant, the environment is unsafe (or staff perceive this), the travel distance is too great (diverse program over an entire county)?

Amount and Quality of Group Work

- List the frequency and duration of in-service meetings, administrative meetings. Is a new program or service necessitating more meetings? (Remember that these cut into the number of visits possible.)

- Is staff returning to the office for informal support from other staff? (This depends on the caregiver; new and inexperienced staff usually want contact with others. The nature of the work may also increase the need for peer consultation on treatment modalities and for peer support; some agencies require all staff back at the office at the end of the day to encourage this peer consultation and decrease the number of team conferences.)

Staff Scheduling. Supervisory skill at scheduling staff impacts on productivity (yes, productivity is a management issue). Consider these areas:

- How is scheduling done; is it poorly planned geographically? For example, staff meet each morning, then drive to a distant locale to complete home visits, then return to the office in the afternoon to "check in." Staff must come to the office before beginning visits, so a caregiver drives from her home, past her first client's home, to the office, checks in, then starts back to the first visit of the day. Consider having staff phone in to document that they have begun the day at the first client's home.

- Is there a specialty program (IV therapy) that covers a wide geographic area with staff expected to cover the entire area? Perhaps that's acceptable in one agency; another agency may wish to hire contract staff that live near the client.

- Do staff live near their service area? Are caregivers purposefully assigned to areas other than where they live; consider reevaluating this if it occurs in the agency.

- Review the assignments that inexperienced and qualified staff receive. Determine whether there are differences in the assignment (there should be) and what they are. Do managers assign underqualified or overqualified staff to cases (e.g., new staff assigned a complex client or an expert staff working with clients they find unchallenging). Assuming that there is a choice of staff in a geographic region, assess how cases are assigned, taking into account an already full caseload, vacations, and other variables specific to the agency. Is staff being used effectively? (More on this later.)

Unnecessary Activities. Review the caregiver's day (following a staff member for a day; asking him to identify redundant activities), to identify where staff is involved in non-direct care activities:

- Answering phones is a major time waster for caregivers. This is an especially troublesome problem with a small agency--who covers when the secretary goes to lunch? Consider call forwarding to another site, use of an answering service (costly and bad for public relations during working hours, overall not the best choice), use of an answering machine, or a part-time secretary, typist, or clerk to cover busy times (early morning, lunch).

- Do nurses and therapists stock their own bags? It may be easier to provide staff with a check-off sheet listing supplies needed, which can be turned in, and supplies can be packaged by a paraprofessional or office staff member for each staff to pick up the following day.

- Is staff providing services that can be done by other professional or paraprofessional staff? Is therapy staff providing counseling that could (and should) be done by social worker staff; are RNs completing morning care that aides could be doing? Look beyond those exceptions to the rule and consider the time that professional staff spend doing other than the skills they've been trained to do and gain satisfaction from. (This is one of the more difficult areas to correct.)

Other. What agency-specific factors impact on the way staff do their job? Is there a seasonal workload change, are admissions highest in the winter months with slack time in the summer, or just the reverse? Track the visits done by month over the past two years to determine the agency's workload changes. Consider reevaluating the number of full-time positions needed and the use of vacations, compensation time, etc., for full-time staff when there is less work than staff. Look at part-time and contract staff for peak times.

Staff Factors

Experience. Experienced staff makes more visits (per unit of time) than inexperienced staff (if this isn't so in the agency, there is a problem!). Expect experienced staff to be more efficient in their use of time. Assuming that the caseload mix is similar, are your experienced staff seeing more clients and making more visits than less experienced caregivers? What is the difference in visit time between experienced and less experienced staff? If visit time is the same, does that mean that experienced staff are seeing the most complex clients?

What does "experienced staff" mean? A productive staff member may have skills such as:

- Ease in charting

- Greater expertise with assessing client needs and goal setting

- Ability to deal with flexibility (the new staff member often complains of "no guidelines")

- Expert in health assessment

- Expert in counseling and therapeutic conversations (the staff member is able to not get overinvolved in social or financial aspects of care and can effectively delegate roles to other professionals).

When does a staff member become "experienced?" Each agency has a different expectation and should manage staff and caseload appropriately for the new and seasoned staff member. Determine your best staff and make a list of why they're good, then (and this is the key), determine how you encourage these behaviors in others.

Length of Service with the Agency. All staff need time for orientation. What is the expected time for staff to become fully functional? Is prospective staff made aware of these expectations in preemployment interviews and during orientation? Do managers assist new staff in developing expertise in efficiency as well as in the traditional aspects of providing home care services? Determine at what point you expect a full contribution by staff (two months, six months, one year?).

Morale and Motivation. Is there good, average, or poor morale among staff? Although many variables cause changes in morale (perhaps the frantic pace of change in the home care industry), consider the agency management style and follow through in the staff. Poor management can cause poor morale and a decrease in motivation in staff, which often can result in decreasing productivity. Carefully analyze the changes that have occurred in the agency within the last six months to one year, and look at the managers' response and their interaction with staff, perhaps everyone needs some morale building.

Other. Miscellaneous occurrences can impact on productivity: illness in staff, leave of absences, and vacations (the agency is paying vacation pay and paying other staff, part-time or contract, to cover the caseload during the vacation period). Identify other factors in the agency that impact on productivity and add them to this list.

The bottom line is that, to maintain productivity, you need qualified staff that stay! Staff and managers are involved in the day-to-day operation of an agency, and staff generally take their cues for performance expectations from management. Therefore, maybe the productivity issue is a management issue and not just an employee issue. Doesn't management (first line supervisors and up) have the power, leadership, and control over many of the factors just described as affecting productivity? Managers have the responsibility to organize the work environment and encourage growth in staff (increasing motivation!), thereby improving the efficiency and quality of services provided (that's increasing productivity). Therefore, productivity involves all levels of management and clinical staff!

Determine Current Productivity. What is the productivity standard in your agency? Is there an expectation that staff will provide a certain number of visits per time period? The productivity standard established should be unique to each discipline and to each program. The variables discussed earlier are unique to each agency, therefore any productivity standard will reflect the characteristics (type of agency, philosophy, financial expectation, etc.) of that agency.

Let's assume that the agency has a standard in force. Are staff members aware of the standard and involved in completing the standard that is expected? Often the staff will know that "six visits per day" is the standard and that that averages out to 30 visits per week, but will not be clear that these visits are to be reimbursable, meaning that the agency can bill and receive payment for the visits. Staff may assume that as long as they log six visits per day they are meeting the productivity standard, even though, of the six visits, one was to a client without the ability to pay and the second was to a client who was not home. The staff member provided four reimbursable visits that day, even though six homes were visited. The standard that is established should delineate whether all visit types are included (reimbursable and nonreimbursable). Reimbursable visits may include those paid for by Medicare, Medicaid, third-part payors, grants, and donations.

Use the information listed in the last section to identify the factors (specific to the agency) that impact on the productivity of staff. Then determine the current productivity of staff, using the following guidelines. (If available, consider computer analysis of this information.)

1. Determine baseline data (categories) to indicate what defines:

- An experienced staff (more than three years experience?)

- Oriented to agency (service more than three months?)

- Contract, part-time, full-time staff

2. For a week selected at random (preferably nonvacation, without extra heavy admissions, etc.) determine the following for each staff discipline (e.g., speech therapy, nursing):

- Basic information (name, discipline, experience, type of employment)

- Number of visits done in a specific time frame, daily and weekly (You are determining the present productivity now, analysis of the specifics of the visits can be done later.)

- Evaluate the visit and travel sheet to note:

  - Was the visit reimbursable or nonreimbursable (Count only reimbursable visits in determining productivity, unless otherwise noted by the agency.)

  - Visit was completed or client not home

  - Travel distance between visits (Is staff determining the most efficient travel route? Do they drive greater distances than necessary, or is client care mandating early morning or late afternoon visits (could a contract staff do these visits?)

  - Travel time between visits. Is inner city travel taking as much time as travel to and from a rural area? (In other words, should geographic areas be reassigned, or are there extra slow or extra speedy drivers?)

  - Visit length, matched with the type of visit (MCH, adult care)

  - Visit was an admission, recertification, an emergency, a discharge, or any other criterion that indicates either the expectation of a longer or shorter visit

  - Time spent in other activities: telephone calls to physicians, clinic personnel, communication with families, return calls to clients, gathering supplies. Staff should be completing a travel sheet documenting visits and mileage; it can be adapted to include the above information (to keep extra paperwork down). These can be turned in weekly for this initial review, later monthly review should suffice.

3. Determine, using this information tabulated over a five day period, the "productivity" or "output per unit of input" for each staff member, then combine by discipline to determine an overall figure. (Number of visits divided by five days equals the number of visits per day.) Beware of combining dissimilar programs to determine this overall figure: staff who do postpartum visits may achieve a higher visit rate than those working within the hospice program and should have higher productivity expectations. Use the overall figure as a guide, and compare it to the staff productivity in different programs, varied geographic areas, and various employment statuses.

4. Ask these questions when analyzing the information:

- Are certain geographic areas more difficult to service than others? (Less clients in the area, greater distance between, geographically isolated, specific factors: bridge, tunnel that causes delays?)

- What type of visits take the least and most time? Do more analysis to see why. Use the staff to assist here, they can identify the complexity involved, and identify roadblocks to the provision of care (managers can then determine if support services can help to remove unnecessary barriers).

- Is the visit length different between PT, contract, and FT staff? Are contract staff (paid by the visit) hurrying through the visit, or are they the most efficient of the staff? (Note: Many agencies pay FT, PT, and contract staff by the visit, so determine whether these are important data for the agency. Perhaps of more significance is whether the visit length is different between experienced and new staff).

- What circumstances may have skewed the data? What occurrences caused the information to represent inaccurately what is happening in the agency? (Increase in sick leave, increase in number of emergency visits or admissions during the sample week)

- What does the staff make of the data? Staff members should be able to describe why the results of the review look as they do, since they provide the day-to-day service and are the most involved in complexities of the provision of services.

- What are the characteristics of the staff with the highest productivity? Are productive staff members those that managers evaluate as being less than thorough clinicians, or those that would be expected to be. What characteristics do these staff members have; why are they productive? A "profile of a productive employee" is one who is "well qualified for the job, is highly motivated, has a positive job orientation, and interfaces effectively." (Riddell 1981)

The Next Step

The purpose of this chapter is to provide a method for evaluating the current productivity for all or a segment of the staff who provide direct service to clients. It involves analyzing the environment that the staff works in, looking at the type and quality of staff working in the agency, assessing what is included in a home visit, and having a good idea of what makes a staff member productive in the agency.

The next step is to determine, using fiscal data, the productivity standard necessary to meet expenses and generate revenue over expenses (make a profit). Indirect costs (supplies, overhead, etc.) and direct staff costs are matched to income generated from billable visits to determine the total cost of doing a home visit (Levy 1979). The information is further analyzed to determine the number of visits necessary to cover the cost of agency operation, and second, the number and types of visits necessary to generate a predecided percentage of revenue over expenses. This is defined as the number of reimbursable visits per staff per unit of time (the standard).

The standard, considered the benchmark, or guide (the expected level of work) should be unique to each discipline; therapy visits per day may be different from expected RN visits. There are several ways to develop the standard, and examples are given in the case studies that follow. References at the end of this chapter also provide an review of how to determine a productivity standard for the agency (Levy 1979; Rozelle 1977).

Having determined what current productivity is and what the productivity standard is, evaluate whether there is a need for a productivity improvement program. If the current productivity does not equal or exceed the standard established for agency viability, then a productivity improvement program is essential. Likewise, if staff productivity cannot increase without a decrease in quality, a productivity improvement program is also needed (to assess and organize those people and things that impact on caregivers' time). Perhaps the productivity standard is being met, staff morale is high, management is totally efficient, and the quality of client services is good, then there is not need for a productivity improvement program.

A productivity improvement program (Bermas 1984) includes: (1) a systematic education of all personnel about the relationship between productivity and agency viability (staff should understand the budget and the cash flow process); (2) an assessment of the total operation (in addition to the review of personnel, which has already been partially completed); (3) the establishment of adequate staffing and performance measurement (yes, productivity does involve having appropriate job descriptions and performance evaluation tools; and having the appropriate number and type of staff, in the field and in the office); (4) development and implementation of incentives for increasing productivity (managing for excellence, etc.); and (5) continual evaluation of the standard of productivity for revision or clarification.

In summary, remember the basic assumptions when evaluating productivity; it's not done in a vacuum; improving only one component of an agency will not increase overall productivity: consider an agencywide program; involve all staff, particularly direct caregivers, in planning and evaluating the productivity of an agency; remember that management holds the key to effective productivity, through effective supervision and the ability to create environments that challenge and motivate staff.

The Diagnosis and Treatment of Community Health Productivity Problems*

Linda Weinberg and Lynda C. Brubaker

Introduction

Community health agencies are operating under severe financial constraints. Because of the regulations set by the Health Care Finance Administration, productivity be-

---

* Excerpt from a Master's Thesis of the same title submitted to the University of Pennsylvania, Philadelphia, PA, 1986.

comes even more important for the agency's survival. One additional daily visit from each staff nurse may make the difference between financial stability and economic vulnerability.

In order for the nurse to make a daily additional visit, management must be able to diagnose and treat their own distinctive productivity problems. As with all diagnoses, certain tests must be performed to confirm or rule out the problem.

These tests should include both objective and subjective matter. With available economic formulas, it is within an agency's means to calculate visits, productive and nonproductive hours, total visit time and nonvisiting time. This should be just the first step in the agency's differential diagnosis.

From the economic data, it is possible to detect if there is a difference between expected productivity levels and the actual productivity levels. From the subjective data, it is possible to detect any problems concerning retention or motivation of the staff.

The next diagnostic step is to gather subjective data from the staff. There are several ways to obtain this information: informal discussions with staff about problems they may be experiencing; formal discussions with staff; and anonymous surveys that reveal what the staff "perceive" as problems that prevent them from obtaining desired productivity levels. The staff's perceptions of the problems are important in diagnosing the problem and assisting the economic data on productivity.

Nursing productivity studies have been primarily hospital-based. Community health nurses are not physically bound by the four walls of a hospital or clinic. This physical freedom and the unique nature of visiting nurse work presents certain problems when one is looking at agency productivity.

There are several reasons why a staff nurse's productivity level may be down: does he shop at the local stores when he is supposed to be visiting patients; how much time does he actually spend for his breaks or lunches; does he get so overwhelmed by the lack of organizational skills that inertia takes over?

These questions need to be answered in order to diagnose productivity problems properly. It is the combination of both subjective and objective data that will lead to a more realistic diagnosis and treatment.

It is our belief that there are certain discriminating factors that are unique contributors to community health agency productivity. We believe that these productivity factors do not operate the same as in a hospital or clinic setting.

Review of the Literature

As early as 1924, community health nursing administrators have been concerned with the number of visits per day, costs per patient visit, quality of nursing care delivered, and a system that would quantify these data. Grettner (1924, 3) was concerned with the "meager amount of material available in public health nursing agencies." The report stated that "until we know the simple facts of what constitutes the nursing load, the frequency of care to the various types of cases, and the outstanding results of such care, we cannot plan intelligently for future development." (Grettner 1924, 3) The members of the commission did not use the term productivity in the report.

It has been 62 years since the abovementioned report was printed. A current review of the literature suggested that limited research has been done in the area of productivity within community health nursing organizations. Nursing has been slow to develop an objective interest in productivity. The emergence of the Diagnostic Related Groups (DRGs) has identified the importance of productivity and the cost containment benefits to the attention of the health professional.

Most of the literature that has been written about nursing productivity from 1966 to 1974 has been concerned with settings such as hospitals, ambulatory clinics, and doctor's offices. Thirty-three percent of the studies in nursing productivity has been sponsored by hospitals, 27% by universities, 21% by private sources, and 17% by government funding (Jelinek and Lyman, 1976). Visiting nurse agencies have suffered from a chronic lack of funds. Unless these agencies, whether in the private or public sector, have sponsorship from outside sources, funding for research activity has been restricted to a minimum.

Historically, written material has helped us to understand that visiting nurse administrators have been concerned with productivity issues. Financial constraints that have previously discouraged productivity research in visiting nurse agencies have today encouraged the very same studies on productivity.

One of the first attempts to quantify and describe how visiting nurses spend their time was written by Charmaine L. Kissinger (1973). Visiting nurse activities were divided into eight categories: (1) written communication; (2) preparation for visit; (3) telephoning; (4) discussion; (5) conference; (6) patient activity; (7) miscellaneous; and (8) travel. Eight nurses were randomly selected and were observed for an eight and one-half hour day by the observer. The nurses were all employed in a large urban visiting nurse agency. Only one geographical district was chosen for this study.

After compiling the data, Kissinger found that 40% of the nurses' time was spent in recordkeeping, 10% in travel, and 13% in patient-related care. Kissinger noted that "although the primary objective of the agency was the provision of direct nursing care to the community, the majority of the nurses' time was spent in other than direct service." (1977, 114) She added that the study was an initial effort to measure both the effectiveness and efficiency of community health nurses.

Another study by Cross, Northrop, and Strasser (1983) identified how community nurses spend their time. They divided the visiting nurse activities into six categories. One hundred and nine nurses participated in the self-reported time study for one week. These nurses were assigned to six county health centers that served both individuals and families. Forty percent of the nurses' time was spent in patient care. Less than 6% was spent in travel.

Bonstein and Mueller (1985) were not only concerned with time studies. They attempted to incorporate definitions of productivity, obstacles to productivity in home care, calculations of productivity, and launching productivity improvement programs. Their article demonstrated a step-by-step method of calculating productivity visits per day. The explicit economic formula was limited in the community health literature. The authors recommended several steps that could be taken by the agency managers to help the staff improve productivity.

The *Easley-Storfjell Instruments for Caseload/Workload Analysis* (See Chapter 15) were developed at the University of Michigan to "provide a summary description of a community nurse's case and workload, to serve as a basis for case assignment (number, type, personnel), and to diagnose problems in caseload management." (Easley-Storfjell 1979, 1) The time allocation sheet contained a time utilization sheet based on a monthly or yearly accumulation of data. The data were descriptive in nature.

Krayne (1982) surveyed a staff of nurses, aides, and therapists in a home health agency. The staff viewed the following variables as those that most limited patient visits: severity of patient's illness, living conditions, and inclement winter weather. Since these variables were difficult to control, the author concluded that managers should concern themselves with "ways of reducing office time and of using that time efficiently and in a more productive manner." (Krayne 1982, 22)

1985 Survey Findings

The purpose of a recently completed study was to identify those factors that affected productivity in one home health agency in 1985. A total of 18 nurses in one home health agency were selected at random to be followed during the course of a day.

On the day of observation, each nurse was informed that the 8.5-hour work day was to be recorded in five-minute intervals by the researcher. Eight different categories of activities (and their appropriate subheadings) were recorded.

The time study was adapted from Kissinger's work in 1973. For the purposes of our survey, 38 categories were used (see Table 9-2).

Results of the Time Study. There were no statistical differences related to the amount of activity time spent by nurses irrespective of their geographical differences. As demonstrated by means and standard deviations, there was as much difference between the individual nurses as there was among the three groups.

Eight one-way ANOVAS were run using the Apple MacIntosh "Statworks" program. The independent variables were city, suburb, and rural geographical areas. The dependent variables were the eight classifications of activities: (1) written communication; (2) preparation; (3) telephoning; (4) discussion; (5) conference; (6) patient care; (7) travel; and (8) miscellaneous. Table 9-3 demonstrates time percentages spent by nurses according to geographical location.

Discussion and Implications of the Time Study. This study demonstrated that there were no significant activity time differences among the geographical subgroupings of city, suburban, and rural nurses.

Community health nurse managers have traditionally computed daily visit expectations based upon geographical considerations. Patient load had determined the amount of paperwork for each nurse. As demonstrated by this sample study, geographical considerations should not have the same importance in determining daily visit expectations at this visiting nurse agency.

The researchers believed that the individual management style of each nurse was the keystone of individual productivity. Individual productivity determined agency productivity. The researchers recommended that community health nurse managers should begin to focus upon the following areas of concern:

1. Office environment and its conduciveness for both the completion of necessary paperwork and the enhancement of individual growth.

2. Ongoing recognition programs for both staff and managers.

Table 9-2. Time study categories with identified variables.

Written Communication

1. Recording visit content by writing
2. Recording visit content by dictating
3. Completion of Medicare and Medicaid forms
4. Completion of initial assessment
5. Securing medical or nursing records
6. Completion of necessary doctor, home health aid requests, and miscellaneous forms.

Discussion

1. Supervisor
2. Home health aide
3. Physical therapist, occupational therapist, speech therapist, masters in social work, staff nurse
4. Medical records personnel
5. Others

Preparation for visit

1. Securing necessary equipment for visit
2. Daily routine preparation
3. Procedure review
4. Research relevant to patient visit
5. Miscellaneous

Travel

1. Travel to and from patient's house
2. Travel back and forth to the agency
3. Looking for parking space
4. Miscellaneous

Telephoning

1. Patient family
2. Physician
3. Calls to or within the agency related to patient concerns
4. Other health agencies or institutions
5. Provide transportation or arrange services for patient
6. Miscellaneous calls

Miscellaneous

1. Time sheet
2. Coffee and lunch break
3. Staff meeting
4. Car maintenance

Conference

1. Supervisor
2. Home health aide
3. Interdisciplinary aide
4. Nursing team

Patient

1. Therapeutic care
2. Assessment of patients needs
3. Teaching or demonstration care
4. Other

3. Recognition of the important contribution that external and internal locus of control exert on individual productivity levels in community health.

4. Scrutiny of individual nursing management styles and problem-solving methods.

Table 9-3. Percentage of time spent by all the nurses during an 8.5-hour work day according to geographical location (n=18).

Location	WC	Prep	Tele	Disc	Conf	Pt	Trav	Misc
	(%)	(%)	(%)	(%)	(%)	(%)	(%)	(%)
City (n=6)	21.7	8.2	3.9	4.1	5.9	30.9	15.3	10.0
Suburb (n=6)	20.4	5.0	3.7	7.2	2.6	29.7	19.8	11.6
Rural (n=6)	17.6	4.1	4.2	2.1	5.6	26.5	26.5	13.4
All (n=18)	20.0	5.7	4.0	4.5	4.7	29.0	20.5	11.6

Abbreviations used: WC, written communication; Prep, preparation; Tele, telephone; Disc, discussion; Conf, conference; Pt, patient; Trav, travel; Misc, miscellaneous.

By utilizing the time study, the employee survey, and the above guidelines, community health nurse managers could begin to diagnose and treat their productivity concerns.

References

Benefield, L.E. Productivity. In Home Health Care Management, ed. L. Benefield. Englewood Cliffs, NJ: The Brady Company, in press.

Bermas, N.F. 1984. The positive side of productivity for ambulator care management. Journal of Ambulatory Care Management 7(8): 1-4.

Bonstein, R.G., and J. Mueller. 1985. Improving agency productivity. Caring 4(11): 4-9.

Cross, J., C. Northrop, and J. Strasser. 1983. How community health nurses spend their time: A study report. Nursing and Health Care. 4:314-317.

Department of Health, Education and Welfare. 1976. A review and evaluation of nursing productivity. Health Manpower References, DHEW Publication #77-15. Bethesda, MD: Department of Health, Education, and Welfare.

Easley, C., and C. Storfjell. 1979. The Easley-Storfjell instruments for caseload/workload analysis. Ann Arbor, MI: University of Michigan Press.

Federa, R.D. and T.W. Bilodeau. 1984. The productivity quest. Journal of Ambulatory Care Management 7:5-11.

French, W. 1982. The personnel management process 200-202. Boston: Houghton Mifflin Co.

Grettner, L. 1924. Report of commission to study visiting nursing. Instituted by the National Organization for Public Health, NY, NY: Metropolitan Life.

Griffin, E. 1986. Developing staffing patterns to increase productivity yet retain quality and flexibility. In Book of Abstracts and Presentation Outlines, The Second National Nursing Symposium on Home Health Care ed. L. Daniel and A. Blaha. Community Health Nursing Area, University of Michigan, Ann Arbor, MI.

Holzer, M., ed. 1982. Public Productivity Review 6(3): 155-240.

Jelinek, R., and D. Lyman. 1976. A review and evaluation of nursing productivity. Washington, DC: Government Printing Office. DHEW Publication HRA 77-15.

Kissinger, C. 1973. Community nursing administration: Quantifying nursing utilization. *Journal of Nursing Administration*. 3(5): 42-48.

Krayne, L. 1982. *Home health agency staff survey of variables affecting number of visits per day.* Sewickley, PA: Sewickley Home Health Agency.

Levy, G. 1979. Productivity for home health services. *Home Health Review* 2(2): 24-29.

Linn, N. and S. Karsten. 1982. Managing public health productivity—the art of taming conflict and chaos. *Public Productivity Review* 6(3): 170-183.

Olson, V. 1983. *White Collar Waste, Gain the Productivity Edge.* Englewood Cliffs, NJ: Prentice-Hall.

Orefice, J.J. and M.C. Jennings. 1983. Productivity—A key to managing cost per case. *Healthcare Financial Management.* August: 20.

Poor, R. 1970. *4 Days, 40 Hours, and Other Forms of Rearranged Workweek.* Cambridge, MA: Bursk & Poor.

Riddell, A.J. 1981. Productivity: A dirty word in the voluntary non-profit agency? *Home Health Review* 4(1): 13-20.

Roscow, J., and R. Zager. 1983. Punch out the time clocks. *Harvard Business Review.* March-April 1983: 30.

Rosenberg, G. 1983. *Issues of the workplace.* Workshop given May 5, 1983. Kennebunkport, ME, National Council of Alternative Work Patterns.

Rozelle, G.J. 1977. Productivity management for cost containment in a home health care agency. *Home Health Review* 1(1): 23-31.

Skeler, J.L. 1981. Flexible work hours gather momentum. *U.S. News and World Report* Sept. 28, 1981: 76-77.

State of Maine, Department of Personnel. *Memorandum 4-83, Alternative Work Schedules,* p. 3.

Werther, W.B. 1983. Nontraditional work schedules: Their use in the health care setting. *The Health Care Supervisor* January: 11-20.

Chapter Ten

Labor–Management Relations

Jessie F. Igou

"Institutions are often thought to be the bricks and mortar of their buildings, which are easily seen. In reality, people are the institution. If they leave, the institution no longer exists. What is important for any institution, therefore, are the interactions, support, feelings, frustrations, challenges, and hopes which come from the people who constitute it. The combination of these elements form the institution's climate" (Lockart and Werther 1980, 103). The characteristics of this climate influence the relationship between labor and management and impact upon the effectiveness of the health agency. This climate also influences whether or not staff feel the need for a union. Administration must therefore be alert to the climate and be aware of and practice ways to enhance a positive relationship with nursing staff. How management responds to employee needs, requests, and concerns will be a major determinant of climate and will produce a positive environment if needs are met. It is a major task for administration to find a "balance between people's needs and organizational needs. . ." (Lockart and Werther 1980, 132) for such a balance will create and sustain an organization that is effective and vital.

Conceptual Framework

The home health agency should be viewed from a systems theory framework in which both labor and management are seen as vital units of the system. There must be interdependency among the units if the agency is to be effective. The agency as a whole has a need for unity and each of the units must cooperate. This cooperation will build cohesion among the units which will enhance the effectiveness of the agency. Labor and management need to view themselves as a partnership in which everyone works for the patient's benefit.

Factors Influencing the Labor Relations Climate

Authors have identified various factors which influence the labor-relations climate of an organization and methods for enhancing the positive relationship between labor and management. These will be discussed in this chapter.

Zacur has identified environmental factors, both internal and external, which influence the labor-relations climate of an organization. While these organizations have been primarily acute care hospitals, it is possible that the same factors would be important in a home health agency. The external factors are identified as: (a) laws such as the 1947 Taft-Hartley Act which guaranteed the rights of representation and collective bargaining with a nonprofit employer; (b) professional organizations such as the American Nurses' Association which has attempted to improve economic status of nurses; (c) the state of the economy which has put pressure on female employees to request and demand increased salaries and has focused attention on the comparable worth issue; and (d) public sentiment regarding health care professionals (Zacur 1982, 6).

The internal factors identified by Zacur are: (a) the organizational climate; (b) the organizational administrators; (c) the nurses' roles; and (d) the nurses' views (Zacur 1982, 6). If the organizational climate is one which tolerates change and new ideas, as opposed to being repressive, the labor-management climate may be positive and vital. If administration is parochial in its approach to managing human resources, lacks sensitivity to internal conditions encountered by staff, fails to recognize the professional issues of concern to nurses, and refuses to negotiate or discuss certain issues, the environmental climate will not be healthy and will reduce the effectiveness of the staff. Another factor affecting the labor-relations environment may be how decisions are made and policies determined. If agencies are administered through a bureaucratic organizational structure and process and policies are issued from administration without any participation from caregivers, the environment may be conducive to collective action. Nursing staff cannot be viewed as functionaries at the lower end of the hierarchy without any participation in decision making if their contributions to the attainment of agency goals are to be maximized. Ginzberg has suggested that because nurses are influenced and affected by conditions in the environment, management needs to maximize opportunities for them to succeed, should carefully match people to jobs, and should provide maximum support to nurses in these positions (Ginzberg 1966, 126). Levitan, Mangum, and Marshall (1981, 390) indicate that the organizational climate and administration should be secure and certain since "uncertainty breeds frustration and dissatisfaction." Another important factor in determining environmental climate is the sense of fairness exhibited or practiced by administration (Gregorich and Long 1980, 105-111). This perhaps more than any other factor will promote a sense of collective action.

How nurses view their roles and responsibilities within the organization and their perception of the nursing profession will influence the labor relations climate of the organization. These views and perceptions are influenced by factors such as length and type of education. As nurses receive increased education with a more professional orientation there appears to be increased dissatisfaction with an environment which does not acknowledge professional autonomy (Zacur 1982, 24). Home health nurses need to be involved in decision making regarding patient care and this must be fostered by administration. In a study by Meyer (1970, 26), job security, social esteem, autonomy, self-realization, job and salary satisfaction, chance for advancement, membership in ANA, beliefs about union power, and feelings toward authority were some of the variables studied in relationship to nurses' attitudes toward collective action. Those specific variables found to be significantly related to a positive attitude toward collective action were "(1) lack of autonomy, self-realization and security, (2) low predisposition to submit to authority, (3) ANA membership, (4) low salary satisfaction, and (5) lack of belief that trade union power was too great." Further analysis revealed that when respondents in the study perceived the organizational climate as more autocratic, their need deficiency scores increased significantly and mean collective action attitude scores were significantly higher. Another study by Alutto and Belasco (1972, 224) indicated that those nurses who were most militant and pro-strike were younger nurses with a low feeling of organizational commitment and strong dissatisfaction with their career. According to Zacur (1982, 74), the primary condition within a hospital that precipitates a nursing militancy or pro-strike attitude are the attitudes of the administrators when they utilize a bureaucratic approach in dealing with human resources and fail to recognize the professional concerns and abilities of the nursing staff. These management approaches breed resentment and appear to initiate militant or strike behavior.

Ginzberg (1966, 72) indicates that individuals have a value orientation and a preference system in their work. These are based on needs, goals, and values. Management, therefore, needs to be aware of preference systems and to assist nursing staff to achieve goals and meet needs within this framework.

Four value orientation categories have been derived empirically and can be used as guidelines by management to identify employee types and their general value orientation (Ginzberg 1966, 75-77). The four types are: (a) individualistic; (b) leadership; (c) social; and (d) ideological. The individualistic type has a great need for autonomy and is always striving for the same. This type wants to be free from strict direction and interference, choosing to structure his own activities, while making optimal use of individual capacities in the work setting. The leadership type has an orientation toward building and maintaining relationships with others, having authority over others, directing and leading others, and being more involved in the organizational structure. The basic orientation of the social type is to be a member of a group or team and to be accepted by group members. Individuals of this type strive for group esteem. They have no intention or desire to become boss and derive satisfaction from the social context of their work. Ginzberg states that "next in importance to earning a living wage is a satisfactory working relationship" (1966, 36) and the worker "strives to improve the conditions under which he spends so much of his time and his energy" (Ginzberg 1966, 36). The greatest numbers in the work force are of this type. The last category, the ideological type, is committed to a system of ideals or ideas and has as a goal to serve a higher value than meeting personal needs. These individuals seek autonomy not for themselves but for the cause. While these four types are not mutually exclusive, most individuals exhibit one stronger orientation which management could identify and use to promote individual well-being and subsequently organizational well-being.

It would appear that any home health agency which is attempting to promote positive labor-management relations should concentrate on identifying internal and external environmental factors which affect the organizational climate. Attempts should be made to understand the nurses' perceptions, needs, and value orientations so that both individual and organizational needs can be planned for and met.

Communication and Interpersonal Skills

Communication and interpersonal skills, vital to promoting helping relationships, possibly aid in creating effective labor-management relationships. Scott (1962, 170) proposes that the health of an organization depends upon successful communication or the imparting of information to all employees. If the home health agency is viewed as a system, then communication can be viewed as a linking process, binding together the various system units (management and labor). Rothstein (1958, 34) states "Organization presupposes the existence of parts, which considered in their totality, constitute the organization. The parts must interact. Were there no communication between them, there would be no organization but merely a collection of individual elements isolated from each other."

Communication networks should exist in the organization. These networks are decision centers interconnected by channels of communication. A feedback system is crucial for the network as it helps to maintain balance among all components of the system. Change can occur and the system can self-regulate when feedback is received.

Davis (1958, 228) states "Communication is the process of passing information and understanding from one person to another." This implies that communication does not occur unless the receiver understands the transmitted information. The greater the degree of understanding by the receiver, the more likely the receiver will be to behave and act so that organizational goals are attained (Scott 1962, 173). Thus, communication is viewed as a manager's tool for accomplishing agency goals.

The focus of communication has shifted from being persuasion- and conversion-oriented to being understanding- and negotiation-oriented (Cushman 1980, 27). Talking and discussing provide both labor and management the opportunity to understand and accept diverse points of view and alternate solutions to a problem which then allows for the successful negotiation of a solution.

For a positive relationship to occur between labor and management, both parties must practice effective sending and receiving skills. Both verbal and nonverbal channels can be used to send messages. However, the majority of messages are sent without words, conveyed with body language, facial expressions, gestures and body movements, eye contact, tone of voice, use of silence and other behaviors. Individuals must constantly be alert to the congruency between their verbal and nonverbal messages. Verbal messages are meant to convey ideas as well as feelings. An important component of verbal messages is to ask for reactions or verbal feedback to assure that the intent of the words is being understood by those receiving them.

Receiving skills are as critical to effective communication as are sending skills. Primary skills in receiving messages are observing behavior and active listening. An active listening response consists of a feeling component and a content component (Gerrard, Boniface, and Love 1980, 137) as the receiver attempts to understand not only what the sender is saying but what he is feeling. The sender does this by concentrating and asking reflective questions. This aspect of communication indicates interest in the speaker, communicates acceptance, builds trust, and assists the person to develop problem-solving skills. It is important that both labor and management take the time to learn, practice, and participate in actively listening to each other.

Both the effective sending and receiving of messages requires that clarification occur. Eliciting feedback from all parties generates understanding between labor and management.

The interpersonal skills of showing respect, empathizing, and developing trust can assist in promoting a positive labor-management relationship. "Showing respect means conveying the attitude that the client has importance, dignity and respect" (Spadley 1985, 273). Respect should be conveyed both by labor and management through tone of voice, recognition of valuable ideas, and the manner in which people are addressed. Empathizing is a skill that can be used by all individuals to show that they are attempting to understand feelings expressed by others. This skill also encourages the sharing of concerns. Developing trust is critical if individuals are to work effectively with each other. Management and labor can develop trust for each other by showing acceptance of each other and treating each other as partners and by having open discussions to share feelings. Candid discussions can be part of a labor-management committee approach discussed elsewhere in this chapter.

Various reasons for communication breakdown exist but most can be traced to the following (Scott 1962, 196):

1. The nature and functions of the human language

2. Purposeful misrepresentation

3. Size of the organization

4. Lack of acceptance

5. Failure to understand.

Distortion and filtering are severe and frequent problems in the communication process. Distortion occurs because messages sent up and down in an organization have to be interpreted by receivers. Because the human language is so complex and can be interpreted differently, the message can be distorted as it gets interpreted by various individuals. Management can minimize distortion be asking for feedback from receivers to see if the content of the message is interpreted as intended. The existence of social barriers or social distance or a difference in thinking between staff and management can also create distortion. Scott (1962, 198) suggests that most communication breakdown occurs because subordinates and boss do not agree on obstacles and problems faced by the subordinate. He recommends empathy as one method by which social distance between different levels of employees can be overcome. If managers can project themselves into the framework of the employees, then any messages sent by managers will more likely be received and understood by the employees.

Filtering produces communication breakdown by deliberate misinterpretation of a message. This occurs primarily in upward communication as subordinates send to managers the material they feel will be most accepted. Filtering includes both commission and omission of information.

As an organization increases in size and complexity, management becomes buried in communication to which response is impossible. Optimum flow of material is necessary if managers are to communicate successfully with staff, so that irrelevant information should be monitored and handled by middle management personnel.

Timing and short-circuiting are other serious communication problems related to the size and complexity of the organization. Information needs to be released at the appropriate time and to be received by all employees at the same time or in a sequential order. Short-circuiting occurs when someone is missed in the communication chain who should have been included. An employee's status may be lowered and angry feelings result when an employee doesn't get the necessary information at the appropriate time.

Communication breakdowns also occur because staff lacks acceptance and understanding of the conveyed information. Even though staff may receive the appropriate material at the right time, the staff may choose not to accept it for various reasons, which include: (a) incongruency in reality between sender and receiver; (b) ambiguous or unclear message; (c) the receiver may not have faith in the sender (low credibility); and (d) incongruency between the content of the message and the receiver's value-need system. As ambiguity of the message increases, as the credibility of the sender decreases, and as conflict between message content and value-need system of the receiver increases, the less likely the receiver is to accept the information (Scott 1962, 204). These are all affected by the receiver's perception of reality so that the manager should work first to understand and change the receiver's view of reality of the situation. Teamwork has been recommended as a mechanism for effectively changing an individual employee's view of reality and thus promoting acceptance of the information.

The last cause of communication breakdown is the lack of understanding by receivers who inaccurately translate the symbols used in communication. Scott (1962, 207) suggests that a "climate for understanding" can be established by management by (1) planning for communication; (2) tailoring the information to fit the employee's frame of reference; and (3) listening to what employees have to say. This last step can be carried out in a nondirective interview between staff and management which will generate information on needs, complaints, and employee goals. The manager acts as a sounding board only, gathering information that will allow him to respond to the needs of staff.

Problem Solving

Creative problem solving is another management tool for promoting a healthy labor-management relationship. The use of conceptual models such as an open systems model assists in improving interdepartmental communications (Golightly 1981, 215). Use of a model serves as a discussion point as information flows from one area to another and discussion occurs between components of the system, between the problem solvers and those who are affected by the solution. This method enhances effective communication which then facilitates the problem-solving process.

Three levels of problem solving exist in an organization such as a home health agency: the individual process, the group process, and the organizational process which contains several groups. The Nominal group approach, the Delphi problem-solving method, and brainstorming can be used by groups to solve problems creatively. Certain factors which affect group problem-solving are: (1) the problem information held by the group; (2) the extent to which the group accepts that there is a need for action; and (3) the extent of congruence between goals of the individual members and the goals of the group (Vroom and Yetton 1976, 626-643).

Organizational problem solving is much more complex than the individual or group process due to the increased number of environmental and personal variables involved. As more individuals are involved, the potential for conflict increases. Objectives for organizational problem solving must be very explicit, providing a framework for goal-directed behavior.

Many situations exist in a home health agency which are complex with many variables interfacing and contributing to the situation. In approaching these situations it seems appropriate to identify all the contributing factors that interface so that a reasonable problem statement and a solution can be formulated. Exhibit 10-1 il-

Exhibit 10-1 The Funnel Analogy

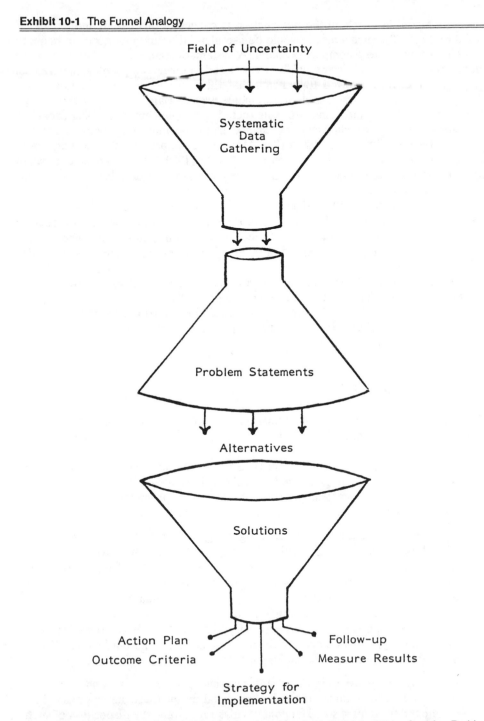

Field of Uncertainty

Systematic
Data
Gathering

Problem Statements

Alternatives

Solutions

Action Plan

Outcome Criteria

Follow-up

Measure Results

Strategy for
Implementation

Reprinted with permission of Aspen Publishers, Inc. from C. K. Golightly 1981. *Creative Problem Solving for Health Care Professionals*, p. 60. Rockville, MD: Aspen Systems Corp.

lustrates a model in which all the information is collected, processed, and expanded (Golightly 1981, 60). Such a model would be useful as labor and management begin to formulate a solution to a complex problem. A systematic gathering of data is done to produce issues, facts, and givens which are analyzed to formulate problem statements. The middle funnel is inverted to indicate that there are many problem statements rather than just one, and that problem statements may overlap.

As these problem statements are constructed, a people-centeredness approach is emphasized. This approach facilitates change from the manager's perspective and recognizes the contributions of the worker. Management must indicate a willingness to help and to work with the work group. Golightly (1981, 61) indicates that when management begins to pay attention to the work group, the out-of-balance state begins to change and improve.

After data have been collected and processed, definition of the problem and all its parameters can be done in small groups. A large group can be divided into smaller groups to address specific issues. Use of such a model with group involvement fosters employee involvement, promotes ownership, and accelerates group acceptance (Golightly 1981, 62).

After the data have been collected and analyzed and alternatives generated, some time should elapse before solutions are recommended. The work group, in identifying the best solution, should consider how a specific solution contributes to the agency objectives, the cost in dollars, time needed to implement the plan, and the feasibility of the solution (Golightly 1981, 69).

General Recommendations

Various authors have made recommendations on how to promote a positive labor-management relationship. These include:

- Establishing a patient care committee. Such a committee should be comprised of all categories of caregivers and should provide a forum for discussion of general concerns regarding patients. This approach promotes a team concept, creative problem-solving, and involvement in decision-making.

- Establishing some mechanism for recognizing nursing staff's professional contributions. A variety of positive reinforcements can be used to reward and thus motivate organizational commitment and performance. The rewards can range from monetary compensation to citations to verbal recognition only. An important criteria is that the reward be perceived as valuable by the employee, which necessitates that such programs be designed with input from the employees themselves. It seems necessary to define what nurses perceive as professional recognition and how it can be achieved. This would indicate to management what motivational methods to use.

- Encouraging a policy of informal staff meetings between nurses and supervisors. Communication can be facilitated during these meetings as input is solicited from nurses and feedback is given regarding the disposition of such suggestions. Critical components of such meetings should be a two-way communication process, much information and praise given, and an emphasis on positive reinforcement and possibilities rather than constraints (Zacur 1982, 76-77).

- Using career counseling to promote professional commitment. Zacur (1982, 76) states that "a long-term developmental approach to staff nurses and their careers can foster organizational commitment and decrease interest in militancy as a means to professional recognition." Administration has a responsibility to ensure that career needs of individuals are maximized, that nurses have the skills and knowledge necessary to perform their jobs, and that they have the opportunity to utilize these skills. This can be accomplished by staff and administration engaging in joint planning.

- Providing orientation update sessions. These sessions provide employees with information about current developments and future plans and allow nurses to share perceptions with management (Gregorich and Long 1980, 108). Problems can be presented during these sessions, but this is done in a positive, constructive atmosphere.

- Filling front line supervisory positions with the best possible people and providing education for them to increase their effectiveness. Individuals hired for these positions should demonstrate excellent interpersonal skills, communication skills, and labor-relations training. Personal attention should be given by the supervisor to all employees, especially those with great needs. The literature indicates that an organization must meet the needs as perceived by employees or the union will come along, meet these needs, and win approval of the group (Cangemi, Clark, and Harryman 1980, 114). It is suggested that the supervisor's treatment of employees is a critical factor in establishing a positive labor-management climate (Lockhart and Werther 1980, 104).

- Preparing an employee-oriented publication. Items concerning employees should be incorporated into the publication, along with pictures and praise. Controversial and threatening messages should not be included.

- Supporting of athletic and recreational programs or social events sponsored by employees.

- Designing an acceptable suggestion system.

- Developing a plan for rewarding loyal dedicated employees who have demonstrated commitment to the agency.

- Developing a system to audit and identify feelings, opinions, and needs of employees. This system provides information which can be used to initiate action to meet employee needs and facilitate movement in accordance with employee goals. Creating a more positive environment requires a proactive behavior by management and allows actions to be taken before, not after, a crisis situation occurs.

- Fostering a cooperative environment. "Cooperating is largely a matter of consultation between the two sides" (Werther and Lockhart 1980, 156). Cooperation is sometimes difficult to achieve because both labor and management harbor fears and misconceptions based on past experiences. A cooperative relationship can begin when either side is in a desperate situation and needs help. Favors are given and reciprocation is expected. These requests form the beginning of a cooperative environment. Such an environment can also be initiated by having a formal suggestion plan in which employees can be consulted and encouraged to give suggestions. Jointly sponsored athletic, recreational, and social events provide the opportunity for each side to have a mutually satisfying interaction, reevaluate opinions of each other, and build teamwork. In order for labor-management relations to be positive, adversarial relationships must be abandoned; each side must view the relationship as a cooperative and a helping one, and each side must agree to consult the other before taking action.

- Establishing an employee relations program. This program must be perceived as equitable and consistent by staff. This applies particularly to wages which must be perceived as satisfactory. If this occurs, the employee relations program and management will have credibility. Nonunionized agencies need to act as though a third party is standing by, judging their actions for fairness and consistency. Agencies should have as part of their employee relations program a philosophy which recognizes the need of both labor and management. Specific components of such a philosophy include:

  - Management should recognize staff needs and all actions should consider these needs.

  - Staff must respect management's need for efficiency and effectiveness.

  - Problem solving should be a joint endeavor between staff and management.

  - Cooperation is the most viable long-term strategy for ensuring agency success.

  - Survival of the agency is paramount (Werther and Lockhart 1980, 159).

- Establishing a position of employee relations manager. The primary role of such a person would be to act as management's conscience, reminding management of their commitment to an employee relations program. The employee relations manager serves as the "expert" in resolving employee relations problems, designs two-way communication systems, and assists both parties in utilizing these systems to promote positive interactions and mutual understanding.

- Providing for a formal grievance procedure. "Union leaders have stated publicly that the best defense against union organization is an effective grievance procedure" (Gregorich and Long 1980, 109). Having a formal grievance procedure in a nonunion setting provides a mechanism for release of pressure, assurance that employee grievances will be considered, an avenue for communication, and also, a stimulus for discovering needs and implementing change. For the grievance procedure to be successful, members of management who have decision-making responsibility in a grievance must be credible, fair, and impartial. Second, employees must have an advocate available to assist in preparing and presenting a grievance. All employees should be encouraged to use the grievance process, without fear of reprisal or being labeled as a troublemaker.

- Establishing a Labor Management Committee. This committee is usually found in an agency which has a collective agreement for the purpose of discussing issues not covered in the collective bargaining process (Hemsworth 1978, 6). It also facilitates communications between management and select members of the bargaining unit in the following ways:

  - Allowing employees to share concerns and suggestions regarding agency services.

  - Identifying employee concerns that do not qualify for the grievance procedure and are not within the scope of the supervisor.

  - Providing a mechanism for nursing staff to give input to administration on their policies and procedures.

  - Providing a sounding board for management to get input from staff.

  - Encouraging a feeling of unity throughout the agency in responding to problems.

  - Facilitating a clear and consistent interpretation of the collective bargaining agreement (Centre County Home Health Service Labor Management Committee 1984, 1).

The composition of such a committee is usually an equal number of management and nursing personnel. Management can be represented by the Executive Director, Personnel Director, Nursing Manager, or a member of the agency's board. Members of the collective bargaining unit would represent the nurses.

One agency (Centre County Home Health Service, Bellefonte, PA) which instituted a Labor Management Committee discussed the following issues as part of the monthly agendas, over a period of a year: recruitment of nurses and supervisors; physical plant, including telephone work stations; the need for a nursing support group; charting procedures; agency finances; new services; agreement with local hospital; increasing referrals from special hospitals; employee handbook; and communication patterns.

Some amount of time was spent discussing communication patterns. Staff would hear comments made by management which they perceived as derogatory and resulted in angry feelings and low morale. Discussions centered around how to prevent this from happening and how to establish open, candid communication between management and staff.

Collective Bargaining

Another way in which the labor-management environment is influenced is through collective bargaining. Historically, attempts at collective bargaining were met with resistance by nurses who felt it was not professional to withhold services from patients. The conflict of professionalism versus unionism existed and prevented nurses from bargaining with employers. However, the trend has changed and unionization is now an acceptable way to assure that employers recognize and discuss the economic and professional needs of nurses.

The National Labor Relations Act of 1935 was the first piece of social legislation which required that employers engage in collective bargaining with employees. However, employees in nonprofit health care organizations were not protected by this federal law to engage in collective bargaining. Not until 1947 when the Taft-Hartley amendment to the National Labor Relations Act was passed, could such employees organize. This legislation enabled health care workers to enter the mainstream of American labor to promote their own professionalism and unity.

The American Nurses' Association (ANA), formed in 1896 as a professional organization committed to quality patient care, approved collective bargaining for nurses in 1946. At this time, ANA approved collective bargaining to secure protection for nurses and to assure the public that adequate amounts of high quality nursing care would be available to all sick people (Kruger 1961, 699). Thus began an era when collective action was accepted as one way to assure professionalism. In 1950, however, the ANA members approved a policy that no strikes would occur as this would be inconsistent with nurses' professional responsibility to patients. In 1966, the ANA Commission on Economic and General Welfare determined that changes were necessary in the economic security program and rescinded the "no strike" policy.

During the 1970s, ANA mounted an aggressive campaign to support the nation's nurses in collective bargaining activities. The number of persons covered by collective agreement increased significantly, indicating that ANA was working to advance the economic and general welfare of nurses.

Hemsworth (1978, 20-21) outlines what nurses have gained through collective bargaining:

1. Professional strength through unity

2. The legal right to voice concerns for patient care and professional improvement

3. The right to contribute to the decision-making process through negotiations

4. Improved benefits, including job security

5. The right to challenge rules through the grievance procedures.

These gains have been primarily attained through presentation of a unified approach and negotiation.

Although collective bargaining can be viewed as an infringement of management prerogatives and an interference of the employer-employee relationship, nurses have continued to choose such activities as a way to affect employment conditions and to determine and control their practice.

Summary

In a home health agency, management must strive to create a healthy work environment in which labor-management relationships are positive. Management must be sensitive to perceived staff needs and to ways to meet these needs. Programs should be designed to maximize all employee contributions to the program. Both labor and management must work together using a team approach, effective communication and problem-solving skills, and consulting with each other in an atmosphere of fairness, respect, empathy, and trust. A variety of methods can be used by management to assure that labor-management relations are positive, that quality patient care is achieved, that employee welfare is maximized, and that organization goals are met.

References

Alutto, J.A., and J.A. Belasco. 1972. *Determinants of attitudinal militancy among nurses and teachers.* Bethesda, MD: ERIC Document Reproduction Service, ED 063 635.

Cangemi, J.P., L. Clark, and E. Harryman. 1980. Differences between pro-union and pro-company employees. In *Labor relations in nursing,* ed. C.A. Lockhart and W.B. Werther, Jr. Wakefield, MA: Nursing Resources.

Centre County Home Health Service Labor Management Committee. 1984. *Minutes of Meeting, May 23, 1984,* p. 1.

Cushman, D. 1980. Organizing campaigns: An analysis of management's use of communication techniques, suggestions for union strategy. In *Unionization and the health care industry: Hospital and nursing home employee union leaders conference report,* Nov. 29-Dec. 1, 1978, ed. R.J. Peters, H. Elkiss, and H.T. Higgins, pp. 24-31. University of Illinois at Urbana-Champaign: Institute of Labor and Industrial Relations.

Davis, K. 1958. *Human relations in business.* New York: McGraw Hill.

Gerrard, B.A., W.J. Boniface, and B.H. Love. 1980. *Interpersonal skills for health professionals.* Reston, VA: Reston Hall Publishing Co.

Ginzberg, E. 1966. *The development of human resources.* New York: McGraw Hill.

Golightly, C.K. 1981. *Creative problem solving for health care professionals.* Rockville, MD: Aspen Systems Corporation.

Gregorich, P. and J.W. Long. 1980. Responsive management fosters cooperative environment. In *Labor relations in nursing,* ed. C.A. Lockhart and W.B. Werther, Jr. Wakefield, MA: Nursing Resources.

Hemsworth, M.J. 1978. *Nurses in collective bargaining.* Ann Arbor, MI: University Microfilms International.

Kruger, D.H. 1961. Bargaining and the nursing profession. *Monthly Labor Review* 84 (July 1961): 699.

Levitan, S.A., G.L. Mangum, and R. Marshall. 1981. *Human resources and labor markets: Employment and training in the American economy,* 3rd ed. New York: Harper & Row.

Lockhart, C.A. and W.B. Werther, Jr. 1980. *Labor relations in nursing.* Wakefield, MA: Nursing Resources.

Meyer, G.D. 1970. *Determinants of collective action attitudes among hospital nurses: An empirical test,* Ph.D. Dissertation, The University of Iowa.

Rothstein, J. 1958. *Communication, organization and science.* Indian Hills, CO: Falcon's Wing Press.

Scott, W.G. 1962. *Human relations in management: A behavioral science approach.* Homewood, IL: Richard D. Irwin, Inc.

Spradley, B.W. 1985. *Community health nursing: Concepts and practice,* 2nd ed. Boston: Little, Brown & Co.

Vroom, V.H. and P.W. Yetton. 1976. *Leadership and decision-making: Basic considerations underlying the normative model.* In Concepts and controversy in organizational behavior, 2nd ed., ed. W.R. Nord. Pacific Palisades, CA: Goodyear Publishing Co.

Werther, W.B., Jr., and C.A. Lockhart. 1980. Collective action and cooperation in the health professions. In *Labor relations in nursing*, ed. C.A. Lockhart and W.B. Werther, Jr.

Wakefield, MA: Nursing Resources.
Zacur, S. 1982. *Health care labor relations: The nursing perspective.* Ann Arbor: University Microfilms International Press.

Chapter Eleven

Personnel Management and Issues for Home Health Administration

Jerry L. Sellentin

The most important resource we have is the human resource. The successful management of human resources can result in employee satisfaction, commitment, increased efficiency, and improved productivity. To achieve successful management of an organization's human resources is more than having a "concern for people" or having a Personnel Department that handles "people" problems. Today, organizations are learning to give employees the same priority they have for capital and equipment. Human resources are the crucial factor that makes everything work effectively.

History

The early history of personnel obscures the importance of personnel function to management. Until the 1960s, the personnel function was viewed as a recordkeeping unit that handed out 25-year tenure pins and coordinated the annual company picnic (Foulkes 1975, 71-72).

"In the past," says John L. Quigley, Vice President of Human Resources, Dr. Pepper Company, "the personnel executive was the 'glad hands' or 'back slapper' who kept morale up in a company by running the company picnic, handling the United Fund drive and making sure the recreation program went off well."

The late 1960s and early 1970s were turbulent years for health care in general and management departments in particular. Among the external influences affecting personnel management in health care were:

- Enactment of the 1964 Civil Rights Act which mandated equal employment opportunity and had a significant effect on selection, testing, performance appraisal, promotion, demotion, equal pay for equal work, and nondiscrimination in matters of employment.

- Enactment of other federal legislation such as OSHA which forced attention on safety in the work environment, and ERISA in 1974 affecting benefits administration.

- Increased unionization in hospitals began in the late 1960s and was supported with passage of the 1974 Nonprofit Hospitals Amendments to the Taft-Hartley Act (Robbins and Rackick 1986, 21-22).

The era of the new worker, self-fulfillment seeker, government regulation increases, and critical productivity challenges has brought a new responsibility to the personnel function. This is perhaps the greatest change in the personnel function that has occurred in the last decade (Cook 1984, 19). Thus, the personnel function is proactive in monitoring and improving the employment climate.

Peter Drucker states, "Above all, the Personnel Department will have to redirect itself away from concern with the cost of employees to concerns with their yield." The greatest change ahead for the personnel function may be its mission. The Personnel Department, as we know it, dates back to World War I, to a time when nine out of ten employees were "labor" doing undifferentiated, unskilled work. Then, "labor" was a "cost" and the first job of personnel was to keep costs down. But in today's business, at least three out of ten employees fit the "labor" category. The rest do highly differentiated, and in most cases, specialized work. They are not "labor," they are "resources," and resources have to be managed for optimum yield rather than for minimum cost (Drucker 1986).

Key Functions for Human Resources Management

Another view of the importance of controlling employee costs is seen with a survey conducted by the Fleming Associates, Inc. Executive Search Consultants. Two hundred sixty-nine top human resources executives were asked the question, "What critical issues or pressure points will have the greatest impact on you while performing your job responsibilities from now until the end of 1985?" This question was followed by a list of 24 issues on which the respondents were asked to indicate individual importance on a scale of one (lowest priority) to ten (highest priority). See Table 11-1.

The results of this survey reemphasize the concern with the fundamental issue of cost control. It also reveals a growing concern to improve communication. Employee communications is the link by which management enrolls the worker as a valuable part of the organization's team.

Personnel management is a set of activities that must be managed. All organizations with people in them must deal with specific personnel activities of staffing, work analysis, training and development, appraisal, compensation, maintenance, and union relations. Notice that the definition emphasizes the personnel activities, not who performs them (Mathis and Jackson 1985, 11). Personnel management is conducted at all managerial levels. Therefore, all managers are responsible for personnel issues.

Staffing

A foundation of personnel management is interviewing and hiring, choosing the right person for the right job. Hiring the wrong person can be costly in terms of both money and time. The aim is to choose the best candidate from a group of applicants. Often, personality or appearance influences us. Sometimes we hire someone who is over-qualified or we may neglect to make certain the applicant has the necessary qualifications, skills, or eduction to do the job.

There is no foolproof method for interviewing and selecting, often it is a "gut feeling." Until the person is on the job and performing as required, you don't know if you have been successful in your interview. Choosing the right person requires thorough

Table 11-1. Following are the results of the survey with comparison for 1982 and 1983:

Pressure point	1984/1985 Average Critical Value	1984/1985 Ranking	1982/1983 Ranking
Controlling costs of employee benefits programs	8.52	1	2
Employee communications	7.60	2	4
Compensation planning and administration	7.57	3	3
Productivity improvement programs	7.55	4	1
Upgrading management training and development programs	7.38	5	5
Organizational development programs	7.36	6	6
Management succession planning	7.14	7	7
Improving employee morale	7.05	8	8
Human resources information systems	6.45	9	9
Quality improvement programs	6.41	10	10
Recruitment of midlevel and senior management talent	6.27	11	11
Promotional opportunities for female and minority employees	6.09	12	13
Union avoidance programs	6.05	13	12
Recruitment of midlevel and senior technical or engineering personnel	5.74	14	15
Administering health and accident prevention programs	5.53	15	19
Improvements of employee benefits program	5.38	16	17
Compliance with OSHA/EEOC and other governmental regulations	5.18	17	18
Recruitment of entry-level management talent	5.13	18	22
Reducing employee turnover	4.62	19	20
Labor relations and contract negotiations	4.54	20	16
Employee relocation costs	4.44	21	14
Outplacement counseling	4.13	22	23
Employee willingness to relocate	3.76	23	21
Union decertification programs	2.24	24	24

Reprinted with permission from Fleming Associates.

preparation which includes asking the right questions and listening effectively to the responses of the applicant.

The following questions can help you in your selection process, further questions for each category can be developed to fit the level of the job for which you are interviewing.

Work History

Tell me about your last job.

What did you enjoy doing most (least) on your last job? Why?

What did you admire most about your boss?

What would your ideal job be?

Do you enjoy work?

Education

What courses did you take?

How well did you do?

Why did you select your course of study?

What extracurricular activities did you enjoy most?

How will your education help you perform the job you are applying for?

Attitudes and feelings

Describe yourself—your accomplishments, strengths, and why you feel you would succeed in this position.

What would the people who work with you say about you?

What are your biggest weaknesses?

What are your ambitions?

What else do you think I should know about you and your qualifications?

These sample questions focus on past behaviors and require an applicant to discuss their qualifications, skills, experience, education, and attitudes as they relate to the job.

A critical understanding of Equal Employment Opportunity laws, regulations, and court cases is mandatory to be an effective interviewer. In the interview process, this relates to the questions you can and cannot ask. Table 11-2 reviews 17 areas as to how EEO applies to the hiring process.

Table 11-2.

Subject of Inquiry	It is <u>not</u> discriminatory to inquire about:	It <u>may be</u> discriminatory to inquire about:
1. Name	a. Whether applicant had ever worked under a different name	a. The original name of an applicant whose name had been legally changed b. The ethnic association of applicant's name
2. Birthplace and residence	a. Applicant's place of residence, length of applicant's residence in Nebraska and/or city where employer is located	a. Birthplace of applicant b. Birthplace of applicant's parents c. Birth certificate, naturalization or baptismal certificate
3. Race or color	a. General distinguishing characteristics such as scars, etc.	a. Applicant's race or color of applicant's skin
4. National origin and ancestry		a. Applicant's lineage, ancestry, national origin, descendants, parentage or nationality b. Nationality of applicant's parents or spouse
5. Sex and family composition		a. Sex of applicant b. Dependents of applicant c. Marital status
6. Creed or Religion		a. Applicant's religious affiliation b. Church, parish or religious holidays observed
7. Citizenship	a. Whether the applicant is in the country on a visa, which permits him to work or is a citizen	a. Whether applicant is a citizen of a country other than the United States
8. Language	a. Language applicant speaks or writes fluently	a. Applicant's mother tongue, language commonly used by applicant at home
9. References	a. Names of persons willing to provide professional or character references for applicant	a. Name of applicant's pastor or religious leader
10. Relatives	a. Names of relatives already employed by the Company b. Name and address of person or relative to be notified in an emergency	a. Name and address of any relatives of applicant
11. Organizations	a. Applicant's membership in any union, professional service or trade organization	a. All clubs, social fraternities societies, lodges, or organizations to which the name or character of the organization indicates the race, creed, color, religion, national origin, sex or ancestry of its members
12. Arrest Record and convictions		a. Number and kinds of arrests and convictions unless related to job performance

Table 11-2, continued.

Subject of Inquiry	It is *not* discriminatory to inquire about:	It *may be* discriminatory to inquire about:
13. Photographs		a. Photographs with application before hiring b. Resume with photo of applicant
14. Height and weight		a. Any inquiry into height and weight of applicant, except where it is a bona fide occupational requirement
15. Physical Limitations	a. Whether applicant has the ability to perform job related functions	a. Whether an applicant is handicapped, or the nature or severity of a handicap
16. Education	a. Training an applicant has received if related to the job applied for	a. Educational attainment of an applicant unless there is validation that having certain educational backgrounds (i.e., high school diploma or college degree) is necessary to perform the functions of the job or position applied for
17. Financial Status		a. An applicant's debts or assets b. Garnishments

Source: Human Relations Department, Omaha, Nebraska. Reprinted by permission.

The next major impact of the hiring process in the 1990s will be the use of computers in the selection interview. To overcome subjectivity and personal biases, the computer will be used and will be effective, especially, as it relates to asking the proper questions and determining what the applicant really meant by their response.

Job Analysis

The process of determining the duties and skills required for performing jobs in an organization is referred to as job analysis (Mundy and Noe 1984, 76). What is the worker doing? In most cases, each job, like its job holder, is unique and the requirements and control of each job must be understood to perform other personnel functions satisfactorily. It is also important as it relates to productivity of the worker and the impact of how compensation decisions relate to job analysis. Gathering information about the job would include the following questions.

Sample Questions For Data Collection in the Job Analysis (Gordon 1986, 36):

1. What tasks does the job comprise?

2. What does a typical workday look like?

3. What is the frequency and duration of each job activity?

4. How complex is each job activity?

5. What job activities are related and how are they related?

6. How much supervisory responsibility does the job entail?

7. To whom does the job holder report?

8. What budgetary responsibilities does the job include?

9. What qualifications are required of job holders?

10. What mental and physical demands are placed on job holders?

11. What expectations do supervisors and co-workers have of the job holder.

12. What outcomes reflect acceptable job performance? Outstanding job performance?

Compensation

Pay is important to the worker and the organization. Part of the importance of pay is whether or not a person is receiving what he thinks he should receive. Compensation refers to every type of reward that individuals receive in return for performing organizational tasks. An employee may see compensation as a return for services rendered or a reward for satisfactory or meritorious work.

Pay systems are designed to attract and retain competent workers, reward individual performance, maintain consistency by paying employees with similar responsibilities similar pay, cost control within goals established by the company, and to conform with various state and federal wage and salary laws and guidelines.

Compensation systems need to be developed to reinforce the mission and strategies of an organization. To do this, it is necessary to keep in mind the organization's culture, values, and external factors such as the economy, market, laws, regulations, and labor unions. To maximize compensation systems, organizations are moving toward programs which provide pay for performance. The performance appraisal system has defined standards which relate to performance.

Planning

As more and more emphasis is placed on planning, as opposed to reacting, the personnel function should address personnel needs to internal and external changes. Emerging "trends" centering around the need to have a linkage with strategic and business issues include:

- A strong desire to influence individual performance.

- An overwhelming concern for the management of business change.
- An intense line management orientation.
- A recognition of the need for effective planning.

Training and development

Training is a set of activities designed to increase an individual's skills, knowledge, or experience, or to change an individual's attitude. Development refers to preparing individuals to assume higher levels of responsibilities or different responsibilities. Training and development will become increasingly important with a shortage of technical and professional employees in health care along with a flexible work force, newer technology, consumer expectations, and competition. Cross-training will be a high priority to meet changing service demands.

Labor Relations

Employees have joined together so that, as individuals, they do not have to stand alone against the power of an employer.

Today, unions are struggling against a tough economy and other ills resulting in a decline in unions in the manufacturing industries. As a result, unions are developing among professional employees, and government workers because of concerns related to job security and working conditions.

Human Resources needs to diagnose and correct problems in such areas as wages and salaries, staffing, benefits, safety, discipline, management techniques, and job security.

The November 1986 *Personnel Administrator* in an article by L. James Harvey highlights nine major trends which will affect the health care industry as follows:

1. Increasing importance of the human resource function.

2. A move toward centralized policy and control and decentralized operations.

3. Increased management development.

4. Increased automation and Human Resource Information Systems development.

5. Human Resource program integration.

6. Move to merit and accountability.

7. Increased concern for employee attitudes.

8. Increased concern for organizational culture and values.

9. Increased and broadened productivity improvement programs.

References

Cook, F. 1984. *Human resource director's handbook.* Englewood Cliffs, NJ: Prentice-Hall, Inc.

Drucker, P. F. 1986. Goodbye to the personnel department. May 22, 1986 *Wall Street Journal.*

Foulkes, F. K. March-April 1975. The expanding role of the personnel function. *Harvard Business Review.*

Gordon, J. R. 1986. *Human resource management A practical approach.* Newton, MA: Allyn and Bacon, Inc.

Mathis, R. L., and J. H. Jackson. 1985. *Personnel human resource management,* 4th ed. St. Paul, MN: West Publishing Company.

Mundy, R. and R. M. Noe, III. 1984. *Personnel: The management of human resources,* 2nd ed. Newton, MA: Allyn and Bacon, Inc.

Robbins, S. A., and J. S. Rackick. July-August 1986. Hospital personnel management in the late 1980s: A direction for the future. *Hospital Health Services Administration.*

Chapter Twelve

Staff Development in a Home Health Agency

Joan Reynolds Yuan

> Nursing is a progressive art, in which to stand still is to go back. A woman who thinks to herself, "Now I am a full nurse, a skilled nurse, I have learnt all there is to be learnt." Take my word for it, she does not know what a nurse is, and never will know. She has gone back already. Progress can never end but with a nurse's life.
>
> *Nightingale 1914*

The concept of furthering one's education is an age-old one in nursing. Traditionally, it has been an important area in community health agencies. Currently, education and staff development are vital to the existence of any community or home health agency. In this era of high tech-high touch home care, an extensive knowledge base, sharp technical skills, and appropriate attitudes are necessities for providing quality care to patients, families, and communities, preventing litigation, and remaining in business. With a view to the individual, one considers personal and professional growth, stimulation, motivation, and increasing or maintaining competence. In viewing an agency, one considers the necessity for providing quality care to clients. To accomplish this, a qualified staff must be employed. With advances in theory and technology, education is necessary to ensure understanding and competence.

Ongoing education is mandated by regulatory and accrediting bodies such as the National League for Nursing (NLN). The National League for Nursing in its *Administrative Handbook for Community Health and Home Care Services* advises that education be a cyclic, ongoing process (NLN 1984).

The Medicare Conditions of Participation mandate education. This is evidenced by these sections:

Section 405.1221. "The administrator . . . employs qualified personnel and ensures adequate staff education and evaluations." (Department of Health, Education, and Welfare 1973, 18980)

Section 405.1224. "The registered nurse . . . participates in inservice programs . . ." (Department of Health, Education, and Welfare 1973, 18981)

Section 405.1225. "The qualified therapist participates in inservice programs." (Department of Health, Education, and Welfare 1973, 18981)

Section 405.1226. "The social worker participates in inservice programs. . ." (Department of Health, Education, and Welfare, 1973, 18981)

Section 405.1227. "Home health aides . . . are carefully trained. . ." (Department of Health, Education, and Welfare, 1973, 18981)

To assist in the task of accomplishing the goals of education in a home health agency, staff development and its educational components will be addressed. "Staff Development is a process consisting of orientation, in-service education, and continuing education for the purpose of promoting the development of personnel within any employment setting consistent with the goals and responsibilities of the employer" (ANA 1984, 5). According to NLN's Administrative Handbook (NLN 1984, 233), "Staff development involves planned employee growth and change that allows the agency to increase its abilities to provide effective and efficient care to the community served."

Central to the staff development program in a community or home health agency is the philosophy that will guide its actions. According to the American Nurses' Association's (ANA) *Guidelines for Staff Development*, components to consider in the development of this philosophy are:

1. The staff development program is an essential component of the agency.

2. The philosophy and objectives of the staff development program reflect the philosophy and objectives of the agency.

3. Administration and staff share the responsibility to support and promote learning experiences to ensure current knowledge and practice.

4. Each employee shares the responsibility with the employer to identify needs and to seek ways to meet these needs.

5. A role of the staff development supervisor is to facilitate the implementation of standards, policies, and procedures through planning, conducting, and evaluating learning activities (ANA 1978).

The title of the person responsible for staff development will vary from one organization to the next. Such titles may include director of education, nursing supervisor, or staff development supervisor. In this chapter, the person responsible for staff development will be referred to as the staff development supervisor.

Clearly stated goals consistent with the philosophy give direction to the staff development supervisor. These may include:

1. Fostering a climate in which the staff members identify their learning needs and seek ways to meet these needs.

2. Facilitating constructive working relationships with an interdisciplinary committee in planning, implementing, and evaluating staff development programs.

3. Designing a staff development program which facilitates the attainment of standards of care.

4. Conducting a staff development program relevant to the learning needs of staff and the goals of the agency.

5. Assisting the staff members to acquire the knowledge and skills necessary to perform their job requirements.

6. Using the expertise of other professionals in providing learning opportunities.

7. Promoting an environment conducive to learning that contributes to job enrichment and personal growth of the employees (ANA 1978).

Responsibility and accountability for improving nursing practice through staff development lies with the employer and the employee (ANA 1978). The roles and responsibilities of the staff, administration, and staff development supervisor will be addressed.

Roles and Responsibilities of the Individual Employee

The role of individual staff members involves active participation in educational programs and endeavors. In ANA's *Guidelines for Staff Development*, the responsibilities of the individual employee include, but are not limited to the following:

- Identify learning needs. Take the initiative to seek out learning opportunities both within and outside the agency to meet these needs.

- Make learning needs known to the appropriate sources.

- Share information obtained from learning activities.

- Seek opportunities to apply new knowledge and skills (ANA 1978).

Roles and Responsibilities of Administration

The achievement of the educational mission of the agency ultimately rests with the agency administrator. Administrative support is vital to the success of the educational program. In ANA's *Guidelines for Staff Development*, the responsibilities of administration include but are not limited to the following:

- Establish policies related to continuing education participation by personnel.

- Assist personnel in the identification of learning needs.

- Provide opportunities for learning experiences; provide time and finances for staff to attend educational programs outside the agency when appropriate.

- Provide opportunities for the sharing of new information.

- Provide recognition for participation in continuing education programs.

- Evaluate changes in performance.

- Evaluate the effects of the staff development department on the quality of health care.

- Seek resources to provide reference materials (ANA 1978).

Roles and Responsibilities of the Staff Development Supervisor

The role of the staff development supervisor in a home health agency is complex. Responsibilities include continuing education, in-service education, and orientation of employees. Depending upon the size and educational philosophy of the organization, the staff development supervisor may be responsible for an agencywide staff development program for all employees. This position requires a blend of educational, clinical, and administrative knowledge and expertise. It is commonly filled by a nurse with a master's degree. Depending upon the structure of the organization, this person reports directly to the executive director or the director of professional services. The staff development supervisor may not have line responsibilities, but power is inherent in the role. In many organizations, this supervisor by virtue of his educational background, experience, and knowledge of the organization, has the authority for decision making in the absence of the executive director and the director of professional services. During orientation he is the first to determine if a new employee is suitable for the organization. He is responsible for the development, education, and training of nursing supervisors. He must be able to address the long-term educational needs of the employees (Stevens 1980).

ANA's *Guidelines for Staff Development* (1978) advise that the responsibilities of the staff development supervisor include but are not limited to the following:

- Establish and use the assistance of an education committee. It is advisable that this committee is interdisciplinary.
- Contribute to the development of the philosophy, objectives, policies, and procedures related to staff development.
- Participate in establishing program priorities.
- Provide leadership in formulating the philosophy and objectives of the staff development program in accordance with that of the agency and identifying necessary funds to maintain a budget.
- Identify the learning needs of the employees.
- Plan the offerings, communicate the plans for the programs, and encourage and foster participation.
- Implement the plan to meet learning needs.
- Evaluate results of the staff development program.
- Participate in counseling employees about their educational needs.
- Participate in research activities and evaluate reported research findings for application to staff development programming.
- Develop and maintain a record system to document achievement of program goals.
- Pursue professional growth and development.

Evaluation of the staff development program is a continuous process to appraise effectiveness. Information gathered in this process can be used for future planning.

According to ANA's *Guidelines for Staff Development* the following criteria may be utilized in evaluating the staff development program:

1. Administrative support is present.

2. Program is consistent with the philosophy.

3. Qualified personnel, adequate facilities and resources are available.

4. Allocation of funds to accomplish program goals.

5. Periodic review of program content and goals.

6. Recordkeeping system is maintained.

7. Utilization of adult education principles.

8. Appropriate utilization of community resources and other health disciplines (ANA 1978).

Formal Education

In this era of high-tech home care, and economic restrictions, the need for highly skilled professionals with a broad knowledge base is evident. Many agencies require a BSN or that a registered nurse be working toward a BSN for entry into the organization. The need for specialists in clinical and administrative areas is growing; hence, the need for graduate education. Personnel policies should include provisions for furthering one's formal education. This can range from having time off and flexible scheduling to attend classes to taking a leave of absence or a sabbatical. This encompasses undergraduate as well as graduate education.

Within the personnel policies, educational leave may be addressed as follows:

- Requests for time off or leave for educational purposes will be submitted to the executive director for individual consideration. A maximum of two hours per week with pay will be made available, as possible, for full-time employees. Additional time may be taken without pay or accrued vacation time used.

- Seniority will not be affected by educational leave.

- No time benefits will be accrued during full-time educational leave.

- Anniversary date will be adjusted according to length of leave.

- Employee will assume full cost of hospitalization during a leave of absence.

- Scholarship fund: Grants to applicants for approved part-time study shall not exceed $1200.00 per fiscal year for graduate studies and $900.00 per fiscal year for undergraduate studies. Fund is available to all staff for academic study that is job-related.

Sabbatical leave: After each seven consecutive years of service, an employee may apply for a sabbatical leave of two months with pay in addition to regular vacation. The sabbatical leave is for educational purposes. Time from one seven-year period may not be carried over to a second seven-year period. A two-month period may be divided.*

Among the benefits to an organization of utilizing the sabbatical are employee retention, stimulation of employees, development of employee talent, and increased commitment to the organization. However, the organization must cope with finding temporary replacements and reentry into the organization (Curran 1985).

Continuing Education

One component of staff development is continuing education. In ANA's *Standard's for Continuing Education in Nursing*, continuing education is defined as ". . . those planned educational activities intended to build upon the educational and experiential bases of the professional nurse for the enhancement of practice, education, administration, research, or theory development to the end of improving the health of the public." (ANA 1984, 5)

The staff development supervisor controls the budget for the continuing education programs. Since funds are not endless, there must be a determination as to how much money is allotted for each person. To get as much for the educational dollar as possible, other avenues should be investigated. Affiliating educational institutions may allow a free conference for an agency staff member in exchange for using the agency as a site for student experience. Participation in a planning committee and a cooperative effort with a providing institution can be another way that the agency can have staff attend a conference free of charge or at a discounted rate.

Many good continuing education programs are available throughout the country. Information regarding the continuing education programs can be posted for staff perusal. The individual staff member files a request to attend a conference. Depending on the conference, staffing, and budget, the request is granted or not granted by the staff development supervisor. Although time off to attend a conference is costly, not to mention the cost of the conference itself, it is usually most helpful for the professional to meet with colleagues from other organizations and broaden one's scope. Attending conferences outside the institution often increases job satisfaction as well as ultimately having a positive effect on patient care. It is often valuable to have the individual report the findings from the conference to his colleagues.

It is important that accurate records are kept. The supervisor will maintain records of the conferences attended by members of all disciplines. In addition, a record is kept in the personnel folder.

If an agency is planning to provide continuing education courses, guidance can be obtained from the following ANA materials: *Standards for Continuing Education in Nursing* (1984) and *Continuing Education in Nursing: An Overview* (1979). These are available through the American Nurses' Association, 2420 Pershing Road, Kansas City, MO 64108. In some areas of the country, continuing education programs are not readily available. Independent study and self-learning modules can help fill this void. (See *Self-Directed Continuing Education in Nursing* (1978), available through ANA.)

---

* Adapted and reprinted by permission of the Visiting Nurse Association of Eastern Montgomery County, Abington, Pennsylvania.

In-service Education

In-service education has been defined in ANA's *Standards for Continuing Education in Nursing* as "...activities intended to assist the professional nurse to acquire, maintain, and/or increase competence in fulfilling the assigned responsibilities specific to the expectations of the employer" (ANA 1984, 5)

To have a viable in-service program it must be backed by the administration. It is the responsibility of the staff development supervisor to assess the educational needs of the employees. A regularly administered needs assessment tool is helpful. In-service education can be required in several different areas (Stevens 1980). Preparatory education such as a physical assessment course may be required. Supplemental education such as management theory may be necessary. Maintenance education for CPR certification, new product education, or new procedure education many times is indicated. Remedial education for foundational support is another area that is addressed by the staff development supervisor.

Planning the in-services is the responsibility of the staff development supervisor with the assistance of the interdisciplinary education committee. It is recommended that a long-range 12-month plan be made. However, this must be flexible, as new products, new procedures, and new needs arise throughout the course of the year. In planning in-services, one must consider the cost of providing the in-service, including the cost of the instructor, materials, and the time of the staff. It is important to remember that the time that the staff spends in in-service must be deducted from the time spent on reimbursable patient care activities. Consideration must be given to utilizing the least amount of time required to accomplish the task adequately. For example, CPR recertification may be given to two staff members in one-hour increments, rather than four staff members in two-hour increments. If the staff is recertified in one-hour increments rather than two, an additional hour becomes available for reimbursable patient activities.

The characteristics of the adult learner is another important area for consideration in planning in-services. Adult learning principles have been defined by ANA as "Approaches to adults as learners based on recognition of the individual's autonomy and self-direction, life experiences, readiness to learn, and problem-orientation to learning. Approaches include mutual, respectful collaboration of teachers and learners in planning, diagnosing needs, formulating objectives, designing sequences, and evaluating learning. Learning activities tend to be experiential and inquiry focused." (ANA 1984, 15) For example, an in-service on diabetic management would include hands on experience with a glucose-monitoring device.

Resources to consider utilizing for in-services include the agency's staff. An adult nurse practitioner may teach physical assessment. A physical therapist may teach proper body mechanics or chest PT. A social worker may discuss community resources available. Staff attending conferences can have valuable information to share. Schools of nursing can be another valuable resource. State school extensions may have staff such as a nutritionist that is available as an educational resource. Community resources such as the American Cancer Society can be utilized. Manufacturers of equipment such as colostomy supplies, ventilators, glucometers are often utilized.

Implementation should be carried out in accordance with written policy. The in-service should take place in an appropriate meeting room. If the agency does not have sufficient space, arrangements can be made with a local church, library, or school.

The staff development supervisor will keep attendance records of the in-services. Individual staff members will maintain educational program records to be collected annually and kept in the personnel file.

Evaluating educational programs is not an easy task. A written content evaluation is one method. The result of education is an increase in knowledge or skill. The quality assurance program can be utilized to assess the effects of education on patient care. According to ANA's *Guidelines for Staff Development*, the following criteria can be utilized in the evaluation of educational offerings:

- Offering is relevant to the learning needs of the individual, health needs of the consumer, and goals of the agency.

- Principles of adult education are used.

- Persons knowledgeable about the content area are involved in planning, conducting, and evaluating the program. Objectives include expected measurable outcomes for the learner.

- Teaching methods are appropriate for achieving the objectives.

- Adequate facilities and resources are available.

- Records are maintained.

Orientation

Orientation has been defined in ANA's *Standards for Continuing Education in Nursing* (ANA 1984, 5) as ". . .the means by which new staff are introduced to the philosophy, goals, policies, procedures, role expectations, physical facilities, and special services in a specific work setting. Orientation is provided at the time of employment and at other times when changes in roles and responsibilities occur in a specific work setting."

The staff development supervisor has the responsibility to orient new employees to the organization as a whole. He orients new nursing personnel to the nursing service department. Depending on the structure of the organization he may be responsible for specific orientation to other departments as well. In a general orientation, the new employee is introduced to the physical setting, specific work area, and personnel. The philosophy, purpose, and goals of the organization are addressed. The spirit of the organization is discussed. For example, this is a team effort. Each job is important to the functioning of the organization. The attitudes of all staff members are important in a service organization. In this highly competitive era, one must be aware of the treatment of the consumer. A lesson can be learned by looking at the orientation process at organizations like Disney where attitudes toward the consumer are of paramount importance. The administrative policies and procedures are reviewed. Orientation to the specific job is provided either by the staff development supervisor or an expert member of the staff. See sample orientation form for a nursing department (Exhibit 12-1).

Exhibit 12-1.

Visiting Nurse Association Of Eastern Montgomery County

Orientation Program

Name:_____ _____ Date of Employment:_____

Position:_____

	Date	Signature
Day One: Field Observation with Staff		
Day Two: I. Orientation to Agency Policies		
A. Introduction to VNA-EMC		
1) Philosophy		
2) Organizaiton		
a) Organization Chart		
b) Functions of Board and Board Committees		
c) Relationship of Nurse to Agency Board of Directors		
3) Introduction to Office Personnel & Facilities		
4) Sources of Financial Support. (United Way, County Commissioners, Boroughs & Townships, Fee for Service)		
5) Geographic Area Served		
6) Scope of Services: Total Program & Services Provided		
B. Personnel Policies: Review & Discussion		
1) Payroll Procedure		
2) Schedule of Pay, Time Hours of Work		
3) Auto Insurance /Reimbursement		
4) Dress Code		
5) Insurance Benefits		
6) Reporting Illness		
7) Staff Inservice Meetings, Outside Activities & Advanced Individual Educational Opportunities		

Exhibit 12-1, continued.

VNA of EMC
Orientation Program   Page 2

	Date	Signature

Day Two, cont'd:

    II. Relationship of Nurse to Other Members
        of Staff: RN's, PT, OT, ST, MSW, HHA's

        A. Individual Responsibilities & Relationships

        B. Coordination of Services

    III. Field Assignments: Days & Type of Patient
         Services

    IV. Criteria for Admission of Patients to VNA

        A. Skilled Care vs Non-skilled Care

    V. Discussion of Referral Sources

        A. Hospital: Social Worker, Discharge
           Planner, Liaison

        B. Doctor

        C. Family

        D. Social Agencies

        E. Staff

    VI. Relationship of VNA-EMC to Other Agencies
         & Organization

        A. Contractual Agreements with Home
           Care Departments

        B. Contractual Agreement with Other Agencies

        C. Contractual Agreement with Homemaker
           Home Health Agencies

Day Three: I. Funding Sources: Discussion of the
         Requirements of the Following Funding Sources:

        A. Medicare

        B. Medicaid

        C. Blue Cross

        D. Home Care Departments

        E. Private Insurance

        F. Veterans Administration

Exhibit 12-1, continued.

VNA of EMC
Orientation Program

	Date	Page 3 Signature

Day Three, cont'd:

    I Funding Sources, cont'd:

        G. Self Pay
           1) Full Pay

           2) Part Pay/Fee Adjustment

           3) No Charge

        H. Discussion of Health Promotion
           Patients

    II Instructions on Use of Day Sheets

    III Discharge of Patients from VNA

        A. PMU's

        B. Discharge Codes

    IV Regulations Governing Home Health Aides

        A. Type of Care Provided

        B. Supervision of Care

        C. Necessary HHA Forms

Day Four: I Format for Documentation of Services
           Provided to Patient

        A. Instructions on Use of Problem Oriented
           Record (POR)

        B. Practice Formulating Problem

        C. Charting for Home Care Patients

        D. Charting for Hospice Patients

        E. Charting for Patients from
           Palliative Care Unit

        F. Charting for Contract Agency

        G. Completion of Necessary Forms for
           Admission to Service

        H. Recertification of Patients

Exhibit 12-1, continued.

VNA of EMC
Orientation Program

| | | Page 4 |
| | Date | Signature |

Day Four, cont'd:

    I   Format for Documentation of Services
        Provided to Patient, cont'd.

        I. Discussion of all other Forms
            Utilized in the Agency

        J. Discussion of Paper Flow

    II Orientation to Dictation

    III Review of Medical Policies and
         Standing Orders

    IV Review of Policies and Procedures

    V Discussion of Professional Ethic

    VI Explanation of the Role of Supervisor
         and the Methods Which Will be Used
         for Evaluating Performance and
         Identifying Needs

Clinical policies and procedures are reviewed with the professional staff. In the nursing department, the nurse completes a skills check list (Exhibit 12-2). This allows for individualization of the orientation program. It enables the staff development supervisor to identify the learning needs of the new employee and it enables the new employee to request a review of clinical skills that have not been fully developed.

Documentation is an area of concentration in the orientation process. Accuracy in documentation is necessary for both quality care and reimbursement purposes. A preceptor arrangement with an experienced community health nurse and a newly employed nurse can be valuable. It is important for the staff development supervisor not only to review the orientee's documentation, but to make home visits with the new nurse to assess his ability to function as a community health nurse and allow for questions and discussion.

Orientation to a new position within the agency is another area addressed by the staff development supervisor. This becomes important as staff nurses move into supervisory positions. Management training can be done in-house or at area institutions. Many consultants are available for this purpose. This is a vulnerable time for the employee and support in the new role is essential.

Skills Checklist for Community Health Nurse Orientees

NAME: _____ DATE: _____

Activity	Prior Experience When/Where	No Prior Exper.	Rev. Pro.	Satis. Perf.
I Problem Oriented Method of Recording				
a) Completes Nursing Assessment Problem				
b) Establishes Appropriate List				
c) Establishes Plan of Care and Completes Flow Sheet				
d) Writes Pertinent SOAP Notes				
e) Writes a Discharge Summary Based on Problem List				
II Routine Procedures				
a) Male Catheterization				
b) Female Catheterization				
c) Insertion of Supra-pubic Tube				
d) Care of Gastrostomy/Jejunostomy Tube				
e) Insertion of N/G Tube				
f) Tube Feedings				
g) Insertion of Kao-feed Tube				
h) Use of Enteral Feeding Pumps				
i) IV Therapy: 1) Insertion				
2) Maintenance				
j) Care of Subclavian Catheter To include irrigation of tube and sterile dressing change				
k) Hyperalimentation				
l) Use of Parenteral Feeding Pump				
m) Oxygen Therapy				
n) Cropharyngeal/Nasopharyngeal Suctioning				
o) General Respiratory Care				
p) Tracheotomy Care				
q) General Ostomy Care				
r) Management of a Diabetic Patient				
s) Wound Care/Dressing Changes				
t) EKG				
u) Supervision of Ancillary Personnel				

Documentation of orientation must be provided. This is necessary for both new employees and employees that have changed positions. The employees will sign the orientation forms as well as their job description. This will remain in the personnel file.

Many organizations will maintain a library for staff use. Often, this is the responsibility of the staff development supervisor. Requests for new books and journals are submitted to the staff development supervisor. He oversees the library budget and maintains adequate records. It is particularly helpful to have a library that includes literature related to community health and home care for staff members who are attending school and doing research.

Education in a community or home health agency is viewed not just as a requirement, but as a necessity and an integral part of an organization concerned about the provision of quality care.

References

American Nurses' Association. 1978. *Continuing education in nursing guidelines for staff development.* Kansas City, MO:ANA

American Nurses' Association. 1984. *Standards for continuing education in nursing.* Kansas City, MO:ANA

Department of Health, Education, and Welfare. 1973. Conditions of participation for home health agencies. *Federal Register* 38:18978-18983. Washington, DC: Government Printing Office.

National League for Nursing. 1984. *Administrator's handbook for community health and home care services.* New York: National League for Nursing.

Nightingale, F. 1914. *Florence Nightingale to her nurses.* London:MacMillan & Co.

Stevens, B. 1980. *The nurse as executive.* Rockville, MD: Aspen Systems Corporation.

Chapter Thirteen

Community-Based Long-Term Care: Preparing for a New Role

David M. Eisenberg and Emily Amerman

Introduction

Directing health or social service organizations in an era of fiscal conservancy and heightened budgetary constraint challenges managers' every waking moment. As government and private payors shift costs and tighten reimbursement policies, the truism that "form follows finance" is brought home anew. Reimbursement policy and economic incentives have a profound impact on the delivery of service by home health care providers, indeed, by all providers. Nevertheless, it would be a serious error to allow our vision of service delivery to be limited by current regulatory parameters.

A tremendous demographic and cultural shift is silently occurring; one which will have a major effect on home health care. The number and proportion of older Americans is increasing dramatically. The number of people over the age of 75 is expected to double between 1980 and the year 2000. People over the age of 75 are more likely than younger persons to experience one or more chronic illnesses and other disabling conditions which interfere with their ability to function independently. They are more likely to be at risk of institutionalization in a nursing home or to be in need of ongoing health and social services. As a result of this surge in numbers of disabled older people, the current heavy investment in acute health care services is likely to be balanced by an increasing emphasis on long-term care. The demand for long-term care services will compel policymakers and providers to respond. Ultimately, home health agencies will provide greater and greater proportions of service to patients with needs outside those currently defined as "skilled care."

The combination of increasing demand for long-term care and the interest by governments and private payers in substituting long-term home care for institutional care where clinically and economically feasible, bodes well for home health agencies. The growth in demand for community-based long-term care will create both an opportunity and a challenge for home health agencies in the next decade. For the past four years, home health agencies in Philadelphia have had this opportunity. This chapter describes the "Philadelphia Model" of community-based long-term care and the critical role home health providers play. To place the model in context, current trends in long-term care policy and program are outlined. In concluding, the chapter offers observations and recommendations which may assist home health administrators in planning and competing for involvement in community-based long-term care programs.

263

Long-Term Care Defined

For decades, "long-term care" has referred to a place, or facility, where chronically ill, old people are cared for until they die. The reality is that for every older person in an intermediate or skilled care facility, there are two people who look the same, living in the community. Thus, approximately 5% of those over 65 are in a nursing home at any one time; another 10% who need comparable levels of long-term care are at home. This is due to the fact that the largest provider of long-term care services is the American family. Studies continually demonstrate that about 80% of all long-term care is performed by family caregivers, despite myths to the contrary. Families are caring for a "pool" of highly impaired older people that create ongoing, every-increasing demand for long-term care.

More recent definitions of long term care refer to a systematic plan of care provided over an indefinite time period to chronically ill, functionally disabled adults, most of whom are old. Since many older people have multiple health and social service needs, and since they may not remain medically stable, long-term care must cut across service delivery systems (health, mental health, aging), as well as levels of care. Long-term care consumers may need acute care in a hospital, then restorative care at home, rehabilitation over an extended period, and then maintenance or custodial care. They may need institutional care or they may be cared for at home. The goal of long-term care is to promote the highest level of independent functioning possible in the least restrictive setting, while attending to the client's preferences and assuring his or her safety.

Current Policy and Program Trends

Despite the rapid increase in the number of persons needing long-term care and a high level of interest in community-based care, federal and state investment remains limited almost entirely to institutional care. Only 1 to 2% of the Medicare and Medicaid budgets are spent on home care; almost none on long-term home care. At all times, there is a pool of highly impaired older people residing in the community that forms the basis of the ever present demand for institutional care. Yet the current cost of institutional care is staggering. The Commonwealth of Pennsylvania, for example, during fiscal year 1985, spent almost 10% of its entire state budget on institutional long-term care. As the old-old double in number, policymakers have a powerful incentive to develop a range of long-term care options that are less costly than nursing home care, or face doubling the current investment in institutional care.

The notion of community-based long-term care is not new. For the past 15 years, the Health Care Financing Administration (HCFA) has been experimenting with community-based long-term care for older people at risk of institutionalization. From 1980 to 1985, the federal government financed a nationwide study on the viability of in-home long-term care called The National Long Term Care Channeling Demonstration. Currently, the Reagan Administration is examining private methods of financing community-based long-term care in the form of privately purchased long-term care insurance and medical IRAs. HCFA is studying the efficacy of Health Maintenance Organizations (HMOs) with long-term care benefits added, called Social Health Maintenance Organizations or "SHMOs." Several organizations are designing Continuing Care Communities (CCOs) for older people of more modest means than those initially targeted by CCCs. One foundation is financing "continuing care without walls," whereby participants will receive both in-home long-term care benefits to enable them to remain at home as long as possible and access to nursing home care should such a need arise. Finally, Pennsylvania and other states are continuing experimentation with nursing home "diversion" programs. In these demonstrations, a subset of people applying for and identified as clinically eligible for nursing home care are given the option to remain at home, assisted by a case manager and provided with home health care and other services, at a cost to the state that is lower than the cost of a state-subsidized nursing home bed.

Nationwide, the majority of community-based long-term care demonstrations rely on a model with two principle components: (1) case management, which includes assessment, development of a plan of care, arranging for services, regular follow-up and monitoring of services, and periodic reassessment of the client's needs; and (2) the provision of a range of concrete services which include, at a minimum, home health services, personal care and home management (homemaker) services, heavy cleaning and minor home repairs, home-delivered meals, adult day care, and transportation.

Emerging from practical experience, and increasingly confirmed in the literature, is the fact that nurses and social workers are the two disciplines most appropriate to direct the provision of community-based long-term care. The interrelationships between medical history, current health status, functional capacity, cognitive status, emotional well-being, family relationships and the physical environment are complex and demand the knowledge and skills of both nursing and social work. Nurses or social workers may be selected to provide case management; the best service delivery models use both.

The Area Agency on Aging: A Partner in Service Delivery

Area Agencies on Aging (AAAs) were mandated by the *Older Americans Act* of 1965. Numbering over 600, they form a nationwide network of planning and service agencies focused on the well-being of older citizens. Their major responsibilities include planning, advocacy, program development, and the prudent purchase of services. AAAs prepare an annual Area Plan delineating demographic trends, projected service needs, gaps in service, and priorities for program development and service delivery in their planning and service area. Each year, a fixed allocation of federal and state money, derived from several funding streams, is made to each AAA, with which they are to carry out their plan. AAAs fund a wide array of services for older people including senior center nutrition and recreation programs, health screening and promotion programs, and services to home-bound people, such as home-delivered meals, homemaker, and chore services. In their role as advocate for older people, AAAs often fund employment programs, legal services, and public education programs on issues related to aging. AAAs also may host a nursing home ombudsman.

In their role as "prudent purchaser," AAAs develop specific program standards and specifications for services. Since they are not usually direct service providers, they endeavor to create and encourage a climate of healthy competition between providers. Whenever feasible, AAAs select service providers on a competitive basis so that all potential providers in the service area have the opportunity to seek public funding to deliver services to AAA clients. Providers are selected on the basis of written proposals, price, in-person presentations, and other criteria. This process promotes high quality of care and simultaneously keeps prices down.

As public purse strings have tightened and public policy has become even more budget-driven, a new role has emerged for AAAs: that of "gatekeeper." With public resources both costly and scarce, states are becoming increasingly interested in the AAA's capacity to conserve resources by (a) assuring that the most needy people are served and (b) using scarce and costly resources prudently. The AAA is viewed by policymakers as a logical choice for gatekeeper because of its ability to assess need and allocate resources, without being affected by the economic incentives that drive the behavior of provider agencies. Provider agencies have incentives to prescribe their particular service, and prescribe it in amounts and ways that increase revenue but decrease burden and expense. AAAs, who are one step removed, are in a more objective position to determine client eligibility and to conserve public dollars. Organizations naturally view patients' needs in terms of the solutions they have most readily available—whether or not other approaches to care may be better. In the early days of the AAA network, AAAs commonly allocated blocks of funds to homemaker agencies, for example, and permitted those agencies to identify needy clients and prescribe service. AAAs found that providers tended to serve fewer clients with larger blocks of hours of service than judged necessary. On the other hand, control of client assessment and care plan development by case managers employed by the AAA has led to an increase in the number of clients served, an increase in the choices of delivery patterns, and a reduction in average client cost.

AAAs then, become the point of access to publicly financed service, and in the minds of some policymakers, are in a position to control that access consistent with larger policy goals. In some states, the AAA network is the basis for the expansion of publicly funded, community-based long-term care benefits. The Philadelphia Model is an example of this new role for AAAs.

The Philadelphia Model

The AAA for Philadelphia County is the Philadelphia Corporation for Aging (PCA). Since 1982, PCA has hosted a community-based long-term care program called Community Care Option (CCO). PCA receives state lottery funds to maintain a caseload of very frail adults in their own homes. In order to be eligible for CCO, each client has been assessed by PCA's Pre-Admission Assessment Program and judged to be in need of at least intermediate level (ICF) nursing home care, but "divertable" to home care. Home care is feasible because of willing family caregivers and the availability of an enriched array of health and social service support through CCO. CCO provides case management as well as home health care, homemaker, home-delivered meals, adult day care, chore service, mental health evaluation and treatment, transportation, respite care, and other related services.

A PCA assessor does a global, multidimensional assessment of the client's health, functioning, mental status, morale, environment, social supports, and resources (personal, social, and financial). A careful assessment of caregiving efforts by informal supports is included and reflected in the subsequently individually tailored care plan.

The case manager determines the type, amount, scope, duration, and pattern of delivery of the service to be provided. Case managers are vested with responsibility for orchestrating all services noted on the care plan and monitoring the client's overall care. Case managers periodically reassess the needs of their clients and caregivers, and monitor the performance of service providers.

Case managers purchase service on behalf of the clients on their caseload in accordance with the specific tasks and schedule in the care plan. Every day a client is on the "active" caseload, funds are encumbered with which to purchase services. Case managers can spend up to 45% of the daily Medical Assistance (MA) reimbursement rate for a nursing home bed. In 1986, this was about $24.00 daily. Funds are earned on a client-day basis, but controlled on a caseload basis. Case managers are responsible for maintaining their aggregate caseload cost at or below the 45% cap. They are permitted to shift funds between clients as long as the total caseload expenditure is "below cap." This ability to treat clients differentially has a powerful effect on case manager behavior. They allocate resources with caution, recognizing that preserving a cushion of dollars permits them to respond more fully if a client temporarily needs more intensive, and therefore costlier service. Case managers have strong incentives both "to serve and conserve." They quickly become prudent purchasers of service on behalf of their clients and, invariably, keep their caseload expenditure level below the cap. This occurs despite the fact that some of their clients may be using resources temporarily at twice the level of the cap.

In addition to planning, authorizing, and orchestrating service delivery for clients, case managers perform functions historically associated with social casework. They counsel families and negotiate with them about caregiving tasks. They provide short-term problem-oriented counseling. They arrange access to entitlements, housing, and protective and legal services when necessary. They serve as a general source of information and as a "one-stop shopping" resource for questions or problems facing clients and their families. Our analysis of their job responsibilities suggests strongly to us that social work is a necessary prerequisite for the job of case manager.

CCO case management staff consists of 12 social workers organized in two teams of six. Given the number and complexity of health problems faced by our clients, nurses could also be an intelligent choice for case managers, but we selected the more generalist social workers for line staff, choosing to employ community health nurses at the supervisory level. In our judgement, case managers' clinical responsibilities are more akin to social casework than nursing. But nursing expertise is critical and must be easily available. Each team of social workers has a social worker and a nursing supervisor. The CCO nursing supervisors are responsible for adding nursing perspective to clinical decision making and to the overall program design and operation. They review assessments and make recommendations concerning individual client needs. they represent the goals and objectives of the program to providers and conduct orientation sessions for health subcontractors. They assist in development of contract specifications for health services and in monitoring the performance of health care providers. They identify training needs of case managers in the area of health care assessment and service delivery, and they provide or arrange training. The CCO nurses essentially define the relationship between CCO case managers and home health providers.

The provision of health and social services by multiple organizations usually involves end-to-end relationships, (as when a discharging hospital refers for home care), or parallel service delivery without collaboration, as when one agency provides counseling and another provides medical transportation. Interactive relationships between different providers is atypical; but in the provision of long-term care, it is a necessity.

Between May 1982 and March 1985, over 1000 older adults were served in Philadelphia by the CCO program. Analysis of service utilization by clients showed that the principal expenditure was for homemaker service. As would be expected, community-based long-term care clients need high levels of personal care and home support (shopping, cooking, cleaning). At any time, about 95% of these clients were receiving homemaker service. The second most frequently used service was nursing care. Approximately three-quarters of the clients were in receipt of nursing at any one time. About 17% of the service budget was expanded for nursing service. All other directly controlled services were utilized at comparatively much lower rates. By far, the critical professional dyad in CCO is the social work case manager and the providing home health nurse. While all service providers must seek prior authorization from the case manager in order to initiate or change the delivery of service to a client, in the case of home health services, case managers exercise administrative authority over service provision while relying heavily on the clinical judgment of the nurse or other home health professional. Case managers rely on their subcontractor nurses for frequent updates on client condition and guidance on plans of care. The experience of reporting to case managers is a new one for home health nurses, but the level of conflict between CCO staff and home health subcontractors has been surprisingly low from the outset. Nurses sometimes find the need to get prior authorization to visit cumbersome, but case manager involvement has its benefits, too.

Medicare and other third-party payors have progressively narrowed the role of the home health nurse. Nurses often complain that they have to discharge clients when they have serious needs remaining, because care is no longer reimbursable by Medicare. In CCO and similar long-term care programs, nurses can remain involved to provide care for chronic, "non-skilled" problems. Physical therapists, occupational therapists, and other professionals can carry out plans of care that extend beyond rehabilitation to maintenance. Gains established in rehabilitation can be maintained by visits to reinforce exercises or other behaviors. Medicare reimbursement is used when visits are covered; where not, lottery funds are utilized. In either case, collaboration and the sharing of progress notes with the case manager takes place.

Several other aspects of the case manager and community health nurse collaboration should be highlighted. The capitated approach to financing care and the case manager control over spending creates cost consciousness among providers as well. In the CCO model, home health professionals become sensitized to the economic consequences of providing service. For example, nurses who are aware of the cost of consumable medical supplies use them differently than their colleagues who are not attending to cost. Providers become conscious of the cost of the care they are giving and assist case managers in their efforts to be prudent, recognizing that unused resources are available for use when necessary later on. Another benefit is that when nurses identify client needs in the normal course of their duties, which they or their agency are unable to meet, they can contact the case manager and immediately enlist a powerful ally in addressing those needs. Lastly, but no less important, providing ongoing care to long-term care clients is physically and emotionally exhausting. Home health nurses have the assurance that they are not solely responsible for the welfare of their patient; they can readily share their clinical and emotional burden with their case manager colleague. Joint home visiting, case conferencing, and peer support has strengthened service delivery in many difficult case situations.

Becoming a Long-term Care Provider: Observations and Recommendations

Since 1977, PCA has been selecting providers annually, using a competitive bidding process. PCA has been competitively selecting home health providers since 1982. PCA has received proposals from many home health agencies, has experienced a wide range of provider behavior, and has worked closely with eight different home health subcontractors. The selection process used by PCA includes a written proposal, an oral presentation, submission of references, and a weighted list of criteria by which judgments are made which result in the selection decision. Price is a major concern but not the overriding one. Selection decisions revolve around factors such as: demonstrated experience in home health care delivery, history and reputation of the agency, current patient census (Medicare and others), past performance, conceptual understanding of the long-term care program and the special characteristics of service delivery in long-term care, the longevity and experience of nursing and rehabilitation staff, and responsiveness as a prospective subcontractor.

The differences between long-term care and skilled care are important to understand before entering into a contract. Long-term care is different from skilled care in several significant ways. Rather than a focus on diagnosis and treatment of medical problems, long-term care assumes a chronic condition and a degree of permanent (if not progressive) disability. Long-term care is therefore principally concerned with functioning and the way a person lives and operates within his environment. Ideally, long-term care services create a prosthetic environment within which a functionally disabled person can live as independently as possible. A second difference between long-term care and skilled care is apparent when analyzing the tasks involved in the care. Eighty to ninety percent of long-term care in nursing homes, for example, is either personal care or tasks like laundry and housekeeping, provided by paraprofessionals. The role of the physician points to a third difference. For most people receiving long-term care, daily oversight by a physician is unnecessary. What is needed is organization, coordination, and supervision of paraprofessional caregivers by health and social service professionals. Physicians are critical to the provision of long-term care but are not central.

A final difference between long-term care and skilled care which must be clearly understood is the nature of the clinical problems presented and the characteristics of the clients served. Although we have clients ranging in age from 18 to 103, the vast majority are over 80. While many are "skilled" intermittently, about half the nursing care provided is custodial; i.e., skill care, catheter care, etc. Some professionals, by dint of focus or personality, prefer to tackle reversible, or unambiguous problems. For example, orthopedics and general surgery are more straightforward than family medicine or psychiatry. For the latter two disciplines, the very definition of the presenting problem or hoped for outcome may be ambiguous by nature or difficult to articulate. Most long-term care clients suffer from multiple chronic conditions or impairments. At a minimum, the professionals who serve them must be able to tolerate ambiguity, comparatively limited gains, and the eventual decline of most of their patients. Professionals do best who are mature, thrive on complex problems, appreciate small signs of progress, and enjoy extended relationships with their patients. Home health agencies serving long-term care patients will need to take this into account as they select and train personnel.

Good agencies are rightfully proud of their track record, and past performance is an important ingredient in selection. To the extent becoming a subcontractor, providing long-term care, or interacting closely with a case management entity are new experiences, past performance does not take the place of a well-informed commitment to the new program by the bidding home health agency. Prospective bidders should be sure they understand what is being asked for, and be sure that their agency is committed to the new program requirements and whatever adjustments will need to be made. We have had contact with agencies that wish to generate additional revenue as a subcontractor, but steadfastly refuse to consider different ways of operating from their tried and true traditional approaches. Such organizations may provide high quality care but they make unsuitable partners in a new enterprise. The relationship invariably ends up conflictual and frustrating for all parties.

At the other end of the same continuum are organizations that have developed as temporary staffing agencies. Typically proprietary, they have a comparatively less developed vision of good service and agency mission as a community caregiver. They often present a posture which communicates: "we will be happy to serve you in any way you require, as long as you pay us." The motivation of these organizations is clear and their flexibility is appreciated, but their apparent lack of internal performance standards shakes our confidence.

New financing arrangements, combined with the special nature of long-term care patients' needs are likely to propel providing home health agencies into highly interactive relationships with gatekeepers and other providers. This too may be a new experience for agencies, requiring a conscious commitment and careful orchestration of effort to achieve success. In the Philadelphia model, it is the AAA that identifies eligible clients, assesses them for service need, develops the care plan, and then arranges for the provision of home health care as part of a larger care plan which the AAA controls. Where long-term care benefits are financed by private payors, a similar gatekeeping and allocation function is likely to exist outside of the home health provider. As such, participating home health agencies have two clients where before they only had one. They must serve their patient, but also serve the needs of the gatekeeping agency which has overall case management responsibility. Thus, concomitant with the development of this new long-term care market, there may be a diminishing of previously enjoyed autonomy on the part of the home health provider.

The question for agencies contemplating the provision of long-term care is the same question we pose in provider selection. Will they be able to grasp the complexities of the new enterprise and perform the clinically and administratively challenging tasks required? A successful bidder must strike an adequate balance between dedication to an agency mission and performance and productivity standards and a position of flexibility and openness to new ideas and program requirements. In our experience, working with agencies of very different identities, voluntary, religious, and proprietary, that balance has been struck successfully.

Part IV

Clinical Issues that Impact on Administration

Chapter Fourteen

Documentation

Elissa Della Monica

Documentation is one of the ultimate challenges facing home health care administrators today. The numerous changes in the health care environment have placed greater emphasis on documentation. With the institution of the hospital prospective payment system, patients are being discharged "quicker and sicker." The increase in the acuity level of patients has necessitated clear, concise, accurate documentation with evidence of coordination of the multiple services needed to care for the patient.

Changes in the interpretation of the *Medicare Home Health Agency Manual* (1966) has resulted in the need for explicit, descriptive documentation of homebound status, clinical status, and teaching protocols. The institution of the new Physician's Plan of Treatment (HCFA forms 485, 486, and 487) (Reprint 1971 24M3-22M42.4) which must be completed and signed by the physician and sent to the fiscal intermediary with the claim for services rendered, places even greater emphasis on the professional's responsibilities for documentation. The fiscal intermediaries are reviewing 100% of the physicians' orders prior to reimbursing the agency for services provided. Nurses, therapists, and social workers are now directly accountable for reimbursement. In effect, poor documentation can impact negatively on the financial stability of an organization.

In this chapter, home health care documentation and recordkeeping are discussed in their entirety. The regulatory bodies governing home health care are examined, with specific focus placed on the documentation requirements of Medicare. Other topics discussed are: the components of clinical record, reasons for documentation, problem-oriented medical records system of charting, and use of flow sheets. Upon completion of this chapter, the reader will possess a basic knowledge of home health documentation and recordkeeping.

The Changing Health Care Environment

As alluded to above, the delivery of health care is engulfed in an era of change. The major impact came in 1983 with the passage of the Tax Equity and Fiscal Responsibility Act which mandated the Department of Health and Human Services to institute the system of prospective reimbursement. This resulted in patients being discharged from hospitals in the acute or early recovery phase of an illness. The need for home care services increased as patients were discharged from hospitals requiring intensive levels of home care services.

At the same time, Medicare (the principal source of funding for many home health agencies) noticed a dramatic increase in home health care expenditures.

"Medicare payments rose from $1.1 billion in 1982 to more than $1.3 billion in 1983." (Jacob 1985,16) In 1988, it is predicted that Medicare will exceed $3 billion for home health care. This increase in home health expenditures was the result of two factors. The government, with the passage of the Omnibus Reconciliation Act of 1981, allowed proprietary and private not-for-profit agencies to apply for Medicare certification. The passage of this act introduced competition into the home health industry, resulting in a dramatic increase in numbers of agencies. The increase in numbers of agencies, all vying for the Medicare patient, coupled with the increased need for home health services caused this sudden increase in home health care expenditures.

The Health Care Financing Administration (HCFA), in its analysis of the situation, has attributed the increase in expenditures to overutilization of services, i.e., services that are not reasonable and necessary to the care of the client. This fact, in conjunction with the federal government's attempts to decrease Medicare costs, has resulted in new Medicare guidelines and new interpretations of the Medicare home health agency manual. These new regulations, i.e., HCFA forms 485, 486, and 487, and more stringent interpretations of the existing regulations necessitated a dramatic increase in the need for perfect documentation. Now more than ever the old cliche, "If it's not documented it's not been done," takes on even greater emphasis as physicians' orders, progress notes, flow sheets, assessment forms are being closely scrutinized by the fiscal intermediary for homebound status, accuracy in completion of forms, and reasonable and necessary provision of services prior to reimbursing an agency for skilled visits.

Throughout the country, agencies are experiencing an increase in medical and technical denials, all based on lack of supporting documentation of homebound status, skilled needs, etc. The importance of documentation cannot be stressed enough. It is not only required to discuss the care rendered to a client and the clinical status of the client, but it is also required to receive payment for services. It is imperative that home health administrators recognize the impact of documentation on the survival of the organization.

Regulations Governing Home Health Care Documentation

All Medicare-certified home health agencies are governed by the Medicare Conditions of Participation (DHEW 1973). An agency is certified as a Medicare provider based on the agency's compliance with the conditions. There are various conditions that govern home health care documentation. During their annual Medicare Certification Review, all agencies must show that they are in compliance with the standards.

The Conditions of Participation contain numerous standards which direct an agency's clinical record policy (DHEW 1973).

Condition 405.1201: "General"

This condition speaks to the existence of a record. "Clinical records shall be maintained on all patients, in order to participate as a home health agency."

Condition 405.1202(d)

This condition defines a clinical note. "A dated, written notation by a member of the health team of a contact with a patient containing a description of signs and symptoms, treatment and/or drug given, patient's reaction, and any changes in physical or emotional conditions."

Condition 405.1221: "Organization, Service, Administration," Standard 405.1221(g)

"All personnel providing services maintain liaison to insure that their efforts effectively compliment one another and support the objectives outlined in the Plan of Treatment.

(i) The clinical record or minutes of case conferences establish that effective interchange, reporting, and coordinating patient evaluation occur.

(ii) A written summary report (see 405.1202 and x) for each patient is sent to the attending physician at least every 60 days."

This standard establishes the agency's responsibilities in the coordination of services. There should be evidence in a clinical record of coordination between disciplines and coordination through the various levels of authority. Documentation of case conferences are an absolute must in all clinical records.

Condition 405.1223: "Acceptance of patients, plan of treatment, medical supervision"

Standard 405.1223(a) Plan of Treatment. The plan of treatment developed in consultation with the agency staff covers all pertinent diagnoses including:

(i) Mental status.

(ii) Types of service and equipment required.

(iii) Frequency of visits.

(iv) Prognosis.

(v) Rehabilitation potential.

(vi) Functional limitations.

(vii) Activities permitted.

(viii) Nutritional requirements.

(ix) Medications and treatments.

(x) Any safety measures to protect against injury.

(xi) Instructions for timely discharge or referral.

(xii) Any other appropriate items. (Examples: Laboratory procedures and any contraindications or precautions to be observed.)

The physician refers a patient under a Plan of Treatment which cannot be completed until after an evaluation visit. The physician is consulted to approve additions or modifications to the original plan.

Orders for therapy services include the specific procedures and modalities to be used and the amount, frequency and duration. The therapist and other agency personnel participate in developing the plan of treatment."

Standard 405.1223(b): Periodic Review of Plan of Treatment. "The total Plan of Treatment is reviewed by the attending physician and agency personnel as often as the severity of the patient's condition requires, but at least once every 60 days. Agency staff promptly notify the physician of any changes that suggest a need to alter the plan of treatment."

Standard 405.1223(c): Conformance with Physician's Orders.

"(i) Drugs and treatments are administered by agency staff as ordered by the physician.

(ii) Nurse and therapist immediately record and sign oral orders and obtain the physician's countersignature.

(iii) Agency staff check all medicines a patient may be taking to identify possible ineffective drug therapy or adverse reactions, significant side effects, drug allergies, and contraindicated medications and reports any problems to the physician."

Condition IX (405.1228): "Clinical Records"

"A clinical record is maintained in accordance with accepted professional standards and contains:

(i) Pertinent past and current findings.

(ii) Plan of Treatment.

(iii) Appropriate identifying information.

(iv) Name of physician.

(v) Drug, dietary, treatment, and activities ordered.

(vi) Signed and dated clinical and progress notes (clinical notes are written the day service is rendered and incorporated no less than weekly).

(vii) Copies of summary report to the physician.

(viii) A discharge summary."

Standard 405.1228(a): Retention of Records. "Clinical records are maintained for five years after the month the cost report for which the records apply is filed with the intermediary, unless State law stipulates a longer period of time. Policies call for retention even if the agency discontinues operation.

If the patient is transferred to another health facility, a copy of the record or abstract accompanies the patient."

Standard 405.1228(b): Protection of Records. "Clinical record information is safeguarded against loss or unauthorized use. Written procedures govern use and removal of records and conditions for release of information. Patient's written consent is required for release of information not authorized by law."

Hospital-based home health agencies are required to comply with the Medicare Conditions of Participation and the standards for home health care services as outlined in the Joint Commission on Accreditation of Hospitals (JCAH 1985). Hospital-based agencies are reviewed by JCAH as part of the hospital's accreditation process. Similar to the Conditions of Participation, the JCAH standards address the existence of a record, contents of a record, discharge report, authorization to release information, plan of care, progress note, retention of records, and coordination of services. The standards are listed below (JCAH 1985).

Topic	Standard
Existence of record	Home Care Services: Standard IV ". . . an accurate medical record shall be maintained for every patient receiving services through the home care program."
Contents of record	Home Care Services: Standard IV "Medical requirements for home care patients include at least the following: • Designation of the physician having primary responsibility for the patient's care. • Information on the composition of the patient's household, and the name of the person who will assume responsibility for his care if such is required. • The suitability/adaptability of the patient's residence for the provision of required health care services.

Topic	Standard
	• Signed and dated progress notes, copies of all summary and transfer reports, a discharge summary."
Discharge report	Home Care Services: Standard IV
	"Upon discharge from the home care program, a discharge report including a summary statement, disposition and, if applicable, referral."
Plan of care	Home Care Services: Standard IV
	"A written patient care plan that conforms with the physician's orders shall be developed for each home care patient. The patient care plan shall include reference to at least the following:
	• All pertinent diagnoses, prognosis, including short- and long-term goals (objectives) of treatment.
	• Types such as nursing, other therapeutic and/or support services.
	• Frequency of services to be provided, including any medications, diet, treatment, procedures, equipment and transportation required.
	• The patient's functional limitations.
	• Safety measures, sociopsychological needs of the patient.
	This serves as a summary report to the physician every 60 days."
Progress notes	Home Care Services: Standard IV
	"Signed and dated for each home visit, including a description of signs and symptoms, treatment, and/or medications rendered. Patient reaction, any change in the patient's condition and any patient family instruction given shall be documented."

Topic	Standard
Retention schedule	Medical Record Services: Standard 9.1.2 "Medical records are to be retained dependent upon the need for their use in continuing patient care and for legal (State Statute of Limitations), research and educational purposes."
Transfer and Referral	Home Care Services: Standard IV "Copies of transfer reports are part of the record, referrals are indicated in disposition portion of discharge summary."

The National League for Nursing (NLN 1987), has established an accrediting process for home health agencies. Unlike the others, NLN accreditation is not mandatory. Agencies applying for NLN accreditation must complete a self-study report verifying compliance with standards as outlined in the manual. The self-study report is reviewed by an expert panel of administrators. A site visit by a few members of the panel is conducted to verify accuracy of the self-study report. During the site visit, the administrators conduct a thorough review of the clinical record system. They conduct their evaluation based on the standards listed below (NLN 1985,25-27,29):

Topic	Standards
Existence of record	Criterion 15: " . . . service records are maintained for each client."
Content of record	S-15.1 "The service record of each client includes: reason for service diagnoses, client/family data base problem list, medical orders, plan of care, progress notes, documentation by all disciplines providing service, written summaries, discharge summary."
Discharge report	S-15.1 "Discharge summary is included in service record for each client."

Topic	Standards
Authorization to release information	S-15.5
	"Policies indicate need for client's permission to release confidential information."
Plan of care	S-15.1
	"The service record of each client includes: plan of care with short and long term goals."
Progress note	S-15.1
	"The service record of each client includes: timely progress notes dated and signed by person providing service."
Retention schedule	S-15.4
	"Record retention and protection policies are in accordance with applicable laws and regulations and insure confidentiality."
Record review	S-15.6
	"There is a mechanism for regular review and updating of the record format to assure ease and simplicity in use and to reduce duplication of data."
	S-17.5
	"Utilization Review performed using records. Random sample of client records appraised determining adequacy/appropriateness of services."

In analyzing the documentation requirements of these three organizations, it is interesting to note the similarities. Conditions of Participation and JCAH contain detailed descriptions of the content of the clinical record, the content of the plan of treatment, and the content of the progress note. The NLN standards address these issues; however, the emphasis is on the quality of the clinical record and the quality of the care rendered as specified in the record review standard.

Clinical Record Policy

As previously stated, the prime resource for funding for agencies is Medicare. Hence, the Conditions of Participation are the primary tool from which agencies develop the documentation policies. Clinical record and documentation policies are a must for all home health agencies. The clinical record policy addresses protection and retention of records, contents of the clinical record, requirements for written plan of treatment, requirements for verbal orders, and reference to record review policy. The clinical record policy is specific to the agency and describes the system of documentation that an agency is utilizing. The record policy is one that should be strictly adhered to, as it will form the basis on which your documentation system is reviewed. During the Medicare certification process, an agency will be reviewed to verify compliance with its own policies, i.e., if the policy states verbal orders will be signed and incorporated into the chart in two weeks, then it better be done.

It would behoove an administrator to develop a clinical record policy that does not place restraints on the agency. The policy should describe what is actually occurring in the management of the clinical record system. Time limits for return of forms from physicians should be avoided, as forms are frequently lost or delayed in the physician's office or mail. However, agencies should strive to get all verbal orders and plans of treatments signed and incorporated into the record within two weeks. All other agency forms, progress notes, assessment forms, etc., should be incorporated into the record within one week. An example of a clinical record policy is found in Table 14-1. The policy is specific to the agency, as it describes the various forms that constitute the clinical record system. The policy clearly describes the agency's procedure for protection and retention of records. The policy indicates that the agency is in compliance with the Conditions of Participation.

Table 14-1

Objective: To maintain clinical records for each patient in accordance with the policies of the agency.

I. Requirements: All clinical records for each patient shall be filed in an individual folder and receive consideration of the following standards:

A. Protection and retention of records

 1. Clinical records may be made available only to authorized personnel.

 2. No record, or portion thereof, may be released without written consent of the patient, family or authorized individual.

 3 All records must be retained for a minimum of seven (7) years in a protected area to safeguard against loss or unauthorized use. Records of minors are to be retained until age 21 (plus an additional seven (7) years). Records may be stored off premises as of November 1982.

 4. A transcript is made available in the event of transfer to another authorized agency.

 5. Records will be retained in an available, safe storage area under the responsibility of the executive director and board of directors. If agency is dissolved, the State Department of Health will be notified of date of dissolution, location of records, and responsible person.

*Reprinted with permission of Visiting Nurse Association of Eastern Montgomery County, Abington, PA.

Table 14-1 continued.

6. Clinical records are maintained in a central file in numerical order. These records are to remain in the office. Flow sheets, medication list and master file input card may be taken on home visits. Under specific circumstances, such as a case conference, an individual record may be taken from the office with prior approval from the immediate supervisor.

B. Contents of the clinical record: Contains past and current pertinent data

1. Master File Input Card: Contains appropriate identifying information and physician's name and telephone number.

   ● Card is taken on home visits and becomes a permanent part of the record on discharge.

   ● A duplicate copy of the card is kept in the clinical supervisor's cardex folder while patient is open to service.

2. Nursing, Therapy and Medical Social Service Assessment Forms: Contain pertinent, past findings and a current clinical assessment of patient's status.

   ● Completed on admission and readmission.

3. Family Information and Summary of Service Form: Contains pertinent family information plus a summary of client's admission and discharge dates.

4. Nursing Diagnosis and Problem List: Contains list of nursing diagnoses and goals for each individual problem.

5. Clinical Notes

   ● Current progress notes dated and signed.

   ● Clinical notes are segregated on colored paper for ease in identification of disciplines.

6. Physician's Plan of Treatment: Contains a summary report to the physician on admission and every 60 days thereafter.

   ● The POT is revised by the agency personnel and reviewed by the attending physician once every 60 days.

   ● Additions or changes in the POT are confirmed with a verbal order.

7. Patient Authorization and Release Form.

8. Medication List: Contains computerized form listing name of medication, dosage, frequency and route, indications, side effects, interactions.

   ● Form is completed on admission and updated as needed.

9. Discharge Summary:

   ● Completed by all disciplines.

10. Clinical record also contains written communications, conferences, and reports to and from other participating organizations and from agency professional personnel.

11. Other Charting Systems:

    ● The agency will comply with charting guidelines as specified by contracting agencies.

C. Record Review

1. Quarterly Review. See "Quarterly Record Review Policy."

2. See "Annual Evaluation Policy and Procedure."

Reasons for Documentation

The routine daily activities of a community health nurse consist of approximately 35% of time spent on documentation and 65% of time spent on patient care. As nurses, whose primary focus is the care of the patient, the amount of time spent on documentation seems to be counterproductive to the care of the patient. Despite the frustrations felt by many community health nurses, the importance of documentation cannot be overemphasized.

Why do we document? There are multiple reasons for documenting. However, a primary reason that comes to the mind of home health administrators is reimbursement. Documentation is the method through which the patient's need for home health services is presented (Jacob 1985,17). Ineffective, poor documentation could jeopardize the financial stability of the organization. Medicare and other third-party payors require documentation to be submitted with the claim for services prior to reimbursing the agency. The documentation must objectively inform the reviewer of the clinical status of the patient, inclusive of a description of the services being provided.

Medicare requires that a signed Physician's Plan of Treatment be submitted with the claim. The Plan of Treatment is a universal form developed and distributed by the Health Care Financing Administration. The form is commonly known as HCFA (Form 485) Physician's Plan of Treatment, (Form 486) Medical Update and Patient Information, (Form 478, Addendum 1973, 24M3-24M42.4). The forms contain all the necessary data elements for a Physician's Plan of Treatment as outlined in the Conditions of Participation. The forms were developed to elicit specific information to enable the reviewer to make Medicare coverage determinations. The reviewer will closely analyze the form for inconsistencies in the clinical picture, i.e., is the diagnosis consistent with the treatment? Is the treatment a simplified procedure that can be safely performed by a nonskilled individual? Is the patient homebound? Do the clinical diagnosis, treatment, and services ordered support the statement on homebound status? If the reviewer detects any inconsistencies in the Plan of Treatment, the determination may be made that the care was not reasonable and necessary or that custodial care was rendered and deny the claim as a medical denial.

If the reviewer detects inconsistencies in the reason for homebound status, the claim will be denied as a technical denial. There are a few other reasons that an agency may receive a technical denial. A denial will be received if HCFA Forms 485, 486, and 487 are not completed accurately, i.e., all sections of the forms must be completed, frequency and duration must be stated on all disciplines, orders for increases and decreases in services must be recorded, and orders must be present to cover all services provided.

A technical denial is received if a determination is made that the patient is not homebound, the physician's orders do not cover services rendered, and if the form is completed incorrectly. Home health aide visits are denied technically in conjunction with medical denials received for nursing, physical, and occupational therapy or speech pathology.

The difference between a medical and technical denial is that a medical denial can only be received if a determination was made that care was not reasonable or necessary or that custodial care was provided. An agency will be paid for a medical denial if they are under presumptive waiver status. The waiver of liability provision was developed by HCFA to allow agencies to be paid for services when they, in good faith, were not aware that services being provided were not reasonable and necessary. Medicare presumes that if your error rate is less than 2.5%, the agency could not have known that they provided unnecessary care. Hence, they will reimburse the agency for the denied visits. Presumptive waiver status is maintained if the agency has less than 2.5% medical denials in a quarter. This is calculated by using the following formula (Medicare Home Health Agency Bulletin 86-23):

$$\text{Denial Rate} = \frac{\text{\# visits denied minus \# visits technically denied}}{\text{Total \# visits for all processed claims minus \# visits technically denied}}$$

If the results are greater than 2.5%, the agency no longer qualifies for presumptive waiver status. Hence, the agency will not be paid for medical denials.

Aside from the Physician's Plan of Treatment, Medicare and other third-party payors frequently review progress notes, assessment forms, and verbal orders. Quality documentation should include observations written in both clinical and measurable terms (Jacob 1985,17). This enables the claims reviewer to assess changes in the patient's condition. Descriptive, accurate documentation is essential to assure reimbursement. As previously stated, the professional caregiver is directly accountable for reimbursement. It is only through the mechanism of documentation that an agency receives payment for services.

The second reason for documenting is to prove that quality care was rendered. In home care, the clinical record is the primary tool for assessing the quality and appropriateness of care. The clinical record is a mechanism of proof that the practitioner provided quality services.

An agency evaluates for quality via the quarterly record review. The agency is responsible for developing criteria or standards on which to base the clinical record review. The criteria should be well-defined and stated in measurable terms. The clinical record will be evaluated to verify compliance with the established criteria. (Refer to chapter 18.)

Good documentation reflects good care. If the required data do not appear in the clinical record, the quarterly record review may show deficiencies in the care provided to the patient. Remember: Care that is not documented is presumed not to have been done.

The third reason for documentation is to show evidence of the coordination of services and continuity of care. Charting shows how several disciplines arrange for continuity and comprehensive care without duplication of services (Stanhope and Lancaster 1984,792). The medical record gives members of the health care team a way to communicate with each other. This is accomplished through the development of problem lists and the formulation of care plans. Short- and long-range goals should be identified to indicate expected outcomes for each discipline. In addition to overall care goals, each discipline should maintain specific short- and long-range goals to guide their care plans (Jacob 1985,18).

A care plan gives direction to patient care by showing the goals that have been set for a patient and giving clear directions for helping staff to achieve these goals. The plan of care and progress note provide for continuity of care in informing other professionals what has been accomplished in the care of the patient. It also informs the caregiver of the plans for future visits.

The coordination of services is documented in the progress note. As previously addressed in the Medicare Conditions of Participation, all home health agencies are required to show evidence of coordination of multiple services. This is accomplished by the performance of and documentation of conferences. A multidisciplinary team conference must establish that there is effective intercoordination of the plan of care. These conferences should include all disciplines involved in the care of the patient with reference to goals and expected outcomes.

There should also be evidence of coordination of services from administrative to supervisory to clinical staff. Coordination between supervisory and clinical staff is documented during patient care conferences and should include reference to current status of the patient, changes in the plan of care, ability to achieve the goals as stated in the plan of care, and plans for discharge. The administrative staff may also get involved in a clinical case conference when there is an issue that cannot be resolved at the clinical level. It is imperative that a progress note be documented with evidence of anticipated plans and expected outcomes.

During the Medicare certification visit, the reviewer will request evidence of coordination of services at all levels. It would behoove all agencies to monitor documentation of coordination of services very closely, since it is explicitly outlined in the Conditions of Participation.

The fourth reason to document is that it is a requirement of all professionals involved in the care of patients. Standard I of the ANA Standards of Nursing Practice (ANA 1973) addresses documentation:

> "The collection of data about the health status of the client/patient is systematic and continuous. The data are accessible, communicated and recorded." Rationale: "Comprehensive care requires complete and ongoing collection of data about the client/patient to determine the nursing care needs of the client/patient. All health status data about the client/patient must be available for all members of the health care team."

Good documentation also establishes the professional's and the agency's credibility. If a chart is poorly written and lacks appropriate terminology and measurable terms, it gives an unfavorable impression of the skill and knowledge of the professional caring for the patient (Jacob 1985,18). Hence, hospitals, physicians, and community agencies may be reluctant to refer patients.

The fifth reason for documentation addresses the liability issue. As previously stated, professional caregivers are required to show evidence of the care that was rendered. The Medicare Conditions of Participation, JCAH and NLN regulations all speak to the necessity of physician's order prior to initiating care and throughout the service period. Professional caregivers are required to report all changes in the patient's medical status to the physician. The caregiver may be held liable if there is no evidence of communication with the physician and there is no evidence of verbal orders to cover changes in the original plan of care.

Home health care workers are also accountable to the Medicare program in documenting provision of skilled services mandated by the federal regulations. An agency may be held liable for fraud and abuse if they cannot demonstrate through documentation that skilled services were provided to a homebound patient and that services were reasonable and necessary to the care of the client.

At all times, agencies must be prepared for an unannounced visit from the Medicare certifier to certify an agency for participation in the Medicare program, or an unannounced visit from the fiscal intermediary to conduct a coverage compliance review. The primary focus of these reviews, particularly coverage compliance audit, is to conduct an intense review of the clinical records to verify compliance with the federal regulations. State Medicaid reviewers may also conduct unannounced visits per the state statutory regulations. It is imperative that home health administrators be aware of the quality and appropriateness of their staff's documentation, as they are ultimately responsible for deficiencies that may be found.

The Key to Successful Medicare Documentation

The key to successful documentation lies in the caregiver's ability to paint a picture of the patient for the Medicare reviewer. This will enable the reviewer to understand the reason services were rendered to the client. The reviewer's first introduction to the patient is the Physician's Plan of Treatment. The plan of treatment must contain enough information to enable the reviewer to make a coverage determination. As discussed, most agencies are using the standard Medicare certification and plan of treatment forms developed by the Health Care Financing Administration. There are three separate pages to the HCFA form. Form 485 is the actual Plan of Treatment and is the only form which must be sent to the physician for signature. HCFA Form 486 is the Medical Update and Patient Information form. This form is completed by the agency to provide Medicare with supplemental information which will enable the reviewer to make the coverage determination. HCFA Form 487 is an addendum for additional writing space in completion of the forms.

There are a few key factors in completing the forms to Medicare specifications. The diagnosis must be a clear diagnosis which conforms in terminology with that of the International Classification of Diseases (ICD9) published by the U.S. Department of Health, Education and Welfare. The primary diagnosis listed should be the primary reason for which the patient is receiving home health services, which may be different from the primary diagnosis listed on the referral. Other diagnoses should be listed in order of importance. Qualify the diagnosis by stating "unstable," "acute," or "uncontrolled." All diagnoses and surgical procedures should contain an ICD9 code with date of onset and exacerbation. (A note of caution: Avoid chronic diagnoses in which there is a reasonable probability that skilled intervention will not affect a change in the patient's clinical status, e.g., organic brain syndrome.)

The treatment orders should be listed per discipline. The orders must be clear and specific to the diagnosis, indicating frequency and duration. Example: SN: 3 x per week x 3 weeks/2 x per week x 3 weeks/1 x per week x 2 weeks.

1. Vital signs every visit.

2. Catheter change: #16 French q 4 weeks and prn x 2 visits for catheter obstruction.

3. Teach medications and 4 gram sodium diet.

Orders for medication should include dosage, frequency, and method of administration. (N) new or (C) changed should be listed after the medication. This indicates to the reviewer the medications for which the patient will need instruction and review.

Goals, rehabilitation potential, and discharge plan should be specific to the diagnosis. Summary of clinical findings should summarize the clinical status of the client on admission to service and, on recertification, summarize the status of the patient over the last 60 days. The physician's signature must be an original signature; a stamp of the physician's signature is not acceptable.

Form 486 Medical Update and Patient Information further qualifies the physician's orders. This form functions as a prospective document in which the caregiver projects the number of visits and a retrospective document in which the caregiver explains, in Section 15, changes that have occurred in the last 60 days. It is imperative that Section 15 (Updated Information: New Orders/Treatments/Clinical Facts) be completed in detail explaining changes in orders, addition of a discipline, and changes in clinical status. The Medicare reviewer closely reviews this section with the expectation that it will describe what has occurred in the care of the patient over the last 60 days. Remember!!! Do not forget this section. Numerous claims have been denied when caregivers have failed to update Section 15.

In Section 17, Form 486, caregivers must document the reasons for being homebound. Once again, be explicit in explaining homebound status, especially if the diagnosis may not necessarily make the patient homebound. For example: "Experiences severe loss of breath in performing all activities/transfers bed-to-chair only," "ambulates with moderate assist 15 feet first floor," "unable to use steps." The reason the patient is homebound should correspond with the diagnosis and the services ordered.

In summary, the Physician's Plan of Treatment and Medical Update are the reviewer's first introduction to the patient. The form should be objectively reviewed by nursing supervisor prior to being sent to the fiscal intermediary. The fiscal intermediaries are accepting no errors in the completion of the form. Be clear, concise, and explicit in your documentation.

Documentation of Skilled Care

The Initial Visit

As previously stated, nurses, therapists, and social workers must document evidence that the patient is in need of skilled care. The initial evaluation is documented on assessment forms specific to each discipline. In addition to the assessment form, an agency may or may not require a clinical note. This initial evaluation documentation is very important as it contains a brief description of the event or accident which renders the patient homebound and in need of skilled services. The initial nursing note should contain: "(1) Pertinent findings of the nurse's physical assessment, (2) Identification of the need for instruction, observation and/or treatment, (3) Review of medications including a preliminary assessment of the patient's understanding of the purpose and signs and symptoms of reaction to the medication, (4) Identification of the need for home health aide services by identification of goals, (5) Anticipated frequency and duration, and (6) Homebound status." (Webb 1986)*

The physical and occupational therapy evaluation notes should contain: "(1) Gradient evaluation which identifies the areas of deficiency, (2) Identification of short- and long-range goals, (3) Specific therapy program to be initiated, (4) Frequency and duration of visits, (5) Homebound status." (Webb 1986)

The speech pathologist's evaluation should include: "(1) Type of test used in the examination, (2) The identified speech disorders, (3) Identification of short- and long-term goals, (4) The specific therapy program to be initiated, (5) Frequency and duration of visits and a list of teaching tools given to the patient for practice and reinforcement, and (6) Homebound status."

The social service evaluation should include: "(1) The persons from whom pertinent information is elicited, (2) Patient's participation or lack of participation in the discussion, (3) Overall plan of action, and actions to be initiated after the evaluation and before visiting the patient again, (4) Short- and long-range goals, (5) Frequency and duration, (6) Homebound status."

After completion of the initial assessment and evaluation, which may or may not be done on a standard assessment and evaluation form, the caregiver is expected to document a clinical note on each visit. The clinical note is a dated, written notation by a member of the health care team on the contact of a patient. The note contains a description of signs and symptoms, treatment and drugs given, patient's reaction to the treatment, effects of medication, and changes in physical or emotional condition (Webb 1986).

Documentation of instructions given to the patient must also appear in the clinical note. Instructions should be broken down to a specific drug, diet, treatment, exercise, etc. Instructions should continue until patient and family demonstrate the ability to perform the treatment independently or until the patient and family verbalize understanding of medication side effects, etc. Once you have documented the patient's understanding of the instruction, etc., further instruction will not constitute a need for ongoing skilled care. Remember: Be specific in your documentation of instructions and do not repeat once the client has become independent.

Skilled Nursing

Skilled observation and evaluation visits must be thoroughly documented. The nurse must show evidence of changes in the patient's clinical status with notification to the physician of the changes that have occurred. Skilled observation and evaluation visits are usually covered for three weeks unless there are significant changes in the patient's clinical status. The nurse should attempt to chart negatively. Describe in descriptive terms such things as the size, depth, and width of the wound, the color and odor of the exudate, the color of the sputum, the congestion of the lungs, the girth of the abdomen, responses to medications, and severity of pain. Skilled observation and evaluation visits are important to the care of the client. In order to insure reimbursement for

* Reprinted by permission.

these visits, the nurse must document all changes in the patient's status and all changes written by the physician on the Plan of Treatment (Engelbrecht 1986,11).

Documentation of direct skilled care, i.e., catheter changes, treatments, injections are more simple, as nurses are accustomed to documentation of specific tasks. Once again, be specific, describe the length and complexity of the treatment. The reviewer will be monitoring the complexity of the care to see if it could be done by a nonskilled caregiver, i.e., the family or home health aide. Treatments that require daily care over an extended period of time may not be covered. It is imperative that the nurse attempt to teach someone the procedures for performing the treatment.

Skilled Therapy

The skilled therapy clinical note should contain an assessment of the patient's clinical status from the therapist's viewpoint: an evaluation of progress or regression since the last visit, the specific therapy modality that was carried out during the visit, response of the patient to the exercise and therapy during the visit, a statement indicating you are working toward accomplishment of goals, and a list of new problems that the therapist has discovered on the visit. The therapist's documentation must reflect the degree of motion lost and the degree to be restored. Distances that the patient ambulated must be recorded in feet and the degree of independence in transfer must be explicitly described.

Speech Pathology

Repetitive drills are not covered. The therapist must document the response of the client to therapy using percentages, degrees, and number of repetitions.

Medical Social Service

As stated in the Medicare Home Health Agency Manual, "Medical Social Service must contribute significantly to the treatment of the patient's medical condition." (1966,153D) The medical social service clinical note must contain a detailed description of the social problems which are affecting the patient and contributing to the instability of the disease process. The social worker is expected to describe how intervention can improve the overall status of the patient. The documentation must contain the actual steps taken by the social worker to resolve the problem, the outcomes of the social worker's intervention, and plans for future intervention. Social service visits are generally provided at a maximum of two to four visits per patient. Clear, concise, explicit documentation is needed for coverage of medical social service visits.

Home Health Aide

In general, home health aides are not required to document in a narrative note. It is customary procedure for a home health aide to document on a worksheet outlining the home health aide's responsibilities. The nurse is expected to develop the home health aide plan of care which directs the aide's activities. The nurse is required to supervise the home health aide on an every-two-week basis and update the plan of treatment as needed. The supervision note should be documented in a clinical note and must include instructions to the home health aide on the plan of care, the home health aide's understanding of the plan, and ability to perform the necessary functions. The nurse should also include the plans for the future and anticipated plans for a change in aide schedule or discharge of aide service.

Another key issue for reimbursable documentation is homebound status. The reason that the patient is homebound must be discussed on admission and at least weekly thereafter. All disciplines involved in the care of the client should speak to the homebound status with a description of why the patient is homebound. Generalized weakness is not a reason for homebound status. Functional limitations should be clearly described and stated in measurable terms. One discipline must be careful to support another discipline's statement on homebound status. For example, nurses and home health aides must not make statements contradictory to the therapist's statements. Nurses and aides may indicate that the patient is ambulating without difficulty, when the therapist is providing service for gait dysfunction. The nurse's statement may disqualify therapy services. Documentation of coordination via multidisciplinary case conferences would alleviate this problem.

Remember, the key to successful documentation lies in the caregiver's ability to describe explicitly why the patient needs home health services and how home health services will improve his overall clinical status. Document negatively, charting objective facts. At the completion of your documentation, ask yourself: "Was the care I provided to this patient reasonable and necessary? Did I perform care that was ordered by the physician? Does the clinical note indicate that the patient was homebound?" All these questions must be answered to insure reimbursable documentation.

Use of a Problem-Oriented Medical Record System

The agency at which I am employed has been using a problem-oriented system of documentation for many years. Prior to this we were using a source-oriented system of documentation in which all disciplines randomly documented their progress in a narrative format. The agency eventually discovered source-oriented documentation provided little to no structure for the clinical staff in working toward a common goal.

The problem-oriented system allows for an organized system of providing care (Weed 1970). All information is associated with the problem to which it relates. The system is based on four components: (1) The development of a data base, i.e., assessment, initial evaluations; (2) the development of a problem list; (3) the development of the initial plan; and (4) the progress note.

How the System was Implemented at the VNA of Eastern Montgomery County

The data base is formulated from the initial assessment and evaluation visit. From this the nurse develops the problem list utilizing the nursing diagnosis of the National Conference Group (Kim and Moritz 1981). Goals are stated and patient outcomes are listed per nursing diagnosis. The initial plan is developed based on the identified problems. Each problem is numbered and addressed in the form of a SOAP note. Thereafter, all entries in the progress note will address a specific problem and be stated in SOAP form. SOAP refers to Subjective Data, Objective Data, Assessment, and Plan. (Refer to Chapter 16.)

In conjunction with the basic system, the agency has developed standardized flow sheets. The flow sheet contains specific parameters and interventions that direct the care of the patient in an organized fashion. They provide structure and guidance to clinical staff and foster continuity of patient care as all staff are following the same plan of care. Flow sheets also allow the practitioner to have a picture of the clinical status of the patient over a course of time. Changes in vital signs, lung sounds, bowel sounds, can be evaluated on a per-visit basis and compared with previous visit reports. Flow sheets may also contain treatment orders which instruct the staff on the specific care of a wound, an ulcer, etc. All standardized flow sheets provide additional space to allow for additional individualization of the treatment plan.

As we found, flow sheets describe clinical status of the patient, treatments, and instructions provided. Staff are not required to document a SOAP note on each visit. SOAP entries and a progress note are required a minimum of one time per week and when it is necessary to address a problem in greater detail than is permitted on the flow sheet. All SOAP entries must restate the name and number of the problem. Temporary problems are addressed in the progress note in SOAP formation. Flow sheets are not required on temporary problems.

After discussing the many advantages of flow sheets, I would be remiss if I did not speak of a disadvantage. The major problem that we have encountered with flow sheets is that many third-party payors (private insurance carriers) do not accept flow sheets as documentation for a visit. They will only accept clinical notes as proof that a visit was made. Hence, all insurance patients have a clinical note per visit. Despite the duplication, staff members insist on using the flow sheet, because they feel it enables them to maintain continuity of care. Although I feel flow sheets are an excellent tool for the visiting staff, it is imperative that they be used in conjunction with a weekly clinical note. (Refer to Chapter 16 for an example of a standardized flow sheet.)

Problems are deleted as they are resolved. On deletion of a problem the nurse must indicate the goal attainment stated in patient outcomes. Eventually, by discharge from agency service, all problems should be resolved. If problems are not resolved, they should be addressed indicating why goals were not obtained.

The problem-oriented system of documentation has proven very successful at our agency. Our staff utilize it without difficulty and place great value on the flow sheets. Flow sheets may be taken to the home with the nurse so that the nurse has data on the patient's clinical status at all times with which to compare current findings.

Thus far, this system of documentation has survived the Medicare certification review, and the NLN accreditation review. This system is recommended for all home health agencies, since it enables the staff to provide goal-directed patient care.

Medical Record Department

Our agency utilizes a centralized filing system for storage of medical records. Active charts are kept in a Centrex circular file and shelf to allow for easy access to the charts. Discharged charts from the previous year are stored in a separate filing cabinet. All other discharged records are stored off the premises. Per the agency policy, all charts must be kept for seven years. Charts are filed in numerical order utilizing a color-coded numbering system. This allows for quick identification of the clinical record. The department is staffed by certified record technicians and medical record clerks. The clinical staff is not permitted to access charts without completing a requisition slip. Staff may request a portion of the chart, the flow sheet, or the entire chart. Charts are not permitted to leave the office. However, flow sheets and medication lists are permitted to be taken to the patient's home. In general, staff members are discouraged from handling the clinical records.

The agency has realized numerous benefits as a result of the tight controls of the medical record system. In general, charts are rarely misplaced or misfiled, forms are incorporated into the charts on a timely basis, and charts are maintained in proper order. The indirect benefits associated with a well-run medical record department are: (1) decrease in stress of visiting staff, since less time is spent on clerical activities; (2) assistance to the supervisory staff seeking patient information; (3) decrease in time spent on quarterly record review, since charts are completed and forms are filed in order; (4) improved efficiency in day-to-day operations of the clinical staff; and (5) reassurance in knowing that the charts are ready for an unannounced certification review.

As administrators, who are forever conscious of the cost of maintaining a department, one must consider the many benefits of a medical record department. As stated in this chapter, documentation via the clinical record is the method through which an agency's services are judged to be reimbursable or nonreimbursable. Based on this fact, it behooves an agency to incur the expense of a medical record department.

Summary

To summarize, quality reimbursable documentation requires the commitment of the entire agency. This commitment must transcend all levels of employees from the chief administrative officer to the visiting staff to the clerical support staff. All levels of employees should be aware of their responsibilities in the documentation process. As one of their primary responsibilities, administrators must educate staff members on the complexities of documentation. In today's health care environment, successful documentation is the key to an agency's survival.

References

American Nurses Association. 1973. *Standards of nursing practice*. Standard I. Kansas City, MO: ANA.

Commission on Professional and Hospital Activities. 1978. *International classification of diseases: Clinical modification, ICD-9-CM,* vols. 1-3. Ann Arbor, MI: Commission on Professional and Hospital Activities.

Department of Health, Education and Welfare. 1971. *Medicare home health agency manual.* (5:71). Washington, DC: Government Printing Office.

Department of Health, Education and Welfare. 1973. *Conditions of participation for home health agencies.* 38(135):18978-18982. Washington, DC: Government Printing Office.

Engelbrecht, L. 1986. Engelbrecht on documentation. *Home Health Journal* March 1986:11.

Jacob, S. R. 1985. The impact of documentation in home health care. *Home Healthcare Nurse* 3(5):16-20.

Joint Commission of Accreditation for Hospitals. 1985. *Accreditation Manual for Hospitals.*

Kim, M. J., and D. A. Moritz, (eds.) 1981. *Classification of nursing diagnosis: Proceedings of the third and fourth national conference.* New York: McGraw-Hill.

Medicare home health agency bulletin #86-23. August 15, 1986. Philadelphia: Blue Cross of Greater Philadelphia, Medicare Division.

National League for Nursing. 1987. Accreditation Criteria, Standards and Substantiating Evidences. Publ. No. 21-1306. *Criterion* 15:S-15.1-S-15.6,p.25-27.S-17-5 p. 29.

Stanhope, M., and J. Lancaster. 1984. *Community health nursing.* St. Louis: C. V. Mosby.

Webb, P. 1985. *Seminar on home health care documentation.* Spring House, PA: Home Health Development Corporation, Inc. (Reprinted with permission.)

Weed, L. 1970. *Medical records, medical education and patient care.* Cleveland: Case Western Reserve University Press.

Chapter Fifteen

Patient Classification Systems

Patient Classification Systems for Home Care

Joanne Tully Cossman

Quantification of nursing requirements in acute care environments received its impetus from the nursing shortage of the 1950s. Nurse staffing and work measurement research resulted in attempting to analyze patient problems to determine amounts of time nurses needed to care for each problem and patient. Consequently, nurses received their assignments on the basis of patient requirements rather than on daily census and numbers of beds. Nurse managers in hospitals and other acute care settings have long recognized this need to allocate nursing resources based on objective evidence of the patient's requirements (Ballard and McNamara 1983, 236).

Since the early 1970s, health professionals in various settings have been attempting to establish patient classification systems. Patient classification systems may be broadly defined as "the grouping of patients according to some observable or inferred properties or characteristics and quantification of these categories as a measure of the nursing effort" (Johnson, 1984).

The classification schemes developed have been based on different viewpoints:

Administrative	Looking at amounts and kinds of care needed and level of practitioner
Clinical	Assessing the scientific principles of care needed
Research	Attempting often to combine both the administrative and clinical view to encourage valid and reliable data and applications.

Developing a classification system requires four elements:

1. A method of grouping patients or the classification categories

2. Guidelines describing the way in which patients are to be classified, the frequency of classification and the method of reporting the data

3. The average amount of time required for care of a patient in each category and

4. A method for calculating required staffing and required nursing care hours (Giovannetti 1979, 4).

The two categorizing methods most frequently used are: factor evaluation and prototype evaluation. "Factor evaluation" entails rating patients individually in terms of the independent elements of care each needs. Each element is then weighted by a score, each patient's scores summed and then placed in a category based on total numerical value. "Prototype evaluations" compare a patient's condition to a category containing a broad description of care requirements. Each patient is then classified into the category he most closely resembles (Giovannetti 1979,4).

Since classification systems developed, they have become key management instruments. Any department or organization must develop a definitive, accurate model, which must be tested and found to be a valid, reliable, workable, dependable, accurate system, adaptable to computerization, and easily monitored.

A reliable measuring tool is one that gives consistent results on repeated applications. It is the determination of the "precision" of the tool, but two major factors can affect the consistency of the results: a variation inherent in the method of applying the tool and observer error. Both of these points need careful consideration when developing a patient classification system. The validity of a measuring tool refers to the extent to which the device actually represents reality.

Even though validity and reliability are always discussed together, they are very different concepts that must be dealt with in the development of an accurate classification scheme. Discussion of reliability and validity testing can be sought elsewhere.

Until recently, few cost accounting and reimbursement mechanisms have made substantial effort to either capture the real nature of the magnitude or the complexity of home health care patient needs.

The literature reveals that the earliest attempts to identify patient needs in a quantifiable, operational, and comprehensive fashion have come from within hospital settings. It is in those acute care environments that the four basic elements and the three viewpoints mentioned earlier have more frequently been able to develop, survive, and prove useful.

Home health care settings, until recently, have not felt the pressing need for patient classification systems whose goals generally are to determine how much effort is required per patient, and the character and cost of those services.

In the home health care services, few patient classification systems have been published to date.

Elizabeth A. Daubert (1979) approached quantifying and qualifying a patient's home care needs utilizing a patient classification system based on rehabilitation potential. Designed and implemented at the Visiting Nurse Association of New Haven, Connecticut, patients were placed in one of five categories that predetermined objective measures of outcome. The system served as a quality assurance program tool, assessed the patient's actual functioning level at the time of discharge from service, and applied to all home health care professional services. The major intent of this system is to provide the answer to the question, "What difference does home health service make in the patient's health status?" This system is discussed in detail elsewhere in this publication.

DeLanne Simmons, Executive Director of the Visiting Nurses Association of Omaha, Nebraska, in the mid 1970s received funding from the Division of Nursing, DHEW. This funding was offered to develop a classification of client problems addressed by nurses in a community health setting. The result was a manual: *A Classification Scheme for Client Problems in Community Health Nursing.* In this scheme, nursing and nonnursing problems were differentiated, as well as individual and family health problems and actual versus potential problems. The nursing problems categorized included risk factor, etiology, and laboratory tests, all referred to as descriptors rather than as signs or symptoms. Uniform names for each problem were developed through the grouping of descriptors and resulted in four categories of problems: environmental, psychosocial, physiological, and health behaviors. The Omaha data base and classification scheme has been tested at multiple sites, refined, computerized, and is being utilized as an agency planning and documentation tool by many agencies across the country.

Costs of care gained great emphasis in 1980 when Young and Fisher presented an analysis of Medicare program charges incurred during episodes of illness or per case for inpatient hospital stays, skilled nursing facility admissions, and home health agency care. One of the major questions addressed by this analysis was "what patient characteristics influence the utilization of these three services?" At a time when hospitals were under tighter cost controls and home health was of growing interest, this analysis found that episodes of illness using hospital care were substantially cheaper than all others. The analysis raised further questions, specifically:

- Can posthospital care services substitute for inpatient hospital care?

- What are the decision-making factors that influence the selection of services for an episode of illness?

- Should costs incurred on a per case basis include costs of food, housing, and opportunity costs for family caretakers?

It is clear, even at this date in the literature, that home health care must provide increasing accountability and documentation and answer these vital questions.

In February 1982, Fobair reported the findings of a reimbursement study group determining if cancer patients require more time from a home health care agency prospective. This study considered only amounts of nursing time spent with the patients on home visits and the amount of education, team collaboration, and desk time spent by nursing staff to care for these patients (Fobair 1982).

Ballard and McNamara (1983) studied home health agency patients for factors predictive of the quantity of nursing service and total home health agency service required particularly by cardiac and cancer patients. Utilizing the health status score, measuring deficits in daily activities and nursing problems as predictors, they were able to predict the need for total agency visits and resource utilization. A significant limitation cited in their study was the lack of complete and consistent recording practices among agencies, lack of standard definitions and guidelines for similar closure of records to indicate lengths of stay (Hardy 1984,26-27).

In 1984, home health agency executives began to write about experiences attempting to utilize known classification systems to accomplish more effective home health agency management. Hardy (1984) examined four broad categories of home care patients, using four nursing diagnoses to determine significance among the number of visits, duration of care, and combinations of other variables. Though no statistical significance was found among the study group, the author did suggest that using nursing diagnostic categories as well as acuity levels can effectively identify and predict nursing resources needed.

Nursing diagnosis was also reported as a potential determinant of nursing resources in home health care and has been used by Cell, Peters, and Gordon (1984) and Harris, Santoferraro, and Silva (1985) as a problem identification and charting mechanism.

Harris has been able to correlate nursing diagnosis, International Classification of Disease (ICD-9) coding, and the Daubert New Haven VNA System (Daubert 1979) with resulting identification and predictors for costs on a per visit, per case basis. This appears to be the most substantial presentation in the literature.

The need for a tried and true patient classification system in home health care is clear. As evidenced by the literature, home health agencies themselves have been struggling with this issue and have made some true gains since the early 1970s, long before federal reimbursement initiatives became more structured.

From all the data gathered, it is believed that the most successful home health classification schemes must address most, if not all of the following characteristics:

1. Accessible and Usable

   The system should "flow" within the workload of all staff involved, clinical and administrative, and must be simple, flexible, and easy to use with other tools. For example, if whatever methodology was developed can be incorporated into an organized, systematic, workable, documentation-charting-reporting mechanism, it will probably be more utilized. A system that saves recording time through objectivity and organization can eliminate lengthy, verbose process recordings and guide staff toward the development of individualized patient care plans and interventions. Also, there is no benefit to a system that applies to only one discipline.

2. Reliable and Valid Tools

   Any system must always pass the test so as to limit inter- or intrarater variables as well as the tests for validity.

3. Identifying Patient Care Needs and Services

   A descriptive system which can objectively assess a patient's needs for services and deliver an outcome which predicts types of services and intensity of services to be delivered can be a powerful management tool. "Predicting" based on objectivity is what must be done to accommodate future regulatory demands. A system chosen to "work" for home health care must not be applicable to only one service but must be able to be applied by all potential services involved in a patient's care.

4. Acuity Based

   This is a most difficult area within which to gain objectivity. Hospital classification systems have struggled with finding determinators of illness. In home health an accurate objective multifaceted assessment tool has been the most accurate approach to patient problem identification which can lead to determination of acute or nonacute condition status and subsequent "grouping."

5. Workload-Staffing-Productivity Determination

   All three of these characteristics are measurements vital to a home health administrator. An acuity-based system predicting patient problems should give an indication of the intensity and type of service required for a given patient. Accumulation of that data can serve as a management tool for determination of case assignment (number, type, personnel), and may diagnose caseload management problems (productivity issues).

6. Reporting

   A key tool for any agency administrator is the management report, the analysis of which may be vital to agency planning. Measurement is vital whether it relates to patient outcomes, recording time, in-home visit times, or payor mix. A classification system should allow reporting beyond the traditional (geography, age, sex, race, diagnosis, and payor source) in order to identify more precisely and to plan more specifically for the health needs of the patient population. It is also important to obtain objective evidence concerning the effectiveness of the services provided on an individual as well as group basis, therefore contributing to quality.

7. Cost Associations

   If most of the characteristics listed are met by a developed system, costing (given cost accounting mechanisms of today) should be feasible. Cost limits and capitation contracts can risk the stability of an agency which reflects on costs incurred. A patient classification system can be integral in those predictions particularly if it addresses average mix of service personnel and subsequent costs by diagnosis, problem, or similar groupings.

8. Computerization

   Dictation and transcription is now a workable solution to time efficiency in relation to documentation. Tools are needed to improve patient services, not burden staff during their care. Professional and nonprofessional tasks need to be spent in direct care. Management time must be economized as well and a system that provides clear data for analysis can only enhance planning and decision making.

Administration of a home health agency is becoming more and more complex and a greater challenge. Faced with cost issues, particularly the recent cost limit regulations, as well as the economic climate of the nation and public scrutiny, it is not surprising that attention has turned to identifying a valid, reliable, objective patient classification system; one that can be integrated into a quality assurance program, direct staffing levels, type and intensity of services, and project and monitor costs of care provided.

Given the history of the development of the classification schemes for home health agencies, there is considerable belief that the work that has been done addressing various problem areas, is a valuable beginning in the effort to develop successful comprehensive systems.

A Patient Classification Outcome Criteria System [*]

Elizabeth A. Daubert

Community-based home health agencies, such as Visiting Nurse Associations, official public health nursing agencies, and hospital-based home care programs, have long grappled with the task of developing reliable, valid ways to measure the quality of services they provide. For the most part, past efforts have been confined to assuring that a high level of quality care is rendered by periodically evaluating the agency's organizational and management structure and by maintaining a method of record review (Daubert 1977). These quality assurance activities can, and do, produce indicators concerning the quality of care provided to patients and families. However, neither provide objective evidence to answer an equally important question, "What difference did agency service make in a patient's health status?"

With increasing frequency real and potential consumers of service, federal and state legislators and regulators, as well as third-party payors are asking for hard data that home health services do, indeed, make a difference in a patient's health status. The answer to this question lies in the development of an assurance tool which has the capacity to objectively evaluate patient outcome: the status of a patient at the time of discharge from agency service. An outcome measurement module is a must for any good quality assurance program (Bailit et al. 1975; Bloch 1975).

Outcome measures, using medical diagnosis, acuity levels, or for specific health disciplines, are fairly common in acute and long-term care facilities. The incidence of outcome-oriented systems currently operating in home health agencies, however, is still the unusual rather than the usual. Designing a system that will provide objective evidence of the quality of care provided by home health care agencies is not an impossible task; however, two problems identified by Aydelotte (1973) immediately appear. These are the difficulties in describing the effect of care an agency hopes to achieve and the problems of identifying the specific population group(s) served by a home health care agency.

Attempts to define outcome criteria for each home health discipline, or according to medical diagnosis, are fraught with problems for several reasons. For example, five of the six traditional home health services, specifically nursing, social work, physical, speech, and occupational therapy, are independent disciplines, which means each service functions with complete autonomy in a patient situation. Therefore, the efforts of each discipline are distinct and measurable. However, the sixth discipline, home

* Adapted by permission of *Nursing Outlook* from Vol. 27(7):450-454, "Patient Classification System and Outcome Criteria," Elizabeth A. Daubert. 1979, American Journal of Nursing Company.

health aide service, is neither an independent discipline, nor is it autonomous. Instead, it is a totally dependent discipline because it always functions as a supplement, or an extension of either nursing, physical therapy, or speech therapy service. In order to write measurable outcome criteria, each service discipline must be able to stand alone in a service setting; each must be independent. Also, the ultimate measure of patient outcome is not which service, or mix of services, is provided. Rather, the final measure of the effectiveness of service is the outcome, the actual functioning level of a patient at time of discharge from service. This is the reason why it is not practical for a home health agency to use outcome criteria according to each discipline provided.

It is equally not practical or effective to use patient diagnosis as a basis for developing outcome criteria for an agency-based home health program. It might be feasible if all patients within an agency's population have only one diagnosis, but the average patient admitted to an agency's illness service program has three or more diagnoses. When one deals with a patient population with multiple diagnoses, outcome criteria based upon patient diagnosis becomes an impractical, unwieldy approach. Such a method would mean that not one but multiple sets of outcome criteria would have to be applied in each patient situation. The paperwork alone would be time-consuming and cost-prohibitive. The pitfalls of using either the service discipline or a medical diagnosis approach can be avoided by classifying patients by groups according to each group's rehabilitation potential. Of greater value, the intent of such a system is met because the characteristic that is measured is the outcome, the end result of the care. The following is an example of an outcome measurement system which has the proven capacity to measure patient outcome, the status of a patient at time of discharge from home health agency service.

The Patient Classification Outcome System

The Patient Classification Outcome (PCO) System developed in 1977, is a formal method of measuring patient outcome that is based upon classifying all patients admitted to an agency's home health care program, regardless of the number of diagnoses per patient or the mix of agency services given, into one of five patient groups according to each patient's rehabilitation potential. Each of the five patient groups is specifically defined to provide clarity and uniformity for assignment of patients to a particular group. In addition, each group has an identified ultimate program objective and a separate set of subobjectives. All service program objectives, both ultimate and subobjectives, are based upon the premise that the phrases "Service Program Objectives" and "Patient Care Goals" are synonymous. Justification for such a conclusion is based upon the following definitions: Goal: an aim; the end toward which effort is directed (Webster's 1975,493), and Objective: an aim, or end of action; a goal (Webster's 1975,791).

For each patient group a specific ultimate program objective as well as a separate set of program subobjectives have been identified. Each ultimate program objective and set of subobjectives apply to all six home health care service components (nursing, home health aide, physical, speech, and occupational therapy, and social work). And finally, each set of program objectives becomes the criteria, or standards, that are used to judge the effectiveness of an agency's home health care program on the health needs and problems of its patient population. All applicable subobjectives for each patient group must be met in order to verify that the ultimate goal has been accomplished for each patient.

Patient Groups and Objectives

A delineation of the five patient groups as well as a set of corresponding objectives, both ultimate and subobjectives, is as follows.

Patient Group I. Patients with acute, nonchronic, episodic-type disease or disability (for example, wound infections, fractures, pneumonia, poor nutritional habits, gastrointestinal disorders, uncomplicated surgical procedures, gestational diabetes, gestational hypertension) who will return to pre-illness level of functioning.

Ultimate Program Objective for Group I. Patient will either: (1) achieve complete recovery from illness or, (2) patient's immediate health need and problem which prompted admission to service (e.g., proper use of crutches, walker, etc., or need to learn correct technique re: dressing change) will be eliminated.

Program Subobjectives for Group I.

    a. Patient will demonstrate capacity to return to preepisodic level of functioning.

    b. Patient will demonstrate the ability to independently manage the patient's personal care needs.

    c. Patient and family will demonstrate the ability to assume responsibility for any ongoing medical supervision.

    d. If indicated, patient and family will demonstrate an understanding of the prescribed diet.

    e. If indicated, patient and family will demonstrate an understanding of the prescribed medication regimen.

    f. If indicated, patient and family will demonstrate the ability to independently perform prescribed treatments and exercises.

    g. If indicated, patient and family will demonstrate knowledge of important safety measures.

    h. If indicated, patient and family will demonstrate knowledge of available community resources.

Patient Group II. Patients with EARLY STATE CHRONIC disease(s) or disability(ies) (for example, cardiac disease, diabetes, C.V.A. with no residual or slight hemiparesis, C.O.P.D., arthritis, hypertension) who are experiencing an acute episode of illness but have the potential for returning to preepisodic level of functioning.

Ultimate Program Objective for Group II. Patient and family will manage chronic health problem(s) without ongoing agency service.

Program Subobjectives for Group II

a. Patient will demonstrate capacity to return to preepisodic level of functioning.

b. Patient and family will demonstrate the ability to independently manage the patient's personal care needs.

c. Patient and family will demonstrate the ability to assume responsibility for maintaining ongoing medical supervision.

d. If indicated, patient and family will demonstrate an understanding of the prescribed diet.

e. If indicated, patient and family will demonstrate an understanding of the prescribed medication regimen.

f. If indicated, patient and family will demonstrate the ability to independently perform prescribed treatments and exercises.

g. Patient and family will recognize signs of significant physical or emotional changes as well as the need to communicate these changes to the appropriate health care provider.

h. If indicated, patient and family will demonstrate an understanding of the restrictions imposed by the illness or disability.

i. If indicated, patient and family will demonstrate knowledge of important safety measures.

j. If indicated, patient and family will demonstrate knowledge of available community resources.

Patient Group III. Patients with either: a, INTERMEDIATE STAGE CHRONIC disease(s) or disability(ies) who, even though a return to pre-illness level of functioning is not possible, will have the potential for increasing their level of functioning and will eventually function without agency service(s); or b, ADVANCED STAGE CHRONIC disease(s) or disability(ies) (for example, cardiac disease, C.V.A. with hemiparesis, arthritis, C.H.F., amputation of a limb, blind diabetic) who do *NOT* have the potential for increasing their level of functioning but, who, because of assistance provided by family member, will eventually function without agency service(s).

Ultimate Program Objective for Group III. Patient will be rehabilitated to his maximum level of physical, emotional and social functioning and patient and family will manage chronic health problem(s) without continued agency service(s).

Program Subobjectives for Group III.

a. Patient and family will demonstrate the ability to independently manage chronic health problem(s).

b. Patient and family will demonstrate some improvement in ability to function independently.

c. Patient and family will demonstrate the ability to independently manage the patient's personal care needs.

d. Patient and family will demonstrate the ability to assume responsibility for maintaining ongoing medical supervision; and

e. If indicated, patient and family will demonstrate an understanding of the prescribed diet.

f. If indicated, patient and family will demonstrate an understanding of the prescribed medication regimen; and

g. If indicated, patient and family will demonstrate the ability to independently perform prescribed treatments and exercises.

h. Patient and family will demonstrate the ability to recognize signs of significant physical or emotional change as well as the need to communicate these changes to the appropriate health care provider; and

i. If indicated, patient and family will demonstrate an understanding of the restrictions imposed by the patient's illness.

j. If indicated, patient and family will demonstrate knowledge of important safety measures.

k. If indicated, patient and family will demonstrate knowledge of available community resources.

Patient Group IV. Patients with ADVANCED STAGE CHRONIC disease(s) or disability(ies) (for example, advanced heart disease, neurological problems, severe arthritis, organic brain syndrome, fractures, G.I. disorder, C.V.A. with residual hemiplegia, cancer, pernicious anemia) who can only be maintained at home because of ongoing agency service(s).

Ultimate Program Objective for Group IV. Patient will be maintained at home as long as possible with ongoing agency service.

Program Subobjectives for Group IV.

a. Patient will receive agency service at the level and intensity needed and within normal limits of the agency to provide such services.

b. Patient and family will demonstrate ability to manage the patient's personal care needs, with or without agency assistance.

c. Patient and family will demonstrate the ability to assume responsibility for maintaining ongoing medical supervision.

d. If indicated, patient and family will demonstrate an understanding of the prescribed diet.

e. If indicated, patient and family will demonstrate an understanding of the prescribed medication regimen.

f. If indicated, patient and family will demonstrate the ability to perform prescribed treatments and exercises.

g. Patient and family will demonstrate the ability to recognize signs of significant physical or emotional change as well as the need to communicate these changes to the appropriate health care provider.

h. If indicated, patient and family will demonstrate an understanding of the restrictions imposed by the patient's illness.

i. If indicated, patient and family will demonstrate knowledge of important safety measures.

j. Complications and regression will be prevented as far as possible.

k. If indicated, patient and family will demonstrate knowledge of available community resources.

Patient Group V. Patients with END-STAGE illness (for example, terminal C.O.P.D., cancer, renal failure, cardiac disease, cirrhosis).

Ultimate Program Objective for Group V. Patient will be maintained at home during the end stage of illness for as long as possible with agency service.

Program Subobjectives for Group V.

a. Patient will receive agency service at the level and intensity needed and within normal limits of the agency to provide such service.

b. Patient and family will demonstrate ability to manage the patient's personal care needs, with or without agency assistance.

c. Patient and family will demonstrate the ability to assume responsibility for maintaining ongoing medical supervision.

d. If indicated, patient and family will demonstrate an understanding of the prescribed diet.

e. If indicated, patient and family will demonstrate an understanding of the prescribed medication regimen.

f. If indicated, patient and family will demonstrate the ability to perform prescribed treatments and exercises.

g. Patient and family will demonstrate the ability to recognize signs of significant physical or emotional change as well as the need to communicate these changes to the appropriate health care provider.

h. Patient's pain and discomfort will be controlled to the extent possible.

i. Patient and family will receive emotional support as needed.

j. Patient and family will be allowed to express feelings about dying.

k. Patient and family will receive assistance as needed to prepare for death.

l. If indicated, patient and family will demonstrate knowledge of important safety measures.

m. If indicated, patient and family will demonstrate knowledge of available community resources.

n. If indicated, family will receive support during the mourning period.

Patient Admission

Every patient admitted to an agency's home health program, even if it is a second or third admission, should be assessed and entered into one of the five patient groups. This process begins, usually following the initial visit, but no later than the third home visit. At that time, the primary caregiver (nurse or therapist) matches the patient's medical diagnosis(es), all identified health needs and problems presented by the patient and family, and the primary caregiver's assessment of the patient and family rehabilitation potential to the typology, or definition, and set of objectives for each patient group. The patient group which fits the patient situation is then selected.

Second, the primary caregiver indicates the selected patient group in the goal section of the patient's record. Because the ultimate program objectives and patient care goals are synonymous phrases, the objective for the selected group then becomes the long-term program service goal toward which all subsequent action is directed, regardless of the mix of disciplines supplying service to that patient.

Third, the primary caregiver records all applicable subobjectives listed for that particular patient group in the patient's care plan. Because the applicable subobjectives are considered minimum goals, the patient care plan will also contain additional action goals tailored to the individual situation. An example may help.

> A 68-year-old, married man with a seven-year history of atherosclerotic heart disease and a one-year history of diabetes mellitus, which is controlled by daily insulin and a prescribed diet, was referred for agency service upon hospital discharge following a partial colectomy that was performed to remove benign polyps. Following surgery, Mr. A developed a secondary wound infection which was subsequently incised and drained.
>
> Mr. A was referred to the home health agency for monitoring of his wound and instruction for him and his wife in daily dressing changes of the draining wound. During the first home visit, the primary nurse thought Mr. and Mrs. A were of average intelligence and both seemed willing to learn the dressing procedure. Mr. A's insulin injection technique was assessed as safe and adequate, however, his understanding of the need for daily urine testing and diabetic foot care was limited. In addition, he was not adhering to a two-gram sodium-restricted, low cholesterol, 1800 calorie diabetic diet. In assessing his rehabilitation potential, the primary nurse judged Mr. A as having the capacity, with Mrs. A's assistance, to eventually manage his chronic health problems without ongoing agency service.

By matching the above patient data with the definition and the set of objectives for each patient group, the primary nurse selected Group II as the appropriate one for

Mr. A. To enter Mr. A into the system, the primary nurse selects the appropriate patient group, indicates it on the care plan, and incorporates and customizes all applicable subobjectives listed for a Group II patient in the patient action plan portion of the record. Had the above patient needed the involvement of any special therapy services such as physical, speech, occupational, or social work, the primary nurse would have discussed the selection of the patient group with the involved therapist(s) or social worker.

The terminology used in the statement of each subobjective does *not* stipulate that the patient and family will do, will accept, or will adhere to the stated action; e.g., patient and family will follow prescribed diet. Rather, each stated subobjective specifies that a patient and family will demonstrate an understanding of, will demonstrate an ability to, will demonstrate knowledge of, etc.

The rationale for such terminology is based upon two factors. First, the recognition that besides the provision of therapeutic care, another major function of every professional caregiver is to teach, to give a patient and family the knowledge they need to either lessen or eliminate their presenting health needs. Second, it is beyond the realm of the community-based professional caregiver to actually modify, much less control patient and family behavior. It is essential that all patient care personnel who use this system have a clear understanding and acceptance of this principle.

At the same time, however, it is recognized that some patient and family members will indeed modify their behavior as the result of the primary caregiver's teaching regimen. Whenever behavior modification is evident, a brief, concise description of the modified behavior should be documented in the patient record. For example, "patient and family verbalized all elements of therapeutic diet and weekly food intake chart substantiated fact."

As ongoing service is provided, the patient record must contain documentation that subsequent action was taken on each applicable subobjective as well as a description of the patient and family response. Furthermore, all applicable subobjectives must be attained in order to determine upon discharge from service that the program goal was accomplished.

Each time a patient is discharged from an agency service, a discharge summary form is completed. Included on this form is specific information such as patient name, length of service, diagnosis(es), service program goal, goal accomplishment, reason for discharge, total visits made by each discipline, cost of each service discipline, as well as payment source and total cost of all services provided. The original copy is forwarded to the agency's statistical department, while the carbon is placed in the patient's record. (See Exhibit 15-1 for a sample of the form.)

Advantages

Besides accomplishing its primary purpose—the development of a method to identify and measure patient outcome—the system has several other advantages. For instance, it:

Saves Staff Time and Reduces Paperwork. The PCO system saves staff time and reduces paperwork because it reduces recording time. It also helps professional patient care staff with decision-making concerning long-term service goals for each

Exhibit 15-1.

DISCHARGE SUMMARY FORM ___/___/___

NURSE/THERAPIST COMPLETES BOXED AREAS ☐ ONLY; ALL OTHER AREAS TO BE COMPLETED BY CLERICAL ST

Pt. Name	_____	Town _____	C.T. _____
	Last First	No.	No.

Patient Number _____

First VNA Visit __/__/__ Last VNA Visit __/__/__ Total Length of Service _____ days) Circle months) One

Primary Dx. _____ | Total Number of Dx. | _____
Code

Payment Source: Primary _____   Secondary _____
                         Code   Code(s)

| SERVICE PROGRAM GOAL | (Check one)

☐ Group   I - Will eliminate health problem/need.

☐ Group II - Will learn to independently manage continuing health problem(s).

☐ Group III - Will learn to function at maximum level.

☐ Group IV - Chronically ill patient will be maintained at home with VNA assistance.

☐ Group   V - Patient with end-stage terminal illness will be maintained at home as long as possible.

| SERVICE GOAL ACCOMPLISHED | (Check one)   ☐ Yes   ☐ No

| REASON FOR DISCHARGE | (Check one box ONLY)

☐ Service program goal accomplished   ☐ Pt. moved

☐ Pt. hospitalized   ☐ Refused to obtain M.D. appointment

☐ Pt. admitted to a nursing home   ☐ Refused continued service

☐ Pt. died at home.   ☐ Obtained service from another source

☐ Refused to provide financial data   ☐ Cont'd service need H.H. Aide; no payment source

Total Visits Made: _____ _____ _____ _____ _____ _____
                    Nsg.   P.T.   Soc.W. Sp. T. O.T.   HHA hrs./visits
                                                         (delete one)
Cost of service: $_____ $_____ $_____ $_____ $_____ $_____
                   Nsg.   P.T.   Soc.W. Sp. T. O.T.   HHA

TOTAL COST OF ALL SERVICES: $_____

Upon completion, the white copy is forwarded to the Statistical Clerk, the pink copy is filed in the patient's record, and the yellow copy is forwarded to Billing Department.

patient. In addition, each set of subobjectives serves as a helpful guide, or check list, for staff as they organize and develop patient care plans. Finally, the discharge summary form also reduces recording time.

Expands an Agency's Statistical Information System. Statistical data compiled by most agencies are usually limited to a breakdown of patient population by geographical location, age, race, sex, primary diagnosis, and payment source. Because the patient classification system provides a breakdown of patient population according to patient groups based on each patient's rehabilitation potential, the system also gives an agency access to descriptive data that more precisely define the specific health needs and rehabilitation potential of its patient population. The system can be used by an agency of any size because the data can be collected either manually or by computer.

Assists an Agency To Establish Measurable Objectives For Its Home Health Program. Because the system has the capacity to collect data concerning the number of patients, according to patient group (who fell in the "Goal Accomplished" as well as the "Goal Not Accomplished" categories), an agency can use these data to determine measurable objectives for its illness service program.

For instance, in one agency where the system has been operational for several years, the system's annual statistical report form produced the following findings for the 1985 service year:

	Goal Met %	Goal Not Met %
Group I	84.3	15.7
Group II	85.8	14.2
Group III	76.8	23.2
Group IV	82.5	17.5
Group V	89.8	10.2

Agency personnel can use the above percentage figures as a basis for establishing measurable objectives for its illness service program for the 1986 service year. Depending upon circumstances, agency personnel might adjust the 1985 data either upward or downward when setting measurable objectives for each patient group for the 1986 service year.

Assists an Agency To Assess the Delivery of Service. By providing objective evidence concerning the degree of effectiveness of its services on the population served, an agency will know its "success and failure rate." For example, the system will generate on an ongoing basis a breakdown of the number of patients in each group for whom the service goal was accomplished, the success rate, and the number of patients in each group for whom the service goal was not attained. For the latter, the system also provides a breakdown of the reasons why the service goal was not accomplished, such as patient hospitalized, patient died, patient and family refused continued service, and so forth. Such data can help an agency assess its current methods of delivering service and plan corrective action where needed.

For instance, if there are an inordinate number of "patient and family refused continued service" reasons, an examination of these patient records may uncover specific weaknesses in the agency's current method of delivering service. Subsequent action can then be taken to strengthen, or eliminate, these areas of deficiency. Or, if many patients were discharged because their continuing need was for home health aide service only, and these patients could not afford to pay for ongoing aide service and no third-party coverage existed to pay for continued service, these data could be used to validate the need for funding from sources such as United Way, private foundations, or municipal and state governments. The result might be expanding the agency's home health aide service with additional funds.

Helps to Forecast Future Staffing Patterns. The data can also be used to estimate future staffing needs and for appropriate use of various kinds of patient care personnel. For example, if the number of patients admitted to Group IV showed a steady increase each year, then an agency might adjust its staffing ratio by employing greater numbers of home health aide personnel and less professional staff.

Provides Data Concerning the Mix of Personnel and the Cost of Service. The system has the capacity to produce descriptive information related to the average mix of service personnel and the subsequent cost by patient group or patient primary diagnosis. This information can be used by the agency in interpreting its service to the community and to third-party payors.

Harris et al. (1985,276-282;279) at the Visiting Nurse Association of Eastern Montgomery County, Abington, PA, used a modification of this PCO system and identified the following average lengths of stays and costs associated with nine disease entities (See Table 15-1[*]).

Validating Reliability

The fact that the primary caregiver enters a patient into the system upon patient admission and, at time of patient discharge from service, determines whether the service program goal was accomplished or not accomplished might be considered a weakness, a major flaw in the system. Therefore, to eliminate this concern and in so doing to insure the reliability and validity of the system, the following criteria should be added to an agency's method of record audit: Service program goal, documentation regarding subobjectives, and the discharge summary.

The addition of these items will ensure that the record contains evidence to substantiate that at time of discharge the correct patient group was selected. And if the primary caregiver indicated that the goal was accomplished then the action plan, service record, and narrative portion of the record should contain evidence that (1) the appropriate actions were listed and taken on each applicable subjective identified for

---

* Reprinted with the permission of Anthony J. Janetti, Inc. from "A Patient Classification System in Home Health Care" by Marilyn D. Harris, published in the Sept./Oct. 1985 issue of *Nursing Economics.*

Table 15-1

Major Disease Category	No.	Average Length of Stay (Days) on VNA Service	Average Number of Visits	Average Time In Hours	Average Cost per Case
Neoplasms	400	33	14	16	$808
Respiratory	121	34	12	9	630
Gastrointestinal	193	19	6	3	296
Neurologic	66	41	18	13	940
Endocrine	132	32	13	5	613
Renal	51	36	13	13	707
Circulatory	590	36	15	9	734
Skin/Subcu- taneous	76	29	13	8	660
Musculo- skeletal	75	43	18	10	913
	1,704			Average Cost for Sample = $700	

the selected patient group, and (2) the record contains a description of the patient and family change in knowledge, understanding, and behavior which occurred during the course of service.

By adding the above criteria to an agency's record audit process, the need to establish a separate system to monitor the reliability and validity of the system is avoided.

In summary, the Patient Classification Outcome System is operational and working well in several agencies in various sections of the United States. It has proven to be a valid method to identify and measure patient outcomes. The secondary benefits derived from its use have helped to improve the efficiency and effectiveness of an agency's home health care program.

Classifying Patients Using a Nursing Diagnosis Taxonomy

Donna Ambler Peters

The idea of patient classification is not new. It can be traced back to the beginning of modern day nursing when Florence Nightingale placed the most acutely ill patients in a ward nearest the nurses' desk and the least ill furthest from the desk (Giovannetti and Thiessen 1983). Today, the end product of the grouping of patients is known as a patient classification system which is used in nursing to calculate staffing needs and more recently to cost out nursing services. As popular as patient classification systems are, however, other classifications are also used in the profession of nursing. Classification of nursing diagnoses for example has been stimulated recently by the convening of National Conferences on the Classification of Nursing Diagnoses in the early 1970s and the more recent formation of a group to develop, refine, and promote a taxonomy of nursing diagnostic terminology (NANDA). This portion of the chapter will examine the concept of classification as it applies to patient classification systems and nursing diagnoses, and how a nursing diagnosis taxonomy can be used for clinical and administrative management of a home health agency. Although the NANDA taxonomy of nursing diagnosis is popular, this paper will discuss the Omaha Patient Classification Scheme since it is a nursing diagnosis taxonomy specific for community health.

Classification Theory

Scientific inquiry has two major objectives: (1) to describe particular phenomena in the world; and (2) to establish the general principles by which the phenomena can be explained and predicted. In order to develop the explanatory and predictive principles, scientifically useful concepts are required. These useful types of concept formations are: procedures of quantitative ordering, comparative ordering, and classification (Hempel 1952). The classificatory concept depicts a characteristic(s) which any object in the domain under consideration must either have or lack. It is an either/or situation. Ordering concepts on the other hand, attribute a value to each item in the domain providing a gradation of the characteristics. Stated another way, the characteristics used in an ordering concept are criteria of precedence and coincidence while the characteristics used in a classification concept are criteria for class membership. The value of the characteristics in an ordering concept may be numerical—giving a quantitative ordering (relative values)—or simply ordinal. These concept formations are explained by the theory of classificatory procedures and systems (Hempel 1965; Sokal 1974).

In a patient classification system, the class to be divided is "patients" and the subclasses are groups of patients with a required need for care. In actuality, the concept used is a comparative ordering because the amount of care required falls on a continuum rather than in the dichotomy of requiring care or not requiring care. The characteristics used for placing a patient in the appropriate level on the continuum are usually critical indicators of care which depict greater or lesser needs for care. The greater the needs for care, the higher the level in which the patient is placed. However, in usage, the procedure has been called a classification.

In a nursing diagnosis taxonomy, the class to be divided is "nursing diagnoses" and the subclasses are the signs and symptoms which a patient may exhibit. These essential characteristics determine membership in the subclass (i.e.; either the patient has the diagnosis or doesn't). The subclasses are not on a continuum and there is no value (either relative or numerical) assigned to any of the diagnoses. Thus, this procedure is defined as a classificatory concept rather than the comparative ordering which is used by patient classification systems. In addition, because it is the class of "nursing diagnoses" which is being divided, and not "patients" as in a patient classification system, a patient having more than one nursing diagnosis may appear in more than one category (i.e., patients are not placed in mutually exclusive categories.)

Patient Classification Systems

A patient classification system is a "generic term used to describe a variety of methods for grouping or categorizing patients according to their perceived requirements for nursing care" (Giovannetti and Thiessen 1983,1). Categorization can be based on natural classifications (patient characteristics) or artificial classifications (critical indicators of care). There are three basic elements to a patient classification system (Exhibit 15-2): (1) a procedure for grouping patients which includes the frequency of classification and the means of reporting these data; (2) a quantification of the nursing care resources associated with each category of care; and (3) a method for calculating staffing for required nursing hours. Such a system can be used to monitor productivity levels, to predict and justify staffing needs in the budgetary process, and to provide a basis for nursing charges (Alward 1983). It must be emphasized, however, that such a system justifies cost only and cannot justify the care.

Logically, it is reasonable to expect that staffing levels based on a patient classification system will have a positive relationship to the quality of care. However, in practice, three problems are evident: (1) the existence of a patient classification sys-

Exhibit 15-2. A Patient Classification System.

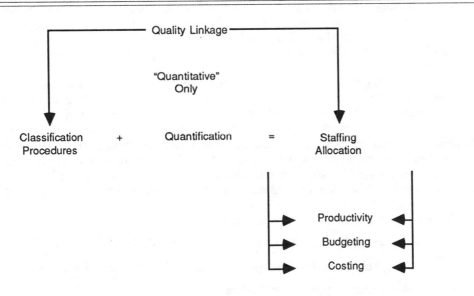

tem does not guarantee adequate staff; (2) there is no guarantee that nurses will or can perform in the manner ascribed in the system; and (3) the staffing levels obtained by a patient classification system represent only the quantitative aspect of the complex system of patient care (Brown 1980; Giovannetti and Thiesson 1983; Jones 1984). Thus, it is not surprising that attempts to correlate staffing levels with quality assessment scores have been largely unsuccessful (Giovannetti and Thiesson 1983; Sienkiewicz 1984).

Nursing Diagnosis Taxonomy

A nursing diagnosis taxonomy is simply the classification of nursing diagnoses. The nursing diagnoses which comprise the taxonomy could be derived either deductively or inductively. In order to be derived deductively, a distinct group of actual and potential health conditions which are amenable to nursing intervention must exist. Currently, however, there is no consensus on defining these conditions but rather several models exist, each providing a different orientation to nursing. Nursing diagnoses derived inductively are based on a description of clients' health problems as they are encountered in practice. Developing a taxonomy of these diagnoses is one way of describing the domain of nursing and thus communicating the nature of that service both to other nurses and to those outside the profession such as patients, other professionals, auditors, and legislators (Roy 1975).

A nursing diagnosis taxonomy for community health nursing was developed by the Visiting Nurse Association of Omaha (Simmons 1980). This taxonomy is consistent with the general and comprehensive practice of community health nursing which includes the following tenets: (1) it is not limited to a particular age or diagnostic group; (2) it is continuing, not episodic; (3) it uses a holistic approach for health promotion, health maintenance, health education, coordination, and continuity of care; (4) it recognizes the influence of social and ecological issues; and (5) it utilizes the dynamic forces which influence change (ANA Standards of Community Health Practice 1974; Simmons 1980).

The 44 nursing diagnoses included in the taxonomy were arrived at empirically from the practice of the community health nurses employed by the visiting nurse agency. The diagnoses are organized by the four broad domains addressed by community health nurses (environment, psychosocial, physiological, and health behaviors). Each diagnosis is described by a list of signs and symptoms, i.e., general statements condensed from assessment data which are patient-specific and are used to arrive at the problem label (diagnosis). For example, one of the problem labels in the health behaviors domain is "Nutrition: impairment." The descriptors for this problem label are:

1. Weight 10% more or less than average

2. Lacks or exceeds established standards for daily caloric intake

3. Lacks or exceeds intake of one or more essential food groups or nutrients

4. Lacks or exceeds appropriate fluid intake

5. Improper feeding schedule for age

6. Emaciated or obese

7. Other.

Finding one or more of these signs or symptoms on assessment would indicate presence of the problem "Nutrition: impairment." The problem may be an actual or potential one. The patient may be defined as an individual, family, or group. For example, if a person were more than 10% over weight due to poor personal eating habits, it would be an actual individual problem. However, if the person were dependent on the family to buy, prepare, and bring the food to the bedside, the problem would be a family problem. If this same person were currently an appropriate weight but the family was feeding the patient an extreme number of calories for the patient's activity level, it would be a potential family problem.

The Omaha Classification Scheme not only provides nursing diagnoses and specific descriptors for each diagnosis, but also general goals and specific, attainable patient behaviors (Exhibit 15-3). For each problem label, the goal of prevention, improvement, or maintenance is attached. This expected outcome (goal) is then augmented by phrases which describe patient responses and serve to validate the achievement of the expected outcome (Cell, Peters, and Gordon 1984; Simmons 1980).

Clinical Management

Patient classification systems by definition are more of an administrative tool rather than an aid to clinical management. Some improvement in nursing care plans and chart documentation has been seen where classification data are obtained from these documents. However, the critical indicators of care used in patient classification systems are inadequate criteria for evaluating the quality of care received until a relation-

Exhibit 15-3. Omaha Classification Scheme

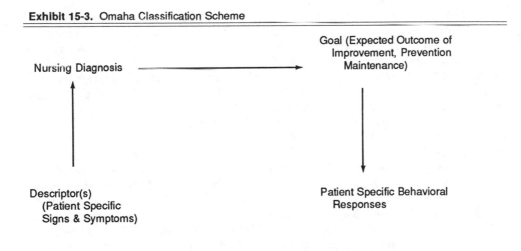

ship between these indicators and the progress of the patient's condition has been established (Aydelotte 1973).

Using a classification of nursing diagnoses, however, directly focuses on the care of the client. Nursing diagnosis is the pivotal factor in the nursing process which is central to community health practice and all nursing actions. Structurally, the nursing process is adapted from the scientific approach to solving problems. It consists of four steps: assessing, planning, implementing, and evaluating. The end point of the assessment stage is the nursing diagnosis. If there is no nursing diagnosis, then there is no reason to continue to the other components of the process.

Using a nursing diagnosis taxonomy inductively derived from community health practice actually defines that practice. Therefore, because the Omaha Classification Scheme defines community health care, when used correctly it provides for the planning, organizing, and prioritizing of that care. It allows for the sifting and sorting of information in an organized fashion. It actually provides a building block for care; the more difficult and time-consuming the case and the more extenuating the circumstances, the more problems will be identified from more domains. By identifying the subsequent problems, the nurse is able to communicate in a logical, concise way to her superiors, auditors, and others that this is a difficult case and more time is needed.

It is the classification of the nursing diagnoses which facilitate the organizing and prioritizing of care. The physiological domain, for example, generally provides the structure for those nursing interventions which are closely aligned with the medical regime. However, as any nurse working in home health care knows, it is those problems that are often the easiest to handle. The diagnoses under the other three domains are the ones that are often the most difficult and time-consuming. For example, the definition of the health behaviors domain states that these problems require personal motivation on the part of the client, thereby indicating resolution of the problem may be more difficult (Simmons 1980).

Utilizing the Omaha Scheme to show the sequencing of care allows nurses to define and adequately document the complexity of care inherent in these other domains. For example, a tuberculosis patient may be referred to an agency for monitoring and streptomycin injections. The nurse may begin by using the diagnosis of "respiratory impairment" (physiological domain) to follow the patient's physiological state. However, upon assessment it is found that the patient is not taking his medication regularly and is also consuming an excessive amount of alcohol. The diagnosis of therapeutic regime noncompliance, prescribed medications (health behavior domain) may then be added and a care plan developed to inform the patient of the consequences of not taking the medication and of mixing the medication with alcohol. On subsequent visits, the situation may be no better, so interventions are revised to include family counseling and the involvement of other community agencies. Eventually it is decided that the underlying problem is really alcoholism and a third diagnosis (substance misuse, also from health behaviors domain) is identified and a relevant plan of care developed. Thus, there is a clearly sequenced description of what was done in this case and how it required both changes in interventions and also subsequent identification of additional nursing diagnoses from another domain. Additionally, the use of the patient-specific behaviors in the scheme (Exhibit 15-3) provided the guideposts to evaluate whether or not the interventions made a difference in the patient's condition.

Once community health care is defined, it can then be communicated to each other, to supervisors, to the patient and to other health workers. Finally there is a way to remove the stereotype that home health care nurses teach diabetics to give insulin, insert foleys, or remove fecal impactions for patients on Friday afternoons. Providing hospital discharge coordinators, staff nurses and others with a list of the 44 nursing diagnoses in the taxonomy provides a means for understanding home health care nursing. Thus, it is easier for these people to discern what type of patient is appropriate to refer for home care. Also, the standard nomenclature provided in the Omaha Classification Scheme means the same thing to anyone reading the chart which facilitates both communication and understanding. This means that no longer is it necessary to spend a half an hour explaining to the weekend nurse about the case she has to see; now, in just a few minutes, she can read the chart and understand the meaning of the terms and care to be provided. Also, no longer do supervisors and auditors have to pursue thick charts trying to identify and evaluate the care rendered. Instead, use of the standard diagnoses allows anyone to follow the professional caregiver's movement through the problem-solving nursing process.

Documentation, an important form of communication, improves with the use of the Omaha Scheme both because the scheme provides objective terminology rather than subjective verbage and because it provides a unifying and organizing framework for care and therefore also for documentation. In an exploratory study done in New Jersey to determine the effectiveness of the Omaha Classification Scheme in improving the community health nurse's ability to identify patient health problems, it was found that after using the scheme for six months, there was an overall improvement in charting patient information. This study involved three test agencies and four control agencies. Test agency staff members were educated in the use of the Omaha Scheme, control agencies were not. Data were gathered using both pretesting and posttesting of staff and auditing of discharged patient charts. The charts were scored as a percentage of criteria met for each step in the nursing process. From pretest to posttest audits, an average net change for the experimental group which implemented the Omaha Classification Scheme, over the control group which did not implement the scheme, was 11% (Cell, Peters, and Gordon 1984). The scheme was originally designed to be used with any documentation system used by an agency whether problem-oriented or narrative, flow sheets or encounter forms, or any other format which a given agency used (Simmons 1980). In practice, however, it has been found that most agencies, at minimum, change their assessment form so that the information is organized using the four domains. It is also usually discovered that the assessment information required for using the scheme is more comprehensive than that found on the agency's current form. Therefore, the form is upgraded to become more comprehensive.

Improving documentation in community health is important because current documentation is inadequate. This inadequacy not only impacts on the ability of an agency to supervise staff clinically, but also impacts on reimbursement, regulations, and research. For example, it is widely known that if chart documentation is inadequate or inappropriate, reimbursement will be denied. However, equally as important is the threat of prospective payment. Alternative prospective payment plans are currently being evaluated based on current documentation. If documentation does not reflect what is being done, the basis for payment will be wrong. Furthermore, the current inconsistencies and ambiguities in the data being collected leaves agencies and the industry at the mercy of the Health Care Financing Administration's (HCFA) mandates as they affect reimbursement. There is no sufficient data base to show the impact of these mandates. Finally, research in community health has been very agency-specific. Inadequate common denominators in charting have made it difficult to collect data across agencies which would improve the ability to generalize the findings, to the industry at large rather than just within the agency where the study was conducted. The problem has been so pronounced that HCFA implemented the famous "485" standard data collection forms not only to foster more consistent Medicare coverage decisions and minimize payment for noncovered services, but also to provide for the gathering of data on a nationwide basis which could be used to establish a prospective payment system (Grimaldi 1985).

Documentation is also the base for a quality assurance program within an agency; more consistent and comprehensive data provide a better foundation for monitoring care. It is important however, that the scheme be used consistently. Inconsistent or improper use of the Scheme will give inaccurate or incomplete data which may not reflect the caregiving efforts. Therefore, a process audit tool to monitor usage of the Scheme is advisable as part of a quality assurance program. Such a tool has been developed by the Quality Assurance Subcommittee of the Home Health Agency Assembly of New Jersey, Inc. This tool is based on the steps of the nursing process (see Exhibit 15-4 for a sample section) and is applied to discharged patient records. Nurses whose records do not meet the established standards are counseled on their use of the Scheme.

Outside of a formal quality assurance program, just implementing the Omaha Scheme can improve quality within an agency. It makes the nurse ask critical questions: What data do I need to make a comprehensive assessment? Why am I visiting this case? Do I need to continue visiting? Is this a problem I can do something about or is it best handled by another discipline or another agency? It also forces agency ad-

Exhibit 15-4. Process Audit Tool

Criteria	Standard		
	Met	Unmet	Exception
Interventions			
A. Interventions are documented for each identified problem label.			
B. Interventions are modified for identified problem labels when patient outcomes are not being met.			

ministration to examine policy to determine if there are existing policies or procedures which impede the team concept of care or which hamper efficient patient-oriented care. For example, in one agency, usual procedure was to refer cases to the social worker using a referral form. The social worker did not have access to the patient chart. It became apparent after implementing the Omaha Scheme that not only did the social worker need access to the chart but she also needed more intimate communication with the nurse since they often were working on the same patient problem and a common (supplemental) plan of care.

Administrative Management

Patient classification systems are valuable management tools for staffing, budgeting, monitoring productivity, costing, and program planning. Historically in home health care, however, classification has been more for the purpose of quality assurance rather than resource allocation or costing. This is expected since the Medicare law of 1965 assured optimal payment to all providers and made no effort toward cost containment. The law, however, was accompanied by certification regulations which set forth standards for quality aimed at limiting participation in the program to those facilities that provided at least minimum care (Kurowski 1980; Mundinger 1983). Thus, the motivation for enhancing quality was greater than the motivation for efficient use of resources. Today, in this cost containment decade the picture is different. With home health care agencies caring for more patients, sicker patients, more high technology patients, and at the same time facing cost containment regulation including the possibility of prospective payment, efficient resource allocation and costing of services is paramount. In response to this "increase in technical services but fewer financial resources pinch," research has already begun in home health care to discover possible critical indicators of care for a patient classification system which will predict resource consumption (Ballard and McNamara 1983; Hardy 1984; Sienkiewicz 1984), but what needs to be explored is the possibility of using a nursing diagnosis taxonomy as the basis for categorization of patients since such a system already exists, and this system defines the essence of home health care. Following are some advantages in using such a system.

Patient Classification Systems are used for program planning. The Omaha Scheme provides the necessary information as a management tool for program planning. Analysis of specific nursing diagnoses addressed by nurses within a given agency allows the agency to systematically devise and revise their programs according to patient and community needs (Simmons 1980). It gives the agency the necessary data to interface with other community agencies and leaders for solving suprasystem problems such as identifying nutritional needs of patients that are not being met by the local food program.

Ideally, categorization of patients would also link quality care to the reimbursement or costing of care, although current patient classification systems are limited in their ability to accomplish that (Exhibit 15-2). The Omaha Scheme as a nursing diagnosis taxonomy for community health both defines reimbursable nursing care under Medicare (facilitation of the Medical treatment plan) and provides for a holistic assessment of the patient (Pankratz 1985). Thus, it provides for high quality nursing care at home while at the same time surviving in this world of regulation and cost containment. To prove the viability of this statement, a small unpublished pilot study was done by myself in 1985 on 41 Medicare patient records in two separate home health agencies to determine if the goals associated with the identified nursing diagnosis were being achieved under current Medicare law. Charts were selected from the total patient population for 1984 from these two agencies. Criteria for chart selection included: (a) Medicare payment, (b) normative discharge (i.e., improved health status), (c) nursing as the primary service used, and (d) inclusion of the nursing diagnosis of Integument: impairment. This diagnosis was used as a tracer. The findings indicated that proper use (as determined by the Process Audit Tool. Exhibit 15-4) of the Omaha Scheme for planning, documenting, and evaluating care allowed the attainment of 96% of the predetermined client goals before the patient was discharged. Unfortunately, the study also showed that often the scheme was not being used at its maximum resulting once more in inadequate documentation of home health care activities (Table 15-2).

Patient Classification requires the use of critical indicators of care or essential characteristics for use in classifying patients. The Omaha Scheme has been evaluated

Table 15-2. Nursing Diagnosis Analysis Number and percentage of nursing diagnoses identified and outcomes met by agency

	Agency A (VNA) (N = 102)		
Problems identified	Problems not identified	Outcomes met at discharge*	Outcomes not met at Discharge*
76 (74.5%)	26 (25.5%)	64 (84.2%)	12 (15.8%)
	Agency B (Hospital-based) (N = 61)		
41 (67.2%)	20 (32.8%)	39 (95.1%)	2 (4.9%)
	Complete charts from both agencies (N = 6)		
27 (16.6%)	N/A	26 (96%)	N/A

*Could not be determined for unidentified problems.

for its possible contribution to the essential characteristics which have an effect on nursing workload. In a study by Peters and Mechanic (in press), it was hypothesized that the quantity of nursing care demanded would be a function of the patient's living arrangements and support system, age, sex, ability to perform activities of daily living, prior source of care, presence of surgical intervention, and nursing diagnosis. All the variables except the nursing diagnosis had been measured in previous studies. This study consisted of 68 patient records from two home health agencies. The records were drawn from the total patient population of these agencies for 1984 using a random numbers table. The inclusion of nursing diagnoses with the variables from previous studies helped to account for 41.9% of the variance in RN visits. Ballard and McNamara (1983) who did not use nursing diagnoses were only able to explain 31.9% of the total variance. In addition, the only variables to enter the regression equation for intensity of nursing visits (number of nursing visits to length of service) were nursing diagnoses. This may indicate that certain problems identified by nurses are especially predictive when examining the intensity of service rendered to patients. Such a finding is important since reimbursements and technological reforms have led to more intense services being provided to home care patients.

Another study (Martin and Scheet 1982) also indicates that the classification of nursing diagnoses may be an important tool for examining costs of home health care. This study found that the number of nursing diagnoses and race were significant in predicting length of agency service.

Evidence is mounting that nursing diagnoses play an important part in the provision of home health care and in allocating resources (money and personnel) for that care. A nursing diagnoses taxonomy per se, however, cannot be used as a patient classification system because it categorizes nursing diagnoses not patients. Thus, patients may not be placed into mutually exclusive categories. In addition, a nursing diagnoses taxonomy uses the classificatory concepts of class membership, while a patient classification system uses the ordering concepts of precedence and coincidence. For example, a patient to be classified in a patient classification scheme would be evaluated using established critical indicators of care and then be placed into a level based on the importance or weight (more or less important than other critical indicators) of the critical indicators connected with that patient's care. Nursing diagnoses within a taxonomy could be used as the critical indicators of care for placing a patient into a level. However, to utilize them in this fashion, the assumption must be made that only the primary nursing diagnosis is considered in order to avoid the complications of having more than one diagnosis. Then, all the nursing diagnoses would need to be weighted in relationship to each other. For example, does a patient with the primary diagnosis of Integument: impairment require more nursing resources and therefore cost more than a patient with the primary diagnosis of Nutrition: impairment? Work has begun on examining relative costs, resource consumption, and intensity of nursing diagnoses (Harris et al., in press) but it is insufficient to determine the feasibility of such a weighting. In addition, work needs to be done on examining the ramifications of using only a primary nursing diagnosis. Alternative considerations are the utilization of groups of nursing diagnoses, if clusters of similar diagnoses appear in practice, or the use of numbers of diagnoses rather than specific diagnosis. Each alternative has its limitations and needs to be explored through research in practice settings.

Conclusion

The home health care market is expected to almost double in the next five years. Sixty percent of the current market is primary nursing service. Thus, nursing has a vested interest in the future growth and direction of home care (Mershon and Wesolowski 1985). Use of a nursing diagnosis taxonomy is valuable in defining, organizing, directing, and communicating this care. It provides the bases for quality and clinical management of care. Its use, however, as a management tool for staffing and costing is limited because it does not place patients into mutually exclusive categories. However, preliminary research studies indicate that such a taxonomy does provide useful information in allocating resources. Thus, the challenge becomes to develop a patient classification system incorporating a nursing diagnosis taxonomy. Such a blending would provide a system that not only measures costs and staffing levels but also includes the qualitative issues of care. If the nursing taxonomy system also included measurable patient outcomes as the Omaha Scheme does, the patient classification system based on a nursing diagnosis taxonomy would also have the ability of incorporating an evaluation measure for monitoring change in a patient's condition based on nursing interventions. Such a system would then have the additional potential of justifying care as well as costs.

Caseload and Workload Analysis In Home Health Care

Judith Lloyd Storfjell, Carol Easley Allen, and Cheryl E. Easley

Introduction

The successful management of nursing caseloads and workloads is essential to the survival of home health agencies as regulations become more complex, competition increases, and more acutely ill patients are referred to home care as a result of prospective payment systems that encourage alternatives to institutionalization. The home care manager is required to increase efficiency and provide a broader range of services while, at the same time, reducing administrative overhead.

The Easley-Storfjell Instruments for Caseload/Workload Analysis (CL/WLA) were designed to give home health care managers tools to obtain strategic information for planning, monitoring, and evaluating field staff activities simply and effectively. These instruments have been used successfully throughout the United States and Canada by a variety of community health and home health agencies since 1977.

The CL/WLA were developed to meet the following criteria:

1. To facilitate supervisory process. The chief purpose was to assist nursing supervisors in assignment of cases, identifying caseload problems and patterns, and to provide a format for supervisory conferences. By jointly performing ratings on a periodic basis, caseload/workload analysis can easily be combined with other nurse-supervisor activities.

2. Simple to use. Some patient classification systems devised for community nursing settings, such as home care, contain too many variables or require lengthy

analysis which discourages adequate use of the tools and could possibly affect their reliability. CL/WLA was kept extremely simple in order to be easily understood by all levels of personnel. Rather than taking extra time from a supervisor's busy schedule, they should, in fact, reduce the amount of supervisory time required. While these instruments were originally designed for manual use, a format for microcomputer application has also been developed.

3. Flexible. CL/WLA were designed for use in a variety of staffing patterns including team nursing and individual caseloads. In addition, they can also be adapted for use in many types of community health agencies as well as for other professionals carrying caseloads.

4. Include both acuity and time requirements. Both the complexity of care and the time required are considered. These two variables are seen as the key indicators in appropriate staffing and productivity planning.

5. Provide summary data. Data may be summarized and quantified by various categories including individuals, teams, districts, and agencies.

6. Compatibility with other tools. While the information derived from CL/WLA is valuable in its own right, it can be augmented by data derived from other common analyses such as costs per unit and time studies.

7. Provide management information. Some management uses of CL/WLA include projecting and evaluating staffing needs, developing a database for prediction of nursing care demands, and revealing trends in care delivery over time.

The two major components of the system, caseload analysis and workload analysis, are defined as follows:

Caseload analysis is a summary of the characteristics of cases carried by a particular professional nurse, technical nurse, or nursing assistant.

Workload analysis is a summary of all activities required of home health nursing employees, including caseload responsibilities.

Description

The Easley-Storfjell process for analyzing a caseload and workload encompasses four steps. First, every case handled by the staff nurse is analyzed to predict the number of visits required per month to accomplish patient and nursing goals and also to determine the complexity of nursing care requirements. Second, after cases are rated, they are charted on a graph and the total of monthly visits required by the caseload is calculated. Third, the time required for duties other than home visits is determined. Finally, all of the above data are summarized and the number of visits required by the caseload is compared with the number possible according to the workload.

Exhibit 15-5. Easley-Storfjell Instruments For Caseload/Workload Analysis.

CASELOAD ANALYSIS GUIDELINES
Time Determination

1. Monthly or less; only one visit.
2. Bi-weekly.
3. 1-2 times per week.
4. 3-5 times per week.

NOTE: Extensive follow-up or lengthy visits (over 1-1/2 hours)–add one time level.
Brief visits (under 1-1/2 hours)–subtract one time level.

Difficulty Determination

Assign the highest numerical categorical rating (most difficult) in which the case meets two or more of the criteria.

Based on: A. Clinical Judgment
B. Teaching Needs
C. Physical Care
D. Psycho-Social Needs
E. Multi-Agency Involvement
F. Number and Severity of Problems

1. **Minimal:**

A. Requires limited judgment, use of common sense, observation of fairly predictable change in patient status.
B. Requires basic health teaching.
C. Requires none or simple maintenance care.
D. Requires ability to relate to patients and families.
E. Requires limited involvement of only one other agency/provider.
F. Few or uncomplicated problems.

2. **Moderate:**

A. Requires use of basic problem-solving techniques, ability to make limited patient assessments.
B. Requires teaching related to common health problems.
C. Requires basic rehabilitation or use of uncomplicated technical skills.
D. Requires use of basic interpersonal relationship skills.
E. Requires limited involvement of two other agencies/providers.
F. Several problems with limited complexity.

3. **Great:**

A. Requires use of well-developed problem-solving skills enhanced by comprehensive knowledge of physical and social sciences, ability to make patient and family assessments.
B. Requires teaching related to illness, complications and/or comprehensive health supervision.
C. Requires use of complicated technical skills.
D. Requires professional insight and intervention skills in coping with psychosocial needs.

Exhibit 15-5, continued.

    E.   Requires extensive involvement of at least one other agency/provider or coordination of several agencies/providers.

    F.   Several complicated problems

4. **Very Great:**

    A.   Requires use of creativity, ability to initiate and coordinate plan for patient or family care, use of additional resources and increased supervisory support, ability to make comprehensive patient and family assessment.

    B.   Requires teaching related to unusual health problems or teaching/learning difficulties.

    C.   Requires knowledge of scientific rationale which underlie techniques and ability to modify care in response to patient/family need.

    D.   Requires ability to intervene in severe psychosocial problems.

    E.   Requires extensive coordination of multiple agencies/providers.

    F.   Numerous or complicated problems requiring augmentation of the knowledge base.

Step One. Difficulty and time are seen as the most important variables in assessing the level of nursing care required and the amount of work time needed. The tools were therefore devised to allow separate and combined assessments in both areas.

Time required is assigned a rating from "1" to "4" with the lowest rank given to cases requiring one visit per month. The actual requirements associated with the time ratings can be easily adjusted according to actual agency patterns.

Difficulty of care determination is based on assessing six variables covering the scope of the care requirements: (a) clinical judgment required; (b) teaching needs; (c) physical care needs; (d) psychosocial needs; (e) multiagency involvement (coordination of care); and (f) number and severity of problems. The difficulty variables have again been assigned into four categories from minimal to very great. Descriptions of the nursing care requirements for each criterion by level of difficulty are shown in Exhibit 15-5. These difficulty levels may also be correlated to the levels of nursing practice and ancillary support frequently available in home health care settings.

It was found that the way to handle the actual rating of cases was through a joint conference between the supervisor and staff member. This process offers an opportunity for a generalized caseload review and a weeding out of cases. During this conference, more accurate information regarding the current status of the patient can be obtained and care plans and goals identified. At the same time, the cases are listed on the *Caseload Analysis Roster* (See Exhibit 15-6) along with ratings for time and difficulty. Space has also been provided for recording the length of time a case has been open and the agency priority, program, or diagnosis.

Step Two. The time and difficulty ratings are then charted on the *Caseload Analysis Graph* (Exhibit 15-7) for a graphic representation of the caseload. This chart, more

Exhibit 15-6. Easley-Storfjell Instruments For Caseload/Workload Analysis

CASELOAD ANALYSIS ROSTER

Name _____ Position _____ Date _____

Case Number/Name	Weeks	Priority/ Program/ Diagnosis	Time	Difficulty	Total
1.					
2.					
3.					
4.					
5.					
6.					
7.					
8.					
9.					
10.					
11.					
12.					
13.					
14.					
15.					
16.					
17.					
18.					
19.					
20.					
Totals					
Averages					

Exhibit 15-7. Easley-Storfjell Instruments For Caseload/Workload Analysis

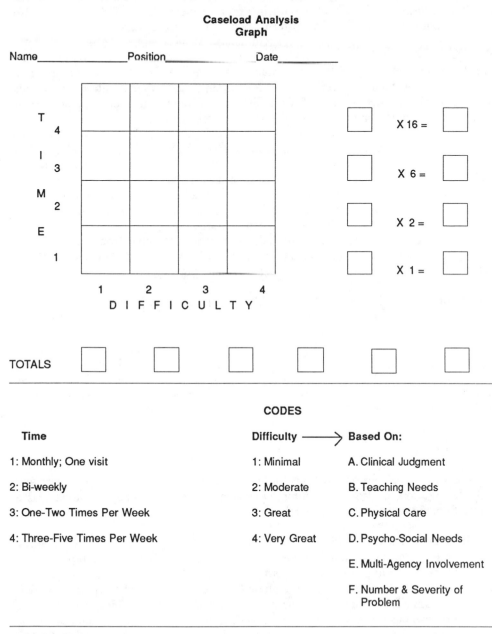

**Caseload Analysis
Graph**

Name_____Position_____Date_____

CODES

Time	Difficulty ⟶	Based On:
1: Monthly; One visit	1: Minimal	A. Clinical Judgment
2: Bi-weekly	2: Moderate	B. Teaching Needs
3: One-Two Times Per Week	3: Great	C. Physical Care
4: Three-Five Times Per Week	4: Very Great	D. Psycho-Social Needs
		E. Multi-Agency Involvement
		F. Number & Severity of Problem

© COPYRIGHT 1979
 Form ES 22

than any other portion of the CL/WLA has been beneficial in assisting the individual nurse to "see" the caseload. This instrument is designed to facilitate calculation of the number of visits required each month in order to meet caseload demands. It also depicts a pattern of the difficulty clustering of a particular caseload.

Step Three. Seldom does a staff nurse have 40 hours a week to devote to home visits and necessary follow-up. Other assignments and responsibilities also require time commitments. A dilemma often develops for the supervisor when additional programs are added without increasing staff. By analyzing staff time available, the supervisor is able to document staffing needs and alteration of assignments.

The *Time Allocation Worksheet* (Exhibit 15-8) allows a calculation of the time needed for the range of activities that characterize the nurse's total workload. Personal time, supervisory activities, special assignments, community service activities, and typical community nursing categories such as supervisor and nurse conferences, hospital liaison, and meetings have been included. But here again, in keeping with the flexibility designed into the system, agencies may modify this tool to provide a realistic representation of their specific workload components.

When the time needed for scheduled activities is subtracted from the total time available, the time that may be devoted to home visits is revealed. This includes time actually spent in the home, travel, charting, and follow-up activities.

Step Four. Finally, the caseload and workload time demands are summarized on the *Workload Summary Sheet* (Exhibit 15-9). The number of home visits each nurse can make is calculated by dividing the total time available by the time needed for each home visit. The time per visit allowed can be determined by doing actual time studies or using specific agency productivity standards. A comparison of the number of visits required by the caseload demands with the number of visits possible based on the workload analysis reveals whether an excessive number of visits is being required or if additional visits are possible.

Implications

CL/WLA has numerous applications for home health administrators, supervisors, and staff. In addition, it also has a potential impact for the home health industry as a whole. Some implications of its use follow.

Administrative Uses. It is important for managers to project and evaluate staffing needs and to determine nursing costs based on a method that encompasses the comprehensive nursing resource demands in a home care agency. Cost-effectiveness determination for nursing should not be based on the bare bones of technical care that the use of medical diagnosis alone would provide. By compiling data on the comprehensive nursing resource demand, staffing needs in a particular agency can be compared with the use of time and the types of service being delivered (Allen, Easley, and Storfjell 1986).

Through repeated analyses, trends in service delivery may be ascertained. Data provided by workload trends for the entire agency may be used to justify budgetary al-

Exhibit 15-8.   Easley-Storfjell Instruments For Caseload/Workload Analysis

TIME ALLOCATION WORKSHEET

Name _____   Position _____   Date _____

TIME AVAILABLE (Monthly, Yearly)   _____

TIME UTILIZATION;

1. Personal Adjustments:
    a. Annual Leave/Holiday   _____
    b. Coffee Breaks   _____
    c. Other _____   _____   _____

2. Supportive Activities:
    a. Supervisor/Nurse Conference   _____
    b. Staff Meetings   _____
    c. Inservice Education/Workshop   _____
    d. Committees _____   _____
    e. Other _____   _____   _____

3. Special Assignments:
    a. Classes _____   _____
    b. Hospital Liaison_____   _____
    c. Field Advisor_____   _____
    d. Other_____   _____   _____

4. Field Activities (Community Service):
    a. Committees/Meetings _____   _____
        _____   _____
    b. Schools _____   _____
    c. Clinics _____   _____
    d. Other _____   _____   _____

TOTAL SCHEDULED TIME   _____

TIME AVAILABLE FOR HOME VISITS, CHARTING & FOLLOW-UP   _____

Exhibit 15-9. Easley-Storfjell Instruments For Caseload/Workload Analysis

CASELOAD/WORKLOAD SUMMARY

Name _____ Position _____ Date _____

	TOTAL		AVERAGE

A   Caseload

1.   Total cases _____

2.   Time factor _____   _____

3.   Difficulty factor _____   _____

4.   Total points _____   _____

5.   Average weeks open   _____

6.   Optional categorical analysis   % of caseload
     (priority/program/diagnosis)

_____   _____   _____

_____   _____   _____

_____   _____   _____

_____   _____   _____

B   Time (monthly, yearly)

1.   Total time available _____

2.   Scheduled time _____

3.   Time available for H.V.'s _____

4.   Time per home visit _____

	Monthly	Yearly

5.   Number of H.V.'s possible   _____   _____
     (divide 3 by 4)

6.   Number of H.V.'s required
     by caseload _____

7.   Number of H.V.'s to new
     referrals _____

8.   TOTAL required H.V.'s
     (add 6 and 7)   _____   _____

9.   Excess H.V.'s required
     (8 larger than 5)   _____   _____

10.   Additional H.V.'s possible
      (5 larger than 8)   _____   _____

11.   Average mileage (optional)   _____   _____

Exhibit 15-9, continued.

CASELOAD/WORKLOAD SUMMARY

Name _____ Position _____ Date _____

| | TOTAL | | AVERAGE |

A   Caseload

1.   Total cases

2.   Time factor

3.   Difficulty factor

4.   Total points

5.   Average weeks open

6.   Optional categorical analysis   % of caseload
(priority/program/diagnosis)

_____

_____

_____

_____

B   Time (monthly, yearly)

1.   Total time available

2.   Scheduled time

3.   Time available for H.V.'s

4.   Time per home visit

| | | Monthly | Yearly |

5.   Number of H.V.'s possible
(divide 3 by 4)

6.   Number of H.V.'s required
by caseload

7.   Number of H.V.'s to new
referrals

8.   TOTAL required H.V.'s
(add 6 and 7)

9.   Excess H.V.'s required
(8 larger than 5)

10. Additional H.V.'s possible
(5 larger than 8)

11. Average mileage (optional)

locations for nursing staff. In addition, comparisons can also be made between service trends and agency goals and priorities.

CL/WLA differs from other productivity methodologies because it takes into account the level of nursing care required as well as time. In addition, time utilization is individualized by assessing all time commitments other than home visits. In this way many of the pitfalls encountered by assigning "average" productivity standards to specific individuals are avoided. If desired, visits required by the caseload and the number possible according to the workload can be calculated on a monthly basis and compared to actual performance.

Supervisory Uses. The use of CL/WLA allows supervisors to base hiring decisions on projections of the nursing care demands of the agency's caseload. The difficulty profile of a caseload may indicate a need for staffing adjustments, thus providing the level of nursing staff competent to provide appropriate care while avoiding underutilization of the skills and educational preparation of any individuals on the nursing team. In this way, nursing costs are managed effectively, based on hard data which justifies the budgetary requirements of the required nursing staff mix.

In addition to general staffing uses, the tools are especially beneficial in the supervision of individual nurses. They have been used primarily in individual conferences in order to plan and adjust assignments. A concentration of high difficulty cases may signal a nurse's need for additional supervisory support or training, while a caseload difficulty rating lower than the nurse's skills may be the key to restlessness or low morale. The average length of time cases are open should alert the supervisor to those nurses who either carry cases too long or close them too quickly. Staff development needs can be identified by both individual and aggregate data. For example, if a particular nurse has a high percentage of clients with a diagnosis of cerebral-vascular accident, continuing education in rehabilitation may be important.

The CL/WLA may be especially valuable when transferring cases from one nurse to another or in the orientation of new staff or new supervisors. As home care agencies increase their use of part-time staff to improve flexibility, it becomes more and more necessary to have a readily available method of allocating cases among a varying group of nursing staff at any given time. The time and difficulty ratings provide this capability.

Staff Uses. This systematic analysis allows nurses to organize their activities, streamline caseloads, and to obtain a realistic picture of workload demands and expectations, all of which lead to greater efficiency, more appropriate time utilization, and increased cost effectiveness.

Many studies have shown a correlation between job satisfaction and turnover as well as between satisfaction and absenteeism. It is clear that improvement in employee morale is cost-effective. Individual staff members can benefit when a realistic caseload and workload has been defined and goals for service are delineated. Staff development needs can be identified by both individual and aggregate data.

Industry Uses. Standards for nursing care based on professional ideals and goals must be established in home care. The model of care that will be recognized in home care nursing is critically influenced by the shape of the patient classification system and the overall dimensions of the workload determination that is deemed appropriate by those public and private agencies that fund home care activities. In addition to facilitating supervision, assisting staff with time management, and providing pertinent data for administrators, the Easley-Storfjell tools can provide the home care industry with hard data necessary to rationalize comprehensive nursing resource demands while demonstrating efficiency in management of personnel and budgets.

Conclusion

Home health nursing managers are increasingly being required to document both the quality and the quantity of care being provided by their staff. The Easley-Storfjell instruments provide a more refined method of analyzing the home health nurse's caseload and workload providing valuable information for various levels of agency personnel. Although the tools have not been stringently tested for reliability and validity, experience has proven them useful to administrators, supervisors, and staff in various types of community health agencies.

References

Allen, C. E., E. Easley, and J. I. Storfjell. 1986. Cost management through caseload-workload analysis. In Shaffer, F., ed. *Patients and purse strings: Patient classification and cost management.* New York: National League for Nursing.

Alward, R. 1983. Patient classification schemes: The ideal vs. reality. *Journal of Nursing Administration* 13(2):14-19.

American Nurses' Association. 1974. *Standards of community health nursing practice.* Kansas City, MO: American Nurses' Association.

Aydelotte, M. 1973. *Quality assurance programs in nursing: Definitions and problems.* Presented at Connecticut Hospital Association Workshop, Hamden, July 1973 (Mimeographed).

Aydelotte, M. R. 1973. State of knowledge: Nurse staffing methodology. In Levine, E., ed., *Research on nurse staffing in hospitals.* Frederickburg, VA: Division of Nursing.

Bailit, H., et al. 1975. Assessing the quality of care. *Nursing Outlook* 23:152-159.

Ballard, S., and R. McNamara. 1983. Quantifying nursing needs in home health care. *Nursing Research* 32(4):236-241.

Bloch, D. 1975. Evaluation of nursing care in terms of process and outcome: Issues in research and quality assurance. *Nursing Research* 24:256-263.

Brown, B. I. 1980. Realistic workloads for community health nurses. *Nursing Outlook* 28:233-237.

Cell, P., D. A. Peters, and J. B. Gordon. 1984. Implementing a nursing diagnosis system through research: The New Jersey experience. *Home Healthcare Nurse* 2(1):26-32.

Daubert, E. A. 1979. Patient classification system and outcome criteria. *Nursing Outlook* 27:450-454.

Daubert, E. A. 1977. A system to evaluate home health care services. *Nursing Outlook* 25:168-171.

Fobair, P. Do cancer patients take more time? A survey of San Francisco Bay area home health agencies. *Home Health Review* 6(4):17-27.

Giovannetti, P. 1979. Understanding patient classification systems. *Journal of Nursing Administration* 9(2):4.

Giovannetti, P., and M. Thiessen. 1983. *Patient classification for nurse staffing: Criteria for selection and implementation.* Edmonton, Alberta: Alberta Association of Registered Nurses.

Grimaldi, P. L. 1985. PPS for home health services? *Nursing Management* 16(12):16-18.

Hardy, J. A. 1984. A patient classification system for home health patients. *Caring* 3(9):26-27.

Harris, M. D., D. A., Peters, J. A. Smith, and J. Yuan. In press. Cost of home care by nursing diagnoses. *Nursing Economics.*

Harris, et al. 1985. A patient classification system in home health care. *Nursing Economics* 3:276-282.

Hempel, C. G. 1965. *Aspects of scientific explanation and other essays in the philosophy of science*. New York: The Free Press.

Hempel, C. G. 1952. *Fundamentals of concept formation in empirical science*. Chicago: The University of Chicago Press.

Johnson, K. 1984. A practical approach to patient classification. *Nursing Management* 15(6).

Jones, K. R. 1984. Severity of illness measures: Issues and options. *Nursing Economics* 2:312-317.

Kurowski, B. T. 1980. *A cost-effectiveness analysis of home health care: Implications for public policy and future research*. University of Colorado, Denver: unpublished Doctoral Dissertation.

Martin, K. 1982. A client classification system adaptable for computerization. *Nursing Outlook* 30(9).

Martin, K., and N. Scheet. 1985. The Omaha System: Implications for costing community health nursing. In Shaffer, F. A., ed., *Costing out nursing: Pricing our product*. New York: National League for Nursing.

Mershon, K., and M. Wesolowski. 1985. Strategic planning for the business of community health and home care. *Nursing and Health Care* 6(1):33-35.

Mundinger, M. O. 1983. *Home care controversy: Too little, too late, too costly*. Rockville, MD: Aspen Publication.

Pankratz, J. D. (1985). *Serving two masters? Professional standards of care and reimbursable care*. Paper presented at the First National symposium on Home Health Care, Ann Arbor, MI, June 1985.

Peters, D. A., and D. Mechanick. In press. *Measuring home care resource consumption using nursing diagnoses*.

Roy, C., Sr. 1975. A diagnostic classification system for nursing. *Nursing Outlook* 23:90-94.

Sienkiewicz, J. I. 1984. Patient classification in community health nursing. *Nursing Outlook* 32:319-321.

Simmons, D. A. 1980. *A classification scheme for client problems in community health nursing*. Washington, DC: U. S. Government Printing Office. DHHS Publication No. HRA 80-16.

Sokal, R. 1974. Classification: Purposes, principles, progress, prospects. *Science* 185:1115-1123.

Webster's new collegiate dictionary. 1975. Springfield, MA: G & C Merriam Co.

Young, K. M., and C. R. Fisher. 1980. Medicare episodes of illness: A study of hospital, skilled nursing facility and home health agency care. *Health Care Financing Review* Fall:1-23.

Chapter Sixteen

Nursing Diagnoses

Nursing Diagnoses in Community Health Nursing

Carol Ann Parente

The Concept

The concept of nursing diagnoses may initially strike the community health administrator as a tool more appropriate for clinical use. After all, of what use is an "alteration in skin integrity" at budget time? The definition and application of nursing diagnoses would definitely seem more valuable to those who provide direct patient services and their immediate supervisors. The nursing diagnosis concept, however, may prove to be valuable indeed to the administrative team as demonstrated in this chapter and the accompanying example. Discussions of nursing diagnoses in recent literature generally do focus on the clinical uses and benefits. This chapter, however, will attempt to discuss the concept, process, and effects of nursing diagnoses from a community health administrative perspective.

Nursing diagnosis represents the beginning steps of the profession's attempts to define its scope and science. Controversy has swirled around the concept since its inception. The debate continues today regarding the appropriateness of identified diagnoses (Jacoby 1985), the taxonomy selected (Lunney 1982), and even the very idea of diagnoses made by nurses (Shamansky and Yanni 1983). In spite of the debate, or perhaps because of it, the concept of nursing diagnosis has continually gained acceptance over the 13 years since the first National Conference on Classification of Nursing Diagnosis convened in St. Louis.

The concept has become well entrenched at all levels of education and in various fields of practice. Indeed, the American Nurses' Association in their Social Policy Statement of 1980 described nursing as "the diagnosis and treatment of human responses to actual and potential health problems" (ANA 1980). The ANA Standards of Practice for Community Health Nursing further elaborate on nursing diagnoses as derived from health status data and leading to subsequent goals and interventions (ANA 1973). The ANA clearly sees the nursing diagnostic process as a key nursing function and vital to providing quality professional nursing care. In addition, many state nurse practice acts now include the terminology "diagnosis" as part of the defined functions of the professional nurse.

Nursing diagnoses have evolved over several paths during the seventies and eighties. The most commonly accepted format has emerged from the North American Nursing Diagnosis Association (NANDA). This group has evolved from the National Conference Group on Classification of Nursing Diagnoses. The NANDA diagnoses list (Table 16-1) may be used by nurses in all clinical fields. Over the years since the First National Conference on the Classification of Nursing Diagnosis in 1973, the list of diagnoses has been refined slowly from just over 100 diagnoses to less than 50 (Gor-

Table 16-1.

Visiting Nurse Association of Eastern Montgomery County
Abington, Pennsylvania

Accepted Nursing Diagnoses

1. Activity intolerance
2. Ineffective airway clearance
3. Anxiety
4. Alt. in bowel elimination: Constipation
5. Alt. in bowel elimination: Diarrhea
7. Ineffective breathing patterns
8. Alt. in cardiac output: Decreased
9. Alt. in comfort: Pain
10. Impaired verbal communication
11. Ineffective Individual Coping
12. Ineffective family coping: Compromised
13. Ineffective family coping: Disabling
14. Family coping: Potential for growth
15. Diversional activity deficit
16. Alt. in family processes
17. Fear
18. Fluid volume deficit
19. Potential fluid volume deficit
20. Excess fluid volume
21. Impaired gas exchange
22. Anticipatory grieving
23. Dysfunctional grieving
24. Alt. in health maintenance:
      A. Cardiac B. Hypertension
25. Imapired home maintenance management

26. Potential for injury
27. Knowledge deficit: A. Diabetes   B. General
28. Impaired physical mobility
29. Non-compliance
30. Alt. in nutrition: Less than body requirements
31. Alt. in nutrition: More than body requirements
32. Alt. in nutrition: Potential more than body requirements
33. Alt. in oral mucous membrane
34. Alt. in parenting
35. Potential alt. in parenting
36. Powerlessness
37. Rape-trauma syndrome
38. Self-care deficit
39. Self-esteem disturbance
40. Sensory-perceptual alterations
41. Sexual dysfunction
42. Actual impairment of skin integrity
43. Potential impairment of skin integrity
44. Disturbance in sleep pattern
45. Social isolation
46. Spiritual distress
47. Alt. in thought processes
48. Alt. in tissue perfusion
49. Alt. in pattern of urinary elimination
50. Potential for violence

don 1982a,346). This reduction in the number represents the series of conferences and refinements over 13 years. Considering the number of medical diagnoses available, you can see we are just making our first steps into this area.

Nursing diagnoses differ, however, from our medical colleagues' diagnostic categories by defining actual or potential human responses to health problems (Gordon 1976) rather than describing specific disease or illness states. The relationship of nursing to medical diagnoses may in one sense be demonstrated in the problem-etiology-symptom (PES) format of nursing diagnoses as described by Gordon (Gordon 1982a,209). Here, the nursing diagnosis is the problem or first part of the diagnostic statement. The etiology, second in the statement format is shown in relationship to the problem and is often (but not always) the medical illness or treatment. Resulting symptoms form the last part of the diagnosis and further individualize the nursing diagnosis to reflect a specific patient's problem. An example may be: alteration in nutrition, less than body requirements related to chemotherapy resulting in anorexia, and taste changes. The relationship of the nursing diagnosis to the medical diagnosis is one that must be considered carefully by the community health administrator in these days of close scrutiny by third-party payors for reimbursable services.

Another nursing diagnosis group is of particular interest to community health administrators and nursing staffs. The Omaha VNA (Simmons 1980), under a 1977 contract with the Division of Nursing, Human Resources Administration, Department of Health, Education and Welfare, defined and tested a patient diagnostic and classification scheme. Four domains of nursing endeavor, environmental, psychosocial, physiological, and health behaviors, were defined and related diagnoses were elaborated. The diagnostic categories resemble the NANDA list in some areas while defining other diagnoses with more direct community health impact such as income and sanitation deficits. The structure of the diagnosis is somewhat similar to the NANDA format. The Omaha diagnosis is listed first and is individualized for a particular patient by the use of modifiers, which are specific for each diagnosis. The Omaha system was structured initially to be computerized, further enhancing its usefulness to the community health administrator. This built-in computerization allows the administrator to maximize the information available on an agency's population. The NANDA diagnoses and other classification systems may also be computerized as you will see in the accompanying example. (See Chapter 15 for more information on the Omaha diagnoses and classification system.)

Other authors, such as Lunney (1982) and Campbell (1978) suggest variations on the diagnostic taxonomy in response to patient and nursing needs. Of particular concern are the areas of wellness care and the independent versus interdependent actions of the nurse. Most NANDA diagnoses indicate a problem with the patient's health and/or his response to his health. The Omaha system does address wellness or health behaviors to some extent. Unfortunately, wellness care is not fully addressed by the diagnostic labels and equally unfortunately it is not reimbursable in the current third-party payor environment.

Controversial too, is the independent response of the nurse in treating certain diagnostic categories, e.g., the NANDA approved "impaired gas exchange." Many of the physiologically based diagnoses are considered to have interdependent responses that are based on both medical and nursing orders (Kim 1985). Some would argue that nurses do not even have the tools to assess such diagnoses (Jacoby 1985). Gordon's diagnostic manual (1982b) clearly suggests medical referral in such cases that a nurse suspects an interdependent diagnosis, e.g., impaired gas exchange. This particular area is less problematic to the community health administrator since the current atmosphere dictates a signed physician's order to cover any nursing activities. Should, however, the legislative climate change allowing direct reimbursement for nursing activities, these interdependent diagnoses may present an administrative challenge.

The Process

Now that we have described the concept of nursing diagnoses, how do we establish the diagnosis? A larger question also remains: what conceptual framework would give focus and definition to the diagnostic process?

To respond to the first question, Gordon (1982a) notes that nursing diagnosis is both a label and an action. Diagnosis therefore requires a nursing knowledge base and skill in application of the nursing process. The second question may prove to be more difficult to answer clearly in that no one unified framework has been established for the profession. Consideration must then be given to the nursing agency's and the individual nurse's philosophy and the framework that most closely corresponds.

The nursing process involves the methodical examination, definition, and solution of the patient's health problems in relation to nursing. More traditionally, the process is defined as assessment, planning, intervention, and evaluation. The ANA Model Practice Act statement (1980) inserts the diagnostic step directly after assessment in their discussion of the nursing process. The step-by-step nature of the nursing process and the placement of the nursing diagnosis within it help to define and organize the patient's care needs for the staff nurse regardless of the complexity of that patient's problems.

Clearly, the nursing diagnosis is established within the nursing process. The staff nurse, after the initial assessment of the patient, defines problems (the diagnosis) which may be addressed by nursing interventions and which may reflect the instructions of the medical regimen, e.g., knowledge deficit related to two-gram sodium diet. The diet in the example was prescribed by the physician and the nurse's evaluation shows the patient in some way lacks the information to appropriately select that diet. For those nurses who are unfamiliar with the diagnostic categories and their defining characteristics, several pocket-sized manuals are available to help the nurse clarify and select appropriate diagnoses (Gordon 1982b; Duespohl 1986). Following the definition of the nursing diagnosis, the nurse may proceed to plan and implement interventions based on the problem and the goals set by patient and nurse. The final step in the process is the evaluation of the effectiveness of the interventions and indeed the overall plan. This step guides the nurse in revision or adaptation of the plan to meet the patient's needs most effectively.

Selection of a particular diagnosis is based on analysis of the patient's nursing assessment data. The focus and definition of the nursing assessment comes from a conceptual framework. A variety of frameworks is available for the clinical nurse's examination. Some popular nursing frameworks include Roy's adaptation model, Rogers' life process conceptual framework, Neuman's behavioral systems, and Orem's self-care agencies (Riehl and Roy 1980). Many agencies and certainly many individuals use an eclectic approach; some combination of formalized framework and unspoken concepts which guide their practice. An additional factor in considering a practical, conceptual framework for an agency is the demand of third-party payors, since although the patient may have an adaptive or self-care problem, that diagnosis may not represent a reimbursable nursing activity.

Regardless of the framework selected, the nursing assessment must consider all aspects of the patient's care needs. Gordon (1982b) suggests a functional approach and considers 11 health patterns as necessary for a complete assessment in any framework. The health patterns she describes include: health-perception-health-management, nutritional-metabolic pattern, elimination pattern, activity-exercise, cognitive-perceptual pattern, sleep-rest, self-perception-self-concept, role relationship pattern, sexuality-reproductive pattern, coping-stress-tolerance pattern, and value-belief pattern. A sample nursing assessment (Exhibit 16-1) contains functional elements as suggested by Gordon, physical assessment, and historical data.

Once selected, the nursing diagnosis may be documented in a variety of ways. Particularly useful is the problem-oriented method of charting which allows the nurse to address each problem separately and systematically. First described by Weed (1971),

Exhibit 16-1.

Visiting Nurse Association Of Eastern Montgomery County, Inc.
Nursing Assessment

Pt. #_____   Date _____

Name:_____ B.D._____ Age _____

Diagnosis _____ Ht. _____ Wt. _____

_____ B.P. _____P. _____R.R. _____T._____

Allergies:_____   *Code*

        Prosthesis (__)   WNL   Within Normal Limits

Eyeglasses: _____   P   Problem

Dentures: _____   NA   Not Assessed

Hearing Aid: _____   +   Positive

Limbs (Indicate): _____   (-)   Negative

CC: _____   Nurse:_____

Assessment	Code	Describe Or Measure
1. Skin		
a. Color		
b. Condition		
c. Temperature		
d. Turgor		
e. Nails		
2. Eyes		
a. Vision		
b. Condition		
c. Last Eye Exam		
3. Ent.		
a. Teeth & Gums		
b. Throat		
c. Tongue		
d. Hearing		
4. Resp. System		
a. Aids		
b. Chest Config.		
c. Auscultation		
d. Breathing Pattern		
e. Cough Pattern/Secretions		
5. Cardio Vascular		
a. Auscultation		
b. Circulation		
c. Edema		
d. Chest Pain		
6. Reproductive		
a. Appearance of Breast		
b. Breast self exam.		
c. General Appearance of Genitalia		
d. Discharges/Secretions		

Exhibit 16-1, continued.

Assessment	Code	Describe Or Measure
7.Urinary		
a. Bladder Elimination Pattern		
b. Foley Size/Type/Last Changed		
8. G.I.		
a. Abdominal Shape		
b. Bowel Sounds		
c. Elimination Pattern		
d. Nausea/vomiting/& other G.I. Symptoms		
e. Nutritional Status		
f. Difficulty Chewing/Swallowing		
g. Appetite		
h. Feeding		
9.Neuro		
a. Pupils		
b. Speech		
c. Equil. & Coord.		
d. Level of Consciousness/ orientation		
e. Sleep Pattern		
10.Musculo-Skel & Related ADL		
a. Ambulation		
b. Stairs		
c. Dressing		
d. Household Activity		
e. Transfer Activity		
f. Personal Care		
g. Toileting		
h. Assistive Devices		
11.Psycho-Social		
a. Mental Status		
b. Relationships		
c. Affect		
d. Physical Environment		
e. Habits		
f. Language		
g. Literacy		

Past Medical Hx: _____

_____

Past Surgical Hx:_____

Referral to: HHA _____ MOW_____ MSW_____ OT_____ PT_____ ST_____ OTHER_____ the problem-oriented method contains four main components: a problem list, a defined data base, initial and revised plans, and progress notes. For our purposes, the nursing diagnoses are the problems listed and the previously discussed nursing assessment is the data base. Goals or expected outcomes are listed with the problems and diagnoses, and detailed plans are established on the physician's order forms or plans of treatment. Progress notes are formulated using the SOAP method (subjective, objective, assessment, and plan). In this format, subjective data represent the patient's point of view; objective data are the evidence collected by the professional; assessment is the professional's analysis of both the subjective and the objective data; and plan outlines the steps needed to deal with the assessment and the overall problem or diagnosis. (Further discussion of documentation may be found in Chapter 14.)

Flow sheets or some other abbreviated form of documentation, such as check lists, may be used with a narrative description of the nursing diagnoses and the subsequent nursing interventions. Depending on the agency's documentation policies and third-party demands, the nurse may document every visit on the flow sheet while recording a narrative only when changes occur or as mandated by the agency. This combination may prove to be time-saving for the community health nurse while also preserving a graphic flow of the patient's needs. Parameters necessary to measure the patient's progress and the effectiveness of the nursing interventions may be defined individually on the flow sheet for each patient according to their diagnoses.

Standardized flow sheets, which reflect parameters necessary to assess and intervene in specific diagnostic categories, can also be established. The standardized flow sheets may be designed to promote a minimum level of nursing care expected by the agency for a certain diagnosis. Items found on the flow sheets may include: physical data such as vital signs, measurements of a wound, or peripheral edema; instruction needs such as insulin administration and diet instructions; psychosocial data such as affect; and treatment needs such as wound dressing changes or catheter changes. Individualization of the patient's care needs, to reflect his own nursing diagnosis, etiology, and symptoms may be accomplished if the standardized flow sheets have ample space for the nurse to document the patient's specific requirements (Exhibit 16-2). In this manner, the nurse may overcome the tendency to fit the patient to the diagnosis rather than fit the label to the patient. Standardized flow sheets may be designed by the agency staff based on their documentation requirements and care plans related to specific nursing diagnoses. Parameters may be adapted from a variety of sources including clinicians, staff members, nursing texts, and nursing care plan manuals. The National League for Nursing (1975) has published a series of standardized flow sheets which may prove to be an additional resource, although they are organized according to medical not nursing diagnoses. Standardized flow sheets in conjunction with the use of a nursing diagnosis taxonomy may further contribute to the establishment of outcomes in relation to a quality assurance program.

The Effects

The effects of nursing diagnoses may be evident in many facets of community health nursing including administration, clinical practice, and associated research.

This is not to say there are no problems with nursing diagnoses. The taxonomy is often awkward whether the NANDA, Omaha, or other system is used. In addition,

Exhibit 16-2. Flow Sheet #42/43

PT. # _____   NAME _____

PG. _____   DATE OF VISIT 19 ___

DATE	PROB. #	PARAMETERS/ INTERVENTIONS	FREQ.
		Actual/Potential Impairment of Skin integrity	
		Mental Status	
		Continence	
		Mobility	
		Pain	
		Assess Wound: Site	
		Grade	
		Length/Width	
		Color	
		Drainage: Amount	
		Color/Consistency	
		Odor	
		Prevention Measures/Equipment	
		Healing/Response to Treatment	
		Instruct Family in: Position	
		Wound Care	
		S&S of Infection	
		Wound Care:	

CODE BREATH SOUNDS
1. FULL
2. DIMINISHED
3. ABSENT

CODE ADVENTITIOUS SOUNDS
0. NONE
1. RALES
2. RONCHI
3. WHEEZES
4. FRICTION RUB

NEXT VISIT _____
BILLING _____
INITIALS _____

INIT.	SIGNATURE	INIT.	SIGNATURE	INIT.	SIGNATURE

CODES

C	Care	N	Narrative	S	Supervision
D	Discussion	I	Instruction	Gr. 1	Red, Unbroken	Gr. 3	Subcut. Tissue, Necrotic
E	Evaluation			Gr. 2	Break in Epidermis	Gr. 4	Muscle, Bone Exposed

even though there has been over a decade of work on the taxonomy, the language of nursing diagnoses can and will change as nursing further refines the lists and explores the range of our professional practice. Defining characteristics for the diagnoses may not always be clear to the practicing staff nurse and there may be some resulting confusion as to the choice of an accurate and appropriate diagnosis (Dalton 1985). The concurrent assessment and documentation scheme for nursing diagnoses may be cumbersome initially for a staff unaccustomed to the concepts of nursing process and diagnoses. Conversion to a nursing diagnoses system will require considerable staff development efforts. While more recently educated nurses may find the process easy, older staff may be unsure and may need guidance from both staff development and supervisory staffs in both selection of and documentation of a nursing diagnosis. There are also possible legal considerations to nursing diagnoses such as inaccurate diagnoses or misdiagnoses resulting in improper nursing treatment. In actuality, nursing diagnoses represent the labeling of problems nurses normally treat; therefore, nurses would be held accountable for whether the label or diagnosis is attached or not (Gordon 1982a,266).

For the clinical nurse, the advantages of nursing diagnoses include the standardization of the language used to communicate within the profession. The communications link of nursing diagnoses aids community health nurses in validating their practices for themselves, peers, supervisors, and third-party payors. For the community health nurse, the stresses of independent home care and the many documentation requirements associated with third-party payors can contribute to a "burn-out" problem (Marvan-Hyam 1986). The nursing diagnosis, clearly showing the nurse's professional assessment, goals, and interventions may increase professional self-worth. This may be accomplished by helping the nurse view the nursing process as a proactive problem-solving technique rather than merely reactively carrying out the physician's orders. The use of nursing diagnoses in an agency's documentation system can also help to clarify communications among staff members when many nurses are needed to see an individual patient, for instance during weekend or vacation coverage. The nursing diagnosis can help to clarify priority problems, and when standardized flow sheets are used, the covering nurse can quickly and confidently follow the primary nurse's care plan as outlined by the selected parameters. Nursing diagnoses can also facilitate communications between the community and our acute and long-term care colleagues, to promote continuity of the patient's care. The transition between hospital to home and home to independence or other care mode may be eased if the nursing diagnoses are clear, and the goals or expected outcomes are well-defined.

In addition, the use of the nursing diagnosis may assist in a peer review process (Warren 1983). The practice of diagnosing and treating competently can be evaluated by peers reviewing a nursing record including a data base. For supervisory staff, the use of a nursing diagnosis taxonomy by their clinical nurses can assist them in evaluating nursing competence and accountability. The supervisor may review the nurse's competence via joint home visits, patient care conferences focusing on nursing diagnosis selection and treatment, or through chart review. Areas of staff concern may be identified by both staff and supervisors and converted into staff development programs as appropriate.

The usefulness of nursing diagnoses clinically is perhaps most crucial when considering third-party reimbursement. This issue is clearly valuable to the community health nurse and administrator when considering the Medicare regulation stipulating reimbursement for skilled nursing services (DHEW 1966). Nursing diagnosis can, within the HCFA constraints regarding time, homebound status, and patient response or progress, assist in documenting areas where nursing contributes significantly to the patient's care and hence is more likely to be considered skilled.

In addition to the benefits of diagnoses for the clinical staff, the community health administrator can also realize distinct advantages from the use of nursing diagnoses within the agency. The administrator may identify many valuable statistics for the provision of cost-effective, quality care based on the staff's use of the nursing diagnoses. As an example, these statistics may show length of service per diagnosis and cost per diagnosis. How long is the mean service period for the patient with an "alteration in skin integrity?" How much does it cost to care for the average patient with an "alteration in mobility?" What other services are required for a person with a "self-care deficit?" What are the most frequently occurring diagnoses for the agency's population base? Analysis of the accumulated data could prove useful in considering the impact of prospective payments in home health care, in planning services, community programs, and in planning staff expansions or reductions. The example accompanying this chapter demonstrates how one agency is using data reflecting the staff's nursing diagnoses and a patient classification system.

A sound quality assurance program may also be an outcome of nursing diagnoses use. Reviewers can identify the appropriateness of the diagnoses and the accompanying goals, interventions, and outcomes as documented in the chart. The consistency of a nursing diagnosis taxonomy such as Omaha or NANDA helps clarify the patients problems even though the reviewer may see only the chart or a "paper" patient. The clear identification of the goals and outcomes related to the diagnosis helps the quality assurance process determine the effectiveness of the available nursing services and the nurse's coordination of services required by the patient.

A utilization process may also be facilitated by nursing diagnoses statistics gathered on length of service per diagnosis, number and frequency of visits, and number of disciplines involved per diagnosis.

Nursing research could be encouraged within the clinical practice and administrative fields to seek refinements of the diagnostic taxonomies, standardization of interventions, develop levels of acuity or nursing intensity. These and other research efforts may prove valuable to the community health administrator who seeks to retain an edge in the competitive home health care market.

Cost of Home Care By Nursing Diagnosis

Marilyn D. Harris, Carol Ann Parente, Judith Baigis Smith, and Joan Reynolds Yuan

Introduction

The Visiting Nurse Association of Eastern Montgomery County (VNA) is a voluntary, certified, accredited home health agency that provides in-home and community health services for 18 municipalities with a population of 250,000.

The VNA has several programs. The Home Care Program includes six certified services: nursing, physical and occupational therapy, speech pathology, medical social work, and home health aides. During the last fiscal year the staff made approximately

60,000 home visits. The agency has an average of 250 admissions and 150 discharges each month with approximately 600 patients served each month. The Maternal Child Health Program includes home health services as well as well-baby clinics. Two pediatric nurse practitioners have the major responsibility for this program. The Health Promotion Program includes nursing service in senior and child day care centers and homes. It also includes community education. Seven thousand visits are logged each year in these last two programs in addition to those made through the Home Care Program.

Patient Classification System: Background and Significance

The Tax Equity and Fiscal Responsibility Act of 1982 (TEFRA) dramatically changed the way hospitals get reimbursed for inpatient care. Before the passage of this act, Medicare paid hospitals retrospectively for each day of care and ancillary service that its patients received. With the passage of this act, hospitals are paid a flat illness-specific amount that is set prospectively, i.e., before services are rendered. The rationale for a prospective payment mechanism is to encourage hospital efficiency and, therefore, reduce Medicare costs.

The Health Care Financing Administration (HCFA) has been charged with developing strategies that will reduce Medicare costs for home health services and is considering a variety of prospective payment mechanisms which will be based on an as-yet-undecided patient classification system.

Thus, the area of methodological research in nursing that has received a great amount of attention has been patient classification systems (Ballard and McNamara 1983; Daubert 1979; Giovannetti 1979; Hardy 1984; Seinkiewicz 1984). This is not surprising, since the purpose of these instruments is to respond to the variable nature of demand for nursing care in a variety of settings through assessment of patients' requirements for nursing care. Nursing administrators are confronted with assuring provision of quality care which requires adequate staffing, appropriate staff mix, and maintaining staff with sophisticated skills to meet patients' needs. These conditions must be realized under governmental regulations, present economic conditions, public scrutiny, and budget constraints. It is therefore essential for the nurse executive to utilize a tool that can address these issues. One such tool is the Rehabilitation Potential Patient Classification System (RPPCS).

Daubert (1979) described and implemented an RPPCS in a community health agency. Daubert's copyrighted method was developed as one component of a quality assurance program to evaluate patient outcomes.

Daubert's system offers five client categories describing the characteristics of clients assigned to each category. Each category has a set of subobjectives that are considered minimum goals. In this system, the subobjectives must be met in order for the ultimate problem objectives to be achieved.

The VNA has collected statistical and financial data by multiple classification systems for several years. These include: Referral Source, Municipality, Major Disease Category (MDC), the Visiting Nurse Association of New Haven's RPPCS (1980).

A variety of outcome data are generated through our Management Information System (MIS): total cost per case; cost per case by discipline, average length of stay; average number of visits per case, discipline, and RPPCS.

Based on the assumption that reimbursement for home care services will change from a per-visit to another yet undetermined system in the future and that nursing diagnoses rather than medical diagnoses influence the level and amount of services home care patients require, the administrative staff was interested in identifying the cost of care by nursing diagnoses. The staff was also interested in identifying those nursing diagnoses that occur most frequently and those that are included within each of the five goals of the RPPCS and the 23 MDC.

Nursing Diagnoses Data Collection

This project was initiated in July 1985. The first month was used to finalize the computer program with our computer service. Data collection began in August 1985.

The VNA's statistical and financial data are collected on a daily basis. The visiting staff complete a daily report form (Exhibit 16-3). Initial data for all new patients are input into the MIS via a Patient Master Update Form (PMU). (See Exhibit 16-4.) Any changes, additions, or deletions to service are input via a Patient Master Update Form II (PMU II). (See Exhibit 16-5.) The use of the PMU II allows the agency to calculate costs by length of stay by discipline.

In order to collect data by nursing diagnosis, a new "Nursing Diagnosis Discharge Summary" (Exhibit 16-6) was initiated. The top portion of the form includes information relevant to total agency service, i.e., agency name, date form was completed, patient name and number, status, discharge reason, date of discharge, service codes (goal on admission and goal attainment on discharge for the RPPCS), and the start of care date. The remainder of the form lists the 50 nursing diagnoses (Kim 1982) used by the staff. The staff is asked to indicate the percentage of total time spent on each nursing diagnosis and the start and stop dates for each diagnosis. The form also includes four columns that may be used at a later time to quantify each nursing diagnosis.

In order to assign a dollar value to each diagnosis, the total cost of nursing service must be divided by some method. The following options were discussed:

1. Cost to be divided equally among all nursing diagnoses.

2. Cost to be divided by percentage of time spent on each diagnosis by total case. Staff nurses would assign percentage of time to each diagnosis on discharge. This would be subjective.

3. Cost to be divided by percentage of time spent on each visit. Although this would be the most accurate in theory, it could be the least accurate in practice. Example: Staff could forget to identify nursing diagnoses service codes on each visit given all of the other documentation that has to be done to meet billing, legal, and agency standards.

We chose option number two, because we believed that the primary nurse was the person who could assign a percentage to each diagnosis in relationship to the total care provided during the length of stay with the VNA.

The VNA staff uses a Problem Oriented Record System based on nursing diagnoses. Each problem must be addressed and a notation made in the clinical record at

Exhibit 16-3. Daily Report

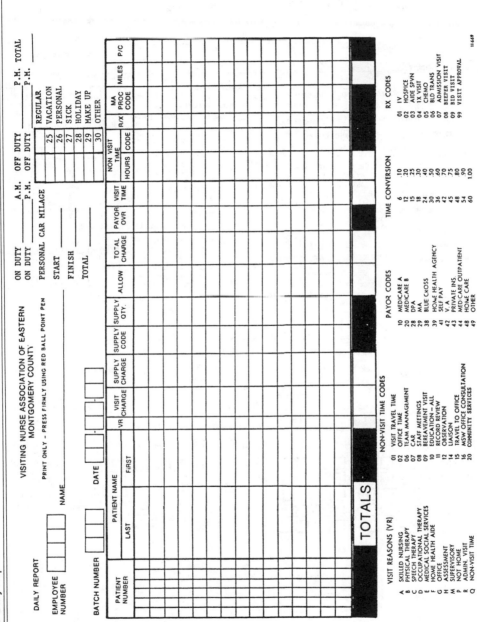

Exhibit 16-4. Patient Master Update

PATIENT NUMBER ☐☐☐☐☐☐   ACTION CODE   3 ☐ NEW PATIENT   5 ☐ CHANGE

SUBSTATION ☐ 0 ☐ 1

☐ A. NAME _____   _____   _____
                LAST   FIRST   M.I.

TEAM ☐☐

☐ B. ADDRESS _____   _____
                STREET   CITY   STATE   ZIP

READMISSION ☐ Y

☐ C. STATUS
   1 ☐ ELIG. REQUEST NEEDED
   2 ☐ WAITING APPROVAL
   3 ☐ ACTIVE
   4 ☐ DISCHARGED

DISCHARGE REASON
1 ☐ DIED   5 ☐ MOVED
2 ☐ PATIENT REFUSED SERVICE 6 ☐ OTHER
3 ☐ NON ACCEPTANCE   7 ☐ NURSING HOME
4 ☐ HOSPITAL

☐☐-☐☐-☐☐ DISCHARGE DATE

☐ D. BILLING   PRIMARY

☐☐-☐☐-☐☐-☐☐ SERVICE CODES

  10 ☐ MEDICARE A   41 ☐ SELF PAY
  20 ☐ MEDICARE B   42 ☐ V.A.
  30 ☐ MEDICAID   43 ☐ PRIVATE INSURANCE
  37 ☐ CHHC   44 ☐ OTHER AGENCIES/HMO
  38 ☐ BLUE CROSS   45 ☐ AMERICAN CANCER SOCIETY
  39 ☐ BOARD OF HEALTH

SECONDARY
A ☐ SELF
B ☐ PRIVATE INS.
C ☐ BC & BS
D ☐ EMPLOYER
E ☐ PUBLIC AGENCY
F ☐ OTHER

☐☐☐☐☐☐☐☐☐☐ MEDICARE NUMBER

☐☐-☐☐☐-☐☐-☐☐☐ MEDICAID NUMBER

☐☐-☐☐-☐☐ PAYOR CHANGE EFFECTIVE DATE

PAY STATUS 1 ☐ NO FEE
             2 ☐ PART FEE
             3 ☐ FULL FEE

INSURANCE DESCRIPTION ☐☐☐☐☐☐☐☐☐☐☐☐☐☐☐☐☐☐☐☐☐☐

☐ E. DOCTOR _____ NO. ☐☐☐☐   START CARE ☐☐-☐☐-☐☐ PLAN ☐☐-☐☐-☐☐

   HOSPITAL _____ NO. ☐☐☐   STAY FROM ☐☐-☐☐-☐☐ TO ☐☐-☐☐-☐☐

   HOSPITAL _____ NO. ☐☐☐   STAY FROM ☐☐-☐☐-☐☐ TO ☐☐-☐☐-☐☐

   RE-CERTIFIED DATE ☐☐-☐☐-☐☐

☐ F. ILLNESS ☐☐☐.☐☐ DIAGNOSIS ☐☐☐☐☐☐☐☐☐☐☐☐☐☐☐☐☐☐☐☐☐☐☐
           ☐☐☐.☐☐ DIAGNOSIS ☐☐☐☐☐☐☐☐☐☐☐☐☐☐☐☐☐☐☐☐☐☐☐
           ☐☐☐.☐☐ DIAGNOSIS ☐☐☐☐☐☐☐☐☐☐☐☐☐☐☐☐☐☐☐☐☐☐☐

EMPLOYMENT RELATED
Y ☐   N ☐

☐ G. PATIENT INFORMATION   REFERRAL
1 ☐ HOSPITAL   5 ☐ STAFF
2 ☐ DOCTOR   6 ☐ COMM. AGENCIES
3 ☐ FAMILY, FRIEND/SELF 7 ☐ NSG. HOMES
4 ☐ OTHER

RACE 1 ☐ CAU
      2 ☐ BLACK
      3 ☐ OTHER
      4 ☐ SPANISH
      5 ☐ ORIENTAL

SEX
M ☐
F ☐

TOWN _____ ☐☐   LIVES ALONE 01 ☐

                    LIVES WITH OTHERS 01 ☐

☐ H. SELF PAY CHARGES

A – ☐☐-☐☐ F – ☐☐-☐☐
B – ☐☐-☐☐ I – ☐☐-☐☐
C – ☐☐-☐☐ N – ☐☐-☐☐
D – ☐☐-☐☐ O – ☐☐-☐☐
E – ☐☐-☐☐ S – ☐☐-☐☐

DATE OF BIRTH ☐☐☐☐☐☐
               MO. DAY YEAR

PHONE ☐6☐1☐7☐ ☐☐☐☐☐☐☐
       AREA   NUMBER

MARITAL STATUS
1 ☐ SINGLE
2 ☐ MARRIED
3 ☐ WIDOWED
4 ☐ OTHER

VISITS TO BE MADE EVERY ☐0☐6☐0☐ DAYS

Exhibit 16-5.

VISITING NURSE ASSOCIATION OF EASTERN MONTG. CO.
ABBY–PATIENT MASTER UPDATE II

EMPLOYEE NAME _____

PT.# _____ NAME _____ DATE _____

DISCIPLINE		ICD9 CODE	DATE SOC BEGINS	DATE SOC ENDS	REMARKS
NURSING	1				
P.T.	2				
SPEECH	3				
O.T.	4				
M.S.S.	5				
HHA	6				
OFFICE	7				

REMARKS: 1=DISCHARGE   2=HOSPITAL ADMISSION   3=DIAGNOSIS CHANGE

20062

the time it is resolved or when the patient is discharged from agency service. There was discussion regarding the assignment of a quantifying goal to each nursing diagnosis. Although this would be ideal it was decided that during the first year, the VNA would benefit more by using goals identified by RPPCS rather than one for each problem based on a nursing diagnosis.

In order to identify specific individuals with specific nursing diagnoses, and to identify outliers, patient names and numbers were built into the data collection system.

All patients admitted to and discharged from nursing service since August 1, 1985, were included in a one-year study. (There were two exceptions: hospice and hospital home care patients. A different charting system was used by these contract services.) The purposes of the study were: to document the cost of care by nursing diagnosis; to identify nursing diagnoses within the RPPCS and MDC; to identify the average length of stay on VNA service; and to identify the average number of visits per case by nursing diagnosis.

Development of Standardized Flow Charts

Prior to beginning the study several preliminary steps were taken including the development of standardized flow sheets (SFS), general assessment sheets for each group in the RPPCS, and corresponding discharge summaries. These SFS encourage

Exhibit 16-6.

FORM 220 **NURSING DIAGNOSIS DISCHARGE SUMMARY**

___/___/___
DATE COMPLETED

AGENCY
NAME _____
PATIENT NUMBER ☐☐-☐☐☐☐ LAST   FIRST

STATUS [4] DISCHARGED   DISCHARGE REASON ☐ (1-7 only)   DATE ☐☐-☐☐-☐☐

SERVICE CODES ☐☐-☐☐-☐☐-☐☐   GOAL ☐

DATE CARE STARTED ☐☐-☐☐-☐☐

		NURSING DIAGNOSIS	% OF CARE	START DATE	CLOSE DATE	OUTCOME 1 MET MAXIMUM	2 MODERATE	3 MINIMUM	4 NOT MET
	1	ACTIVITY INTOLERANCE							
	2	INEFFECTIVE AIRWAY CLEARANCE							
	3	ANXIETY							
	4	ALT. IN BOWEL ELIMINATION: CONSTIPATION							
	5	ALT. IN BOWEL ELIMINATION: DIARREHEA							
	6	ALT. IN BOWEL ELIMINATION: INCONTINENCE							
	7	INEFFECTIVE BREATHING PATTERNS							
	8	ALT IN CARDIAC OUTPUT: DECREASED							
	9	ALT. IN COMFORT: PAIN							
	10	IMPAIRED VERBAL COMMUNICATION							
	11	INEFFECTIVE INDIVIDUAL COPING							
	12	INEFFECTIVE FAMILY COPING: COMPROMISED							
	13	INEFFECTIVE FAMILY COPING: DISABLING							
	14	FAMILY COPING: POTENTIAL FOR GROWTH							
	15	DIVERSIONAL ACTIVITY DEFICIT							
	16	ALT. IN FAMILY PROCESSES							
	17	FEAR							
	18	FLUID VOLUME DEFICIT							
	19	POTENTIAL FLUID VOLUME DEFICIT							
	20	EXCESS FLUID VOLUME							
	21	IMPAIRED GAS EXCHANGE							
	22	ANTICIPATORY GRIEVING							
	23	DYSFUNCTIONAL GRIEVING							
	24	ALT. IN HEALTH MAINTENANCE							
	25	IMPAIRED HOME MAINTENANCE MANAGEMENT							
	26	POTENTIAL FOR INJURY							
	27	KNOWLEDGE DEFICIT							
	28	IMPAIRED PHYSICAL MOBILITY							
	29	NON-COMPLIANCE							
	30	ALT. IN NUTRITION: LESS THAN BODY REQUIREMENTS							
	31	ALT. IN NUTRITION: MORE THAN BODY REQUIREMENTS							
	32	ALT. IN NUTRITION: POTENTIAL, MORE THAN BODY REQUIREMENTS							
	33	ALT. IN ORAL MUCOUS MEMBRANE							
	34	ALT. IN PARENTING							
	35	POTENTIAL ALT. IN PARENTING							
	36	POWERLESSNESS							
	37	RAPE-TRAUMA SYNDROME							
	38	SELF CARE DEFICIT							
	39	SELF-ESTEEM DISTURBANCE							
	40	SENSORY-PERCEPTUAL ALTERATIONS							
	41	SEXUAL DYSFUNCTION							
	42	ACTUAL IMPAIRMENT OF SKIN INTEGRITY							
	43	POTENTIAL IMPAIRMENT OF SKIN INTEGRITY							
	44	DISTURBANCE IN SLEEP PATTERN							
	45	SOCIAL ISOLATION							
	46	SPIRITUAL DISTRESS							
	47	ALT. IN THOUGHT PROCESSES							
	48	ALT. IN TISSUE PERFUSION							
	49	ALT. IN PATTERN OF URINARY ELIMINATION							
	50	POTENTIAL FOR VIOLENCE							

TOTAL ☐

_____
SIGNATURE

documentation of quality care delivered for a specific group of patients with a specific nursing diagnosis by outlining the parameters to be addressed. The use of SFS would also encourage efficiency when documenting care. Nurses would no longer have to write a narrative for each patient visit. Preprinted flow sheets would reduce the time needed to complete charting.

The development of standardized flow sheets was also in response to staff's request for this type of charting format.

To develop the flow sheets, three people, the director of professional services, a nurse practitioner, and the nursing supervisor in charge of the VNA's quality assurance program, spent hours reading the relevant literature and drawing on their experiences in community health nursing. The staff provided feedback on the completeness and practicality of the flow sheets developed by these three.

A general assessment flow sheet was developed for each of the five groups in the RPPCS (See Exhibit 16-7.) This would provide a method to measure the overall program objectives. These five groups also represented the patient's long-range goal.

A pilot study was conducted with four of the staff nurses. The results of this pilot showed that the patients in the study had been placed in the correct group 90% of the time.

The nursing diagnosis flow sheets were developed at the same time that the general assessment sheets were done. Fifteen of the more commonly used nursing diagnoses were selected. The flow sheets were developed with emphasis on the primary nurse's ability to individualize care for each patient. Refer to Exhibit 16-8 for the flow sheet for Actual Impairment of Skin Integrity.

Exhibit 16-7.

General Assessment III
Intermediate/Advanced Chronic: Rehab

Vital Signs: B.P.
                         P.
                         R/T
Breath sounds
Assess edema - Pedal - RT/LT
   Assess nutritional status, Appetite diet instruction
   Demonstrates understanding of diet
Evaluate Elimination Patterns
Assess and instruct medication regimen
   Demonstrates understanding of meds
Assess ability to perform treatments
   Treatment instruction
   Demonstrates ability to do treatments
Assess and Instruct safety in home
   Demonstrates knowledge of safety measures
Assess emotional status and coping mechanisms, provide support
   Patient recognizes physical and emotional changes
   Communicates changes to appropriate professional
Assess and instruct re: restrictions
   Demonstrates understanding of restrictions
   Next M.D. visit

Exhibit 16-8.

Actual and potential impairment of skin integrity

Mental status
Continence
Mobility
Pain
Assess Wound
   Site
   Grade
   Length/Width
   Color
   Drainage
   Amount
   Color/Consistency
   Odor
Prevention measures and equipment
Healing and response to treatment
Instruct family in
   Position
   Wound care
   S&S of infection
Wound care

Objective data such as breath sounds, diet, safety, and subobjective data from the RPPCS were on the general assessment sheet. Data specific to a particular problem were on the nursing diagnosis flow sheet. Yet, some duplication was unavoidable. For example, blood pressure appears on both the general assessment RPPCS form and the "Alteration in Health Maintenance" nursing diagnosis flow sheet. In the future, this type of duplication will be eliminated by inputing the flow sheet directly into the agency's computer system.

The agency utilizes a Problem Oriented Record System. The nursing diagnoses are the problems. The five patient groups in the RPPCS are preprinted on all Problem Lists. Patients are entered into one of these groups on admission to the agency.

A standardized "Discharge Summary" (Exhibit 16-9) was prepared for each of the five patient groups. The subobjectives appropriate for each group match those on the flow sheets. On discharge, the nurse uses this check list to indicate whether the patient or family has demonstrated an increase in knowledge, understanding, or had a behavior change. Goal attainment (outcome) is noted as none, moderate, or maximum. Evidence must be presented in the body of the record to substantiate this outcome. The nurse must address each nursing diagnosis by recording the specific outcome and the date this occurred. If a problem is not resolved, the nurse records the status and date of discharge from agency service.

Exhibit 16-9.

VNA of EMC 　　　　　　　DISCHARGE SUMMARY 111
　　　　　　　　　　Intermediate/Advanced Chronic: Rehab

NAME_____Patient #_____Date:_____

Ultimate Objective: Patient will be rehabilitated to maximum level of physical,
　　　　　　　　　emotional and social functioning; patient/family will manage
　　　　　　　　　chronic health problems without continued VNA service.

| | Nursing Action | | Patient Outcome |
| | | | Demonstration of Increased Knowledge, |
Subobjectives	Assessment	Instruction	Understanding, or Behavior Change
Diet			
Med. Regime			
Treatments			
Safety Measures			
Medical Supervision			
Recognizes Physical/ Emotional Change			
Communicates Change to Approp. Profess.			
Restrictions Imposed by Illness			

Goal attainment is determined by demonstrating that applicable subobjectives were met/
nursing problems resolved. Action must be taken and patient/family must demonstrate
increased knowledge, understanding, and/or behavior change as a result of nurse's
intervention.

Goal Attainment Code: _____#1 Maximum: 　All applicable subobjectives were met/
　　　　　　　　　　　　　　　　　　Nursing problems resolved.
　　　　　　　　　　　_____#2 Moderate: Less than 100% of total goal attainment.
　　　　　　　　　　　_____#3 None: 　　None of the applicable subobjectives were
　　　　　　　　　　　　　　　　　　met/ Nursing problems resolved.

Summary of Services:_____
_____
_____

Problems:
#101 O/A _____
_____
_____

#102 O/A _____
_____

#103 O/A _____
_____

#104 O/A _____
_____
_____

　　　　　　　　　　　Signature:_____

Staff Education

Formal orientation to the new system and use of forms via lecture, slides, and over-heads was also done prior to the beginning of the study. A manual was distributed to each nurse that included sample forms, case studies, and charting guidelines.

The educational process also included practice sessions in classifying patients into the correct group. There was general discussion and questions and answers. These sessions were done in both large and small groups by the administrative and supervisory staff.

Quality Assurance

The correct identification of the RPPCS and nursing diagnoses for each patient are included in the VNA's quality assurance (Q.A.) program. If the patient is not placed in the correct category on admission, the discharge summary cannot be completed since the categories would not coincide. The chart would also receive additional reviews at the time of the record audit if the admitting medical diagnoses did not qualify the patient for a specific group in the classification system.

Several check points are built into the Q.A. program to insure accuracy. On admission each chart is reviewed by the clinical supervisor to determine that the nurse has selected the correct group. Any change from this original grouping must be discussed with the supervisor. The PMUs are reviewed for gross errors by the supervisors on discharge.

The Q.A. program includes a quarterly review of a random selection of both open and closed records. This random selection is programmed into our computer system.

The review format includes questions that had been brought before an expert panel to establish validity. Recommended changes were incorporated into the review check list.

Fifty nursing records are reviewed each quarter based on the number of patients who receive nursing service. One hundred records were reviewed during the six-month study period. Eighty-five records were for patients who were included in this study. The percentage of agreement was 98%. Based on this finding, plus the overall results of the record review process, the management staff has determined that the data reported in this study are valid.

Description of Subjects

Five hundred and forty-one patients were discharged during the first six months of the study. The sample followed the agency's population in that two-thirds were women and a majority were over 75 years of age.

Data Analysis

Six-month data (August 1985 to January 1986) were analyzed. Five hundred and forty-one patients were discharged during this time period. The number of nursing diagnoses per patient ranged from one to six with an average of 1.8.

There are 50 acceptable nursing diagnoses used by the VNA. Thirty-one were identified during data collection. The ten most frequently identified diagnoses are found in Table 16-2 and represent 84% of all diagnoses identified by the staff. The main reason for this finding is probably because most of the diagnoses used are physiologically based and are identified as "Medicare-reimbursable."

The charges per diagnosis ranged from $34 to $451. The average charge was $166.35. Each diagnosis may be only a percentage of the total cost of care for a patient depending on the number of diagnoses identified for that patient.

The ten most expensive diagnoses were identified (Table 16-3) based on a charge of $45 per nursing visit. We speculated on why there were wide price variations among these ten diagnoses. One possibility may be the involvement of other disciplines. For example, a patient with the diagnosis of Impaired Physical Mobility may have the need of other disciplines such as physical therapy and a home health aide. If these services

Table 16-2. Most frequently identified nursing diagnoses

Alt. in health maintenance	224
Self-care deficit	150
Act. impairment skin integrity	113
Knowledge deficit	103
Ineffective breathing patterns	72
	662 = 67%
Impaired physical mobility	61
Alt. in pattern of urin. elim.	49
Alt. in bowel elim.: Constip.	44
Alt. in Comfort: Pain	42
Alt. in nutr.: Less than body req.	35
	832 = 84%

Table 16-3. Most expensive nursing diagnoses

	Charges	Visits	Cases
Pot. impair. skin integrity	$451	17	7
Alt. in cardiac output: Decreased	$359	12	6
Act. impair. skin integrity	$305	11	113
Impr. home maintenance mgmt.	$299	8	14
Alt. in health maintenance	$286	9	224
Ineffect. breathing patterns	$230	9	72
Alt. in parenting	$225	5	1
Knowledge deficit	$201	7	103
Impaired physical mobility	$200	10	61
Ineffect. airway clearance	$197	13	2

are utilized there may be less need for nursing time for this diagnosis. On the other hand, someone with the diagnosis of Actual Impairment of Skin Integrity would use mostly nursing service rather than other therapy disciplines resulting in a higher price than that for Impaired Physical Mobility.

The ten least expensive diagnoses are noted in Table 16-4. This finding may occur since they represent a small portion of the nurses' time. Reasons for this occurrence may be that the nurse is not skilled or comfortable with dealing with such complex psychosocial phenomena like rape-trauma syndrome or ineffectual family and individual coping. Another reason is that another professional such as a medical social worker is available to address these very complicated matters and the nurse refers such patients to another discipline.

Table 16-5 lists the nursing diagnoses with the highest number of visits. It is interesting to note that "Potential Impairment of Skin Integrity" is the diagnosis with the highest number of visits and the most expensive. "Alteration in Cardiac Output" is the diagnosis with the third highest number of visits and the second most expensive diagnosis. "Actual Impairment of Skin Integrity" is the fifth highest diagnosis in visits but it was the third most expensive.

The nursing diagnoses with the lowest number of visits were noted (Table 16-6). The researchers established a minimum of three visits to be included in the data analysis. It can be noted that diagnosis such as noncompliance is included in the list. The nurse may do what can be done and discontinue service if noncompliance persists. Also, these diagnoses are less reimbursable as compared with those with the highest number of visits.

Table 16-4. Least expensive nursing diagnoses

	Charges	Visits	Cases
Rape-trauma syndrome	$34	3	1
Anxiety	$36	8	3
Alt. in bowel elim.: Diarrhea	$39	4	2
Sensory-percep. alt.	$41	3	1
Alt. in nutr.: More than body req.	$63	5	2
Noncompliance	$68	7	3
Ineffect. family coping	$81	15	5
Ineffect. ind. coping	$88	10	11
Alt. in bowel elim.: Incont.	$94	5	8
Self-care deficit	$112	11	150

Table 16-5. Nursing diagnoses with highest number of visits

	Visits	Charges	Cases
Pot. impair. skin integrity	17	$451	7
Ineffective family coping	15	$ 81	5
Alt. in cardiac output: Decreased	12	$359	6
Self-care deficit	11	$112	150
Act. impair. skin integrity	11	$305	113

The most intense nursing diagnoses were also identified (Table 16-7). Intensity level was obtained by dividing the number of visits by the length of stay. When there is continued, concentrated care with a frequent number of visits in a short period of time, there may be decreased flexibility in scheduling staffing visits.

Once again, "Actual Alteration in Skin Integrity" appears on this list in third position. Since this diagnosis was one that appeared on all four tables (most frequent, most expensive, highest number of visits, and most intense), we decided to examine it more closely.

First, outliers for this diagnosis were identified. They were arbitrarily defined by the agency as those cases whose charge exceeded $1,000. Seven cases met this criterion. For example, Case 3 (Table 16-8) reveals a charge of $1700 as compared with the average charge of $305 per case. The most common complication identified in

Table 16-6. Nursing diagnoses with lowest number of visits

	Visits	Charges	Cases
Alt. in bowel elim.: Incont.	5	$ 94	8
Alt. in bowel elim.: Constip.	5	$121	44
Potential for injury	6	$143	3
Knowledge deficit	7	$201	103
Noncompliance	7	$ 68	3
Alt. in tissue perfusion	7	$153	7

Table 16-7. Most intense nursing diagnoses

	Cases
Anticipatory grieving	1
Ineffect. family coping: Compromised	5
Act. impair. of skin integrity	113
Alt. in bowel elimination	2
Alt. in nutr.: More than body req.	2

Table 16-8. Act. alteration of skin and self-care (s.c.) deficit

Cases	Skin	S.C.	Visits	Charges	Rehab. goal
	(%)	(%)			
1	30	70	6	$ 270	Recovery
2	85	15	8	$ 360	Rehab.
3	75	25	38	$1,710	Rehab.
4	20	80	5	$ 225	Rehab.

these cases was wound infections. This finding has quality assurance implications. This is one reason that nursing diagnoses are included in the VNAs record review process.

Second, we discovered that this diagnosis appeared in 12 of the 23 Major Disease Categories (MDC). Table 16-9 lists five of these MDCs. However, there was no specific pattern to the cluster of nursing diagnoses under any of the 12 MDCs. For example, under the MDC of Neoplasm, the nursing diagnosis of Actual Alteration in Skin Integrity appeared four times alone, four times with one other diagnosis (self-care deficit), three times with two other diagnoses (self-care deficit and pain), and 14 times in other combinations.

Reasons for this lack of clustering by medical diagnoses are hypothesized to be: (1) physicians and nurses view the patient from different perspectives; and (2) nursing care is patient-specific and, therefore, diagnoses vary from patient to patient.

The nursing diagnoses within the five goals of the RPPCS were also examined. The patients with this nursing diagnosis reflected a similar frequency of occurrence by RPPCS as the entire sample. The charge by RPPCS goal for "actual impairment of skin integrity" was identified (Table 16-10). In general, the greatest percentage (79%) of patients fall within the "rehabilitation" goal, but this was not the most expensive goal. It was the maintenance level of care that was the most costly to provide.

The total number of visits by rehabilitation goal was also analyzed (Table 16-11). Although a different pattern emerged, once again it was the maintenance level of care that had the most number of visits for this nursing diagnosis.

The maintenance category is still highest on the list for "Actual Impairment of Skin Integrity" when the length of stay is addressed (Table 16-12). But length of stay for the "Terminal Care" RPPCS Goal has increased to almost the same level as that for maintenance care.

Table 16-13 compares data for the five RPPCS goals for patients who had "Actual Impairment of Skin Integrity."

Patients with a "Rehabilitation" goal had more intensive nursing care (Table 16-14). There were almost twice as many nursing visits for this category of patients during the same length of stay as for the "Recovery" group which was the next highest group which needed intensive nursing care.

Finally, the data for the different percentages of time spent for a given diagnosis during the care of a patient were analyzed. Table 16-15 itemizes data for those patients who met their "Rehabilitation" goal on discharge. Although the total percentage of time spent per diagnosis actually ranged from 5 to 100%, only the data in the 25, 50, 75, and 100% of time categories were included here. As would be expected, the less the percentage of time spent on the diagnosis, the less the charge. However, this

Table 16-9. MDCs with act. alteration skin integrity

	Cases	Charges
Neoplasms	25	$235
Injury and poisoning	21	$553
Skin and subcut. tis. dis.	17	$345
Digestive system disord.	16	$224
Circ. system diseases	12	$212

Table 16-10. Act. impairment skin integrity: Charge by rehab. goal.

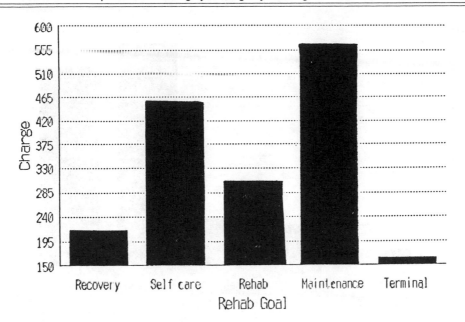

Table 16-11. Act. impairment skin integrity: No. of visits by rehab. goal.

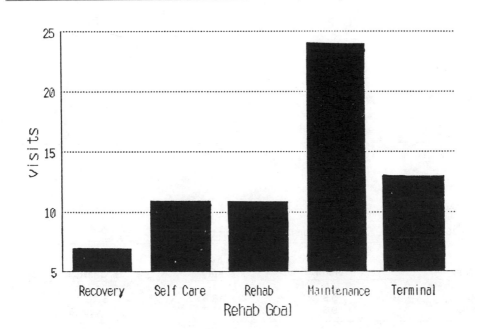

Table 16-12. Act. impairment skin integrity. Length of stay by rehab. goal.

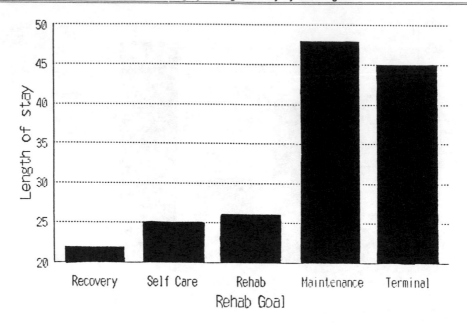

Table 16-13. Act. impairment skin integrity: Rehab. goals.

	No.	Percent	Percent for all nurs. diag.
		(%)	(%)
Recovery	9	8	5
Self-care	7	6	6
Rehabilitation	85	75	79
Maintenance	4	4	4
Terminal	8	7	6

Table 16-14. Act. impairment skin integrity. 100% of visit.

Goal	No. visits	Ave. stay	Charges
Recovery	5.8	18.5	$262.50
Rehab.	9.5	18.7	420.16

Table 16-15. Act. impairment skin integrity

Rehabilitation		Outcome Met	
Visits	No. of visits	Ave. stay	Charges
(%)			
100	9.5	18.7	$420.16
75	10.4	33.2	350.90
50	7.3	28.9	164.42
25	8	33.4	101.25
Aver. for rehab.	11	26	$303.00

same trend is not seen for the number of visits nor for the average length of stay. What is important to note is that there are differences in length of stay, and number of visits based on the percentage of time spent on the diagnosis of Actual Impairment of Skin Integrity, especially in length of stay when it is the only diagnosis addressed and when it is addressed simultaneously with other diagnoses.

Summary

Data on the cost of care by nursing diagnosis has been provided along with the nursing diagnoses in the RPPCS and the MDC. The average lengths of stay and the average number of visits per case by nursing diagnosis have been identified for one VNA.

Ten of the fifty possible nursing diagnoses were used 84% of the time in this six-month study. This could be a function of the current reimbursement system, i.e., Medicare billing forms for patients with these problems are less likely to raise questions on audit by a fiscal intermediary. It could also mean that nurses are dealing with but not documenting other diagnoses. A third reason is that nurses may no longer have time to address all nursing diagnoses. This last reason must be considered from a quality assurance viewpoint. More study needs to be done since it is important that other diagnoses do not go unaddressed in order to evaluate the cost of care by this method.

Valuable information was obtained from the outliers that were identified. Five of the seven outliers for "Actual Impairment of Skin Integrity" had wound infections. If wound infections are a primary diagnosis in other agencies, this information should encourage administrative and supervisory personnel to develop flow sheets and audit forms that would address this particular need. Such standardized flow sheets could contribute to improved quality care, decrease charting time, and identify the kind of care that is the most costly for the agency to provide.

Administrators must always keep alert to potential changes in reimbursement for home care services. Since no homogenous groups were identified during the first six months of data collection, we concluded that nursing diagnoses must be used in connection with patient outcome classification systems. Agency administrators must select a patient classification system that meets their needs and begin to document the cost of care by a method other than the per visit basis.

References

American Nurses' Association. 1973. *Standards of community health nursing practice.* Kansas City, MO: American Nurses' Association.

American Nurses' Association. 1980. *The nursing practice act: Suggested state legislation.* Kansas City, MO: American Nurses' Association.

American Nurses' Association. 1980. *A social policy statement.* Kansas City, MO: American Nurses' Association.

Ballard, S., and R. McNamara. 1983. Quantifying nursing needs in home health care. *Nursing Research* 32:236-241.

Campbell, C. 1978. *Nursing diagnosis and interventions in nursing practice.* New York, NY: Wiley.

Dalton, J. 1985. A descriptive study: Defining characteristics of the nursing diagnosis "cardiac output, alterations in: decreased. *Image: The Journal of Nursing Scholarship* 17:113-117.

Daubert, E. 1979. Patient classification systems and outcome criteria. *Nursing Outlook* 27:450-454.

Department of Health, Education and Welfare (Social Security Administration). 1966. *Home health agency manual* HIM-11, Sect. 204, 14a. Washington, DC: Government Printing Office.

Duespohl, T. A. 1986. *Nursing diagnosis manual for the well and ill client.* Philadelphia, PA: W. B. Saunders.

Giovannetti, T. 1979. Understanding patient classification systems. *Journal of Nursing Administration* 9(2):4-9.

Gordon, M. 1982a. *Nursing diagnosis: Process and application.* New York, NY: McGraw-Hill.

Gordon, M. 1982b. *Manual of nursing diagnosis.* New York, NY: McGraw-Hill.

Gordon, M. 1976. Nursing diagnosis and the diagnostic process. *American Journal of Nursing* 76:1300.

Hardy, J. 1984. A patient classification system for home health patients. *Caring* 3(8):26-27.

Harris, M., C. Santoferraro, and S. Silva. 1985. A patient classification system in home health care. *Nursing Economics* 3(5):276-282.

Jacoby, M. K. 1985. The dilemma of physiological problems, eliminating the double standards. *American Journal of Nursing* 85:281-285.

Kim, M. J. 1985. Without collaboration, what's left? *American Journal of Nursing* 85:281-284.

Kim, M. J. and D. A. Moritz. 1982. *Classification of nursing diagnosis* (Third and fourth national conferences). New York: McGraw-Hill.

Kim, M. J., et al. 1984. *Classification of nursing diagnoses proceedings of the fifth national conference.* St. Louis, MO: The C. V. Mosby Co.

Lunney, M. 1982. Nursing diagnosis: Refining the system. *American Journal of Nursing* 82:456-459.

Marvan-Hyam, J. 1986. Occupational stress of the home health nurse. *Home Healthcare Nurse* 4:18-21.

Rhiel, J. P., and C. Roy, eds. 1980. *Conceptual models of nursing practice.* New York: Appleton-Century-Crofts.

Shamansky, S. L., and C. R. Yanni. 1983. In opposition to nursing diagnosis: A minority opinion. *Image: The Journal of Nursing Scholarship* 15:47-50.

Sienkiewicz, J. 1984. Patient classification in community health nursing. *Nursing Outlook* 32:219-221.

Simmons, D. A. 1980. *A classification scheme for client problems in community health nursing.* DHHS Publication No. HRA 80-16. Washington, DC: Government Printing Office.

Visiting Nurse Association, Inc. Burlington, VT. 1975. *The problem oriented system in a home health agency—A training manual.* New York: National League for Nursing. Pub. no. 21-1554.

Visiting Nurse Association of New Haven. 1980. *Patient classification objective system methodology manual.* New Haven, CT.

Warren, J. J. 1983. Accountability and nursing diagnosis. *The Journal of Nursing Administration* 17:34-37.

Weed, L. L. 1971. *Medical records, medical education and patient care.* Cleveland: Case Western Reserve University Press.

Chapter Seventeen

High-Tech Procedures

High-Tech Home Care

Elaine R. Volk

The introduction of the Medicare Prospective Payment System has brought a tremendous shift of complex home care service needs to the community. The current cliche for this expanded care technology is "high-tech" service. High-tech care has become an all-inclusive term used to describe a variety of comprehensive home services. The word "high-tech" immediately brings to mind images of machines, tubes, pumps, monitors, and solutions. There is no standard definition for high-tech services at the present. The most common modalities on the service market today include home ventilators, IV therapy services, parenteral and enteral nutrition, and Apnea monitor programs. We know as high technology advances, home care experiences parallel growth. As home care administrators we must respond to the complex technological demands of caring for the seriously ill client in the home setting in an effort to meet the community's needs and maintain viability in the growing home care market. The purpose of this chapter is to discuss the development of high-tech services in the community setting.

A review of the rapid process which has led to the emergence of high-tech care in the community reveals that society's quick acceptance of innovative health care regime, advances in life support technology, and the institution of medical cost containment programs has prompted many home health agencies to explore new advanced levels of home care delivery. The current challenge for home health agencies is to meet the demand for a new level of care within the home setting; care which requires a high degree of competency and accountability. To meet this new challenge, the agency must be willing to invest time, money, and energy in goal-directed change and innovative program development. It will take strategic planning for home health agencies to meet the new high-tech needs of the community. The agency's administrative board will need to develop and define key elements of strategic planning to accomplish successful operationalization of a community-based high-tech program.

The initial step in strategic planning for high-tech service is for management to define the agency's mission statement. Most agencies have a well-developed mission. Administrators will want to review their present mission statements to assess whether a high-tech program will work within the organization's code of conduct and ethics. The purpose of a mission statement is to remind management of its social responsibilities to the community and to recognize the potential of the organization to favorably impact the environment in which it operates. Management should have a clear idea about their mission as a home health agency.

The second element of strategic planning involves a review of the environment. The point here is to enable the home health agency to determine which variables will be impacting on the community's environment. An assessment of environmental factors such as sociological, economic, technological, and political composition of your catchment area gives the agency the ability to determine those factors likely to impact positively or negatively the development of community-based high-tech programs. These data enable home health administrators to identify the community's high-tech service needs and quantify financial resources that can support program development. Needs and assessment tools for high-tech care assist agency's management in qualifying high-tech service care programs (Exhibit 17-1). The evaluation tool should be sent to all primary care physicians and care centers in your catchment area. High-tech assessment tools have been developed and are available from a variety of sources. To reiterate, program evaluation assessment tools will direct management to high-tech programs with the highest service needs in their area. The tool assists administrators in forecasting budgetary needs and in identifying potential revenue sources for high-tech programs. The home health agency's management can decide from the assessment where not to incorporate certain high-tech care and refer clients to neighboring agencies prepared to meet the sophisticated client service needs.

Once the need for a specific high-tech program has been confirmed, the home health agency must then define the structure which will enable those needs to be met. The agency needs to develop a multidisciplinary professional advisory committee. The advisory committee should be composed of health care professionals who are experts in knowledge and experience in the specific areas of high-tech services. The purpose of the committee includes: the development, review, and revision of high-tech policies and procedures; review of client records and care plans; and participation in an annual formal quality assurance evaluation of the high-tech program. The size and composition of the committee will vary depending on the area of concentration of high-tech service. The development of a well-structured set of policies and procedures sharpens and delineates the mission of service, eliminates the need for duplication of decision-making and specifies parameters which govern the established objectives of the program. Exhibit 17-2 is a sample description of an IV high-tech advisory committee.

It is important for an agency to have a general course of action, a framework for planning and implementation of high-tech care. A quarterly review of the agency's service goals and objectives is utilized to assess the management's ability to achieve strategic goals. High-tech program goals guide administrators in identifying those problem areas which may have resulted from incompleted planning or failure of the manager to implement current organizational plans. Especially in the area of high-tech service, program development and implementation are essential to the agency's ability to successfully meet the community's high-tech service needs. Your agency may have a limited number of opportunities to assure the community that the high-tech service needs will be met adequately and appropriately. Other agencies proficient in that service will be competing for your market share and may easily penetrate your service area.

High-tech program development may seem overwhelming at first, but the task becomes manageable when program goals and objectives are clearly identified and defined. Program objectives are the agency's quantified expression of a desired outcome for the community. Simply stated the objectives for a high-tech program are the provision of safe and effective home high-tech care. The key to successful planning for high-tech care is the establishment of attainable, well-developed, and measurable ob-

Exhibit 17-1.

Dear:

   In an effort to meet the growing high tech needs of our community, we are collecting data to assess areas for future home care program development

   Please complete the checklist below by (specify date) and return to us in the pre-addressed, pre-stamped envelope. Thank you for your participation.

Sincerely,

Mary Doe, RN
Home Care Director

DEMOGRAPHIC DATA

TYPE OF FACILITY	NUMBER OF PATIENTS
_____ Acute care facility	0-100 _____
_____ Long term care facility	101-200 _____
_____ Intermittent care facility	201-400_____
_____ Skilled nursing facility	401-600 _____
_____ Physicians office	601-more _____
_____ Other _____	Other name: _____ _____

Please indicate the approximate number of community based patients you have or could have provided high tech services in the last year.

_____ Apnea monitors	CAPD therapy _____
_____ IV antibiotic therapy	Home Ventilator _____
_____ IV chemotherapy	IV blood component _____
_____ IV Pain Management	Other: Name Service
_____ Enteral nutrition	and indicate number
_____ Total parenteral nutrition	_____
	_____
	_____

Please indicate present payor mix by percentage. Total percentage must add up to 100%.

Third-party or commercial insurance	_____
PPO or HMO	_____
Medicare	_____
Medicaid	_____
Private Pay	_____
Other: (name source)	_____
	_____
Total	100%

Profession of person completing data:

Administrator _____	Secretary _____
Physician _____	Other: _____ (name) _____
Office Manager _____	
Nurse _____	_____

Exhibit 17-2.

HomeCare		
Subject: Multi-Disciplinary Committee	**Skill Level:** RN LVN: ___x___ HHA: _____	**Page** _1_ of _3_ .
		Section/Number: I - 6
Manual: Intravenous & Nutritional Therapy	HM: _____ PT: _____	**Date Formulated:** 4·1·85
Approved by: *Carol A. Cagno*	OT: _____ Other: ___x___	**Date Revised:**

Purpose: HomeCare shall organize a multi-disciplinary committee for the Home Intravenous and Nutritional Therapy Program prior to program implementation.

Policy:

1. Membership:
   a. Physician
   b. Clinical Pharmacist
   c. Hospital Based Registered Nurse
   d. HomeCare Registered Nurse
   e. Dietician
   f. Discharge Planning Representative (Ad Hoc Member)

2. Meetings:
   a. The committee shall meet prior to commencement of the I.V. program
   b. The committee shall meet quarterly thereafter
   c. Minutes will be documented, dated and maintained in a manner consistent with Utilization Review procedure

3. Organization and Functions:
   a. The committee will be organized as a subcommittee of the Professional Advisory Committee
   b. The committee will review and approve policies and protocols for I.V. and Nutritional Therapy program
   c. The committee will develop an interdisciplinary process to periodically review I.V. and nutritional therapy patient records and care plans
   d. The committee will be requested to review all cases taken for care where admission criteria/protocols were altered or not met
   e. The committee will participate in a formal evaluation of the I.V. and nutritional therapy program at least annually (see Section VIII)

Source: Reprinted with permission from the Hospital Home Care of Greater Philadelphia Administrative Manual.

Exhibit 17-2, continued.

Subject: Multi-Disciplinary Committee	Section/Number: I - 6	Page 2 of 3.
	Date Formulated:	Date Revised: 5·15·85
Manual: Intravenous & Nutritional Therapy		

MEMBER	QUALIFICATIONS	RECOMMENDED RESPONSIBILITIES
Physician	1. Active State License 2. Knowledgable in the management of I.V. Therapy 3. Specialization in a field of medicine related to use of total parenteral nutrition and/or other home I.V. Therapy 4. Active hospital staff	1. Provides consultation for total parenteral nutrition 2. Review and evaluation of I.V. therapy management 3. Utilization review function
Clinical Pharmacist	1. Active State License 2. Additional knowledge of total parenteral nutrition (TPN) Therapy, I.V. Therapy & Chemotherapy*	1. Assists in standardizing and/or altering the I.V. Therapy prescription to meet individual patient needs 2. Compounds solutions 3. Participates in education programs
Registered Nurse (Hospital Based)	1. Active State License 2. Additional knowledge of total parenteral nutrition Therapy and I.V. Therapy*	1. Assists in providing the patient teaching program 2. Verifies skills of patient and significant other
Registered Nurse (HomeCare Office)	1. Active State License 2. Additional knowledge of total parenteral nutrition Therapy and I.V. Therapy/Chemotherapy*	1. Coordinates patient teaching program 2. Provides home visitation for supply delivery and/or patient assessment 3. Maintains contact with primary care physician 4. Provides liaison function between HomeCare and Multi-Disciplinary Committee

(585)

Exhibit 17-2, continued.

Subject: Multi-Disciplinary Committee	Section/Number: I - 6	Page 3 of 3.
	Date Formulated: 4·1·85	Date Revised:
Manual: Intravenous & Nutritional Therapy		

MEMBER	QUALIFICATIONS	RECOMMENDED RESPONSIBILITIES
Registered Dietician	1. Active State License if applicable 2. Additional knowledge of Nutritional Assessment*	1. Participates in patient teaching program as applicable 2. Conducts nutritional assessment for TPN and EN patients and makes recommendations for nutrition prescription components as required by physician

*   Additional knowledge as evidenced by attendance at accredited continuing education courses or has specialized university training in I.V. and/or Nutritional Therapies.

Exhibit 17-2, continued.

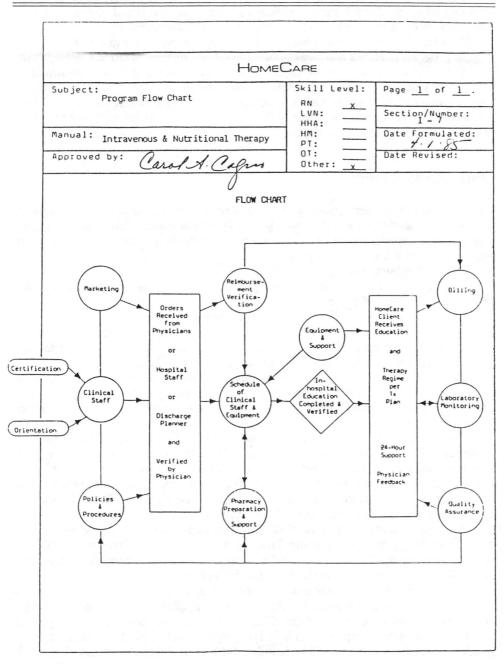

HOMECARE

Subject: Program Flow Chart	Skill Level:	Page 1 of 1 .
	RN x	
	LVN: ____	Section/Number: 1-7
	HHA: ____	
Manual: Intravenous & Nutritional Therapy	HM: ____ PT: ____	Date Formulated: 4·1·85
Approved by: *Carol A. Cafrus*	OT: ____ Other: x	Date Revised:

FLOW CHART

jectives. They provide a continuity of thought and direct the agency in achieving its desired end result. For this reason, objectives must be reviewed and revised on an ongoing, timely basis and used as tools to evaluate client care outcomes.

Agencies involved in planning high-tech services must recognize the agency's overall program strengths and weaknesses. Identifying the organization's strengths enhances the effectiveness of management. It provides administrators with an inventory of areas in which high-tech programs need to be structured that capitalize on the positive capabilities of the organization to achieve the agency's overall objectives. In the same respect, the agency must identify those characteristics which may limit the effectiveness of the program's objectives.

Operational Planning

Having done the strategic planning the agency enters the second phase of implementing high-tech service – the operational phase. Health administrators need to develop plans for manpower and budget requirements, to define the process of delivery, and to implement quality assurance programs.

The agency must have qualified staff to meet the special needs of the high-tech client and caregivers. The type of service provided and geographic specifications will indicate the number of adequate staff for a 24-hour period. The selection of skilled employees will vary depending on the concentration of high-tech service. Agencies may decide to subcontract high-tech nursing care. Administrators should follow the agency's contract procedures and policy on signing high-tech contracts. The liability aspects of care should be considered carefully when service contracts for high-tech care are utilized. Whether you are performing the service yourself or subcontracting the care for high-tech service the personnel must be highly competent and accountable to safely and effectively meet the complex technological needs of the high-tech client in the home setting.

Home health agencies delineate the process of delivering high-tech home care products and service. The process should include a referral or intake procedure identifying potential home care candidates, thorough assessment of the type of high-tech therapy, clients, caregivers, and nurses safety, and guides for administrators in developing an intake admission screen. This intake assessment defines the specific client's care needs. It provides clinical data to support a decision to accept or deny specific clients. Examination of admission criteria assists agencies in selecting clients who can be safely managed at home. Utilization of admission criteria, informed consent, plans of medical treatment, special assay test, and signs and symptoms to observe are critical indicators for successful high-tech home care.

The use of a standard admission screen will assist the agency in selecting appropriate and successful home care clients. Once the client has been identified as a home care candidate, a review of the client's insurance coverage and reimbursement capabilities must be completed. This is typically conducted by the agency or independent contract vendor who will be handling the billing. This step is particularly critical since Medicare and other insurers require specific indicators and conditions to qualify for reimbursement. Most high-tech services are areas presently not covered by Medicare. A supplemental major medical policy usually covers the insured 80 to 100%. A specific insurance verification procedure must be implemented to identify payment source. The agency should develop a fixed limit indigent fund to assist clients with no insurance coverage. The importance of paying close attention to high-tech service reimbursement policies cannot be underestimated. All members in an agency who are involved in the high-tech business must be continually educated on current and changing reimbursement issues.

Education and training provided to the client and caregivers is a crucial component of high-tech care. Education must begin prior to discharge and continue in the home setting. A key factor determining whether a client qualifies for high-tech care often is the client's and caregiver's capability to be effectively trained in high-tech service. Training includes proper use of equipment, supplies, aseptic technique, therapy process, and emergency procedures. Some agencies have established affiliations with primary hospitals to provide skilled personnel for client and caregivers training and education. The utilization of a proficiency education check list provides the agency with a written document of educational goals the client and caregivers have safely and effectively demonstrated.

Hospitals discharge planners and home health agencies should coordinate the acquisition and delivery of appropriate supplies for high-tech service. The supplies should be delivered at least 24 hours prior to discharge to assure the client and caregiver that all necessary supplies are available and working. High-tech supplies can be provided by the agency or from an independent high-tech company. The timing of subsequent deliveries varies between high-tech modality and vendors.

A quality assurance program is an important control mechanism for any home health agency. A functional quality assurance program establishes the process that assures that an agreed level of excellence is achieved in the delivery of high-tech health care. It is a major factor in establishing the confidence that is necessary for clients, physicians, referral agencies, and service providers. Quality assurance is divided into three components: standard development, program process, and evaluation. Quality assurance is an ongoing process. Managers must understand that a break in any part of the process threatens the integrity of the whole process.

Standards of care are the agency's policies and procedures that reflect the level of quality and commitment to excellence the agency has established in the delivery of high-tech care. Standards should be well-defined, attainable and measurable. They must be reviewed and revised on an ongoing timely basis and used as tools to measure and evaluate client care outcome. Home health agencies must keep abreast of new procedures and incorporate those changes into revised standards. High-tech care standards are usually contained in a comprehensive client manual which is easily accessible to all home care personnel. Agencies utilizing contracts for high-tech care must have all parties agree on a standard set of policies and procedures to minimize staff and client confusion. To reiterate the purpose of standards is to maximize the provision of quality care while ensuring that care is provided safely.

The delivery of high-tech care denotes the agency's commitment to the community's complex care needs. To meet those needs the agency must develop a comprehensive educational program. Such a program insures that field personnel will be proficient in the skills necessary to provide quality high-tech care. The staff of registered nurses must be properly prepared in the educational and clinical components of care. Clients must be properly educated to assume responsibility for their medical regime. Educational program components like standard of care change with advanced technology. Home health administrators must develop and revise high-tech education programs to meet the complex demands of the community-based client.

Program Evaluation

The evaluation process involves the client, caregiver, physician, nurse, and the agency. Physician response can be measured by verbal and written evaluation tools. Service satisfaction surveys quantify a physician's evaluation of the effectiveness of the community-based high-tech program. Frequently, the success of a program can be measured by the continuance of referrals for specific high-tech therapies from community-based physicians. Planned interval physician surveys allow home health agencies to measure their ability to meet expected program goals. In the same vein, patient satisfaction surveys elicit positive or negative feedback from former clients to measure success or failure of the agency to meet client's needs.

Patient response is more readily apparent by the fact that client has consented to perform the high-tech service at home and that the client has either successfully completed the therapy or an alternative course of action has been made. A home health agency must monitor client outcome to evaluate the program. The agency must perform quality assurance (Q.A.) activities to measure if the agency has attained the predetermining standards of care. The best way to measure the quality of care employees provide is to make direct, on-site supervision of care. This allows supervisors to assess client's condition, observe caregivers' skills, observe providers' interaction with client and family, and monitor progress toward care goals. Indirect Q.A. tools include patient care conferences, clinical record reviews, and random chart audits.

A combination of direct and indirect monitors offers a whole system of checks and balances that assist the agency with identifying potential problems and taking corrective action. The home health agency must work to ensure that all clients receive the highest quality service possible, while also working to remain competitive in the booming health care market.

Legal Responsibilities

High-tech care delivery carries the same liabilities risk as that for similar therapies in the hospital setting. Nurses in home care programs are not at any higher risk of liability than those who work in acute care settings, because in any liability situations, the nurse's performance is measured against the current standard of practice. Home health agencies must provide protocols and procedures that help define the standard of practice for a given treatment. Home care personnel must work within these guidelines and find them realistic and attainable. The home health agency is responsible for negligent acts of its employees because the agency is responsible for their supervision. The agency therefore assumes vicarious liability. The concept of vicarious liability is similar to the concept of corporate liability. The home health agency like a corporation is viewed as guaranteeing the quality of the product, health care. The agency is responsible for the standard and supervision of homecare provided to ensure that the care is safe and is performed competently. A second legal concept is contributory or comparative negligence.

Some liability cases are ajudicated by the doctrine of comparative negligence. This type of judgment is one in which the court weighs the acts of faults of the medical profession against that of the client on a percentage of faults basis. Settlements are gauged on the percentage of damage the defendant is proven to have contributed to the client. Contributory negligence is a similar legal concept in which the client has been deemed by the court to have aided to the process by which the client has received damages. It is up to the agency to be familiar with current standards of care because, in a liability situation, the agency's personnel performance will be measured against the present accepted standard of care. For these reasons, it is imperative that home health agencies develop, follow, and evaluate standards of high-tech home care.

In any action for negligence the burden of proof lies with the injured party. The four essential elements to any action for negligence are duty, standard, breech, and injury.

Key factors in minimizing liability in home high-tech care are: (1) a physician's order must be obtained stating the exact medical treatment plan; (2) consent must be obtained with the patient's full knowledge and understanding of the procedures and potential complications; (3) the registered nurse administering the therapy must be fully qualified in the specialty; and (4) strict adherence to agency protocol and procedures must be maintained, and the procedure and patient responses to the therapy must be accurately documented in the medical record (Gardner 1986, 96). Although client care may vary from agency to agency, nurses are held liable for meeting the accepted standard of nursing practice for that therapy.

Contract Services

Home health administrators may be unable to provide full high-tech services and decide to use an outside contractor. Contractors may be a licensed health professional or an agency- or community-based service organization. A written contract between said personnel or service should clearly describe the process by which the services will be provided. Selecting a contractor for high-tech should include reviewing service history, references from other contractors, 24-hour, 7-day-a-week availability; review of contractor's personnel and skill level; and quality assurance capability. Exhibit 17-3 is a checklist for evaluating potential high-tech contractors.

Contracts for high-tech service should include: a written specification of service, whether full- or part-time; a clause indicating clients are accepted for care only by the primary care agency; a statement indicating that all contractors are obliged to follow the home care agency's policies and procedures; a statement indicating that contracted services must be written within the scope and limitations of a medical treatment plan; statements defining the method in which services are coordinated, controlled, and evaluated, statements defining procedures for charges and reimbursement; and statements defining the length of contract and definitions of when and how the contract may become null and void. Exhibit 17-4 is a sample contract checklist to help you coordinate and maintain safe and effective contract services.

Exhibit 17-3.

Checklist For Selecting High-Tech Company

_____ Does vendor have skilled personnel to provide education and service?

_____ Does vendor have other high-tech contracts?

     If yes,

        _____ Are other agencies/contractors satisfied with service?

_____ Does vendor have policy/procedure manual describing type of services

     and standard of practices?

_____ Does vendor have 24 hour, seven days a week professional back-up
availability?

_____ Does vendor have well developed quality assurance program?

_____ Does vendor offer full line of products/service such as IV therapy services?

_____ Does vendor have capabilities of one-step shopping (one call for
product/personnel/service)?

_____ Does vendor have evidence of sufficient liability insurance?

_____ Does vendor have professional advisory personnel or mechanism to handle medical
service problems?

In summary, home care services are growing rapidly. Home health agencies must respond to meet the complex needs of the seriously ill client in the community setting. Administrators must keep abreast of new technologies and develop strategic plans to operationalize community-based high-tech programs. Home health care agencies may have limited opportunities to assure the community that high-tech service needs will be met adequately and appropriately. Agencies are seriously competing for the market share to meet this new challenge. The agency must be willing to invest time, money, and energy in goal-directed, innovative high-tech programs. Administrators must respond in developing safe and effective home care programs. They must develop clear program missions and follow that mission to its completion. Home health care is a dynamic process and any disruption in the process threatens the integrity of the whole process. The delivery of high-tech care denotes the agency's commitment to meet the community's complex care needs. As home health care administrators, we must respond to the advances in technology in an effort to meet the community's needs and maintain viability in the growing home care market.

Exhibit 17-4.

Contract Check List To Delineate Services

Does contract include:

_____ Statement declaring patients are accepted by primary home health agency only

_____ Statements defining services to be provided

_____ Statements declaring necessity of contractors to conform to all applicable agency policies including personnel qualifications

_____ Statement(s) declaring responsibility for participating in developing plans of treatment.

_____ Statements defining method in which services will be coordinated, controlled and evaluated by the primary agency

_____ Statements clarifying procedures for submitting clinical progress notes, scheduling of visits, and periodic patients' evaluations

_____ Statement defining procedures for determining charges and reimbursement

_____ Statement(s) defining length of contract, and method of notification if contract to be discontinued

_____ Statement(s) defining reason contract would become null and void

Management of Intravenous Therapy in the Home: A Case Study
Kathi Collins

IV therapy can be managed in the home, although the road is not always a smooth one, for the home health agency or the patient. There are many variables which may impact on the overall effectiveness and success of the therapy, as illustrated by the following case study.

Dr. T. telephoned in a referral for home IV therapy to VNA, a small, but growing suburban home health agency. The patient, who was to get an IV antibiotic via a Heparin lock, had a history of poor resistance to infection, and on two recent hospital admissions had contracted nosocomial infections, complicating his original diagnosis. For this reason, the patient had asked his physician if he might be treated at home, rather that being readmitted to the hospital a third time. Dr. T. agreed to allow the patient to learn to administer the IV antibiotic at home.

Mr. P.M. (a former patient of VNA) was a 60-year-old man who had been an insulin-dependent diabetic for 15 years. Three months previously, he had developed an infected ulcer on his right foot after stepping on a piece of broken glass in his home.

After two hospitalizations and two courses of IV Ancef, his foot was still not healed. Each time it had responded initially to the antibiotic, only to deteriorate again once he went home. The physician had now diagnosed a cellulitis of the entire right lower extremity.

His orders were to start a peripheral IV line and administer Ancef one gram every eight hours. The IV therapy was to last four weeks. Dr. T. also ordered daily wound irrigations of the newly debrided foot ulcer with Dakin's solution. The patient and his wife could be taught both the daily IV care and the wound care. Ms. C., the nursing supervisor who took Dr. T.'s call, warned him that although the nurse could begin teaching the wound irrigations that day, it would probably be the following day before all the preparations for the IV therapy could be completed. The physician was satisfied with that plan.

Ms. C. read in the old clinical record that Mr. P.M. had been disabled for three years with diabetic neuropathy in his lower extremities, which qualified him for Social Security Disability and Medicare. She telephoned his home to explain to his wife that the nurse would only be able to visit on an intermittent basis, and that Mrs. P.M. would need to agree to be the primary caregiver for both the IV and the would care. Mrs. P.M. acknowledged her understanding, and said she wound try to learn anything the nurse thought she could be taught.

After completing the written referral, Ms. C. mentally checked off each of VNA's conditions for acceptance to a home IV antibiotic therapy program that had been met: treatment had been ordered by a physician for a condition considered amenable to such therapy, that could be safely taught to a layperson. The patient and his wife had agreed to assume primary responsibility for the three times daily (T.I.D.) IV infusions once they had received adequate instruction from an IV-certified nurse. The last condition for acceptance was that the patient be on the IV antibiotic for at least 48 hours prior to initiation of home IV therapy. Because of the circumstances, Ms. C. decided to waive the last condition, particularly since Mr. P.M. had received IV Ancef during his most recent hospital stay without any untoward effects, and had no history of any other drug allergy.

After assigning one of the field nurses, Sarah, to make an admission and assessment home visit with Mr. P.M., Ms. C. prepared to select a durable medical equipment (DME) company. VNA was just beginning to expand into "high-tech," and had not yet developed a relationship with any one particular company. She reviewed the promotional literature that had been left by several different dealers. Some of the attributes she thought might be important when choosing were: the company's reliability and speed of service, their ability or willingness to bill insurance for the patient and to waive co-payments when the patient was unable to pay, and their reputation and size. She called a colleague at a larger agency in a nearby urban area and got several recommendations.

She finally chose a large, urban-based firm which was part of a national chain and had been operating in the area for about two years. Ms. C.'s colleague had said the company had a "good" reputation, and Ms. C. felt more comfortable going with an established company which had a national reputation to consider as well as their own individual one.

Ms. C. called the company, and the representative who answered the phone promised to have the necessary supplies in the home early the next morning.

Sarah, the field nurse, visited Mr. P.M. and his wife in their home later that day to further assess their suitability for home IV care. She reviewed the conditions of acceptance with them. They agreed, once they were taught, to accept responsibility for the T.I.D. infusions and heparin flushes. Sarah emphasized that her visits would be intermittent and that she might not be present when emergencies arose, although she could always be reached by phone. She assured them that she or another IV-certified nurse would visit every two to three days to change the IV site. When all these things were understood and agreed upon, Mr. P.M. and his wife signed patient and caregiver's consent forms (See Exhibits 17-5 and 17-6).

Sarah completed her physical assessment, and began teaching the wound irrigation to Mrs. P.M. She found the patient and his wife to have an open and supportive relationship. Although they were apprehensive, they seemed eager to learn and listened closely to her instructions.

The home was quite cluttered and dirty in the main living areas, so the nurse suggested they designate a seldom-used spare bedroom as the "IV room." All supplies would be kept in this room (behind a closed door), and the IV infusions would be administered in this room.

Exhibit 17-5.

Consent For Intravenous Therapy In The Home

I consent to the administration of intravenous therapy in the home by Moorestown Visiting Nurse Association as it is ordered by the physician.

I understand that Moorestown Visiting Nurse Association is a part-time service and I therefore agree to assume the responsibility for the care of _____ in the absence of the visiting certified Registered Nurse from the Agency.

I further understand that if the visiting certified Registered Nurse was not available, I would call the Physician and/or take the patient to the Hospital Emergency Room, if necessary.

Date: _____   Signature: _____

Relationship to Patient _____

Witness: _____

Exhibit 17-6.

Patient Consent For Intravenous Therapy In The Home

I, _____ consent to the administration of intravenous therapy in the home for myself as ordered by Dr. _____.

I understand that intravenous therapy will be administered by the visiting nurse and

_____

    (Care Giver)   (Relationship)

I will attempt to learn and to do as much of my own care as is possible. I will also cooperate and assist other family members or significant others in learning the care I need.

I am aware that a visiting nurse is a part-time service and may not be present at times when emergencies could arise. I will follow written instruction guidelines for care and emergency measures.

I am also aware that I will be responsible for obtaining medication and other prescription items.

I do understand that failure to comply with the terms of this agreement will result in termination of the Moorestown Visiting Nurse Association's services.

Signature: _____

Date: _____

Witness: _____

Date: _____

Before she left, Sarah gave Mr. P.M. and his wife some written protocols to study on administering IV antibiotics at home. She planned to return the following morning and the three of them would administer the first dose of Ancef together.

The nurse arrived as scheduled the next morning, but found that the DME dealer had not yet delivered the supplies. After waiting about half an hour, she called Ms. C., who tried to track down the problem. When she called the DME dealer, Ms. C. was told casually that there had been "some sort of mix-up," and that they would be unable to deliver until that evening, as they did not have a driver who would go that distance (about 25 miles). Ms. C. cancelled the order immediately and quickly called a smaller, local firm that was just starting out, trying to develop new business and was therefore eager to please. After she explained the problem to them, they promised to deliver by lunchtime.

Ms. C. called Sarah back and sent her on to her next patient. Ms. C. then spoke at length with Mr. P.M., who was quite upset at the delay, and certain that each hour he went without the antibiotic brought him closer to losing his leg. It took Ms. C. close to half an hour to reassure him.

Sarah returned to the home a few hours later, just as the supplies were arriving. She began her teaching, and Mr. and Mrs. P.M. learned quickly. After only one demonstration, they were anxious to try it themselves with Sarah providing verbal cues as needed. Sarah planned to visit three times a day until they could go it alone, and then would decrease the frequency of her visits to every 72 hours to change the site of the IV.

After five participatory sessions, Mr. and Mrs. P.M. were able to administer the IV infusion and give the heparin flush independently. At one point about 10 days into the therapy, some of the supplies ran low before anyone noticed. A frantic mid-afternoon call was placed to the DME dealer, asking for a delivery before the close of the business day. The dealer was understandably displeased with the last-minute request, although he did manage to deliver the supplies within two hours. Ms. C. realized that the VNA's responsibility to the DME company was just as important as the reverse. From that time on, supplies were checked each visit and ordered well in advance of when they were needed.

Things progressed smoothly after that. At the end of the four weeks, Mr. P.M.'s foot ulcer was nearly healed, and the IV Ancef was discontinued. Sarah continued weekly visits for three more weeks to monitor the foot ulcer until it healed completely.

Conclusions

Overall, the skilled care rendered to Mr. P.M. was effective. The patient's goals of staying independent and at home were met, as were the professionals' goals of safe administration of the therapeutic regime and wound healing.

From the patient's viewpoint, Mr. P.M. stated on a consumer evaluation form that he was extremely pleased with the service, but that "better choice of a medical supply company initially would have made the road smoother for all of us."

The letter reminded Ms. C. that her unfortunate choice of an unreliable DME company initially resulted in an inconvenience to both the agency and the patient. From an agency viewpoint, there was a loss of productivity of the field nurse on two separate occasions: first, when the original DME dealer was unable to deliver and, second, when the nurse failed to reorder needed supplies. The dissatisfaction of the patient, who was caused needless worry and apprehension, must also be considered. Although things turned out all right this time, the patient might have been dissatisfied enough to look at another agency for the service then or in the future. In today's competitive market, all precautions must be taken to avoid losing patients to your competitors. Maintaining consumer satisfaction is an important task. Considered individually, these points might seem inconsequential, but if these problems were encountered with every home IV case, it could mean a significant loss of manpower, time, referrals, and ultimately, money, to the agency. Ms. C. realized how important it would be in the future for her to develop a good working relationship with one or more DME dealers, and to supervise her field staff closely.

Intravenous care in the home can be managed successfully, if all details are considered carefully, and potential problems identified and dealt with responsibly.

Sending a Ventilator-Dependent Child Home: A Case Study

Karen M. Polise

Billy is an active, personable four-year-old preschooler who spent his first two and a half years of life in a pediatric intensive care unit. At 30 months of age he was discharged home on a ventilator. Over the next 14 months he was successfully weaned from all respiratory support at home. This case study illustrates how the intricacies involved in providing a safe home environment for a ventilator-dependent child can be accomplished.

Neonatology and pediatric critical care have evolved over the last 20 years. The progress in these fields has paralleled the quantum advances in medical technology. Critically ill infants and children are now surviving because of these technological advances. Some of these survivors are left with chronic medical problems and disabilities, with a growing number dependent on some type of technology for their survival. Children who require sophisticated technological support, such as ventilators, have traditionally remained in intensive care units, an environment that is incongruous with normal growth and development. The prolonged hospitalization of these children is occurring at a time when policy-making and reimbursement strategies focus on shorter stays and lower costs. As health care professionals endeavor to meet the spiraling cost of medical care and deal with psychosocial needs of these children and their families, home care of the technology-dependent child has become an option.

Billy, a premature infant born at 32 weeks, developed severe respiratory distress syndrome requiring prolonged mechanical ventilation. As a result, he developed bronchopulmonary dysplasia (BPD), a chronic lung disease that is reported to occur in 7 to 38% of patients with respiratory distress syndrome who are mechanically ventilated. Severe respiratory distress syndrome and the development of BPD is associated with a high mortality rate. As centers develop more expertise in caring for premature infants, the population of children with BPD will increase. Experience has shown that infants who survive the initial insult will show gradual improvement in pulmonary function. During this time, infants with BPD often require some type of respiratory support and have traditionally remained in the hospital. As a result, their development is often delayed. Nurses have recognized that these children require special care to meet their developmental needs as well as care for their medical problems, but an intensive care unit is not conducive to this type of care. Thus, home care has become an alternative.

Billy was placed on a ventilator shortly after birth. Numerous attempts to wean him were unsuccessful. In order to grow and develop, Billy required significant respiratory support. During attempts to wean him all his energy was utilized for breathing and not for growing and developing. A medical decision was made to temporarily discontinue weaning attempts to allow Billy to grow and develop. It was hoped that as he grew he would become stronger and his lung function would improve to allow him to wean. In the interim, with adequate respiratory support and an intensive infant stimulation program, he would progress developmentally.

Billy's parents were actively involved in his care from the beginning. After the critical period of his illness had passed, they became more involved, visiting frequently, learning his care. They often talked about the day when they would be able to bring him home. Once he was stabilized and the decision was made not to pursue further weaning for a while, the idea of taking him home on a ventilator was broached to his parents.

The decision to discharge a child home on a ventilator is an involved one. It is a major endeavor and not every child and/or family are appropriate candidates. The child must be medically stable. He must have a stable airway, sufficient blood gases, and oxygen requirements that can be maintained practically at home, and adequate nutritional intake for growth and development. The family must understand the child's condition and prognosis and be willing and able to care for their child at home.

Mr. and Mrs. P were reluctant at first to take Billy home. They were knowledgeable about the complexity of his care, but unsure if they could provide that care at home. Mr. and Mrs. P were assured that the discharge process could be delayed or even discontinued in the event they felt unable to proceed. This is an important underlying principle in planning for the discharge. The parents must have a thorough understanding of their child's needs in order to make an informed decision. They need to be actively involved and supported during the discharge process and allowed to participate in decision making about home care. A comprehensive discharge plan utilizing an interdisciplinary approach seems to be most effective in planning and preparing for home care of the ventilator-dependent child.

Mr. and Mrs. P began an intensive teaching program to prepare them to care for Billy at home. Since they had been involved in Billy's care from the beginning, teaching proceeded well. Teaching should be comprehensive and include all aspects of the child's care. It is important to document all teaching done and show that the parents are prepared to provide safe care of their child at home. Mr. P worked during the day so his training needed to be done on evenings and weekends. Staffing adjustments in the unit were made to accomplish this. It is recommended that at least two individuals be trained in the care of the child and that they spend 12 to 24 hours providing total care of the child in the hospital prior to discharge.

In addition to the comprehensive education program, there are a number of other discharge considerations that need to be addressed. The first is the funding issue. Who will pay for the care of this child at home? The ventilator-dependent child requires constant surveillance. It is usually unrealistic to expect that the parents will be able to provide 24-hour care at home. Therefore, some supplemental nursing support is usually required. Before any decisions can be made on the amount or type of nursing care, or equipment and supplies, a funding source needs to be found. Most insurance policies have limited home care benefits. In addition, many insurance policies have a lifetime maximum. Children, like Billy, who remain in the hospital for any prolonged period of time often reach their lifetime maximum before they are ready to be discharged. While in the hospital, once insurance is exhausted, children are usually eligible for some type of public assistance. This assistance often ends at discharge because the family income is considered. This was the situation with Billy. By the time Billy was stable enough to be discharged home and his parents had been taught his care, he had exhausted all his insurance benefits. Therefore, even though he was ready to go home there was no funding available to pay for home care. As long as Billy remained in the hospital, his medical costs were covered by Medicaid. Once discharged, his parents' income would make him ineligible for any public funding. This was the same situation that President Reagan addressed in a national speech about a little girl from Iowa. As a result, a special board was set up to grant a waiver to a small number of disabled children who were ineligible for Medicaid due to their parents' income. This waiver enabled these children to receive SSI and Medicaid benefits by waiving the SSI deeming rule on parents' income if: 1. lower Medicaid costs were realized by home-based care; and 2. the quality of home care is proven to be equal to or better than the care provided in an institution. Billy was eventually granted this waiver and was provided funding for home care.

Billy was also enrolled in the Ventilator Assisted Children/Home Program. This is a state-funded program for Pennsylvania residents that provides consultation and supportive services to families and professionals who are involved in home care of a child on a ventilator. In addition, this program provides postdischarge follow-up and a limited amount of funding.

Once funding was established, the other considerations for discharge could be addressed. Equipment and supplies that the child requires at home need to be determined. The physician, respiratory therapist, and nursing staff involved in Billy's care met and prepared an itemized list of all the necessary equipment and supplies. This list specified the manufacturer, model numbers, and sizes of each item. Disposable supplies were determined and a 30-day supply was estimated.

Next, a vendor needed to be identified to provide the equipment and supplies along with follow-up services. Mr. and Mrs. P were given the name of three local vendors in their area who were able to provide the required service. They were then responsible for interviewing each vendor and determining the one they wanted to use. When choosing a vendor for home care there are a number of considerations that need to be examined. Central to this determination is the vendor's willingness to care for a ventilator-dependent child. Other issues that need to be explored are:

1. What insurance or payment plan does the vendor accept?

2. Is there emergency service 24 hours a day, seven days a week, and what is the response time?

3. How often will a respiratory therapist visit the home and what are his responsibilities?

4. Will the company review the use and care of the equipment with the family and home care nursing staff? Do they have written guidelines?

5. What is the preventive maintenance schedule for equipment? If equipment needs repair, who does the repair and does the vendor supply loner equipment?

The P's interviewed and selected the vendor they wanted to use. The company was then given the itemized list of equipment and supplies. The durable equipment, including the ventilators, were delivered to the hospital where they were checked for electrical safety and performance by the biomedical department. It was then used on Billy for a week prior to discharge to familiarize his parents with it and further assess safety and compatibility. The day before discharge all the equipment was picked up from the hospital and delivered to Billy's home along with supplies for 30 days. Everything was set up in the P's home in preparation for Billy's discharge. The respiratory therapist reviewed with the P's and their home nursing staff the function and maintenance of all the equipment. On the day of discharge, the respiratory therapist was at the P's home to assess Billy's adjustment to his home equipment.

Another major decision the P family needed to make was the amount and type of nursing care they would need at home. In most instances, when a child is at home on a ventilator some nursing support is necessary, but it is ultimately the parents' decision. The Ps met with Billy's primary nurse and the social worker to discuss the need for nurses and how many hours were necessary. Every family is different and the amount of nursing support varies depending on family responsibilities (parents' work, other children and complexity of the child's care). The Ps had one other child, Danny, a year older than Billy. Mr. P worked full-time and Mrs. P stayed at home. Billy was on the ventilator 24 hours per day and required frequent suctioning. A nursing time study done in the hospital showed that Billy required about 18 hours of direct nursing care daily, including maintenance of his equipment. The Ps elected to have 16 hours per day of nursing care, one day shift and one night shift. Mrs. P would provide the late afternoon care and Mr. P would assist in the evenings when he returned from work. The P's felt it was important to have some time to themselves as a family without a nurse present.

Nursing care at home can be provided by a registered nurse, licensed practical nurse, and in some cases, a home health aide. It was determined that Billy should have registered nurses because of the complexity of his care. It was hoped that Billy would begin to wean at home and thus would require frequent assessments of his respiratory status by a professional.

It was then necessary for the P's to hire the home care nurses. Nurses can be hired independently by the family or obtained through a nursing agency. This decision is often dependent on third-party constraints. Some insurance companies require families to use nursing agencies. Other funding sources may have a limit on how much they will pay and nursing agencies may be too costly.

While nursing agencies are more expensive, the agency assumes the responsibility for providing appropriately educated and qualified personnel. They also handle all funding and reimbursement issues.

Independent hiring is less expensive, but the family must interview and hire all the nurses. They also have the responsibility for educating, scheduling, and paying the nurses. While this gives the family greater control of personnel, it also results in their assuming an employer role as well as a parental role.

Funding for Billy's nursing care was being provided by Medical Assistance with a maximum dollar amount on the hourly rate that could be paid. This necessitated the Ps to hire their nurses independently. They placed an advertisement in their local paper and were successful in recruiting qualified nurses. Parents often need guidelines when interviewing home nursing personnel. The P's primary nurse assisted them in this process. Some of the important information that needs to be obtained includes credentials, previous employment and experience, and references. Each potential nurse should be questioned about what skills they are proficient in that relate to the ventilator-dependent child's care. It is also important to discuss the number of hours and days the nurse is available to work.

Mrs. P hired two full-time nurses and three part-time nurses. Each nurse came to the hospital for an 8-hour training session with Billy's primary nurse prior to his discharge. This helps assure both the discharging institution and the family that the nurses are competent in providing the care. All of the nurses the Ps had were able to care successfully for Billy. In the case where the primary nurse may feel that one of the home care nurses is not able to provide the level of care the child requires, she will meet the parents to discuss her concerns. Further training may be required or the primary nurse may recommend that the nurse not participate in the child's care.

Home care nurses who come to the hospital for training should have a structured education program set up. There should be specific objectives and goals delineated to make the session valuable.

The home environment should be assessed before discharge to help the family best plan for the care of their child. Some changes in the home environment may be necessary to ensure a safe level of care. The Ps had a small two-bedroom split-level home. Since Billy shared a bedroom with his brother, it was decided to use the family room as his bedroom initially. This would allow his brother to sleep through the night without being disturbed by Billy's care. The electrical wiring was checked and additional outlets were installed in the family room for all of the equipment.

Lastly, the family was assisted in preparing a list of emergency resources and in notifying local essential services that a child dependent on life support equipment was living in the community. These included the gas, electric, and phone company, along with the local hospital and rescue squad. Prior to discharge, Billy's primary nurse, the parents, and the home care nurses developed a home nursing care plan. Exhibit 17-7 is the plan developed for Billy. The home nursing care plan should be evaluated and revised periodically. The parents and home nursing care staff should work together on this. It is useful to specify in the home nursing care plan who is responsible for certain tasks. For example, the Ps delegated the responsibility for changing ventilator tubing and disinfecting equipment to the night shift nurse.

Many studies have documented that families with a sick child in the hospital find it a stress experience which inevitably results in family disruption and disorganization. The Ps reported that Billy's premature birth and subsequent prolonged hospitalization resulted in major disruptions in their life. With the strong extended family support the Ps were able to cope positively with Billy's hospitalization. They became active in his care and were able to establish a loving, nurturing relationship with Billy.

Home care of ventilator-dependent children is a relatively recent phenomenon. There is a limited amount of experience and the research documenting the psychosocial effects of having a ventilator-dependent child at home. The Ps identified a number of new and different stresses as a result of home care. There continued to be a disruption in family lifestyle, although they felt there was less disruption than when Billy was hospitalized. Having a constant flow of persons in and out of their home left little time for privacy or spontaneity. Billy became the center of the family life and other activities (such as Danny's soccer practice) became secondary. Mrs. P found careful scheduling of her activities in coordination with nursing care allowed her more

Exhibit 17-7.

Home Care Plan

Problem	Goals	Assessments	Interventions
Alteration in respiratory status secondary to tracheostomy and tracheomalacia	Billy will have a patent airway and adequate respiratory function.	Observe Billy for signs of respiratory distress: Restlessness Nasal flaring Retractions Cyanosis Tachypnea	1. Maintain patent #2 Portex tracheostomy tube at all times: a. Suction every 2 hrs. and PRN b. Provide humidification via ventilator. When off the ventilator use a heat and moisture exchanger. c. Change tracheostomy tube weekly (Wed.)
	Billy will eventually be weaned from respiratory support.	Check ventilator settings (rate, inspiratory pressure, O_2, alarms) q 2 hrs.	2. Maintain ventilator settings as ordered. Maintain humidifier temperature at 30 ° -34 ° C. Empty H_2O traps PRN.
			3. When going outside or on trips, always take emergency travel bag. Should include: Tracheostomy tube with strings; Endotracheal tube; Portable suction; Resuscitation bag; K-Y jelly; Saline; Scissors and hemostat.
Potential for respiratory infections secondary to tracheostomy.	Billy will be free of respiratory infections and atelectasis.	Assess breath sounds q 4°. Observe for signs and symptoms of respiratory infection: Change in amount, color, order, consistency of secretions. Decreased aeration Fever Chest congestion	1. Follow good handwashing technique. Always wash hands before tracheostomy care. 2. Daily tracheostomy care: a. Clean tracheostomy site with water (half strength H_2O_2 if crusted) daily and PRN. b. Change tracheostomy dressing twice daily and PRN. c. Change tracheostomy strings every morning and PRN. Use reston foam. d. Change tracheostomy tube weekly (Tues.) with sterile technique and 2 caregivers.

Exhibit 17-7, continued.

Home Care Plan

Problem	Goals	Assessments	Interventions
			3. Chest percussion every 4 hrs. while awake. Instilled 1-2 cc NSS PRN for thick secretions.
			4. Maintain clean technique during suctioning q 1-2 hrs. while awake; every 4-6 hrs. while asleep.
			5. Change disposable ventilater tubing every 3 days (on night shift).
			6. Change and disinfect cascade humidifier and non-disposable ventilator parts every 3 days (night shift).
Alteration in growth and development secondary to prematurity and prolonged hospitalization.	Billy will increase developmental skills and reach age appropriate developmental milestones.	Assess developmental skills.	1. Encourage Billy to be independent--allow him to feed self, assist in dressing himself.
			2. Follow posted daily schedule for activities.
			3. Provide play time and encourage developmental skills.
			a. Gross Motor: allow to ride big wheel; walk up and downstairs while providing Billy manual ventilation with resuscitator.
			b. Fine Motor: Encourage use of crayons, using blocks, etc.
			c. Speech: Encourage Billy to vocalize around tracheostomy. Billy knows some sign language.

Exhibit 17-7, continued.

Home Care Plan

Problem	Goals	Assessments	Interventions
			Speak to Billy about his environment. Introduce new things he has not had the opportunity to experience while in the hospital.
			Follow through on speech therapist recommendations. Will receive speech therapy 3 times/week.
Alteration in nutritional status secondary to poor PO intake and new environment.	Billy will gain weight.	Weigh weekly.	1. Provide high calorie, high protein meals with 3 snacks at 10 a.m., 2 p.m., bedtime.
			2. Allow Billy to eat with the family, sitting at table in high chair. Provide favorite foods (peaches, ice cream, pudding).
			3. Encourage Billy to use cup. Do not give him bottle until after meals.
Potential alteration in family functioning secondary to Billy's prolonged hospitalization and complex needs.	Billy will become an active family member. The Ps will be an intact family unit.	Assess family for signs of stress.	1. Allow time for individual attention of Billy and Danny by parents.
			2. Encourage Billy and Danny to play together.
			3. Provide time for Mr. & Mrs. P. to go out by themselves.

flexibility. She occasionally would split her nursing shifts if she had evening activities to attend.

The tasks and issues related to home care of Billy were time-consuming. The first few weeks Billy was home were disorganized and Mrs. P often found herself exhausted. She discovered that by being organized and delegating more tasks to her nurses, she had more time for herself, Billy, and her family.

A major stress factor for the Ps was hiring personnel. Soon after Billy was discharged one of the P's full-time nurses quit. They had difficulty finding another competent nurse and were dependent on the part-time nurses to fill in. As a result, there were many shifts uncovered and Mr. and Mrs. P were providing a lot more of Billy's care. It was during this time that Danny began to exhibit some regressive behavior which added to the Ps' stress. This experience resulted in Mrs. P developing a list of relief nurses that she trained in Billy's care. This enabled her to cover sick calls and vacations.

Besides hiring nurses, locating other services and dealing with service providers created some problems for the Ps. Service providers were not experienced in providing services for a ventilator-dependent child, and thus, the Ps often had to look aggressively for services. Most established programs for handicapped children are specific for a diagnosis and thus Billy had trouble qualifying for certain services.

Some families with a child at home on a ventilator have identified social isolation and alienation as a source of stress. The Ps did not see this as a problem. Family and friends often visited, and as Billy was weaned from daytime ventilation, he frequently accompanied the family on outings, including trips to the zoo and beach.

Mr. P. was concerned about the financial implications Billy's illness presented and its effect on his job. He was a construction worker and much of his work was seasonal. When he was out of work there was no income and they had to depend on savings. Mr. P also identified a number of increased costs they had not expected, the major one being a 35% increase in their electrical bill.

Mr. P expressed concern about the amount of time he missed from work because of Billy's illness and the effect this might have on his job in the future. He also had limited job mobility since the Ps felt it important to remain close to the tertiary care center where Billy's care was coordinated. Other fathers have stated they feel they cannot change jobs because they may lose insurance coverage for their child.

Danny, as previously mentioned, did experience some difficulty adjusting to Billy's homecoming. Since Billy had been hospitalized for almost three years, Danny never really identified Billy as his brother. Once Billy came home, Danny no longer had his parents' undivided attention at home. Mrs. P set aside time to spend alone with Danny in the evening while Mr. P cared for Billy. Danny started kindergarten 10 months after Billy was discharged. The Ps paid special attention to this major milestone in Danny's development. After some initial hesitancy and jealousies on Danny's part, he and Billy became great buddies. Danny enjoyed assuming the "big brother" role.

One of the goals of Billy's home care was to assure his continued development. Prior to discharge he had a comprehensive developmental evaluation. As a result, it was recommended that he have an ongoing rehabilitative program at home that included speech therapy and infant stimulation. Services were coordinated by the local intermediate unit. The comprehensive developmental care Billy received was valuable. A follow-up developmental evaluation done after Billy was weaned and decannulated 14 months following discharge, revealed that Billy was functioning within a normal range of intelligence for his age. Two areas of weakness were note, speech and fine motor control. Billy's language skills had shown remarkable improvement over a three month period after being decannulated, and he was able to speak in four- to five-word sentences. His articulation was still garbled and it was recommended that he continue speech therapy.

Mrs. P was encouraged to continue to work on Billy's fine motor skills by encouraging him to crayon, draw, and use blocks. He was enrolled in a regular pre-school program to further enhance his development.

Our experience has shown that comprehensive preparation and training prior to discharge and ongoing support after discharge usually result in a positive home care experience for the ventilator-dependent child and his family.

References

Furtz, N. 1986. *Informed consent in the home setting.* Boston: Choats, Hall and Stewart.

Gardner, C. 1986. Home IV therapy; Part I. *NITA* 9(2):95-106.

Gardner, C. 1986. Home IV therapy; Part II. *NITA* 9(3):193-203.

Griffith, D. 1986. Keys to quality. *Nursing and Health Care* 1(6):300-303.

Louden, T. L. 1985. Planning your niche in the "high tech" home care market. *Caring* 4(10):20-22.

Shaw, S., J. E. McNamara, and R. Perchand. 1985. Assuring quality and confidence in new home care technologies. *Caring* 4(1):51-55.

Stuart-Siddall, S. 1986. *Home health care nursing administrative and clinical perspectives.* Rockville, Md: Aspen Publications.

Sumser, S. S. 1985. Creating a safe environment for high tech home care. *Caring* 4(1):47-50.

Vnollmueller, R. 1985. The growth and development of home care: From no-tech to high-tech. *Caring* 4(1):3-8.

Wagner, D., and D. Cosgrove. 1986. Quality assurance: A professional responsibility. *Caring* 5(1):46-49.

Weisslein, S. 1984. Home care today. *American Journal of Nursing* 84(3):341-345.

Weisslein, S. 1984. Home health care programs and the law. *Intravenous Therapy News* Nov.-Dec.

Weisslein, S. 1985. *Hospital homecare administrative manual.* Philadelphia, PA: Hospital Homecare of Greater Philadelphia.

Part V

Quality Assurance

Chapter Eighteen

Quality Assurance in Home Health

Components of a Quality Assurance Program

E. Joyce Gould and Nancy DiPasquale Ruane

Assuring the quality of patient care services is a multifaceted operation which is central to the existence of any home care agency. The public holds health care providers accountable for the provision of good care. A quality assurance program is designed to demonstrate and monitor the degree to which an organization's actual performance compares to expected outcomes. There are a number of approaches or methods used to ensure quality and a variety of techniques or tools to measure quality.

Quality Assurance as a Comprehensive Agency Function

Quality Assurance in its broadest sense encompasses all aspects of agency operation including personnel, provision of services, acceptance and discharge of patients, community education, and fiscal integrity.

Personnel

Since a home care agency's "product" is patient care, the skilled performance of all personnel is the most essential ingredient in assuring quality. Considerable attention must be given to recruiting staff. Personnel must have appropriate credentials and the knowledge and skills to provide the services needed or wanted by patients. In addition, staff should have a commitment to service delivery goals which are compatible with the agency's philosophy.

Specific job descriptions should identify all qualifications an individual must possess in order to perform his role successfully. The agency must verify licensure for those professionals who, by state law, must be licensed in order to practice. For all other professional and nonprofessional staff, the agency must verify whatever training or education is necessary in order to perform a specific job. If experience is a prerequisite to enable a staff member to achieve expected performance levels, this must be objectively described and assessed. Finally, there should be an examination of the "fit" between the personal goals of each individual staff member and the agency's mission and philosophy.

Consistent supervision is necessary to ensure compliance with the agency's performance standards. Supervision should also include constructive assistance to modify behavior when performance is less than desirable. Since personal goals and needs change over time, a process of evaluation must be in place. Sometimes, the job must be modified to meet the individual's changing goals. Sometimes, the individual needs to be guided to a new job that meets his needs either within or outside the agency. The criteria should be quality patient care and agency philosophy in decisions that reflect the interest of all concerned parties.

In-service education must be provided to enable staff to maintain skills, to acquire new skills as service needs change, and to acquire new knowledge as it becomes available. (See Chapters 4, 7, and 11 for further discussion on professional standards, clinical competency, and educational issues.)

Provision of Services

Every agency must decide on the types of and intensity of services that it will be able to provide effectively. Fiscal considerations must be addressed at this point to ensure that the agency will have the financial resources necessary to deliver the amount of care the patient requires at the level of quality set by the agency. Staffing must be adequate in terms of numbers and type of professionals and nonprofessionals; staff competencies should be matched to patient need.

Establishing clinical policies and procedures is a critical proactive approach to defining quality care. These procedures must be relevant to the individual clinical setting. Making the procedures available in a useful, practical format will encourage staff to use them as a guide for practice. However, rigid adherence to established rituals can actually be counterproductive in the pursuit of quality. Review and revision is necessary to ensure that procedures comply with current professional standards and practice and allow for individualization of care.

Acceptance and Discharge of Patients

Once the decisions have been made regarding the provision of services, the agency must develop guidelines which identify those patients whose needs they can adequately meet. Clearly, this is an important step in enabling an agency to be successful in meeting the goal of providing quality care.

The agency should have clear discharge criteria. The process for addressing a patient's need in the event that the cost of the care exceeds the patient's financial resources (third-party payor or private-pay) should be addressed in policies and procedures. When the patient requires care that the agency does not provide, it is necessary to establish mechanisms for referral to the appropriate provider.

Community Education

Community education and marketing efforts are designed to provide potential patients and referral sources with information about the services of the agency. The accuracy of this information clearly influences what types of patients seek to be accepted for service.

Fiscal Integrity

Financial viability is an absolute minimum requirement for agency survival. Managing in a way which assures effective and efficient resource utilization in achieving agency goals is an essential part of meeting the public mandate to provide quality care.

The concept of quality to which the agency subscribes is an integral part of all activities: statement of mission, long range planning (business plan), program goals and objectives, utilization review, personnel management, and risk management. Only through such a coordinated and pervasive approach can an agency operationalize its definitions of quality.

Quality Assurance Program

A Quality Assurance Program is a more limited concept which focuses on a set of activities to:

- Define quality in an individual agency.

- Identify criteria by which quality is measured in a specific organization.

- Assemble the resources (people, measurement tools, specific approaches) necessary to design and carry out a quality assurance program.

- Examine performance against stated criteria and standards in a systematic, cyclical manner.

- Propose remedial actions where deviations exist.

- Follow-up to ensure that discrepancies have been corrected.

A quality assurance (QA) program concentrates on the actual delivery of care; that is, identified instances of interaction between the provider and the patient. The QA program must be a two-way activity which sends out information to all agency staff about what is expected in performance and collects information to determine if performance actually matches expectations.

The predetermined criteria and standards reach out to each service that interfaces with the patient. Evaluation is a feedback loop which primarily measures performance and determines if corrective actions have taken place when deficiencies occur. Moreover, information gathered during the evaluation process can also be used to influence the development of criteria and standards.

Exhibit 18-1 is a pictorial representation of this process. The heavier arrows radiating outward from the QA criteria and standards indicate that the QA program should be strongly geared toward giving out information about what is expected. The evaluation process is an important, comprehensive activity which provides information to modify performance when deficiencies occur and to influence the development of criteria and standards.

Exhibit 18-1. Quality assurance program: Two-way activity

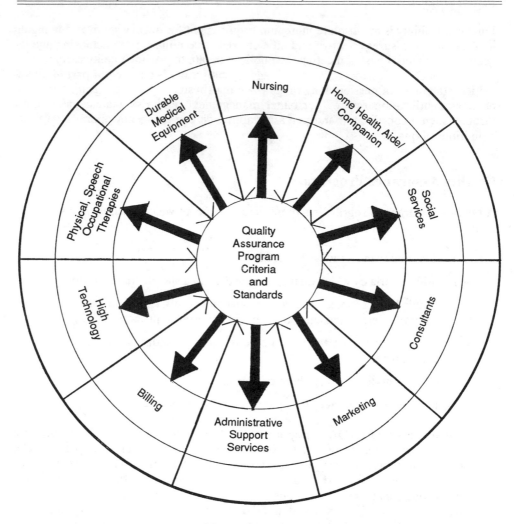

The primary influence on performance is sending out information about expected outcomes for each service. Evaluation is the comprehensive activity which ties all parts of the system together. Feedback from the evaluation process is used to rectify deficiencies in performance and to influence the design of criteria and standards.

Legal and Ethical Issues Related to Quality Assurance

The very term quality assurance may be overly optimistic. In reality, it may be more accurate from a legal standpoint to talk of assessment rather than assurance (Spratt 1984,1). In a litigious society, it is important to establish and communicate to the public the systematic efforts that an agency engages in to address quality issues. All of these activities must be geared "to inspire confidence that the patient is receiving optimal care that meets the highest professional standards within available resources and consistent with achievable goals. The term should *not* imply an absolute guarantee of perfection." (Spratt 1984,1). These efforts need to be documented as well as implemented in order to demonstrate accountability which can withstand legal scrutiny.

Accountability is demonstrated when there is a formal, written program which identifies what standard of care is expected, states how performance is measured, and describes who is responsible for carrying out the program and resolving problems. It is this aspect of a quality assurance program which has fostered the connection between quality assurance and risk management programs. Furthermore, cost-containment efforts directed at decreasing utilization of health care services have the potential of affecting quality care. Therefore, it is important to integrate utilization review activities with quality assurance activities so that a workable balance is achieved between potentially conflicting goals.

The agency has both a legal and ethical duty to protect the patient from health care practitioners whose clinical competence is compromised. However, the quality assurance program is neither a replacement for nor an adjunct to an employee performance evaluation system. Staff need a clear explanation of the purpose of all quality assurance evaluations so that improved patient care is a joint effort of all clinicians and clinical managers. All evaluation findings, both positive and negative, should be provided to staff as a motivator and reminder of the expected level of performance. Using the quality assurance program to discipline errant performers is both inappropriate and ineffective. Punitive actions for continuing poor performance should be handled by the agency's usual disciplinary process.

Patient-specific data collected in carrying out quality assurance activities are considered confidential and should be treated as such. Individual patient permission is not generally required for the agency's quality assessments. However, data must be reported in such a way that they do not provide information which can reveal the identity of individual patients. The purpose of the data collection is to uncover patterns of problems so that strategies can be designed to resolve them. All data collected should be filed separately from the clinical record and should be protected in the same manner.

Inappropriate documentation of performance deficiencies uncovered in quality assessments can adversely affect an agency's liability. The same principles which guide legally acceptable documentation in a patient's clinical record should guide the writing of individual and summary reports of the findings from a quality care evaluation process. Findings should be written legibly, completely, and objectively. Conclusions, if any, must be clearly supported by the data. (See Chapter 14 for additional information on recordkeeping and documentation.)

External Influences on Quality Assurance Activities

No agency functions in a vacuum in the area of quality assurance. It is important to look at activities which will impact on the design and scope of an agency's quality assurance program. These influences can be divided into three categories: general principles which affect all agencies, specific program mandates that agencies choose to meet in order to participate in the program, and voluntary standards that agencies choose to meet in an effort to excel.

General Principles

Professional practice standards apply to all individuals who provide health care services. One of the hallmarks of a profession is its inherent contract with the public to regulate its practitioners. Most professional groups have done this by establishing a code of ethics or standards of practice. Therefore, an agency should acquire a working knowledge of the standards which apply to each professional service it provides. Examples of national organizations which have such standards are: American Nurses Association, National Association of Social Workers, National Homecaring Council (homemakers and home health aides), American Medical Association.

The scope of practice is defined for each professional in state law. Agencies should be aware of which professionals must be licensed in the state(s) in which they provide service. Although there is some consistency in the scope of practice across the country, there are state variations which must be taken into consideration when designing a quality assurance program. Furthermore, professional practice is constantly evolving and influencing the revision of each state's rules and regulations regarding practice.

Current practice is a standard by which all health care providers are measured in the event of litigation. Actions which are consistent with those of other similar, prudent providers in a comparable situation are defensible. Therefore, awareness of quality assurance activities of other home care agencies is necessary to ensure that a specific agency's activities meet the standard of common, current practice.

Specific Program Mandates

First consideration must be given to determining whether state licensure of the agency is a prerequisite to service delivery. There is considerable variability across the country regarding the types of agencies which must be licensed in order to provide services. In some states, licensure is not required for hourly private duty home care services but is required to intermittent skilled services (e.g., Medicare and Medicaid). Some states require licensure for neither hourly nor intermittent services; yet other states require licensure for both types of services. Where licensure is required, an agency must design its quality assurance program to meet initial and renewal requirements for maintaining licensure in order to operate.

Third-party payors frequently mandate specific or general quality assurance standards which must be met in order to provide and receive payment for service to their beneficiaries. Examples of such programs are Title XVIII Medicare, Title XIX Medicaid, Blue Cross, Title V Family Planning, and commercial insurers. When an agency chooses to provide services to the beneficiaries of these insurance and assistance programs, the agency's quality assurance program design and implementation must satisfy the requirements of each third-party payor. Medicare certification, that is, compliance with the Medicare Conditions of Participation for home health agencies, is one of the most widely used criteria; third-party payors as diverse as Medicaid and commercial insurers use Medicare certification as the standard for measuring quality and acceptability. (See Chapter 3 for further information on licensure and Medicare certification.)

Voluntary Standards

An agency may choose to seek accreditation from an outside organization which has established standards for inspecting an organization's performance. The National League for Nursing (NLN) and the Joint Commission on Accreditation of Hospitals (JCAH) both have well-established programs for accrediting home health agencies. For hospital-based agencies, the JCAH standards could be considered quasi-voluntary (Stanhope 1984,222), as accreditation is encouraged by governmental regulations regarding Medicare payment to hospitals.

The standards for accreditation are generally more rigorous than the minimal current level of practice. Thus, both NLN and JCAH go beyond Medicare requirements for quality assurance activities. However, both NLN and JCAH have primarily focused on standards of organizational structure and process. Recent and planned revisions in the standards of both organizations are focusing more on defining outcomes of quality health care. This represents a significant and meaningful shift which will require agencies who seek accreditation to design their quality assurance programs to comply with the revised standards.

Submission of documentation and on-site survey visits are the primary mechanisms used by accrediting organizations to establish compliance with standards. Licensing and certifying organizations use similar methods to determine whether or not an agency has met their standards.

A different type of voluntary mechanism is illustrated by the standards or ethical codes of trade associations. Examples of state and national organizations which have such standards or codes are: National Association for Home Care, Pennsylvania Association of Home Health Agencies, Home Health Assembly of New Jersey, Inc., and American Federation of Home Health Agencies. Each member agency is essentially responsible for establishing and monitoring its own compliance with these standards. Since association members develop these standards, they do represent a method for defining current practice standards which are applicable to the whole agency as opposed to individual disciplines.

In summary, an agency must identify which external influences are relevant to its particular situation. General principles apply to all agencies. Specific mandatory program requirements are ones that many agencies choose to meet. Voluntary standards are strategies that are chosen by a smaller number of agencies.

Internal Influences on Quality Assurance Activities

A crucial factor in any organization's success is its ability to fulfill its self-identified mission. A home care agency must therefore design all activities in light of its statement of mission. The quality assurance program must clearly coordinate with the agency's philosophy which expands upon the mission statement. Program goals and objectives are yardsticks by which to plan and measure success in implementing the stated organizational purpose.

Quality assurance activities primarily focus on clinical care. Administrative responsibilities which closely relate to assuring the quality of care are risk management (RM) and utilization review (UR) programs. These three activities are currently viewed as related (Tobias 1984; Orlikoff and Lanham 1981,54-55; Jackson and Lynch 1985). A successful integration of these three programs will assure quality care of patients and the maintenance of the agency's mission and existence. However, despite some overlap, they retain distinctive and separate foci. Each agency must address how it will integrate or coordinate activities which cover the common areas of concern and how it will meet the individual requirements of each program. (Exhibit 18-2 pictorially represents the area of common concern. Exhibit 18-3 summarizes the primary purpose of each program and how it overlaps with the other two programs).

The common area shared by the Quality Assurance, Risk Management, and Utilization Review programs is the goal of providing "optimal care that meets professional standards within available resources and consistent with achievable goals." (Spratt 1984,1) Successful achievement of this goal occurs when there is a mechanism to establish a balance among the goals of the three programs. Without such coordination, the goals of any one program initiative may become either dominant or neglected.

Exhibit 18-2. Relationship among quality assurance, risk management, and utilization review programs

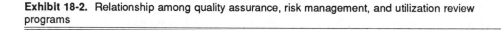

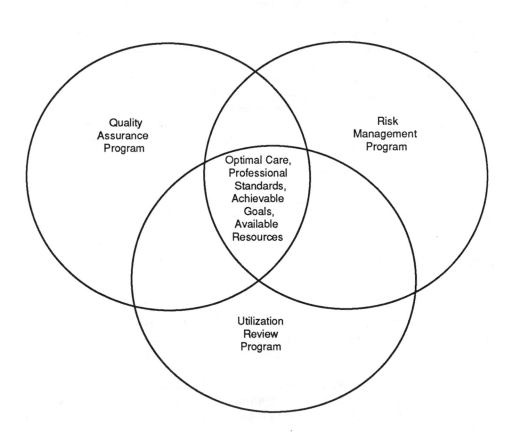

Exhibit 18-3. Primary purpose and overlap of quality assurance, risk management, and utilization review programs.

PROGRAM	PRIMARY PURPOSE	AREA OF OVERLAP
QUALITY ASSURANCE (QA)	Defining, promoting, and monitoring the delivery of quality patient care.	Overlaps with RM and UR in identifying, solving, and preventing instances of less than optimal care.
RISK MANAGEMENT (RM)	Identifying, controlling, and preventing risk of all types.	Overlaps with QA and UR in controlling the potentially compensable event.
UTILIZATION REVIEW (UR)	Defining and controlling costs through cost-efficient utilization of services.	Overlaps with QA and RM in area of controlling the type and amount of service utilization based on established indicators.

Home care agencies now are diversified both in the variety of services they provide and in their corporate structures. An agency must consider its own organizational structure to determine how best to implement a QA program. A large national company with many branch offices has different logistical considerations from an average-sized, community-based agency. If an agency's services range from intermittent skilled care to durable medical equipment to private duty services, it must determine whether it will establish a central, corporatewide QA program or design specific QA strategies appropriate to each distinctive service.

Development of a Quality Assurance Program

A written QA plan is required by many third-party payors and accrediting bodies. An acceptable program includes the following elements:

1. Purpose, goals, and objectives
2. Responsibilities and lines of authority
3. Criteria and standards
4. Evaluation methodologies
5. Data sources
6. Implementation strategies
7. Problem resolution mechanisms
8. Integration with agency operations

9. Evaluation of QA plan

In order to design a plan, it is important to have a working knowledge of a number of concepts which are frequently used in the quality assurance literature. The following definitions serve as a reference for use in answering the questions in this section.

1. *Audit*: A formal examination of clinical records to compare performance against established criteria and standards.

2. *Checklist*: A process evaluation method to determine if there was compliance with a "laundry list" of performance steps for giving good care.

3. *Concurrent audit*: A method to evaluate performance against preset criteria at the time care is being given.

4. *Criteria mapping*: A process evaluation method to assess clinical decision making based on the presence or absence of certain signs, symptoms, patient needs.

5. *Criterion (criteria)*: Variable(s) to be measured.

6. *Discipline specific evaluation*: An assessment of one individual service such as nursing, physical therapy, or medical social services.

7. *Goal*: The desired end toward which activities are directed.

8. *Levels of care and staging*: An outcome-oriented evaluation method to determine severity of medical problem or functional limitations at time of admission as an important factor which influences service utilization and outcome.

9. *Objectives*: Measurable steps toward meeting a goal.

10. *Outcome evaluation*: A method to assess the end result for the recipient of health care services.

11. *Patient satisfaction survey*: A method to determine patients' perception of the relevance and acceptability of care they received.

12. *Peer review*: A process by which health care professionals collegially monitor each other in the provision of quality care.

13. *Plan*: A detailed, orderly procedure for achieving a goal.

14. *Process evaluation*: A method to assess performance of patient care activities.

15. *Program*: A system designed for taking action toward a goal.

16. *Quality Assurance Program (QA)*: A set of activities designed to define, promote, and monitor the delivery of quality patient care.

17. *Reliability*: The degree to which a tool consistently generates the same results when measuring a particular situation.

18. *Retrospective audit*: A method to evaluate performance against pre-set criteria after the patient is discharged.

19. *Risk Management Program (RM)*: A set of activities designed to identify, control, and prevent risk of all types.

20. *Sentinel*: An outcome evaluation method based on an epidemiological approach which monitors all factors which contribute to an identified unnecessary disease, disability, or complication.

21. *Standard*: Specified level of achievement of a criterion.

22. *Structural evaluation*: A method to assess administrative organization, facilities, equipment, range of services, qualifications of health care providers, and patient mix.

23. *Tool or instrument*: A written form used in the evaluation process to identify what data to collect and how to record them.

24. *Tracers*: A process and outcome evaluation method best suited to evaluate care provided to a group of patients by an institution rather than an individual professional. It measures how the parts of the system work together to affect health status.

25. *Utilization Review Program (UR)*: A set of activities designed to define and control costs through cost-efficient use of services.

26. *Validity*: The degree to which a tool actually measures what it is intended to measure.

Each component of the QA plan addresses a set of issues designed to satisfy the demand for accountability. Answering the following questions will be helpful in writing a comprehensive plan which meets external and internal requirements.

I. *Purpose, goals, and objectives*

    A. Is there a clear statement of QA program purpose and goals?

    B. Are there measurable QA program objectives?

    C. Are the external standards that the agency must meet included?

        Consider: State licensure (if applicable)
                       State practice acts for individual professionals
                       Quality assurance programs in comparable agencies

    D. Are the external standards that the agency chooses to meet addressed?

        Consider: Medicare certification
                       NLN accreditation
                       JCAH accreditation

    E. Do they support the agency's philosophy and purpose?

Medicare, NLN, and JCAH do not require specific QA program goals and objectives, but they do specify what must be evaluated. Goals and objectives which reflect the intent of these external standards are helpful in guiding an agency's efforts to satisfy Medicare, NLN, and JCAH requirements.

II. *Responsibilities and lines of authority*

    A. Is the governing body ultimately responsible?

    B. Are representatives of each professional service provided by the agency included in the review process?

    C. Do external bodies require the inclusion of any other discipline?
    (Note: JCAH requires physician involvement. State licensure may also require physician participation. NLN and Medicare regulations permit, but do not require, physician involvement unless an individual agency specifies physician involvement in its policies.)

    D. Is there a clear system to identify responsibilities by collecting data, determining problems and recommendations, communicating findings, acting on recommendations, and following up on remedial actions?

    E. Is there a clear statement regarding who is responsible for carrying out each aspect of QA program? Are these responsibilities reflected in the corresponding job descriptions?

    F. Is there a central committee or individual responsible for coordinating all QA activities and findings?

Medicare, NLN, and JCAH all require a coordinated, logical approach which identifies who is responsible for obtaining information, communicating findings, and acting upon recommendations. Because responsibility is critically and comprehensively examined in the event of litigation, adherence to clearly defined operations which are consistent with prudent professional practice can be effective in reducing liability.

III. *Criteria and standards*

    A. Are they measurable?

    B. Are they valid?

    C. Do they include both process and outcome evaluation methods?

    D. Are they realistic and reasonable?

    E. Are exceptions appropriate?

    F. Is there a process for annual review and revision of the criteria and standards?

    G. Are they relevant to QA program goals and objectives?

    H. Do they measure conformance to the agency's policies and procedures?

There are many tools in the literature for measuring the quality of care. It is often more economical in time and effort to review what is available and choose one that relates to the agency's QA program. If appropriate tools do not exist, adapting existing ones or creating new ones becomes a priority. Tools are used to evaluate identified variables (criteria). The agency should set performance standards which are realisticly based on its own past performance and defensibly based on performance in comparable agencies.

IV. *Evaluation methodologies*

    A. Do methods employed uncover cause and scope of problems?

    B. Are a variety of methods used? (Stanhope 1984, 223-227; Barto 1984,1-5)

        Consider: Concurrent audit
                              Retrospective audit
                              Patient satisfaction survey
                              Tracers
                              Criteria mapping
                              Checklist
                              Structural evaluations
                              Sentinel method
                              Peer review
                              Discipline specific evaluation
                              Literature review
                              Malpractice litigation review
                              Levels of care or staging
                              Process evaluations
                              Outcome evaluations

    C. Are they applicable to all services provided? If not, are the methodologies spelled out for each service?

    D. Are they appropriate to the topics being studied?

    E. Is sampling used? Is it statistically valid?

    F. How is reliability established?

Medicare, JCAH, and NLN require concurrent and retrospective audit. All three specify utilization review and process evaluation. NLN's recent revisions include outcome variables as well. JCAH plans to revise its accreditation standards to address outcome evaluation especially for high risk and high volume patients (McCann 1986).

V. *Data sources*

    A. Are a variety of sources used to identify problems?

        Consider: Clinical records
                              Agency committees' findings and recommendations
                              Incident reports
                              Patient questionnaires and surveys
                              Personnel interviews
                              Studies reported in the literature
                              Letters of complaint or comment
                              Medicare surveyor reports
                              Clinical supervisory conferences

B. Do the sources provide usable data?

Consider: Are the clinical records legible and complete?
Are interview data objective?
Are studies relevant to clinical setting?
Has confidentiality been protected?

C. How are data sources chosen?

Medicare, JCAH, and NLN require clinical record reviews. Medicare requires that ten percent of patients receiving each service are reviewed quarterly. An agency may be doing itself a disservice to limit data collection to the one source required by external bodies. Agency performance and development will be enhanced by systematic assessment of other data sources.

VI. *Implementation strategies*

A. How is quality defined?

B. What tools are used to measure quality?

C. Are the tools appropriate to the stated criteria, standards, and methodology?

D. Who is responsible for choosing the tools?

E. Who is responsible for carrying out the actual assessments?

F. Who receives, approves, and acts on results of assessments?

G. How often are assessments done?
(Note: Medicare requires quarterly clinical record review. Both JCAH and Medicare require review of each patient's treatment plan every 60 days; NLN requires quarterly utilization review and annual peer review and quality audit.)

H. Is there a method to prioritize what will be assessed?

I. Are all relevant disciplines involved?

Medicare regulations focus on structure and process requirements. Both NLN and JCAH are expanding QA to include process-outcome evaluation. The latter strategy combines examination of means and ends; an agency must look at both the path the health care provider traveled and the destination reached by the patient.

VII. *Problem resolution mechanism*

A. What is the process for identifying and prioritizing problems that could have an adverse affect on the quality of care?

B. Is there periodic monitoring to determine the effectiveness of corrective actions?

C. Who is responsible for resolving problems?

D. Are problems and actions aimed at resolution documented in writing? Is documentation objective?

E. Are all appropriate levels of the organization informed of problems and remedial actions?

F. Are all appropriate levels of the organization involved in resolving problems?

JCAH has the clearest statement requiring problem identification and resolution; priorities for assessment and intervention must be those that have the greatest potential for affecting the quality of patient care. NLN requires evidence that assessments yielded at least three recommendations and changes in agency operations during the past year. Although Medicare regulations do not specifically address problem identification and resolution, the Conditions of Participation serve as clear priorities for agency activity; noncompliance with one condition means decertification. Therefore, Medicare-certified agencies must spend considerable time and effort on structure and process evaluation of the agency; this may consume significant energy and resources which fosters a false sense of security that the agency has done enough to assure quality care. Hence, the agency should consider what to do beyond the Medicare requirements to protect its own interest and achieve its goals.

VIII. *Integration with agency operations*

A. Are QA activities integrated with appropriate UR and RM activities?

B. Are educational and training programs provided based on QA findings?

C. Do QA findings and recommendations influence hiring, staffing patterns, and clinical evaluations?

D. Are individuals counseled regarding deviations from expected norms of performance?

E. Are QA performance expectations and assessment results communicated to all staff?

F. Does the community education and marketing program communicate the QA program?

G. Are policies and procedures revised or instituted based on QA findings?

H. Does the orientation program for new employees describe QA program?

NLN standards stipulate specific agency operations that should be addressed based on UR and QA activities. Neither Medicare nor JCAH explicitly specify these interrelationships; however, compliance with each of their standards necessitates such integration of QA activities. Agency management and performance can be enhanced when the QA plan specifies how activities to promote quality care are operationalized throughout the agency.

IX. *Evaluation of QA plan*

A. Is it written?

B. Is it integrated with other agency activities?

C. Is it comprehensive?

D. Is it reviewed and revised annually?
(Note: Medicare, JCAH, and NLN require physician involvement in annual review of agency policies and procedures. State licensure may also require physician involvement.)

E. How effective is the plan in monitoring, evaluating, and problem-solving activities?

F. Does the plan cover all services provided directly and under contract?

G. Does it promote interdisciplinary collaboration?

H. Is it focused on problem identification and resolution which directly affect quality of services?

Clear, written answers to each of the questions in this section will enable an agency to satisfy the QA requirements of Medicare, state licensure, and NLN or JCAH accreditation. Documented compliance with the agency's QA program is necessary to maintain Medicare certification, state licensure, and NLN or JCAH accreditation. (For additional resource information, see Appendix A).

Implementation of a Quality Assurance Program

Quality assurance programs must be tailored to meet the agency's needs and resources. A sophisticated and costly QA program is inappropriate for a small home health agency; a modest widely used method may be inadequate to meet the needs of a large, multiservice agency.

Therefore, start with the agency's present QA plan; evaluate its relevance, practicality, effectiveness, and thoroughness based on the list of questions in the previous section. Then contact other similar agencies to learn what they are doing; this will help in deciding whether or not your program activities are adequate and appropriate. Look at current quality assurance literature, industry trends, and current litigation judgments to project what factors will be affecting QA in general and your agency specifically in the near future. Review your current QA plan to determine its adequacy for meeting these projected changes.

Individual circumstances will also affect how an agency designs its QA program. A new agency will probably choose established criteria and methodology so it can concentrate on meeting at least minimal standards. An established agency may want to prepare for the future by designing innovative strategies which will benefit both its own operations and contribute to the improvement of quality throughout the home care industry. A large multi-unit agency will have to decide what QA program components will be done centrally and what will be done in each unit. Tailoring the QA plan to promote the achievement of agency goals and choosing QA activities which coordinate with organizational operations will yield the greatest benefit.

Summary

The development of an internal quality assurance program is essential to provide quality care and to ensure agency survival in a highly regulated litigious environment. Establishing a written, workable, comprehensive QA plan is a necessary step in demonstrating the level of accountability the public mandates. Each agency must clearly describe and document its own QA activities for regulators and the public. Within the context of current practice, the agency's own needs and goals dictate the design of its quality assurance program.

Quality Assurance Case Study

Marilyn D. Harris

An agency's Quality Assurance Program (QAP) is important for several reasons: to monitor and evaluate the quality and appropriateness of patient care provided by all disciplines; to meet certification, accreditation, professional, and agency standards; to address and resolve identified problems; and to maintain risk management.

A QAP should include all aspects of patient care as well as total agency operations. Characteristics to be evaluated should include the personnel providing the service, the care provided and documented, cost of providing the service, and the patient outcome on discharge from service.

Multiple methods of evaluation should be utilized in a QAP. Examples are: Quarterly Record Review (QRR), Patient Discharge Questionnaires, Physician Questionnaires, Utilization Review (UR), Annual Agency Evaluation.

The QRR is the responsibility of a supervisor at the Visiting Nurse Association of Eastern Montgomery County (VNA). Each month a list of randomly selected names of patients is generated by the computer. This list is the basis for patients' charts to be reviewed each quarter. The charts are assigned to the various disciplines for review, results are tabulated, and a written report given to the staff, the Professional Advisory Committee, and the board of directors each quarter. Exhibit 18-4 is a checklist for nursing and aide services.

A discharge questionnaire (Exhibit 18-5) is sent to a random selection of patients each quarter. These patients are selected from the discharged patients and families who were included in the record review process each quarter. This selection process allows for two viewpoints, those of an independent reviewer and those of the patient and family, on a percentage of charts reviewed each quarter. Discrepancies, if any are noted, are followed up by the supervisor and resolved through discussion with those responding to the questionnaire, reviewer, or VNA staff.

Physician questionnaires (Exhibit 18-6) are distributed to all physicians whose patients require a re-certification of a plan of treatment during one 60-day cycle each year. The supervisor follows up on any comments or suggestions from the physicians. Most often, this consists of providing information on services that are already available through the VNA or its contracting agencies. Each year a substantial number of physicians take time to include comments about the services provided to their patients.

Exhibit 18-4.

VISITING NURSE ASSOCIATION OF EASTERN MONTGOMERY COUNTY

QUALITY ASSURANCE - QUARTERLY RECORD REVIEW

NURSING (HOME HEALTH AIDE)

CLIENT NAME: _____   DATE OF REVIEW: _____

CLIENT CASE NO.: _____   PRESENT QUARTER: _____

PRIMARY NURSE NAME: _____   MONTHS INCLUDED: _____

STATUS OF RECORD: ACTIVE _____

                DISCHARGED _____   SIGNATURE OF REVIEWER

SERVICES INVOLVED:

		YES	NO	N/A	Comments
I	Assessment				
	A. Does the clinical record include assessment of physical, psychosocial, and environmental needs of patient/family?				
	B. Was the nursing assessment form updated upon each new plan of treatment or past each hospitalization?				
	C. Were nursing diagnoses based on assessment factors?				
	D. Did the primary nurse select the correct patient group on admission?				
	E. If the patient's status changed, was the patient group changed accordingly?				
II	Planning				
	A. Were client goals stated?				
	B. Were the nursing parameters specific to the identified nursing diagnoses/problem?				
	C. Was the plan of treatment (orders) current and signed by physician?				
	D. Was the POT completed in accordance with agency policy?				
	E. Were signed verbal orders obtained to cover any change in the plan of treatment?				
III	Implementation				
	A. Was the frequency of nursing visits based on the assessment of the client's needs?				
	B. Was the service provided consistent with the care plan?				

cont'd--

Exhibit 18-4, continued.

VNA OF EASTERN MONTGOMERY COUNTY   QUALITY ASSURANCE - QUARTERLY RECORD REVIEW   NURSING (HOME HEALTH AIDE)

	YES	NO	N/A	COMMENTS
III Implementation, cont'd				
C. Does the record contain evidence that the applicable subobjectives in the patient classification/objectives system were being acted upon?				
D. Did the nurse request consultative services of other disciplines when needed?				
E. Did the nurse regularly supervise the performance of the HHA/LPN?				
F. HHA consistent with client's needs?				
G. Did the nurse demonstrate evidence of his/her coordination of all services?				
H. Did the nurse hold conferences/joint visits with other services when appropriate?				
I. Did the nurse notify the physician/other team members of any significant changes in the client's status?				
J. Were service reports legible, dated, and signed?				
K. Did service reports include: 1. Adequate information regarding the client's current condition?				
2. Specific treatments/instructions given?				
3. The date of the next visit?				
L. Were the following forms present and updated according to agency protocol: 1. Authorization and Release Form?				
2. Medicare Termination letter?				
3. HHA Plan of Care?				
4. Family Information Sheet?				
M. Does the record contain evidence that medications were checked for significant side effects and indications?				
N. In the opinion of the reviewer, were services: Appropriately utilized:				
Over-utilized?				
Under-utilized?				

cont'd--

Exhibit 18-4, continued.

VNA OF EASTERN MONTGOMERY COUNTY   QUALITY ASSURANCE – QUARTERLY RECORD REVIEW   NURSING (HOME HEALTH AIDE

		YES	NO	N/A	COMMENTS
IV	EVALUATION				
A.	Were patient/family responses to nursing intervention documented?				
B.	Were necessary modifications in the care plan made based on the nurse's evaluation?				
C.	If discharged from nursing service:				
1.	Was discharge a logical development of the care plan and client goals?				
2.	Does the record contain a description of the patient/family change in knowledge, understanding &/or behavior as the result of the nurse's intervention?				
3.	Was there evidence of the client's goals having been met?				
4.	Was the discharge summary present and accurately completed?				
5.	Were the nursing diagnoses on the discharge computer summary consistent with those on the problem list?				
6.	Were the service codes (group # and goal attainment) listed on the discharge computer summary consistent with the evidence found in the record?				
7.	Was the physician notified of client's discharge?				

Utilization Review (UR) is closely linked with the QRR process at the VNA. Example: If a reviewer indicates that services are under or overutilized, this chart is reviewed by representatives of the disciplines involved in the provision of care (Exhibits 18-7 and 18-8).

The Annual Agency Evaluation process is the responsibility of the Professional Advisory (PAC) and Agency Evaluation Committees. This process is completed at the end of each fiscal year in keeping with established policy (Exhibit 18-9). A detailed procedure describes the type of reviews to be done, by whom, when and to whom the results are to be reported at various time periods. Some of these activities are done on a monthly basis, others on a quarterly, and still others on an annual basis. Within 90 days of the close of the fiscal year, representatives from board and PAC meet to complete the necessary worksheets. A summary of the evaluation is presented to the PAC and the board of directors for final approval and action. (See Appendix B for additional information and sample review forms.)

Exhibit 18-5.

Visiting Nurse Association Of Eastern Montgomery County
Discharge Patient Questionnaire

1. Who referred you to the Visiting Nurse Association? Doctor _____ Hospital _____
    Friend _____ Patient/Family _____ Other _____

2. What services were provided? Nursing _____ Home Health Aide _____ Physical
    Therapy _____ Speech Therapy _____ Occupational Therapy _____ Medical Social
    Service _____

3. Were there other services you would have liked us to provide? Yes _____ No _____
    If yes, please list: _____

4. Were instructions and/or treatments explained clearly and thoroughly?
    Yes _____ No _____

5. Were your questions answered adequately? Yes _____ No _____

6. Do you feel he/she considered your family's special problems? Yes _____ No _____

7. Were you satisfied with the personnel? Yes _____ No _____
    If no, why not? _____

8. Was the service what you expected it to be? Yes _____ No _____ if no, how did
    it differ from what you expected? _____

9. Did you have the same nurse or therapist each visit? Yes _____ No _____
    If not, did this change in personnel bother you? Yes _____ No _____
    Why? _____

10. When we ended our service to you, did you feel that patient/family needs were met?
    Yes _____ No _____ If not, why not? _____

11. Why was the service discontinued? Condition improved _____ Admitted to the
    Hospital _____ Deceased _____ Other _____

12. Would you use this service again? Yes _____ No _____
    If no, why not? _____

13. Would you recommend this service to others? Yes _____ No _____

14. Were office personnel courteous and helpful to you on the phone? Yes _____ No _____

15. Was there anything you particularly liked or disliked about this service?
    Yes _____ No _____ Please explain: _____

16. What suggestions would you make to improve the services? _____
    _____
    _____

Signature (if desired): _____

Exhibit 18-6.

VISITING NURSE ASSOCIATION
OF EASTERN MONTGOMERY COUNTY

PHYSICIAN'S QUESTIONNAIRE

Your patients have used one or more of the professional services available through the Visiting Nurse Association of Eastern Montgomery County. This agency is pleased to offer these services to you and your patients and it is important for the board of directors and staff to have your comments regarding your experience with the service and personnel. Would you please take the time to complete and return this questionnaire in the enclosed self-addressed envelope. Please comment and make suggestions for improvements you believe would be helpful in making this association more effective in the community.

Thank you for your cooperation in this evaluation process.

Marilyn D. Harris

Marilyn D. Harris, R.N., M.S.N.
Executive Director

Do you feel that you receive sufficient, pertinent information from this agency concerning the patient's status?   Yes_____   No_____

Are you satisfied with the quality of care given by this agency's personnel?
Yes_____   No_____

Is an effort made to individualize the care provided to your patients?
Yes_____   No_____

Is there anything more that should be done for your patients that has been overlooked?   Yes_____   No_____   If so, please comment:

_____

_____

_____

_____

Additional Comments:_____

_____

_____

_____

_____
Signature (Optional)

Exhibit 18-7.

Visiting Nurse Association Of Eastern Montgomery County
Utilization Review

Purpose:
To evaluate the appropriateness of client admissions and discharges, appropriate utilization of levels and types of personnel and over and under-utilization of services.

Objectives:
1. The supervisors will review clinical records due for recertification of physicians' orders every sixty days.

2. The Quality Assurance Committee will review randomly selected clinical records for over and under-utilization of services on a quarterly basis.

Procedure:
1. Clinical supervisors, therapy supervisors, and director of professional services are presented with a computerized listing of patients due for recertification. Following review by the staff, the supervisors review the recertified orders and recertification list and note comments or action on the computerized list.

   The clinical supervisor reviews the case with the staff in an attempt to jointly analyze the ongoing provision of services in keeping with existing regulations.

   The data from the computerized recertification list is tabulated by the medical records department.

2. The Quality Assurance Committee reviews clinical records on a quarterly basis per quarterly record review policy and procedure.

   The Utilization Review Report is completed on cases in which there are questions of either under- or over-utilization. Reports are presented to quality assurance supervisor for further investigation.

3. Based on the above reviews, a summary report is presented to Professional Advisory Committee discussing appropriate utilization of all clinical services.

Exhibit 18-8.

VISITING NURSE ASSOCIATION OF EASTERN MONTGOMERY COUNTY

UTILIZATION REVIEW REPORT

Patient's Name:_____ Record #:_____

Physician's Name:_____ Medicare #:_____

Referral Source:_____ Start of Care:_____

Diagnosis:_____

_____

Skilled Services Ordered: Frequency:

  Skilled Nursing
  Physical Therapy _____   _____
  Occupational Therapy _____   _____
  Speech Therapy _____   _____
  Medical Social Worker _____   _____
  Home Health Aide _____   _____

In the opinion of the reviewer, is there evidence of underutilization:_____

Comment:_____

_____

_____

In the opinion of the reviewer, is there evidence of overutilization:_____

Comment:_____

_____

_____

_____
Signature

Report of Quality Assurance Supervisor:_____

_____

_____

_____   _____
Signature of Supervisor   Signature of Director Professional Services

Exhibit 18-9.

Visiting Nurse Association Of Eastern Montgomery County
Annual Program Evaluation Policy

Definition Of Program Evaluation:

Program evaluation is the systematic collection and analysis of information necessary to assess agency effectiveness, quality, and efficiency relative to accepted performance measures and standards, and to guide agency planning for the provision of health care to those it serves.

Goals Of Agency Evaluation:

A.   To assess and improve the quality of agency programs and services.

B.   To assure the relevance of all agency programs and services to community needs.

C.   To accomplish and maintain overall agency accountability for programs and services.

D.   To document and facilitate the prudent utilization of resources in the operation of agency programs and services.

E.   To achieve and maintain the relevance of agency programs and services to the agency mission.

Uniform Program Evaluation Criteria:

A.   *Scope:*

   1.   The annual program evaluation will include an assessment of all programs and services offered by the agency both directly (i.e., by employed staff) and through contract in a twelve month period comprising the program year.

   2.   The annual program evaluation shall address the following elements of the agency: (I) administration and organization; (II) staffing; (III) programs and services; and (IV) the status of future agency plans bearing on service delivery and/or quality.

   3.   The annual program evaluation will provide for an assessment of the adequacy, appropriateness, effectiveness, efficiency, and competency of health care delivery to agency patients and other service beneficiaries.

B.   *Responsibility:*

   1.   The procedure for the Annual Evaluation specifies which personnel, group or committees participate in the process.

Exhibit 18-9, continued.

2.   The Board of Directors, Professional Advisory Committee, Administration and staff are involved in the evaluation process.

C.   *Required Annual Reviews:*

1.   The annual program evaluation will document and appraise the conformance of agency program operations with policies established by the Board of Directors and approved by the Professional Advisory Committee.

D.   *Format And Organization:*

1.   The annual program evaluation will be presented in a written format indicating those involved, general methods and procedures, specific findings or results, and any comments regarding corrective action or recommendations for further improvement.

2.   The annual program evaluation report will also address the disposition of any specific findings or recommendations presented in previous agency evaluation reports.

E.   *External Feedback:*

1.   The annual program evaluation process will involve a formal method of determining patient satisfaction with the services provided by the agency. Comments should be gathered directly from the patient or their representatives.

2.   The annual program evaluation process will include a means of collecting information on agency program performance from the physicians of patients served by the agency.

3.   The annual program evaluation process will provide for the collection of information from sources such as hospitals, other health care providers, social agencies, and similar entities concerning agency performance in accepting and follow-up with referrals for service when appropriate.

F.   *Integration With Agency Accreditation:*

The documentation requirements for initial and ongoing voluntary accreditation under the National League for Nursing are recognized as fully consistent with above stated criteria. The comprehensive self-study report that is prepared for interim and renewal of accreditation will be utilized for program evaluation purposes for the years covered.

References

Barto, R. 1984. Quality assurance. In *A study guide in quality assurance and utilization review,* ed. R.D. Tobias. American College of Utilization Review Physicians.

Jackson, M.M., and P. Lynch. 1985. Applying an epidemiological structure to risk management and quality assurance activities. *Quality Review Bulletin* 11 (10):306-312.

Personal communication, McCann, B. JCAH, May 27, 1986.

Orlikoff, J.E., and G.B. Lanham. 1981. Why risk management and quality assurance should be integrated. *Hospitals* 55 (11):54-55.

Spratt, C.E. 1984. How one hospital copes with the demands of quality assurance. In *A study guide in quality assurance and utilization review,* ed. R.B. Tobias. American College of Utilization Review Physicians.

Stanhope, M. 1984. Record keeping and quality assurance in community health nursing. In *Community health nursing,* ed. M. Stanhope and J. Lancaster. St. Louis: C.V. Mosby Company.

Tobias, R.B., ed. 1984. *A study guide in quality assurance and utilization review.* American College of Utilization Review Physicians.

Appendix A

Resources For Quality Assurance Plan, Methods, Criteria, Standards, Tools

American Federation of Home Health Agencies, Inc. A national association for home health care providers. Contact the association at: 1320 Fenwich Lane, Suite 500, Silver Spring, MD 20910. (301)588-1454.

Bulaw, J.M. 1986. *Administrative policies and procedures for home health care.* Rockville, MD: Aspen Publishers, Inc. Sections 3000 (Clinical Records) and 6000 (Quality Assurance) provide specific policies, procedures, committee composition and function, task assignments, criteria, and tools for clinical record audit and quality assurance program.

Colorado Association of Home Health Agencies. 1983. *Colorado quality assurance audit criteria.* Englewood, CO: The association. Contains tools for audit of individual case records for 36 different medical diagnoses or problems. Outcome criteria and process parameters for nursing care have been developed for each of the 36 diagnoses or problems. Contact the association at: 7235 S. Newport Way, Englewood, CO 80112. (30)694-4728.

Daubert, E. 1979. Patient classification system and outcome criteria. *Nursing Outlook* 27(7):450-454. Classifies patients into five groups. Each group has an overall outcome objective and subobjectives which can be applied to each of the home health service disciplines.

Florida Home Health Services, Inc. *Patient Care Plans.* A set of care plans for a variety of nursing problems; includes goal of care and outlines the process for nursing care. *Nursing Standards of Care* and *Outcome Criteria* are also available. Contact the agency at: 8181 South Lamiami Trail, Sarasota, FL 33581.

Gould, E.J., and J. Wargo. 1985. *Home health nursing care plans.* Philadelphia: United Medical Services. Includes 49 standardized nursing care plans based on nursing diagnoses. Identifies process and outcome standards for nursing care. Contact publisher at: 5308 Rising Sun Avenue, Philadelphia, PA 19120. (215)329-3550.

Gould, E.J. 1985. Standardized home health nursing care plans: A quality assurance tool. *Quality Review Bulletin* 11 (11):334-338. Describes how one agency developed quality standards for nursing care as part of daily practice.

Gribbon, J. 1985. *American Board of Quality Assurance and Utilization Review: Mini review course.* pp. 5-8. Camp Hill, PA: The Board. Explains JCAH requirements for quality assurance program. Rest of book provides insight into the concerns of a hospital quality assurance program. Contact publisher at: 30 North 36th Street, Camp Hill, PA 17011. (717)737-5660.

Health Care Financing Administration. Conditions of Participation; Home Health Agencies. Regulations No. 5, Subpart L, Sec. 405.1201,1202,1220-1230. Contains the conditions (criteria) and standards an agency must meet to obtain Medicare certification.

Jackson, M.M. and P. Lynch. 1985. Applying an epidemiological structure to risk management and quality assurance activities. *Quality Review Bulletin* (11) 10: 306-

312. Describes use of epidemiological model to determine cause and effect of clinical risk. Application in identifying and resolving problem is provided.

Joint Commission on Accreditation of Hospitals (JCAH). 1986. *Accreditation manual for hospitals, 1986.* pp. 47-55. Chicago: The Commission. Describes standards and characteristics necessary for hospital-based home care agencies seeking JCAH accreditation. Contact publisher at: 875 North Michigan Avenue, Chicago, IL 60611. (312)642-6061.

National Association for Home Care. A national association for home health care providers. Contact the association at: 519 "C" Street, N.E., Stanton Park, Washington, DC 20002 (202)547-7424.

National League for Nursing. 1985. *Accreditation program for home care and community health.* New York: The League. Contains accreditation criteria, standards, and substantiating evidence for obtaining NLN accreditation. Contact publisher at: 10 Columbus Circle, New York, NY 10019-1350. (212)582-1022.

National League for Nursing. 1984. *Administrator's handbook for community health and home care services.* New York: The League. Pub. No. 21-1943. Chapter 5, Evaluation, reviews utilization review and quality audits. Examples of forms from different agencies are provided. Examples cover several individual disciplines as well as entire agency.

Ohmart, M.L. 1982. *Basic home health nursing care plan.* Eureka Springs, AR: Diamond Publishing House, Inc. Includes approximately 100 standardized nursing care plans for a large variety of medical diagnoses and clinical problems. Provides process standards for nursing care. Contact publisher at: 249 Spring Street, Eureka Springs, AR 72632.

Orlikoff, J.E., and G.B. Lanham. 1981. Why risk management and quality assurance should be integrated. *Hospitals* 55 (11):54-55. Compares the goals and functions of risk management and quality assurance. Explains how they overlap and how they are distinct.

Pennsylvania Association of Home Health Agencies. 1985. *Home health service provider standards.* Harrisburg, PA: The Association. Describes criteria and standards for home health agency operation. Optimal and minimal standards and criteria are defined. Contact the association at: 2400 Park Drive, Harrisburg, PA 17110. (717)657-7605.

Rakich, J.S., B.B. Longest, and K. Darr. 1985. *Managing health services organizations.* Philadelphia: Saunders. 308-319. Defines risk management and quality assurance compares the advantages and disadvantages of process and outcome measures of quality.

Shaffer, K., J. Lindenstein, and T. Jennings. 1981. Successful QA program incorporates new JCAH standard. *Hospitals.* 55(16):117-120. Describes integration of quality assurance program efforts to meet new JCAH standard.

Stanhope, M. and J. Lancaster. 1984. *Community health nursing.* St. Louis: C.V. Mosby Company. Chapter 10, "Record Keeping and Quality Assurance in Community Health Nursing," gives an overview of all aspects of quality assurance. Specific tools used to measure nursing quality are listed. Chapter 34, "Home Health Care Nursing," discusses all types of home care services with emphasis on the requirements for Medicare-certified home health agencies.

Tobias, R.B., ed. 1984. *A study guide in quality assurance and utilization review*. Camp Hill, PA: American College of Utilization Review Physicians. The guide has three main sections: Utilization review, quality assurance, and risk management. There are 21 brief articles by different authors. It describes the principles for successfully meeting JCAH hospital standards for quality assurance. Relevant to home care agencies as part of literature review on current practice in QA. Contact publisher at: 30 North 36th Street, Camp Hill, PA 17011. (717)737-5660.

U.S. Department of Health, Education and Welfare. 1970. *Home health agency case record review*. Washington, DC: Government Printing Office. Memorandum No. 10, Vol. II, March 1970. A tool often used in home health agencies to do record audit. Includes form and directions. It is reprinted in Bulaw, J.M. Administrative policies and procedures for home health care.

Appendix B[*]

United Home Health Services
Utilization Review And Quality Assurance Programs

Utilization Review and Quality Assurance are separate but related programs designed to assure that an agency provides effective and efficient care. Activities designed to achieve the goals of the Utilization Review and Quality Assurance Programs are carried out prospectively, concurrently, and retrospectively. These activities are integrated to establish a balance between programmatic goals, thus avoiding care which is excessively costly or of poor quality.

Quality Assurance Program Goals

1. To provide effective, quality care that meets patients' needs.

2. To provide services necessary to enable patients to meet realistic treatment goals.

Utilization Review Program Goal

1. To provide care in such a manner that treatment goals are achieved through efficient utilization of services.

UTILIZATION REVIEW AND
QUALITY ASSURANCE ACTIVITIES

I. *Case Review Conference*
Supervisory Nurse(s) conduct weekly Case Review Conference with each primary nurse and other team members to review the status and design of patient care. The plan of care for each patient is reviewed concurrently and prospectively to ensure that the following objectives are met.

A. *Quality Assurance Program Objectives*

1.   Purpose of visits for following week are planned.

2.   Care by all team members is coordinated.

3.   Progress is being made toward meeting goal(s) of treatment.

4.   Patient's problems and/or progress is reported to physician in timely manner.

5.   Clinical management problems are promptly identified and problem-solving strategies are designed.

---

[*] This section has been reprinted by permission of United Home Health Service

6. Need for consultation and/or referral to other services is identified and implemented.

7. Adequate plans for patient welfare after discharge from agency are made.

8. Care provided is within legal scope of practice and agency policies.

9. Care provided is provided is properly documented.

B. *Utilization Review Program Objectives*

1. Patient requires on-going intermittent skilled care for medically necessary treatment of illness or injury.

2. Frequency of visits for following week is planned.

3. Problems requiring review and/or intervention by Utilization Review Physician are referred promptly.

4. Utilization of services is appropriate to meet patient needs.

5. Avoid unrequired overlapping of services by different members of the team.

6. Plan for timely discharge is developed and implemented.

II. *Clinical Record Design*
The charting system utilizes an original and extensive set of standardized nursing care plans with specific nursing diagnosis, outcome goal, nursing orders, and teaching objectives for the most frequent nursing care problems encountered in this agency. The record is a tool which both facilitates and monitors progress toward meeting the objectives and goals of the Utilization Review and Quality Assurance Programs. This tool is used in all phases of the programs: prospectively, concurrently, and retrospectively.

A. *Quality Assurance Program Benefits.*

1. Represents standards of care for each nursing diagnosis.

2. Defines meaning of "quality care."

3. Provides consistent approach to patient care.

4. Encourages recognition of all nursing problems.

5. Fosters more complete documentation by saving writing time.

6. Documents results of care provided.

7. Identifies specific steps (behavioral objectives) to reach stated goal.

8. Reminds RN what needs to be taught.

9. Allows for teaching only what patient needs to know.

10. Allows for individualization.

B. *Utilization Review Program Benefits*

  1. Indicates when timely discharge is approaching as objectives are met.

  2. Graph-like portrayal of progress/changes/benefits is quickly comprehended.

  3. Avoids useless repetition of teaching.

  4. Pictorial presentation enables identification of variance from expected rate of progress so that plan and/or goal be promptly revised.

III. *Nursing Supervisor Review of Records*
  The nursing supervisor routinely reviews all clinical records at specified intervals. Prospective and retrospective reviews during the actual provision of care enable the agency to monitor compliance with the goals and objectives of both the Utilization Review and Quality Assurance Programs. Records are reviewed at the following intervals.

  A. All admission charts are submitted within two working days for review of planned care and frequency of visits.

  B. All verbal orders are reviewed prior to submission to physician for signature for accuracy, appropriateness and completeness.

  C. All verbal orders signed and returned by physicians are reviewed for additions, deletions, corrections.

  D. All therapists' notes are reviewed weekly for appropriateness of services and utilization.

  E. Every 60 days the record is reviewed for the quality and quantity of services already provided, goals achieved, and the appropriateness of plans for continued care. Any problems are referred to the Director of Patient Services and the Utilization Review/Medical Director.

  F. All discharge charts are reviewed for quality and quantity of services provided. The reason for the timing of discharge is reviewed.

  All deviations from established norms discovered during the above reviews are promptly addressed with appropriate staff to rectify present problem and prevent future recurrence.

IV. *Director of Patient Services Review of Claims and Bills*
  The Director of Patient Services monthly reviews all third-party claims and patient bills for services provided during the previous month. This retrospective utilization review analyzes the pattern of service provision, the frequency of visits, and the type of services provided in relation to the primary and secondary medical diagnosis. All deviations from established norms are pursued to determine if there is an acceptable reason for the deviation. If not, strategies to identify and resolve the problem(s) are initiated.

V. *Clinical Record Review*

The Clinical Record Review is an audit of a random sample of both active and closed clinical records to monitor compliance with goals and objectives of Utilization Review and Quality Assurance Programs and established agency policies. The health professionals conducting this review represent the scope of services of the agency and may be the Advisory Board Members. Initially, the first 100 charts for each service will be audited. Thereafter, at least quarterly a minimum of 10%, but no less than 10 records, will be reviewed.

One percent of the records will be audited twice by nurses, utilizing the Home Health Agency Case Record Review Form. By random selection, a second nurse will audit this one percent without having seen the other nurse's audit. This will provide inter-rater reliability, thorough evaluation, objectivity, plus insulate against bias.

To provide a comprehensive review of charts, it is imperative that other therapists audit records. The therapy evaluation will be achieved in three ways:

1. Each therapist uses a record audit form for therapy services to assist in evaluating charts for appropriateness and thoroughness of patient care provided in therapist's area of expertise.

2. Each therapist evaluates a minimum of 10% of the charts of patients who were *not* referred to their area for therapy. This is done to determine whether the patient should have been referred to their specific service because the patient had an unmet need or could have benefitted from their care.

3. All charts selected for audit will be reviewed by a registered pharmacist for appropriateness of medication regime, possible drug-drug or drug-food interactions, adverse reactions, and unresolved problems amenable to drug treatment.

All audit results are reviewed and discussed by the Professional Activities Committee on a quarterly basis. Recommendations from this committee are directed to the Administrator, Director of Patient Services, Advisory Board, and staff for implementation. Follow-up activities and results are reported back to the Professional Activities Committee at the next meeting.

The Utilization Review Physician/Medical Director quarterly reviews records to determine the appropriateness and adequacy of continuing care.

There is a continuing review of each clinical record for each 60-day period that a patient receives home care services. The summary report and plan of treatment are sent to the patient's physician every 60 days for review and revisions to ensure the adequacy and appropriateness of continuing care.

Yearly, the Advisory Board reviews the methods and tools used for clinical record evaluation to determine whether the tools and methods are appropriate, effective, adequate and efficient.

Audit Procedure

1. The Administrative Assistant randomly selects at least ten per cent of all admissions but no less than ten records, during each quarter for audit being sure that the selected sample is increased to represent ten per cent of patient's receiving each service. One per cent of the records will be audited twice by nurses.

2. The Administrative Assistant notifies, in writing, each nurse and therapist which charts have been selected for audit. The goals of the audit and plan for feedback are included in this memo.

3. The Administrative Assistant arranges for audit of each chart to be completed by a nurse, a physical therapist, an occupational therapist, a speech therapist, a social worker and a pharmacist.

4. The Professional Activities Committee reviews each audit report and makes recommendations. All proceedings are confidential.

5. The Director of Patient Services forwards copies of the minutes of each Professional Activities Committee meeting to the Nursing Supervisor; Directors of Social Service, Physical Therapy, Occupational Therapy, Speech Therapy; the Administrator and the Chairman of the Advisory Board.

6. The Supervisor and Directors disseminate this information to their staffs.

7. The Advisory Board reviews, revises and approves recommendations from the Professional Activities Committee.

8. The Director of Patient Services discusses individual problems with the appropriate Supervisor and/or Director for follow-up with staff. A copy of the audit report is reviewed with individual staff members as indicated.

9. Supervisor and/or Directors report back to Director of Patient Services regarding follow-up done and results accomplished individually or with a group.

10. Follow-up with individual staff members is documented in their personnel file.

Date _____

MEMORANDUM

To: _____

From: E. Joyce Gould, RN, MSN
       Assistant Administrator for Clinical Services

Re: Quality Assurance Program

The Quality Assurance Program of United Home Health Services is composed of a number of activities to ensure that the following goals are met:

1. Effective, quality care that meets patient needs is provided.

2. Services necessary to enable patients to meet realistic treatment goals is provided.

The Case Conference, clinical record design, Nursing Supervisor review of records, and Director's review of bills are activities which are designed to foster the delivery of quality care. An activity mandated by Medicare is a quarterly audit of a sample of open and closed clinical records. This is a form of peer review conducted by health professionals which present the scope of services provided by the agency. The Professional Activities Committee is the group responsible for reviewing the audit and making recommendations.

To enable you to utilize the information from the audit for your own enlightenment and professional growth, the minutes of the Professional Activities Committee will be circulated to you.

For the quarter under review (   ), the following charts of patient's you have cared for will be audited.

Date _____

MEMORANDUM

To: _____

From: E. Joyce Gould, Assistant Administrator for Clinical Services
Re: Audit

Attached please find a copy of the audit report from the Professional Activities Committee. Please circulate information to therapists.

The following specific areas need to be addressed with individual staff members:

_____

_____

_____

_____

_____

Attached are copies of the audit reports to be addressed in this discussion. As part of
the peer review process, the focus of this feedback is to disseminate information
necessary for professional enlightenment and growth.

Please advise me, in writing, of the outcome of your discussions and follow-up. Please
feel free to contact me by phone if I can be of any assistance.

Record Audit of Therapy Services

Patient Record Number _____ Age ___ Sex ____
Agency Admission Date _____ Discharge Date _____
Start of therapist's care _____ Discontinued _____
Therapy provided _____

Code: (NA = Not Applicable; YS = Yes Satisfactorily; YI = Yes/Insufficient;
        NO = None)

Record Review Indicates: NA YS YI NO   COMMENTS

1. Diagnosis(es) or limiting con-
    ditions needing therapy or
    rehabilitation program?

2. Physician's orders for
    therapy?

3. Therapy services in plan of
    care?

4. Therapist gave direct therapy
    modalities?

5. Therapist instructed
    rehabilitation program to:
    a. Patient?
    b. Family?
    c. Household employees?
    d. Nurse(s)?
    e. Home health aide(s)?
    f. Others?

6. Therapist reassessed
    patient's needs on a con-
    tinuum?

7. Therapist arranged for
    devices, equipment, etc.?

8. Therapist reported problems
    (patient or home health aide)
    to nurse?

9. Therapist discussed
    therapy/rehabilitation
    plan of care with physician?

Record Review Indicates:	NA	YS	YI	NO	COMMENTS

10. Recording was appropriate?

11. Phone call to patient within 1
    day after receiving referral?

12. Visit within 3 days?

_____

1. Were therapy services rendered in accord with agency policy? _____

   If not, why? _____

2. Were therapy services appropriate for this case? _____

   If not, why? _____

3. What other services or resources would have benefited patient? _____
   _____

REMARKS: _____

_____

_____

Prepared by _____ of _____ on _____

PATIENT CARE REVIEW FORM SPEECH PATHOLOGY

DATE: _____   PATIENT'S ADMISSION # _____

Upon receipt of referral: YES   NO   COMMENTS

1. was family contacted within
    24 hrs. of receipt of referral

2. was initial visit made within 3
    working days

3. was physician/referral source
    contacted if indicated

4. are initial evaluation and
    treatment goals documented

5. are therapy and treatment
    goals discussed with family

Ongoing therapeutic services:

1. are therapeutic procedures
    relevant to pt's diagnoses

2. are frequency of visits ap-
    propriate

3. are pt's progress and therapy
    goals reviewed and approved
    by physician every 60 days

4. is there ongoing evaluation of
    pt's communication skills

5. is there subsequent modifica-
    tion of goals and procedures

PCRF - SPEECH   PAGE 2

	YES	NO	COMMENTS

6. is each visit documented in
    the progress notes

7. are pt/family educated re:
    promoting functional com-
    munication

8. is there evidence of pt/family
    compliance

9. is there follow through on
    referrals made to other dis-
    ciplines

10. is communication between
    therapist and other health
    care workers documented

Discharge Summaries:

1. was adequate time given to
    pt/fam re: termination of ser-
    vices

2. were reasons for discharge
    discussed with pt/family

3. does discharge summary in-
    clude:

    a. initial status
    b. focus of therapy
    c. discharge status
    d. pt/fam response to d/c
    e. factors influencing d/c

PCRF - SPEECH   PAGE 3

SUMMARY:

_____

RECOMMENDATIONS:

_____

DATE: SIGNATURE:

_____

ACTION TAKEN:

DEPARTMENT OF SOCIAL WORK   PEER REVIEW FORM

Reviewed by: _____

Medical Record # _____   Date case reviewed: _____

YES   NO   N/A

1. *Referral*

    a) reason indicated
    b) reason appropriate
    c) source indicated

2. *Medical Information*

    a) diagnosis stated
    b) medical treatment specified
    c) significant past medical history noted

3. *Social Information*

    a) family constellation noted
    b) living situation specified
    c) education specified
    d) occupation specified
    e) income source specified

4. Are specific *psychosocial* histories or growth and development studies present?

5. *Psychosocial Assessment*

    a) does assessment include an understanding of pt's/family's conception of situa-
       tion
    b) pt's prior level of functioning described
    c) does assessment include an understanding of pt's/family's emotional reactions
    d. are support systems specified
    e. are the problems clearly identified

6. *Plans, Goals and Interventions*

    a) are worker's plans specified
    b) are they appropriate
    c) are the interventions specified
    d) are the interventions related to goals
    e) is mutual agreement addressed

                                                          YES   NO   N/A

7. *Summary*

    a) is outcome stated
    b) are follow up plans specified
    c) are follow plans appropriate
    d) if indicated, was follow up carried out

8. *Miscellaneous*

    a) phone call to patient acknowledging referral within three working days
    b) is there an initial evaluation within three working days or indication why not
    c) progress notes periodic and appropriate
    d) discharge note
    e) is record legible

9. *Comments and Recommendations*

Revised 4/12/85

MEDICAL DIRECTOR'S DOCUMENTATION
FORM OF CHART REVIEW FOR PATIENTS

Patient Chart Number:_____

Date Chart Reviewed:_____

Reviewer Name and Title: _____
(please print)

Reviewer's Conclusions and Recommendations:

1. _____ therapy not needed.

2. _____ therapy should have been ordered.

3. _____ information inadequate in chart to decide.

4. _____ other, specify: _____

5. _____ continued care needed.

If other than number one above is checked, please give reason:

Reviewer's Signature: _____

Therapists' Chart Review Information Sheet

In order to determine that therapy services are provided for all patients who need them, a random review of charts by the various specialty areas is to be done. A minimum of ten percent of the charts of patients who were *not* referred to your area for therapy are to be read. After reading the chart, determine whether the patient should have been referred to your specific service or not.

Fill out the form documenting your review of the chart. Under "Reviewer's Recommendations" check the appropriate box and comment as stipulated on the forms.

Return charts and forms to the Nursing Supervisor.

Adopted 10/3/84

Therapist's Documentation Form of
Chart Review for Patients

Not Receiving Their Services.

Patient Chart Number: _____

Date Chart Reviewed: _____

Reviewer Name and Title: _____
(please print)

Reviewer's Conclusions and recommendations:

1.   _____ therapy not needed.

2.   _____ therapy should have been ordered.

3.   _____ information inadequate in chart to decide.

4.   _____ other specify.

If other than number one above is checked, please give reason:

Reviewer's Signature: _____

Chapter Nineteen

Program and Service Evaluation

Nancy DiPasquale Ruane and E. Joyce Gould

Program evaluation measures effectiveness, a major concern of home health agencies. It is used to project future changes and anticipated agency responses. External and internal constraints and supports influence program evaluation. Information gathering and analysis provide a basis for rational decision making.

Definitions and Characteristics

Program. A program is a structured set of activities, organized to accomplish a goal. It pursues a comprehensive goal with multifaceted objectives utilizing various levels of human potential and resources. A program activates a prearranged plan of operation which acts as an outline of the work to be done by the organization. The viability and progress of a program relies on the effectiveness of its evaluation.

Evaluation. Evaluation is the process of assessing qualities or characteristics of an individual, a program, or an agency as the basis for making a judgment. The emphasis in evaluation is on collecting data designed to delineate the relevant, identifying features of factors under study. It involves a systematic process of determining the extent to which the objectives are achieved. Evaluation starts with quantitative measurement and goes beyond it to include qualitative description and judgment.

The effectiveness of evaluation can be promoted by attention to the following points:

1. Evaluation is a process of analysis.

2. Evaluation is a means to an end and not an end in itself.

3. Evaluation is a method of gathering and processing evidence which may indicate a need for improvement.

4. Evaluation clarifies goals and expected outcomes.

5. Evaluation is a process of determining the extent to which goals and objectives are met.

6. Evaluation is a system of quality control which determines the effectiveness of the program.

7. Evaluation must be utilization-focused to identify what changes must be made to ensure the effectiveness of the program (National League for Nursing 1974, 2-3).

8. Evaluation must be credible.

An evaluation has a sponsor. This is the person or organization, who requests the evaluation and is responsible for its completion. In a home health agency, the sponsor may be the governing body, fulfilling the mandate of certification and accreditation bodies, as well as its desire to provide quality services. There is always an audience for an evaluation. Of course the findings and recommendations are reported to the sponsor, but there are other recipients of the information. The audience varies and may include the program managers and staff, the recipients of the program services, prospective consumers, special interest groups, professional peer groups, and the community served by the agency (Morris and Fitz-Gibbons 1978a, 6).

Evaluation may be formative or summative. Formative evaluation assesses how well the program is going. It is used throughout the duration of a program for the primary purpose of improving the program operation.

Formative evaluation helps to determine if the program is moving toward its goals and objectives. It differs from summative evaluation in timing and audience, which is usually the program management and staff. The emphasis is on improvement as the program continues.

Summative evaluation focuses on assessing the achievement of the goals and objectives of the program. It is done annually, at other specified intervals or at the conclusion of the program period. Summative evaluation determines if the goals and objectives of the program have been attained, and it gives feedback for future planning. It looks at the total impact of the program (Breckon 1982, 166-167).

Program Evaluation. Program evaluation is a set of methods, skills, and individualized interpretation, used to determine the necessity, compliance. and relevance of an agency's goals and activities. It provides a basis for rational decision making for the future. Program evaluation without sensitive adaptation results in sterile critiques and recommendations without vision.

Program evaluation involves the conducting of research within an agency to acquire information that can be fed back to enhance the agency's functioning. It is applied research involving problem solving and strategic action (Rothman 1980, 17). Evaluation research differs from basic research; the latter produces or verifies theories and knowledge and is not aimed at prescribing a solution to a problem. Program evaluation entails such inquiries as: needs assessment, agency mission, statement and beliefs, descriptive information about quality of services delivered to clients, the population served, the tracking of clients, analysis of professional activities, client outcomes, and cost analysis.

Issues

Relationship to Planning. Program evaluation is part of the cycle of program development. The cycle begins with the planning phase, moves through the implementation phase, and is followed by the review or evaluation phase. This last phase of program development is linked directly into the planning phase at which point the cycle is reviewed. (Exhibit 19-1 illustrates this cycle.)

Exhibit 19-1. The cycle of program development

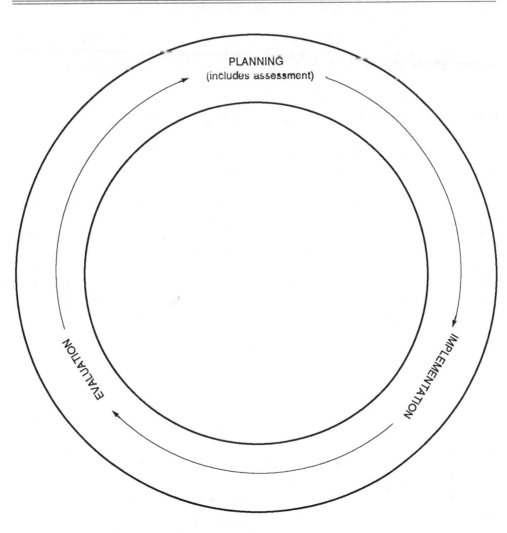

PLANNING
(includes assessment)

EVALUATION

IMPLEMENTATION

The cycle starts with the planning phase, moves to the implementation phase, and then to the evaluation phase, which moves directly into the planning phase. The cycle starts again.

Program evaluation is reactive evaluation for proactive planning. It is like a "mirror image of planning in that it is the process of looking back upon action, making judgment about it in order to provide the necessary information for planning for the future." (Blum 1979, 542) Program evaluation acts like a comet in the heavens. A comet, with energy from its source, has momentum and gains speed as it is propelled through space to fulfill its purpose in the universe. Program evaluation gathers and analyzes data from the program's activities and propels the findings into the future to plan for progressive development. (This concept is depicted in Exhibit 19-2 which also illustrates the Context and Purpose of Program Evaluation.)

Accountability. Program evaluations are conducted to describe and assess the effects of program activity. This information is essential because the agency, through its governing body, is accountable to the community which it serves. The accountability

Exhibit 19-2. Context and purpose of program evaluation

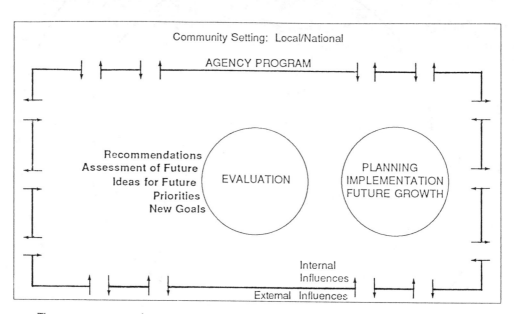

The agency program is an open system which has internal and external influences. The internal influences are contained within the boundary of the agency and impact the program evaluation process.

The agency program output crosses over the boundary into the community—usually local but sometimes national. The external influences lie beyond the agency boundary and impact the agency program and its evaluation by crossing over the boundary.

Internal Influences	External Influences
Agency philosophy and goals	Patient population
Management	Demographics
Staff	Health status and needs
Policies	Economic status
Procedures	Demand for service
M.I.S.	Market competition
	Legislation
	Industry trends
	Third party payors
	Home health associations

includes the quality and extent of the services provided and the funds used to finance the services. In proprietary agencies, the stockholders constitute another group that expect accountability. An effective program evaluation can establish accountability.

Relationship to Quality Assurance. Home health care is very familiar with accountability. It is the common denominator for quality assurance and program evaluation. Both processes are evaluative in nature and are essential to the existence, growth, and development of an agency.

Program evaluation focuses on examining the achievement of the outcome of a set of objectives, activities, and services. This examination leads to recommendations which feed directly into the planning process.

Quality assurance is a proactive set of policies and activities utilized to evaluate the patient care delivery scope and quality. The recommendations from this evaluation usually result in stronger enforcement of procedure or change of procedure.

Influences on Program Evaluation

External Influences

Although program evaluation is designed to assess the appropriateness, adequacy, effectiveness, and efficiency of an agency, it is impacted by forces over which it has little or no control. These forces may be characteristics of the climate of the industry, the population served by the agency, rules and regulations imposed by legislation, and third-party payors.

Industry. The climate of the industry is influenced by numerous factors. Home health care agencies have proliferated overwhelmingly in the last decade, especially in those states that do not require a certificate of need. This has placed agencies in adversarial positions with each other. However, this climate provides support for performing program evaluation and is a strong influence in urging agencies to go through this process. In addition to the increasing number of agencies, future trends of the industry and the economic forecast must be researched and understood since their effect is unavoidable.

This force in the industry has prompted some agencies to go beyond the minimum criteria imposed by Medicare. Many agencies utilize the accreditation services of the National League for Nursing (NLN) or the Joint Commission for Accreditation of Hospitals (JCAH). For hospital-based home health agencies, accreditation by JCAH is not optional but required since the home health agency is part of the hospital organization. Medicare criteria for program evaluation require the assessment of organizational structure and process. The NLN and JCAH, through recent and proposed revisions, have expanded the evaluative emphasis to include standards which concern quality health care outcome statements. This shift requires the agencies seeking accreditation by these bodies to reflect these standards in their programs.

In addition to the above accrediting organizations, the industry has associations which also develop codes of ethics and standards for their membership. Membership in these organizations is voluntary and the codes and standards are developed by the members. Nevertheless, the codes and standards do influence the programs of the member agencies by establishing guidelines for quality programs. Indirectly these guidelines influence the nonmember agencies since they establish informal criteria that are accepted by the industry.

Population Served. The population served by the agency influences the services offered. The demographics, health status, health needs, and socioeconomic levels of the people served by the agency all impact on the type and amount of services that will be utilized by the community. Careful monitoring of population shifts, health statistics, and the economy of the region is absolutely necessary and, therefore, is an item to be considered in program evaluation.

Rules and Regulations. The mandates, imposed by rules and regulations of legislation and third-party payors are the strongest influences on program evaluation. Many states require licensure before an agency can provide any home health services (Warhola 1980, 40). In some states only certified home health programs are required to be licensed. The licensing agency is usually the state government. The licensing criteria require the agency to have program evaluation policies and procedures. The state health department evaluates these programs at specified intervals. Usually the agency must complete a self-study report and experience an on-site visit. The criteria used for this internal report mandate that at least organizational structure and process evaluation be completed. This process is, in itself, a program evaluation.

The third-party payors view program evaluation as a vital indicator of the agency's functioning. Program evaluation is required by Medicare and Medicaid. Blue Cross and most commercial insurers use the Medicare certification criteria as a standard for measuring the acceptability of an agency for reimbursement eligibility. Therefore, in order for an agency to be eligible for reimbursement and survive as a provider, program evaluation must be included in the agency's policies. (The external influences are illustrated in Exhibit 19-2.)

Internal Influences

Influences that the agency develops or can usually control still have an impact on program evaluation. This group includes the agency's philosophy and goals, the quality of its staff, the expertise of the management, and the system of managing all patient information within the agency.

Philosophy and Goals. In the development of an agency, the philosophy and goals, or mission statement, is created initially to give substance to the project. From this statement the agency's founders draw the ideas and direction for the programs. The objectives and policies for the implementation of the programs emanate from the ideas. Directed by the objectives and policies, the program managers guide the staff's activity to provide services. The program objectives, along with the mission statement, give direction to the evaluation, since they are included in the criteria used to measure program effectiveness.

Staff. The quality of the staff members impacts upon program evaluation because they are actors in the performance of the program activity. Inadequately prepared, undereducated staff can lead to ineffectiveness of programs and become a threat to the program's quality. Control of the quality of the staff begins with the job advertisement, continues through the selection process, and is maintained through employer evaluation and staff development.

Management. The expertise of management influences program planning and implementation as well as program evaluation. The quality of management is essential not only to maintain the program's effectiveness, but also to assure that the programs are properly planned. Ineffective managers lead to ineffective leadership and ineffective functioning of staff. The program goals will not be achieved as the evaluation will reveal.

Management Information System. The patient information system is vital to program evaluation. It represents a significant portion of the information that is gathered for analysis in the evaluation process. Therefore, the lack of accuracy and other characteristics of the system influence program evaluation. Tracking of the information can be done by computer or by hand. In either case, the information must become part of the system and monitored at certain checkpoints for accuracy, so that quality and comprehensiveness of care can be demonstrated. (Exhibit 19.2 illustrates the agency program stages surrounded by the internal influences.)

Development of a Program Evaluation System

Since the beginning of the home health care movement, evaluation was an integral part of the fundamental principles and practices of the industry. Evaluation areas are numerous and can be endless. There are relevant issues which must be considered and heeded in approaching evaluation. Investigative areas are selected according to their influences to patients, home health agency management staff, and to the community served by the agency. The focus of the evaluation is also dictated by those regulatory and accreditation bodies that set standards for the industry.

Relevant Issues. By law, the Medicare regulations require certified home health agencies to evaluate their programs. Section 405.1229 of the Conditions of Participation deals with evaluation. This section states the agency must have written policies requiring an overall evaluation of the agency's total program at least once a year. The evaluation must be completed by the professional advisory group of the agency or a committee of the group, along with the home health agency staff and consumers. The professional advisory group includes at least one registered nurse (preferably a public health nurse) and one physician, as well as appropriate representation from the other professional disciplines who administer the scope of services. Overall policy and administrative and clinical record review are included.

The aim of the evaluation is to assess the extent to which the agency's and patient service delivery are appropriate, adequate, effective, and efficient. Each policy and administrative practice and their effect on patient care are reviewed. A report of the evaluation is presented to the governing body for action. The report is maintained as a part of the administrative record.

The agency must have established written mechanisms for the collection of data to assist the evaluation. The suggested data may include: numbers of patients receiving each service offered, sources of referral, number of patient visits, criteria for admissions, reasons for discharge, total staff days for each service offered, number of patients not accepted with reasons. If other data are available, it may be included for it will broaden and strengthen the statistical picture presented. This section also addresses the clinical record review which is accomplished through Quality Assurance and Utilization Review. (Refer to Chapter 18 for information in this area.) The Medicare Conditions of Participation serve as the basic structure upon which an evaluation program for home health agencies can be built (Stuart-Siddal 1986, 36-44).

The JCAH is a private, nonprofit organization whose purpose is to encourage the attainment of uniformly high standards of institutional health care. The manual notes that one of its roles is that of evaluator. All hospital-based agencies are required to have JCAH accreditation. Other home health agencies may choose to request it.

Section 5 of the JCAH Accreditation Manual for Hospitals deals with Home Care Services. Standard 5:3,2 states that the program's policies and procedures are reviewed annually, revised as necessary, and dated to indicate the time of last review or revision. The evaluators are the individuals who are representative of the home care services provided. At least one physician and one registered nurse are among the evaluators. The specific inclusion of a physician as reviewer is unique to this evaluation (Joint Commission of Accreditation of Hospitals, 1986, VII).

Through the National League for Nursing (NLN), the home health agencies participate in a voluntary accreditation process which aims to evaluate and improve the agency's services. The criteria of the Accreditation Program for Home Care and Community Health is compiled by the Accreditation Standards Committee. To quality, the agency must complete a self-study report and experience an on site visit. Written description is presented in the report and concrete evidence must be available for the site visitors.

Criterion 17 states that the provider must evaluate its programs(s) annually. The evaluation includes the assessment of program, service, and practice policies; the quality of care delivered by each discipline; the population served; the services and visits provided; and the client outcomes. The inclusion of client outcomes in program evaluation differentiates the NLN Criteria from the Medicare Conditions of Participation and other criteria. This criterion also states that the agency make the needed modifications in the program's service and practice policies as soon as possible after the review.

Criterion 23 deals with the overall program evaluation plan. It expects the agency to have an overall evaluation plan to include strategic planning and marketing; organization and administrative review; programs and services; staffing policies and practices. This plan should indicate the frequency of each evaluation and the person or group responsible as well as the purpose of the evaluation. The NLN places the responsibility for implementing the evaluation on the governing body or the professional advisory group. There are no specific regulations about membership on the board, but consumer representation is stressed (National League for Nursing 1985a).

Another mechanism that has a part in controlling the quality of care is licensure. Some states have assumed the responsibility for mandatory regulation. The regulations vary from state to state. The criteria are similar to the criteria for Medicare certification with minor variations in each state. Generally, states establish agencies composed of a majority of professionals to set the guidelines for licensure. This process gives the states a means to revoke a license and therefore prevent an agency from continuing in the provider role if compliance with criteria is not met (Spiegel 1983, 417-480).

Considering the nature of the home health care setting, the program evaluation is a mechanism utilized to assure the delivery of quality care. It is difficult and costly to do comprehensive on-site evaluation of the care as it is being delivered. Other methods of evaluation involving staff and patients are employed to measure certain aspects of the agency's program. The staff participates in evaluating of home visits, conducting surveys of other agencies in the area, opinion polling of patients and referral services, descriptive reviews and comparison evaluations. Usually the patients are involved in evaluation by answering opinion or attitude polls and by commenting on care received at specific times by specific health professionals.

Areas to be Evaluated. Program evaluation has four areas of concern: organization, activities, outcomes, and costs. These areas are also known as structure, process, outcome, and fiscal evaluation. Structure deals with the administrative organization, the facilities and equipment, scope of services, the qualifications and profile of the professional personnel, the characteristics of the patient population and the policies and procedures governing patient care. Process involves the activities that were planned to occur in the program. Outcome refers to the program or patient objectives in relation to their attainment. The fiscal area focuses on costs and cost accountability (Dever 1980, 158-159).

Structure may be considered an input measure of the quality of services based on the number, type, and quality of the resources used in the production of the services. Structure is an indirect measure since it does not consider the activities or actual result. Because of this, structure may be considered an inferior area to evaluate (U.S. House of Representatives 1976, 83). However, structure and its relationship to the process and outcomes has sufficient support. Donabedian (1978) supported the evaluation of structure on the assumption that, when an agency that has good structure, good care will follow. The National League for Nursing (1985b), in its accreditation program, pays particular attention to achieving and maintaining an efficient, effective management structure in the delivery of quality care. Therefore, the evaluation of structure continues to be a relevant area of focus.

Process is an indicator of the quality of care used to assess the activities of the multidisciplinary team and the programs in the management of patients. Process measurement documents the activities that comprise a program and the flow of these activities. The specific activities are directed by the agency mission and the policies and procedures that evolve from it. Generally such measures study the degree of conformity with standards and expectations that are established by the peer groups and leaders of the professions (U.S. House of Representatives 1976, 129).

Outcome measures the quality of care in which the standard of judgment is the attainment of a specified result. The outcome of patient care is measured by the parameters set by the health professionals providing the care. These professionals are guided by the standards of their professions and directed by the agency mission, policies, and procedures (U.S. House of Representatives 1976, 116).

Fiscal evaluation looks at planned and actual expenditures. The planned or budgeted expenditures are compared with the actual expenditures. Another aspect to be examined is whether or not the actual activities occurred as a result of the expenditure of the resources. Actual costs and any possible alternative costs are considered. This evaluation may also involve the study of bookkeeping, billing, and banking policies, procedures, and systems.

The sources of information for program evaluation are: the patients and their families or significant others, the patient's clinical record, the analysis of patient statistics, the administrative and organizational documents, community statistics and financial records and reports.

The patients and their families or significant others can influence the program by choosing to accept or deny services. They also play a significant part in the accomplishment of outcomes by cooperating with the health professional. Assessing the patient's reactions, feelings, and judgments about the program are very important to the evaluation of both process and outcome.

The use of the clinical record as a source of information for program evaluation has been reported in literature since the 1960s (Helbig, O'Hare, and Smith 1972). The clinical record reveals information about process and outcome. Along with the analysis of patient statistics, which reveals at the minimum, reasons for admission and discharge, amount and types of services, number of visits, and patients' diagnoses, the evaluator can report a very significant amount of information to the governing body.

The documents related to the administration and organization of the agency give the evaluator information from the agency's philosophy and objectives to the most specific patient care policy. Their information forms the frameworks upon which the program is built and can reveal much about the program's quality.

The statistics, which describe the community served by the agency, are important to the evaluator in developing recommendations. Without knowledge of the community needs, it is difficult to recommend changes and prospective plans for the future.

Financial records and reports assist the evaluator in realizing the cost effectiveness of the program. Cost accountability is as much a reality as professional accountability. Sufficient information about fiscal evaluation is included in every program evaluation so that the governing body can make the correct decision about future programs.

Evaluation Models

To ensure a well-organized evaluation study, an evaluation model is used. Models reinforce conclusions drawn by the evaluator. Without a model, the information presented after an evaluation may be misinterpreted. Typically, the program evaluations performed by home health agencies are summative evaluations. This type of evaluation is associated with the use of a model (Morris and Fitz-Gibbon 1978, 9-11). The summative evaluation, described earlier in this chapter, is the focus of the following discussion and illustration.

Systems Model. The Systems Model of evaluation focuses on the process as a working model or social unit capable of achieving a goal. This model is concerned with attaining objectives, coordinating the functioning of its subunits, maintaining resources, and adapting to the environment. The systems model examines other aspects in addition to the goal. Recognizing that organizations have multiple goals, this model considers single goal attainment in relation to its effect on other goals in the system.

The variables that are described and evaluated are the input, the throughput, and the output. The input refers to characteristics and conditions of the people and of the resources. Throughput refers to human and nonhuman resources and process. Output refers to the product of the system (Stanhope and Lancaster 1984, 215; Schulbert, Sheddon, and Baker 1969; LaParta 1975; Baker and Northman 1979). The systems model is very comprehensive since it considers more elements and describes their interaction with each other.

Structure-Process-Outcome Model. The Structure-Process-Outcome Model by Donabedian was primarily designed for medical care. Since it is applicable to the broader area of health care, today it is a popular method. The definitions of structure, process, and outcome were presented earlier in this chapter. The rationale to structure evaluation is based on the concept that good care is dependent upon good administration, organization, facilities, and providers. Through review of the patient records and direct observation of care, Donabedian believed that an evaluative judgment can be made. The activities performed by the provider of care can be labeled good and competent when viewed in the context of a certain patient. While outcome usually refers to the attainment of a goal for patient recovery, it is also used to convey changes in health status, health-related knowledge, attitude, and behavior (Stanhope and Lancaster 1984, 214).

Goal Attainment Model. The Goal Attainment Model refers to a method for assessing the effectiveness of a program by measurement of the predetermined goals. The components of the goal attainment model are developing objectives, deciding how to measure the objectives, collecting information, assessing the effects, analyzing and interpreting data. Shields (1974) developed an example of the goal attainment model. For each goal, the evaluator examines the categories of wherewithal, structure, operations, and outcomes.

Wherewithal refers to resources, materials, equipment, and physical facilities. Structure includes the organizational framework or the administrative structure, lines of authority, committee linkages, and patterns of communication. Operations pertain to processes and procedures for carrying out program goals. Outcome refers to the attainment and to the level of attainment of the goal (Shields 1974). The criteria applied to the outcomes are: (1) effectiveness or the attainment of purpose, (2) efficiency or cost effectiveness, (3) control or whether unexpected events were associated with the program. The evaluation process was applied to each goal in the program (Stanhope and Lancaster 1984, 215).

Planned versus Actual Performance Model. The Comparison of Planned versus Actual Performance Model compares preprogram-targeted objectives to the actual program performance. Realistic goals are established for the evaluation criteria. The establishment of realistic goals is an important issue. The model assumes that the goals that are established are the best available indicators of the actual accomplishments. It can be used widely and regularly once a plan for the program evaluation is developed (Dever 1980, 68-69).

To summarize, the Structure-Process-Outcome Model, the Goal Attainment Model, and the Comparison of Planned versus Actual Performance Model are the most practical ones for a home health agency to use. Each of these designs may be applied with limited resources and minimal personnel. As a home health agency management tool, program evaluation must demonstrate its worth. The expected results of program evaluation are: benefit increase and cost reduction (fiscal evaluation), increase in efficiency and productivity (structure evaluation), improvement in effectiveness (process evaluation), and documented change in health behavior and status of patients (outcome evaluation).

Program Evaluation Tool. An evaluation tool or instrument is used to identify the information to collect and provides the evaluation criteria. There are numerous tools found in the literature for conducting a program evaluation (National League for Nursing 1984, 331-348; Bulaw 1986, 41-42; Morris and Fitz-Gibbon 1978a, 73-88; Idem 1978, 49-78; Kosecaff and Fink 1982, 66-78). In selecting a tool for your agency's program evaluation, the review of these tools is time and cost-effective. A program evaluation tool is a worksheet which indicates those areas to be evaluated, the time of evaluation, the rationale of the evaluation, and the evaluator.

In designing or selecting a tool, the following guidelines provide direction to evaluate:

1. How well did the program achieve its goals or outcomes?

2. Were the program's activities implemented as planned?

3. How effective were the activities in achieving the goals?

4. Does the program have any unintended adverse or beneficial effects?

5. Is the quantity and scope of service provided sufficient to meet the needs of the program participants?

6. How quickly does the program respond to requests for service?

7. Are patients discharged from the program prematurely?

8. Do the patients or families or significant others, who use the program, consider it satisfactory?

9. What did the program cost?

10. How did social, political, and regulatory factors influence the program's development and impact?

11. How well was the program managed?

12. What is to be changed in the program in the immediate future and in the long-term plan? (Dever 1980, 63; Kosecaff and Fink 1982, 27-64)

In addition to the above guidelines, the following criteria assist in assuring that the assessment by the tool will be valid, accurate, and complete:

1. The tool provides useful information about the program which justifies the collection, analysis, and presentation of the data.

2. The tool addresses the aspects of concern of the governing body and regulatory agencies.

3. The sources of data requested by the tool are sufficiently reliable. There are no biases, exaggerations, omissions, or errors that will cause the tool to become inaccurate or misleading.

4. The tool enables the data to be collected and analyzed in time for the deadline.

5. The tool does not restrain the evaluator from obtaining required information.

6. The cost requirements for the utilization of the tool can be met by the agency.

7. The information that the tool produces can be interpreted clearly as desirable or undesirable (Dever 1980, 63).

8. The tool has validity. Each criterion in the tool is based on expert judgment, past experience, and data from research.

Collection of Information. After considering the development or selection of a tool for program evaluation, thought is given to collecting information or data. This involves numerous and very important techniques. To choose the correct technique for your program, consider these factors.

The technique should:

1. Be acceptable to the governing body and management staff.

2. Be technically sound to collect data which is reliable, valid, and targeted to evaluation criteria.

3. Provide the best data that the budget can afford.

4. Allow sufficient time for collecting and analyzing the data before the deadline (Kosecaff and Fink 1982, 111-112).

The major methods and strategies that are utilized to collect information are:

- Review of organization of agency.

- Critical review of administrative philosophy, goals, objectives, and documents.

- Clinical record review for quality and utilization of services. The quality assurance and utilization review committee reports may be used, or the evaluator may review a sampling of clinical records.

- Patient care policies and procedures review and evaluation, using the current literature of the multidisciplinary health professions as a resource.

- Review of the goals and objectives of each program for attainment and relevancy.
- Critical review of personnel policies, job descriptions, professional qualifications, and activities.
- Reports of Medicare survey, state licensing consultant, or accreditation agency.
- Recommendations from the agency committees.
- Results of patient opinion surveys and patient letters of appreciation and complaints.
- Results of referral source opinion surveys.
- Compilation of any patient statistics which can be acquired from the agency information system.
- Analysis of the proposed and actual budget and the cost report.

Program Evaluation Report. The report is the official record of the program evaluation. Consider the audience of the report so that the style of writing will be understood. Communicate the evaluation findings in a comprehensible way without compromising any qualitative and quantitative details.

A clear and logical evaluation report increases the credibility of the information presented. The report should include:

1. An introduction which briefly describes the program(s) being evaluated, the participants conducting the evaluation, and the approach to the evaluation.

2. The evaluation model and evaluation tool description including any limitations. Attach a copy of the tool if possible. If not, give some sample items. Present information about the reliability and validity of the tool.

3. A summary of all activities performed in the collection of data and what sources were used.

4. The results of any analysis that was done to arrive at answers to the evaluation criteria. Use graphs and other visual presentations where applicable.

5. The evaluation findings, the answers to the evaluation questions, and the evaluator's interpretation of the findings. It is important to point out the strength and weaknesses of a program. It is important to report the limitations of the findings.

6. The recommendations and modifications for the program. Prioritize the recommendations so that they may be readily incorporated into the plan.

7. A report on the sequence of events in conducting the evaluation and recommendation for future evaluation. This may be appended to the report for the governing body and the management team.

A summary, a brief overview of the evaluation report, explains the purpose of the evaluation and lists its major recommendations and conclusions. It contains enough detail to be usable and believable, but is easy to read. The summary may be placed at the beginning of the evaluation as an introduction. Since the summary may be more widely circulated and read than the complete report, it should be prepared carefully.

The evaluation report may begin with a section devoted to background information concerning the program. A description of the development of the program and its purpose sets the evaluation in context. The amount of detail presented is dependent upon the degree of program familiarity of the audience of the evaluation report (Kosecaff and Fink 1982, 111-112; Morris and Fitz-Gibbon 1978b, 15-26).

It is important to emphasize here that the recommendations of the evaluation report must be effectively communicated to the persons responsible for plan development. The evaluation of a program is one of the ways in which the planners get a sense of how their ideas are being implemented. The relevance of what was planned in the past has a significant influence on what is planned for the future. Communication of evaluation findings, so that the planner or planning committee has a better comprehension of program effectiveness, is a vital step in the evaluation process (Blum 1979, 546).

The evaluator(s) can go one step further and present questions about the future to the planners as part of the section on recommendations. These questions can address such subjects as population shifts, prospective payment programs, change in federal, state, or local regulations regarding health care delivery, consumer movements and occurrence of a disaster.

Systematic Approach to Program Evaluation. A program comes into being because an individual, a committee, or other group of concerned persons has an idea for a service that is needed by the community. The idea's creator visualizes a set of goals which, when taken collectively, become the program.

The next phase in the development of the program, after the idea is conceptualized, is the stating of goals. Planning and evaluation are continually interfacing. The evaluative process, which begins operation at the onset of the program is very similar to the planning process in the development of the program.

The first step in the evaluative process is to look at the goals of the program. The goals must be clear, specific, and measurable. They should be people-oriented. They must address program outcomes.

The next step in the evaluative process is to clarify goals. Rewrite any goals that are not measurable, people-oriented, or stated in outcome terminology. It may be necessary to change the stated measurement in the goal to be more realistic or relevant.

The process moves on to goal activation or the implementation of the goals. At this time, the activities of the program are being performed and the patients are receiving the services.

The measurement of the goal effect follows. At this stage, the goal effect is measured through patient statistics and utilization review data.

The final step in the evaluative process is the evaluation of the program. It is the judgment concerning the attainment of the program goals.

The planning for program evaluation is also part of the program plan. It is similar to the evaluative process but is more directive, specific, and task-oriented. The steps in planning for program evaluation are:

1. Identify people as evaluators. Usually program personnel, professional advisory board members, and consumers are included.

2. Conduct preliminary meetings to discuss the evaluation's purpose. A decision is reached to do the evaluation in a specific time period. A time line is drawn to indicate who will evaluate each section of the program in the time indicated.

3. Review of the literature by the evaluators who are external to the program.

4. Determine the methods of conducting the evaluation. What evidence is needed to measure the program outcomes?

5. Conduct the evaluation.

6. Determine what committee or individual will write the program evaluation report, after receiving recommendations from the evaluators.

7. Determine who will compose the planning group, who will carry out the recommendations for change, and how the change will be accomplished.

8. Present the evaluation report to the governing body, planning group, and the community groups. The recommendations are emphasized so that they are not ignored, but received and implemented if possible (Stanhope and Lancaster 1984, 212; National League for Nursing 1984, 332).

Operational Considerations of Program Evaluation

Even though the principles of evaluation are known and the topic is in firm control, a critical aspect of evaluation should be considered. The present climate of the home health industry is embodied with cost containment. Everyone is seeking to prove cost effectiveness in the delivery of home care services. The federal government has awarded grants to study and develop cost-effective care techniques like a prospective payment system. However, it may be erroneous to concentrate solely on dollars. While cost containment is important, we must remember that care of human beings is equally important.

Benefits of the Program Evaluation. The central benefits of a program evaluation are the judgments concerning the attainment of the goals of the program. Through evaluation, the program managers and governing body can determine if the program's purpose is being fulfilled. The feedback which gives information about goal attainment also verifies that the program is effective. This knowledge assists the decision makers in planning for future allocation of funds. Competent monitoring or evaluation of the program enables the decision makers to determine whether the achieved goals can be met in a more cost-effective manner.

Fiscal accountability may be another benefit derived from program evaluation. Funds given to operate a program must be spent for the purposes for which they are given. The accountability of the funds requires more than simple auditing of accounting records. The funding agency may take an alternative approach to monitoring, namely, if certain milestones (structure, process, and outcome) are achieved within the stated budget, it is assumed that the money given to the agency has been used appropriately (Alkin and Solman 1983, 22-25).

Evaluation can make contributions to the store of knowledge about the program, certain professional activities, and consumer needs. This information can be used to market the program through direct marketing and public relation efforts. It can provide a basis of comparison from which to judge the relative quality of good practice. Accumulated information from many evaluations can serve as a basis for conclusion about what sorts of programs work best.

Program evaluation is an intelligent response to controversy. An accumulation of strong data can resolve a situation with diverse opinions. Evaluation also persuades people to pay attention to data concerning what home health agencies are doing. It is the best response to the individuals who continuously push new ideas without substance. Innovations must be tried, but if health professionals never find out which ones are worthwhile, home health agencies will deliver care with a fad-oriented mentality. Each time an evaluation is conducted, additional people acquire evaluation skills. As more people in home health agencies become familiar with evaluation methods, they will be able to collect information and to distinguish valuable effective innovations from ineffective fads (Morris and Fitz-Gibbon 1978a, 14-15).

Special Implementation Considerations. The organization of the home health agency may present specific circumstances that directly influence program evaluation. Most home health agencies have only one site. In these agencies, all administrative, organizational, and direct patient care activities ar found on that site. Some agencies, because of the size of staff or the large geographic area, have multisites. In these agencies, some decentralization is necessary.

In such situations, the decentralization is not merely physical. The home health personnel who work in the site offices and neighborhoods are in the best position to know the problems, needs, and resources within the area served by the site office. Therefore, the personnel from that home health agency site, under the directions of the site administrator, should have the responsibility and the authority for determining and carrying out the details of the daily operations and activities. They function, of course, with the overall agency philosophy, goals, and policies. Capable leaders are placed in the administrative position of the decentralized units. They administer their local programs to the maximum extent feasible.

Program evaluation in the one-site agency is conducted without difficulty since everything to be evaluated is centralized. In the multisite agency, the planning is more tedious. The governing body of a multisite agency has two options. The first is to evaluate the total agency as one site. With this plan, the evaluator(s) must coordinate the data so that each site is represented in the evaluation of each goal in the program. This approach is very difficult to coordinate and requires meticulous attention to assure accuracy.

If the governing body chooses to evaluate each site individually, the evaluator(s) task is less complicated. Also, this approach will enable the agency to do comparison evaluation studies. These studies would yield valuable information about the differences and similarities of the program as it is delivered to different communities.

Program evaluation in a multisite agency is a challenge to the most seasoned evaluator. However, the information that this evaluation yields can be so rewarding that it negates the frustrations of the experience.

Program Evaluation Tool Formats. There are numerous approaches to presenting a program evaluation tool. The following examples present a few approaches. Each format attempts to assess the extent to which the home health care agency's program is appropriate, adequate, effective, and efficient. If you choose to do more research on the topic of tools, please refer to the Bibliography at the end of the book.

Evaluation tool formats are included in the appendix (at the end of this chapter). These formats may be modified as necessary to meet the objectives of the evaluator or the evaluation team.

References

Alkin, M., and L. Solman. 1983. *The Costs of evaluation.* Beverly Hills, CA: Sage Publishers.

Baker, F., and J.E. Northman. 1979. Evaluation of a school mental health clinic. In *Program evaluation in the health field*, ed. H.C. Schulbert and F. Baker, vol. 2. New York: Human Sciences Press.

Blum, H. 1979. *Planning for health.* New York: Human Sciences Press.

Breckon, D.J. 1982. *Hospital health education.* Rockville, MD: Aspen Systems.

Bulaw, J.M. 1986. *Administrative policies and procedures for home health care.* Rockville, MD: Aspen Systems.

Dever, G.E.A. 1980. *Community health analysis.* Rockville, MD: Aspen Systems.

Donabedian, A. 1978. The quality of medical care. In *Health care regulation, economics, ethics, and practice,* ed. P.H. Abelson. Washington, DC: American Association for the Advancement of Science.

Helbig, D., D. O'Hare, and N. Smith. 1972. The care component core. *American Journal of Public Health* 62:540-546.

Idem. 1978. *How to measure program implementation.* Beverly Hills, CA: Sage Publishers.

Kosecaff, J., and A. Fink. 1982. *Evaluation basics.* Beverly Hills, CA: Sage Publishers.

Joint Commission on Accreditation of Hospitals. 1986. Home care services. *Accreditation manual for hospitals.* Chicago.

LaParta, J.W. 1975. *Health care delivery system: Evaluation criteria.* Springfield, IL: Charles C. Thomas.

Morris, L., and C. Fitz-Gibbon. 1978a. *Evaluator's handbook.* Beverly Hills, CA: Sage Publishers.

Morris, L., and C. Fitz-Gibbon. 1978b. *How to present an evaluation report.* Beverly Hills, CA: Sage Publishers.

Morris, L., and C. Fitz-Gibbon. 1978. *How to design a program evaluation.* Beverly Hills, CA: Sage Publications.

National League for Nursing. 1974. *Faculty-curriculum evaluation.* Part II. New York: The League. Publ. No. 15-1530.

National League for Nursing. 1984. *Administrator's handbook.* New York: The League. Publ. No. 21-1943.

National League for Nursing. 1985a. *Accreditation program for home care and community health.* New York: The League.

National League for Nursing. 1985b. *Accreditation program for home health agencies and community nursing services.* Unnumbered leaflet.

Rothman, J. 1980. *Using research in organization.* Beverly Hills, CA: Sage Publications.

Schulbert, H.C., A. Sheddon, and F. Baker. 1969. *Program evaluation in the health field.* New York: Behavioral Publications.

Shields, M. 1974. An evaluation model for science programs. *Nursing Outlook* July, 22: 448.

Spiegel, A.D. 1983. *Home health care.* Owings Mills, MD: National Health Publishing.

Stanhope, M., and J. Lancaster. 1984. *Community health nursing.* St. Louis: Mosby.

Stuart-Siddal, S. 1986. *Home Health care nursing.* Rockville, MD: Aspen Systems.

U.S. House of Representatives Committee on Interstate and Foreign Commerce, Subcommittee on Health and Environment. February, 1976. *A discursive dictionary of health care.* Washington, DC: Government Printing Office.

Warhola, C.F.R. 1980. *Planning for home health services.* USDHHS Publ. No. (HRA) 80-14017, August 1980.

Appendix 1.

Format 1

Evaluation Area with Outcomes	Outcome Met		Corrective Action Needed	Suggested Frequency and Month
	YES	**NO**		
A. Administration				1 x year
1. The governing body maintains relevant articles of incorporation				July
B. Organization				1 x year
1. The CEO keeps the O.C. up to date				July
C. Patient Care Policies				2 x year
1. All patients who fit the admission criteria received care from the agency				March September
D. Nursing Services etc. . .				Annually June

Continue this format until all areas that are to be evaluated are completed.

Appendix 1, continued.

Format 2

Activity with Outcomes	Evaluation Frequency	Responsible Group/Person	Outcome Met	
			YES	**NO**
A. Organizational Structure	Annually	Governing Body or Ad Hoc Committee		
1. Articles of Incorporation	Annually			
2. By laws The governing body reviews the by laws annually	Annually			
3. Agency Philosophy The governing body & staff review the philosophy annually	Annually			
B. Financial Management	Monthly	Finance Committee		

Continue this format until all areas that are to be evaluated are completed.

Appendix 1, continued.

Format 3

Activity with Outcomes	Minimum Frequency	Responsible Body/Person	Comments
A. Organizational Structure	Yearly and prn	Board of Directors	
1. The CEO manages the day to day operation of the agency			
B. Administrative Policies	Monthly and prn	Board of Directors	
C. Financial Management	Monthly	Finance Committee	
1. The controller prepares for the preparation of monthly financial statements			
D. Community Assessment	Annually	Programs Coordinator	
E. Program Services	Quarterly	Professional Advisory Committee Program Coordinator	

Continue this format until all areas that are to be evaluated are completed.

Appendix 1, continued.

Format 4				
Evaluation Area-- List outcomes under category	Frequency	Responsible Committee/ Person	Outcome Met	
			YES	NO

Organization and Administration

A. Organization Chart The CEO keeps the O.C. consistent with the agency operation	Annually	Board CEO		
B. Philosophy & Goals	Annually	Board		
C. Administrative Policies	Annually and prn	Board CEO		
D. Administrative Procedures	Annually and prn	Board CEO		
E. Community Needs	Annually	Board, CEO, Consultant		
F. Financial Management	Monthly	Board and Finance Committee		

Program and Services

A. Program Services	Annually	Board, CEO, P.A.B.		
B. Practice Policies		Procedure Committee		
C. QA / UR		UR Committee QA Committee		

Continue this format until all areas that are to be evaluated are completed.

Appendix 1, continued.

Format 5

Evaluation Area with outcomes under each category	Frequency	Responsible Body/Person	Outcome Met YES NO	Comments
Structure				
A. Organization	Annually	Board		
The CEO keeps O.C. consistent with agency operation				
B. Administrative	Annually			
1. Policies All patients who meet criteria receive care from the agency		Professional Advisory Board		
2. Procedures				
C. Community Needs	Annually			

Appendix 1, continued.

Format 5   (continued)

Evaluation Area with outcomes under each category	Frequency	Responsible Body/Person	Outcome Met		Comments
			YES	NO	
		Structure			
D. Facilities	Annually				
1. Equipment					
E. Staff	Annually				
		Process			
A. Program Services	2 x / year	CEO			
Skilled Nursing		Director of Professional/Patient Services			
HHA					
PT					
OT					
MSS	Staff				
B. Utilization of Services	4 x / year	CEO, Professional Advisory Board			

Part VI

Financial Issues

Chapter Twenty

Insurance

William W. Fonner

The spectrum of property and liability insurance is wide and the elements exceedingly diverse. Moreover, modern society demands heavy use of such insurance. Owning a home, driving an automobile, or operating a business are but a few of many cases in point. Because of this magnitude and diversity, it would be impossible in one chapter to provide a comprehensive means to treat this subject. The basic objective of this chapter is to attempt to instruct the beginner in the basic analysis of risk management and insurance.

As would be expected, terminology presents a major problem in the treatment of a number of property and liability subjects. Many words have the same meaning from one branch of the business to another. We have ended this chapter with basic definitions of the more common terms used by risk managers and insurance advisors to assist you further with analyzing insurance needs.

The basic rule of insurance in the economic and social structure of society is to provide relief for financial consequences of uncertainty. In turn, this relief of financial loss, especially from fear of loss, influences the direction and magnitude of economic and social ventures. Insurance provides relief from the harassing threat of financial catastrophe. Insurance is just one of the many ways in the evaluation method of risk management, but what really is risk?

"Risk" may well be the most heavily used word in insurance terminology. It is a proper topic for inclusion of a discussion of insurance fundamentals. The word risk is often used to refer to the object of insurance. One short and straightforward definition is simply that risk is "chance of loss."

There are many ways of treating risk. They can be briefly summarized by retention, the elimination of loss possibility, transfer of risk, or the anticipation of loss. Insurance is the vice for handling risk, a way in which risk can be transferred.

Three precepts have been developed that might be helpful in risk management. These are: (1) do not risk more than you can afford to lose, or consider the size of the loss; (2) do not risk a lot for a little, or consider profit and loss, and (3) consider the odds of chance of loss.

A problem facing risk managers is the creation of productive relationships with several classes of people outside the health provider. The principal relationships are those with procedures and insurance companies. The most prominent source of discontent stems from cost of service. The producer is responsible for a number of services which include the placement of insurance, marketing of an individual insurance account for both broad coverage and a fair price for the coverage being purchased. There is also a need to be able to coordinate loss control services, review statistics, analyze claims, and monitor claims activities.

It is extremely important to analyze the method of purchasing insurance and the services that can be provided to the health care provider. Most important is who can be made accountable for the services that are required by the health care provider. The second most important relationship in risk management is with the insurance company or companies. During the last two decades it has become increasingly evident that this selection process must be done prudently. Some of the questions that should be asked are what is the financial stability of this carrier? How long has this carrier been in the business of providing the coverages I am going to purchase? What kind of loss control services can this carrier provide for me? What is the method in which they will be rating the coverages being purchased? What are the claim processing and handling procedures? Am I dealing directly with the insurance company or must I deal through my agent or broker? How is the billing process handled? What kind of authority does my agent or broker have with the carrier providing my coverages?

The health carrier is primarily interested in buying protection against catastrophic losses. Unless the probability of loss is so extremely remote as to be ignored, protection is wanted no matter what the probability of loss. If the probability of loss is so high as to make the premiums out of reach, the health care provider may choose to go without coverage.

In respect to losses of less severity with greater expected frequency, if the insured feels his experience will be worse than the average experience on which the rate is predicted, he will have a particularly strong incentive to insure. On the other hand, if he feels his experience will be superior to that of the average, he will be less excited about insuring these relatively low-level loss potentials. The viewpoint of the insurance carrier may be to encourage, through its price structure and underwriting, the prospects with superior loss records.

There are certain prerequisites of insurance. For the insurance mechanism to operate, certain conditions are necessary. Insurance is associated with pure risk. The insured must be in a position where he faces uncertain loss; that is, where he may or may not lose, but does not know which outcome will occur. This condition of facing a possible loss upon the occurrence of a particular contingency is said to give such a person an "insurable interest" in respect to property which he stands to lose. The important consideration in this immediate context is not so much the fine point of what constitutes an insurable interest as the mere recognition that such insurable interest must exist.

The ability to predict is another condition or prerequisite of insurance. The predictions in the long run have to be reliable to permit the insurer's income to exceed total expenses. To meet these requirements there are several subconditions. First, there must be a sufficiently large number of insureds to permit the law of large numbers to operate. Second, individual insureds must be reasonably similar in terms of exposure and the likelihood of suffering a loss. Third, there must be some stability in the pattern of the events being predicted.

Most insurance contracts carry promises of the insurer to pay an expressed or determined amount of money to or on behalf of the insured. Most insured losses and claims have to be expressed sooner or later in monetary terms. Therefore, for the insurance mechanism to work, insurable values must be reducible to monetary units. To be subject to insurance, a given loss potential has to be expressible in a money amount.

For the insurance mechanism to work, the losses must be fortuitous. The thought is merely that the losses must not occur at the discretion of the insured. Even if such events are technically in his control, the insured must not intentionally cause them to happen.

Another condition necessary to insurance is that agreements involving the insurer's promise to pay losses must be enforceable by law. Without enforceability, promises might not be carried out.

Property Insurance

The insurance contract follows a standard format. First, a declaration page identifies the named insured, the policy term, policy number, the insurance company that is providing the coverage, and usually a brief description of the type of coverages or itemization of the coverages that are being provided by the policy and what the premium requirement is for the coverages being provided. Following the declaration page is the review of the actual policy form which specifies the details of the coverage being provided by the contract. This policy form is further subdivided to identify the property that is being covered. This section will specifically describe the property which is covered. The third section contains what is not covered under the policy; this is any kind of property which is being insured which is subject to limitations. The third section usually describes the item that has a limitation and what the limitations are. The following portion of the contract identifies the extension of coverage. This portion describes the conditions for changes in exposure during the policy period, or provides the conditions for extra things which are not specifically described on the declaration page.

The next section describes the perils insured against; specifically how broad the policy is. Next is the exclusion section, a very specific itemization of those things that would not be covered by the policy under either a very broad basis or a very specific basis. The final section of the policy is usually the valuation for which a loss would be settled. This section describes the method in which a loss would be settled—replacement cost, actual cash value, or stated amount.

The standard fire insurance policy is only a part of a complete insurance contract. The policy contains the basic general conditions applicable to any fire insurance transaction. It conveniently serves for the attachment of forms prescribed by building, contents, or both. It also may be adapted to cover consequential losses due to interruption of business, extra expenses resulting from fire or other damages.

The wording of the fire insurance policy is generally described by state law. All companies insuring risks within a state must use a prescribed wording that is standard for that state. The reason for standardization of fire insurance policies is that it greatly reduces confusion on the part of insured as to the coverage obtained. Second, standardization simplifies the adjustment of losses and the reduction of time expense for both the insured and the insurer for promoting relations between them. Third, court decisions are more generally applicable throughout the nation. Such interpretation of standard phraseology reduces the need for litigation in the event of disagreement. Last, a result of standard provisions is that the statistical data on losses and premiums are more valid and meaningful for rate making. It should, however, be noted that we are only talking about the standard fire policy. Many policies can be expanded to include additional perils, additional conditions or coverages which will vary between carriers and should be analyzed for the differences between what different carriers are offering.

Under the standard fire insurance contract, there are basically only three things covered: fire, lightening, and damage removal from the premises. Under the standard insurance policy, the policy insures to the extent of the actual cash value of the property at the time of the loss. Under certain policies, the actual cash value method of loss determination can be expanded to include replacement cost or stated amount (a specific appraised value). The next concept to discuss under a property policy is what constitutes allied lines insurance. Basically, this takes the standard fire insurance contract and expands it to include such things as sprinkler leakage, water damage, earthquake, vandalism, malicious mischief, optional perils, demolition, increased cost of construction, and data processing. Each of these describes alienated lines of insurance to physical property resulting from direct damages caused by the specific perils insured under each of these contracts.

Other types of coverage can be classified as consequential loss coverages which cover secondary losses or losses which result from or are the consequence of direct losses. For example, destruction by fire of your building is a direct loss. However, the result in loss of either rental income or the loss of business is a consequential loss. Consequential losses involved somewhat more imagination than the direct losses, but money is involved in both cases. Consequential money is just as important as the direct loss money.

A broad segment of broad consequential loss insurance is labeled as prime element coverages. These can be described further as losses which the element of time required to repair, rebuild, or replace is of particular importance to the size of the consequential loss. Other than business interruption being a form of consequential loss, there are many other types. Some examples of these are loss of rents coverage, additional living expense coverage, and extra expense coverage.

Another form of property coverages can be described as inland marine coverage. This pertains to the insuring of (1) property in transit over land, and (2) insuring of property that is mobile by nature. The principal function of inland marine policy is insuring against loss to the person who owns personal or commercial goods which are subject to loss away from home or in transit. Many inland marine policies or floater policies provide insurance on scheduled property or equipment. This type of coverage can also be written on a blanket insurance basis, which is unscheduled property.

Liability Insurance

Liability is a hazard of quite another sort for it is purely an artificial creation of law. Insurance designed to protect against liability hazard has characteristics which vary, depending upon the way in which the legal system structures the liability. It is possible to conceive of a legal system that makes no provisions at all for liability of one person to another: persons living under such a system would not need liability insurance. No civilized legal system has a doctrine so extreme. Even in a civilized world, the range of variation is substantial.

The reason for transferring loss that is most important for liability is that the defendant has been negligent. Negligence is conduct that is blameworthy. It produces liability because it creates a greater risk of causing damage.

There are separate elements or requirements that are said to be necessary to establish a cause of negligent actions. They are (1) a legal duty to conform to the standard of the reasonable man; (2) breach of that duty by failure to live up to the standard; (3) actual harm or damage to the plaintiff's interest; and (4) a casual connection between the breech of duty and the harm that is close enough to satisfy certain standards.

A typical general liability policy provides for one or more of the following coverages: (1) bodily injury liability, (2) property damage liability, and (3) medical payments. Also available under a general liability policy can be a large list of scheduled additional liability exposures which can be broken out to include premises and operation, independent contractors, products, completed operations and malpractice, and those specifically described in the liability section of the definitions at the end of this chapter.

One of the main areas for concern in the health care business is medical professional liability coverage. It should be immediately known that all medical professional liability policies are not the same. They vary not only in exclusions and broadness of insurance clauses, but also in company interpretations of the policy.

An important area of concern is professional liability. In particular, coverage for a nonprofit organization should include the name of the institution as well as the named insured's board of trustees, directors or governors, and volunteers, while acting in the scope of their duties.

Workers Compensation

Workers Compensation provides for the payment of medical and indemnity benefits determined according to law for covered occupational injuries or disease incurred by an employee while on the job without regard to the fault of the employer. Inasmuch as workers compensation acts have been passed in most states, benefits provided by a workers compensation policy are prescribed by law and vary by state. The following items are particularly important in consideration of workers compensation laws: (1) persons and employments covered, (2) injuries and disease covered, (3) benefits provided, (4) the administrative system in handling workers compensation, and (5) the method of securing benefits. The law of each jurisdiction must be studied to determine which employee comes within the act.

From the viewpoint of the individual worker, the possibility of having to leave employment because of injury or illness generally presents a greater threat to his well-being than to that of his family. Even relatively nonserious injury and disease may result in medical expense, and the more serious disabilities may cause a reduction or elimination of the worker's income or earning ability.

Automobile Insurance

All insureds are concerned with liability resulting from bodily injury to others or damage to property of others caused by automobiles whether they are owned or non-owned.

The basic policy is designed to provide insurance primarily on described autos. However, through the use of endorsements, the policy lends itself to a multitude of coverage extensions and combinations to make it very comprehensive. It can be expanded to include not only specifically described vehicles, but use of other vehicles, hired vehicles, and nonowned vehicles.

Agents and underwriters look upon the comprehensive automobile policy as one of the most advanced and salable contracts in the market. This policy can protect the insured's liability arising out of accidents caused by the ownership, maintenance, or use of any automobile. The policy should be studied from the standpoint of two general categories from the insured — named insured and the additional insureds. The use of a comprehensive automobile policy can be readily made to include not only the liability for both bodily injury and property damage as a result of an occurrence, but also to include medical payments and physical damage coverage to covered owned automobiles.

Excess Liability Insurance

Since World War II, there has been a growing tendency toward the purchase of separate excess liability contracts. This term is insurance jargon for the insurance liability contract which pays up to a maximum amount the liability claims against an insured, but only to the extent each claim exceeds some specified limit of primary insurance.

An insured cannot pick its claimants. The injured party may turn out to be a professional golfer, entertainer, or rising young executive with a substantial annual income. As a result of negligence, serious medical bills could result in hundreds of thousands of dollars in claim payment.

Furthermore, an insured cannot anticipate what a jury will do. The size of jury verdicts has been growing by leaps and bounds during the last two decades. Based on the information of which so much is unknown, this creates a very uncomfortable feeling for the insured, the producer, and the professional counselor. One of the ways to solve this uncomfortable feeling is the evaluation of an excess liability policy or umbrella liability policy. These types of policies are designed to respond when the primary limits of liability have been exhausted.

Most insurers have loss prevention departments staffed by trained and technically oriented people. The loss control department carries out two major functions: (1) inspection and evaluation perspective of businesses to provide underwriting departments with information needs and to decide whether or not the prospect should be underwritten and, in some cases, what to charge; and (2) education of policyholders in the avoidance of losses. The activity of the property and liability insurance carrier's loss control department is basically the same under every coverage. Essentially, it is to advise the policyholder regarding any condition that might cause injury to persons or property for which the policyholder might be held financially liable.

Summary

It is extremely important to analyze the method of purchasing insurance and the services that can be provided to the health care provider. Administrators and members of the board of directors must ask pertinent questions and receive satisfactory answers concerning the issues related to the types of insurance coverage needed to protect the agency, its governing body and staff, as well as the qualifications of the broker or individual insurance agent.

Glossary

"All Risk" Property Insurance. "All Risk" Property Insurance protects against all risks of direct loss or damage to contents, unless it is specifically excluded by one of the exclusions in the policy. Most Standard Property Policies only provide coverage for either specific perils or hazards, and if a loss is not caused by one of these eight hazards, then the policy will not cover the loss.

Extra Expense Insurance: Extra Expense Insurance pays for the necessary extra expense (over and above normal operating expenses) which must be incurred in order to continue as nearly as possible the normal operation and conduct of business following damage or destruction to real or personal property by a covered peril.

Replacement Cost Coverage: Replacement Cost Insurance eliminates the deduction normally taken for depreciation following any type of insured loss to property.

An Agreed Amount Endorsement: An Agreed Amount Endorsement is an agreement obtained from the insurance company stating that the values for which they are being insured are in compliance with the Co-insurance Clause in your policy. In effect, the Agreed Amount Endorsement waives the Co-insurance Clause in your policy, which relieves you of the burden of proving to the insurance company *after a loss* that you are carrying insurance at least equal to the amount required by the Co-insurance Clause.

Premises-Operations Coverage: Premises-Operations Coverage provides protection for Bodily Injury or Property Damage claims arising out of premises (e.g., someone tripping or falling in your office or job site) and all operations of business both on and away from your premises *except where specifically excluded by definitions, conditions, exclusions, or other clauses which will be pointed out in our proposal.*

Independent Contractors Coverage: Independent Contractors Coverage provides protection in the event that you are sued because of a Bodily Injury or Property Damage claim caused by an independent contractor who is operating on your behalf. However, this coverage does not provide protection for the independent contractor.

Products Liability Coverage: Products Liability Coverage provides protection against any claim or suit brought against you, for Bodily Injury or Property Damage arising out of any product manufactured, sold, handled, or distributed by you. Such claim must 1) occur away from any place of business owned by or rented to you, and 2) the product must physically be in the possession of someone other than an insured.

Completed Operations Coverage: Completed Operations Coverage provides coverage for Bodily Injury or Property Damage occurring after you have completed your job (or a portion of one at a job site) or abandon it. Coverage while you are working on the job is covered by Premises-Operations Coverage.

Blanket Contractual Coverage: The first exclusion in the Standard General Liability Policy states that your ". . . insurance does not apply to liability assumed by the insured under any contract or agreement." Many jobs for which you contract will require that you assume the liability of others. These clauses in a contract which require you to assume someone else's responsibilities are referred to as "Hold Harmless" Clauses.

Blanket Contractual Liability Coverage provides you with protection for any liability of others assumed under any written (or oral) agreement.

Personal Injury Liability Coverage: Personal Injury Liability Coverage provides you with protection against nonphysical types of injury, such as false arrest, libel, slander, defamation of character, and other similar related allegations. If one of your employees apprehends a "thief, caught in the act of stealing" and has this person arrested, your firm could be involved in a suit for false arrest, malicious prosecution, wrongful detention, etc.

Advertising Injury Liability Coverage: Advertising Injury Liability Coverage provides protection for nonphysical types of injuries arising out of an offense occurring in the course of an insured's advertising activities, if such injuries arise out of libel, slander, defamation of character, violation of right of privacy, piracy, unfair competition, or infringement of copyright, title, or slogan.

Premises-Medical Payments Coverage: Premises-Medical Payments Coverage allows you to pay all of the medical bills (incurred within one year of the date of the accident and not to exceed policy limits) because of any injuries that a person may sustain because of a condition in your premises, or because of any of your operations (except products and completed operations). There are a large number of exclusions in connection with this coverage, but basically, it is intended to cover guests who are invited to come on your premises.

Host Liquor Liability Coverage: Host Liquor Liability Coverage protects you from bodily injury or property damage claims arising from the serving or giving of alcoholic beverages to any person in violation of a Liquor Statute (i.e., to a minor or an intoxicated person).

Additional Insured Employees Coverage: The Standard General Liability Policy only protects Officers, Directors, and Stockholders of your company if they are personally named in a suit as the result of activities that further the company's interests. *Additional Insured Employees Coverage* grants the protection of the policy to each and all of your employees, provided your employee is acting on behalf of your business when such a claim occurs. This would remove the possibility of having a loyal employee lose his home and assets because the employee was *personally* named in a suit while involved in company duties.

Extended Bodily Injury Coverage: The Standard General Liability policy does not provide coverage for Bodily Injury claims arising out of *intentional* acts on the part of the insured. Extended Bodily Injury Coverage extends your policy to cover any intentional act by or at the direction of the insured which results in bodily injury, if such injury arises solely from the use of reasonable force for the purpose of protecting persons or property.

Chapter Twenty-One

Budgeting for Home Health Services

Gregory J. Brown

The Budgetary Process

What is the importance of the budgetary process?

The budgetary process obligates management to make an early study of its current and projected operating problems. It instills in the organization the habit of making a thorough and careful study of information before making decisions. When all programs have been coordinated into a well thought-out budget (program), the budget becomes management's written plan for the future. The budget should enlist the aid of the entire management organization so that final decisions represent the combined judgment of the entire organization and not merely that of an individual or small group of individuals. The budget promotes increased coordination of limited financial resources for use by all agency programs. The budget allows current operations to be measured against a financial and statistical model which incorporates management's projections of anticipated operational activity. The steps of the budgetary process include: long-range planning, program planning and evaluation, budget development and budget control.

Long-Range Planning

The long-range planning phase of the budgetary process establishes the environment under which the home health agency will operate. The agency must identify the type of home health agency it will align itself with and establish the agency's statement of purpose. Currently, there are seven categories of home health agencies. In general, they all offer a home health care program. Having been formed to meet either social or financial goals, they are controlled by a governing body whose role is to ensure that the agency fulfills its statement of purpose.

Types of Home Health Agencies

1. Official

2. Visiting Nurse Association

3. Combination

4. Hospital-based

5. Private nonprofit

6. Proprietary

7. Other

Even though the seven types of home health agencies may provide many of the same services, the budgetary process of each category will vary in one way or another. Agencies will budget in a manner that best facilitates their current operating environment. Because I believe the Visiting Nurse Association home health agency can have the greatest number of factors influencing its operations, further discussions will characterize the budgetary methods utilized by such an agency. Home health agencies of other categories would follow a similar budget preparation process, altering the process where required.

Program Planning and Evaluation

One of the most important tasks that the home health agency must accomplish during the budgeting process is to evaluate the effectiveness of all of its existing programs and to ensure that all programs continue to meet the goals and objectives that the organization has established.

The viability of each program should be determined from answers to questions which the agency considers important, i.e.,

1. Has each program met its established goals?

2. Are any changes necessary for the program to be more successful?

3. If the program is to be continued, are there any changes in the demand for that program?

4. Are there sufficient controls established to monitor the program's progress?

5. Can the program generate sufficient revenues to cover expenses or must it rely on alternate sources of funding? If funding cutbacks dictate program cuts, what is the program's rank of importance in relationship to other programs?

6. What risks are there associated with this program?

Budget Committee. To gain a broader base of information about each program, the agency may choose to establish a program review team as part of the budget evaluation process. The program review team should involve as many agency board members and administrative personnel as the agency considers practical. However, the team should not be staffed in a manner that would jeopardize the subjectivity between clinical and financial criteria. The higher the degree of scrutiny that each program receives, the more reliable will be the data from which the upcoming budget will be based. The greater the involvement the board and administrative staff have in the budget review process, the greater the commitment to support the programs under the guidelines established.

Budget Development

During the development phase of the budgetary process, the agency will establish specific parameters under which it will prepare the budget. During this phase, the agency will also establish the time frame for accomplishing the budgetary process. A list of all budget procedures and required items are identified and prioritized in the order of date required. Budgetary assignments are delegated to appropriate personnel or board committees with dates due for completion. The primary focus of this section will be spent dealing with the development of the actual operating budgets.

Operating Budget

Cyclical versus Noncyclical Operating Year. Budget information is usually based upon the time period covered by the operating or fiscal year. The budget is comprised of twelve monthly periods from which comparisons can be made against the actual monthly and year-to-date levels of activity. If the organization operates in a noncyclical environment, i.e., flat or nominal growth projections, the operating budget can be prepared as twelve individual monthly budgets, all presenting identical levels of activity. If the organization operates in a cyclical environment, i.e., seasonal or with specific growth projections, then the annual budget can attempt to reflect these projections by presenting the twelve monthly budget periods in a manner that would coincide with the cyclical or projected levels of actual activity. Presumably most organizations have a planned goal of a favorable growth rate. But as we all are aware, organizations may at times need to project a downward growth pattern. In either case, if this information is known at the time of the budget preparation, then it must be incorporated into the annual budget.

My experience has shown that the utilization of home health agency services are cyclical in nature. The summer months tend to have a less-than-average utilization, while the winter and spring seasons have above-average utilization. While there has not been a home health care season identified, various factors are known to influence when home health care services are utilized. For example, the effects of a severe winter season will tend to produce an increase in the number of patients with muscular-skeletal injuries. Winter also generates patients with influenza and respiratory infection problems. Conversely, there are fewer patients with these problems during the warmer summer months. Summer months generate fewer elective surgery patients because of physician and client vacations. Summer vacations by agency staff also tend to decrease the availability of personnel to perform visits. If per diem help is unavailable to make up for the shortage of visiting staff, patient admissions may have to be delayed or visit frequency for other patients decreased. Immediately prior to and during major holidays, many home health agencies receive an above-average number of referrals for patients being discharged from hospitals and skilled nursing facilities. This may be attributed to (1) families choosing to have the patient at home during the holidays, or (2) elective surgery with a planned recovery over the holiday period. While an agency may find it necessary to consider the significance of noncontrollable utilization factors when making the decision to develop a cyclical or noncyclical budget, that decision would ultimately be made from the data collected while preparing the agency case-mix analysis.

Case-Mix Analysis

After having evaluated the services and programs the agency chooses to provide, the agency must project the cross-section (case-mix) of individuals who would actually utilize the agency's services. The agency can project this level of need from historical data or from a demographic market survey studying population and medical requirement characteristics of potential patients. From these data, the agency must make a crystal ball projection of when and how many units of service will need to be provided to meet the demands of the consumers. Consumers may be: an individual patient, other home health agencies, hospital home care departments, HMOs, PPOs, insurance companies, and even private industries.

While a significant amount of data can be collected on prospective consumers, only a limited amount is required for preparing the actual case-mix analysis.

When the case-mix data are being collected, they should be classified as units of service in each of three catagories: 1) Types of services required; 2) reimbursement resources available; and 3) time frame for services required. Types of services required would be comprised of all of the services the agency chooses to provide, i.e., skilled nursing, physical therapy, home health aide, well baby clinic, and health promotion services. Reimbursement resources would be comprised of all the reimbursement resources patients would utilize to help pay for the services they receive, i.e., Medicare, state assistance program, private insurance, patient pay, no reimbursement source. Time frame would be comprised of the number of monthly operating periods during which the service would be provided, i.e., throughout the year, summer only, from the date a new contract starts.

When sufficient data have been collected, the information is placed onto a matrix format worksheet to observe the units of service required for each category of service offered and the units of service to be paid for by the reimbursement resources available. At this time, it is not important to classify the information by time frame; however, the time frame information is important for planning staffing level changes. (See Exhibit 21-1 for an example of the case-mix analysis worksheet).

The information on the initial worksheet only represents potential clients. Agency administration must further review these data to identify the exact case-mix of clients for which it intends to provide services. For example, if the administration chose not to provide homemaker service to clients who have no reimbursement resources, then the corresponding units of service should be removed from the worksheet. The worksheet should continue to be reworked until it represents what the administration considers to be a realistic representation of the types and units of service to be provided under each program and reimbursement resource.

Because all subsequent budget analysis will be based upon the case-mix analysis, it is important to take the time to review your findings before going much further in the budgeting process.

Productivity and Staffing Requirements. The case-mix analysis indicates the annual projection of the units of service to be provided. This projection of provided services needs to be converted into a staffing requirement. This is done by calculating how many full-time equivalents of each profession it would take to provide the units of service projected in the case-mix analysis. The staffing requirement calculation must

Exhibit 21-1. Example of matrix format worksheet.

Budget Worksheet #___

Service Type	Reimbursement Resources						
	Medicare	Medical Assistance	Private Insurance	Self Pay	Hospital Home Care	Home Health Agencies	Total
Nursing							
Physical Therapy							
Speech Therapy							
Occupational Therapy							
Medical Social Service							
Home Health Aide							
Homemaker							
Total							

also take into account the employment factor and the average-visits-per-day calculation.

Employment Factor

The employment factor is a calculation to project the actual annual productive work hours that are available from staffing a full-time position. The available productive work hours are calculated by taking the annual payroll hours paid to staff; regular hours (skilled visit time, skilled non-visit time, and all nonskilled service time), overtime hours if significant and any types of paid leave time (vacation, holiday, sick). From these annual payroll hours paid, deduct all leave and nonskilled service-related hours paid and divide the result into the total annual hours paid. An analysis of the agency's historical time records will provide data on the average annual leave time taken.

The basic concept for calculating the employment factor is shown in Exhibit 21-2.

If the nonservice time and leave benefit levels provided to an agency's employees are significantly dissimilar, an agency may need to calculate separate employment factors for each service provided. The employment factor calculation has provided two pieces of information: 1) it indicates the amount of time that can be utilized for revenue-generating activity; and 2) it provides a factor from which one can calculate Full-Time Equivalent (FTE) staffing requirements. For example, in Exhibit 21-3, if the services being provided are to be sold by the hour you would take the total projected hours to be provided and multiply them by the employment factor for that service to determine the FTE staffing requirement.

Average Visits per Day

If the services provided are made on an encounter basis and without regard to length of the time spent on the visit, then the staffing requirement calculation must take into account the productivity capacity of the employees. This requires that the agency calculate the average visits per day (AVD) productivity statistic for each group

Exhibit 21-2.

Nursing Employment Factor		
Total annual paid hours		1,950.00
Less paid leave hours:		
Avg. annual vacation	(112.50)	
Avg. sick time usage	(52.50)	
Holidays	(67.50)	
Personal days	(15.00)	
Less nonservice hours paid:		
Administrative functions	(20.00)	
		(267.50)
Available work hours		1,682.50
Employment factor (1950/1682.50)	1.16	

Exhibit 21-3.

Home Health Aide Staffing Requirement

Projected home health aide hours to be sold	25,000
HHA Employment factor	x 1.08
Total payroll hours budgeted	27,000
Payroll hours budgeted/1950 =	
FTE staffing requirement	13.85

---

of service providers. Although many formulas exist, the one used for illustration will be the National League for Nursing productivity calculation . . . (See Exhibit 21-4). The agency's historical time study data are the best source of data to use when making the average-visits-per-day calculations. If historical data do not exist, an agency may wish to survey other home health agencies to obtain average-visits-per-day productivity statistics.

Exhibit 21-5 is an example of how the employment factor and the average visits per day statistic can be utilized to calculate FTE staffing requirements when services are provided on an encounter basis.

When the FTE calculation for each service is identified, a comparison should be made against the existing staffing requirements. If the projected FTE requirements exceed the existing level of staff, positions should be added to the budget. If projected FTE requirements are less than the existing level, a reduction in staff is warranted.

Exhibit 21-4.

NLN PRODUCTIVITY CALCULATION — Home Visits Per Day Per Employee

$$\text{Average visits per day} = \frac{\text{Number of visits during period}}{\text{Number of days available for visiting}}$$

To count visits:

Include: All completed visits by discipline (MCH, health promotion, care of sick, whether or not "billable").

Exclude: not home, not found, supervisory and observation visits (two persons in home) and office visits.

To calculate available days:

1. From attendance records, enter total hours on duty for each discipline on staff level (exclusive of holidays, vacation, time off, sick time. Include weekend time if on duty.).

2. Subtract: nonvisiting service time (in clinics, schools, etc.); time spent in supervision, orientation, etc.; in-service time; and office visit time.

3. Add time spent in home visiting by agency personnel above staff level replacing staff.

4. Divide resultant hours by working hours per day in agency to calculate equivalent full days available for visiting.

Reprinted with permission of NLN from *Productivity Home Visits Per Day Per Employee* © 1979.

Exhibit 21-5.

Projected skilled nursing visits	35,000
Divide by AVD calculation	5.20
Service days required	6,542
Multiply by 7.50 daily work hours	7.50
Service hours required	49,065
Multiply by nursing employment factor	1.16
Total payroll hours budgeted	56,915
Divide by annual work hours	1,950
FTE staffing requirement	29.19

Reductions in staff should be accomplished in a manner that would not jeopardize the provision or integrity of services being provided. Reductions could be accomplished via layoffs, natural attrition, or reducing workweek hours for all or specific staff of the program in question.

Expense Classifications and Departmental Expenditure Budgets

Expense Classifications

Once administration has identified its staffing requirements, it will begin identifying expense categories and preparing departmental expenditure budgets. The goal of expense budgeting is to accumulate, on an accrual accounting basis, records of expenses that will be incurred during the provision of services to patients. Every expense category listed in the agency's chart of accounts will need to be classified as either a direct or indirect expense. Expenses that can be directly identified with a service or program objective are known as direct expenses, i.e., salaries, benefits, conferences, auto allowances. Expenses that cannot be directly identified with a service or program objective are known as indirect expenses. Indirect expenses are also known as overhead expenses. All agency indirect expenses will need to be equitably allocated to each service program to determine the true cost of providing that program. Examples of indirect expenses are: plant operation expenses, administrative services, general and professional liability insurance coverages, marketing, legal and accounting services.

Departmental Expenditure Budgets

The departmental expenditure budget is comprised of three components: 1) direct compensation and benefits analysis; direct contract services analysis; and 2) other direct departmental expenditures analysis.

Since one aspect of the budgetary process is the need to identify the total direct operating cost of each service offered, the departmental expenditure budget should attempt to identify as many direct expenses as is considered practical. This might entail that each direct expense category be expanded so each service program has the same set of direct expense categories. For example, the health insurance expense category would be listed for each service as: nursing health insurance, physical therapy health insurance, homemaker health insurance, and finance health insurance. Salaries would be nursing salaries, physical therapy salaries, homemaker salaries, and finance salaries. An advantage to using this detailed classification process is that it can specifically identify direct cost that would be incurred by a department if it operated at the service volume levels established in the case-mix analysis. A disadvantage to using this process is the time and cost associated with the increased data collection requirements and the volume of data required to be changed if a budget parameter is altered.

Direct Compensation and Benefits Analysis. A detailed compensation and benefit analysis will allow administration to evaluate the direct cost associated with every position within the agency. This information is helpful when doing a cost-benefit analysis evaluating staffing versus contracting for services. The compensation and benefit analysis will list each position required by that department, projected annual working hours, proposed hourly wage, projected annual salary, projected annual cost for payroll taxes, and annual cost of each health and welfare benefit provided.

Payroll related taxes:	*Employee health and welfare benefits:*
FICA	Pension
Unemployment compensation	Life insurance
Workers compensation	Health insurance
FUTA	Disability insurance

Direct Contract Services Analysis. If an agency has done a cost-benefit analysis and has determined that it is to its advantage to utilize contracted services in lieu of hiring additional employees, the cost for the contracted services are considered a direct expense of the department for which the services are provided. Projecting the cost of contracted services for a direct service contractor is usually a matter of multiplying the projected units of service the contractor will perform times the contractor's negotiated charge per unit of service.

Projecting the cost of contracted administrative services can be accomplished by obtaining fixed bids for the contractors services, reviewing historical cost data, or a combination of both.

Other Direct Departmental Expenditures Analysis. The other direct departmental expenditures analysis will list the remaining expenditure categories which can be directly associated with a department, i.e., conferences, seminars and education, uniforms, books and periodicals, auto allowance, auto operating expenses, auto insurance and auto depreciation, direct supply purchases, and any other expense item which can be allocated directly to the department. Other agency expense categories not directly associated with a service department are the indirect cost associated with plant operations and maintenance, and the administrative and general catagories. Within these two expense classification categories, an agency may wish to establish several other functional departments. As stated previously, these categories of expenses are considered overhead and will need to be allocated to each service being offered to arrive at the true cost of providing that service.

Typical plant operation and maintenance expenses:

Heat light and power

Building repairs and maintenance

Janitorial and groundskeeping service

Real estate taxes

Depreciation building

Depreciation furniture and equipment

Typical administrative and general expenses:

Administrative services

Financial services

Data processing services

Medical records and transcription services

Contracted professional services: legal, accounting, marketing

General and professional liability insurance coverages

Allocating Indirect Cost. If an agency is going to provide care to Medicare patients, there are specific guidelines established for allocating indirect expenses to existing departmental expenses. This allocation procedure is known as the Medicare step-down method of cost allocation. Agencies may want to review Medicare Provider Reimbursement Manual Part II — Provider Cost Reporting Forms and Instructions for HCFA Form 1728, to determine the exact parameters which they must follow. While there are alternatives to using the Medicare step-down methodology for cost allocation purposes, i.e., discrete costing, the volume of documentation required by Medicare to support an agency's cost apportionment findings might prohibit many agencies from successfully utilizing discrete costing as an alternate method of allocating indirect costs. For budgetary purposes, most agencies will find it acceptable to allocate indirect cost according to the Medicare guidelines.

Plant operations and maintenance costs are allocated on a square footage basis. This requires that a floor plan for all leased or owned space occupied by agency personnel be prepared, allocating the square footage to a service or department by (1) actual square footage occupied by each employee, or (2) if the employee participates in several activities, division of the employee's square footage by time spent in each activity. The actual cost attributed to each service is calculated by taking the square footage for each service multiplied by the projected cost per square foot.

$$\text{Cost per square foot} = \frac{\text{Total projected plant operation cost}}{\text{Total square footage occupied}}$$

Administrative and general costs are allocated on an accumulated cost basis. If one were to total all direct costs that have been identified with a service; i.e., salaries and benefits, direct departmental expenses, direct contract services, direct costs associated with adjustments and allocations from other departments, this total would be referred to as the department's total direct accumulated costs. When total accumulated costs have been calculated for each service it is possible to allocate administrative and general cost which have not previously been assigned to a service or cost center as a percentage of the total accumulated costs of all services.

When all agency expenses have been allocated to a service program, the agency can determine a per unit cost for each service it intends to provide. This is done by dividing each program's total accumulated cost by the units of service to be provided by that program as indicated in the case-mix analysis. Once the agency knows what the projected cost of providing each unit of service will be, it can project a charge structure and begin making revenue projections and profitability analysis of each service provided.

Revenue Projections

Revenue, like expenses, should be recorded on an accrual accounting basis and by the corresponding service or revenue center established during the preparation of the expense budget. Revenue for home health agencies falls into two major categories: Revenue from Patient Care Services and Nonoperating Sources of Revenue.

Revenue from Patient Care Services

An accurate projection of patient care services revenue must take into account the sources of gross revenue, and any deductions from gross revenue that would represent a less than full-charge reimbursement for provided services.

1) Revenue from Patient Care Services represents gross revenues, measured in terms of the agency's full established rates earned from all services rendered to patients by the various revenue producing centers in the agency.

2) Deductions from patient service revenues represent reductions in gross revenues arising from charity service, contractual adjustments, policy discounts, administrative adjustments, and bad debts (Serluco 1984, IA-4).

Several matrix worksheets will need to be prepared to assist in the cost and profitability analysis. These worksheets will be prepared in the same format as the case-mix analysis — by service by reimbursement source.

Worksheets required.

1. Cost per unit of service — Gross service cost divided by total units of service provided by each service provided.

2. Gross cost of services — Cost per unit of service times case-mix units of service.

3. Charge per unit of service—Projected gross charge for each type of service being offered.

4. Gross charges for services—Charge per unit of service times projected case-mix units of service to be offered.

5. Expected net revenue per unit of service—Gross charge per unit of service adjusted for deductions from patient care services.

6. Net revenue from services—Net revenue from service times case-mix units of service.

7. Gross allowances on services—Gross charges less Net Revenue.

8. Gain or Loss on Service—Net Revenue from services less Gross Cost of services.

Many home health agencies are faced with a reimbursement environment where revenue from fees for service fall far short of the actual cost of providing the services which the agency has stated it will provide. For example, unexpected clinical needs of patients may force program cost to exceed the revenue-generating capacity of the established charge structure. Revising the charge structure to cover the increase in cost may only complicate matters if the new charge structure requirements price the service higher than what consumers are willing to pay. Because this scenario has become a routine occurrence it has become a commonplace practice for agencies to pool unrestricted program surpluses for use by other programs which lose money or have limited income sources. The practice of pooling surpluses is necessary because the typical nonprofit home health agency has stated that its purpose is to provide a wide range of community and public health services to any individual who is in need of a service provided by the organization. Services will also be provided without regard for the patient's ability to pay. If a program is highly desirable, it may be continued even if the funding allocation has been exhausted. The degree to which agencies can lose money on the services they provide depends on the agency's ability to secure other sources of income to supplement the losing programs.

Nonoperating sources of income: Nonoperating sources of income are often acknowledged as a reason why many nonprofit home health agencies have been able to survive in today's health care environment. Home health agencies have come to rely heavily on the funds made available by United Ways, fraternal organizations, public and private contributors, interest income, and the allocations that state and local governments have earmarked for the provision of public health services.

Profitability Analysis

The completion of the worksheets and procedures outlined in the budget development stage will give the agency an idea of how much it will cost to provide services, how much revenue is expected to be received, and how much money the agency expects togain or lose on the services provided. The profitability and expenditure budget analysis worksheets may need to be recalculated until the profitability results meet the financial objectives that were established during the program planning and evaluation process. Although the need to generate profits is obvious, there is the absence of pressure to generate a return on equity like there is in the for-profit home health agency. In the not-for-profit home health agency, year-end profits are often viewed as funds for which other programs or services could have been provided but were not. Frequently, although unfortunate, the absence of the profit motive may also be construed as the home health agency's inability to make a profit.

The measure of success for many agencies is frequently determined by how well the agency did in meeting its program goals and fulfilling the needs of the communities it serves. In essence, the typical home health agency chooses to derive a psychic income from the provision of services to the community rather than work solely for the bottom line profits. However, the current upheaval in the home health care environment is forcing most agencies to strike a more equitable balance between bottom line profits and the agency's psychic income.

Other Budgets

Two additional components required of the budget development process are the Cash Budget and the Capital Acquisitions Budget.

Cash Budget

A cash budget involves detailed estimates of anticipated cash receipts and disbursement requirements coinciding with the twelve monthly periods of the projected budget. The cash budget is an important management tool for monitoring the operating condition of the organization.

Specifically, the cash budget: (1) will indicate the effect on the agency's cash position for changes in service utilization patterns, routine and unusual cash receipt or expenditure items, and the affect of inefficient accounts receivable collections; (2) indicates the cash requirements for capital acquisitions; (3) indicates when cash shortfalls may make it necessary to borrow or utilize credit lines; and (4) indicates when excess cash balances will be available for investment purposes.

Most cash budgets are prepared from cash receipt and disbursement data. Items to be considered when preparing the cash receipt portion of the cash budget would be all anticipated incoming cash from; the provision of patient care services, state and local government allocations, United Way allocations, fund raising revenues, restricted and unrestricted contributions, grant and trust monies received, interest income, proceeds from sale of assets, rental and lease income. Projecting the actual period of time during which the cash receipts are going to be received is difficult because (1) home health agencies encounter problems with accounts receivable collections; (2) the unpredictability of planning contribution receipts; (3) the uncertainty of knowing when private and public allocation funds are going to be made available to the agency.

Expenditure items of the cash budget would be: payroll, payroll-related taxes, employee health and welfare benefits, the cost of operating supplies and operating expenses, capital expenditures, income taxes, and dividends paid to owners.

Expenditure items are easier to project since the majority of a home health agency's costs are payroll-related and would occur in a predictable pattern.

Capital Expenditure Requirement Analysis Budget

The capital expenditure analysis has a twofold purpose: (1) it indicates additional cash expenditure requirements for the upcoming year; and (2) it helps to identify annual cost associated with depreciation and maintaining new capital acquisitions. The capital expenditure analysis will list: purchase priority of item, a brief description of its purpose, potential vendors, the item's cost and its expected useful life. Cost associated with the installation, delivery, and maintenance of the equipment should also be estimated.

Budget Controls

Budget controls are intended to give management the ability to monitor, alter, or limit the degree to which actual agency activity deviates from budgeted activity. Monitoring can be achieved by having the agency's internal financial statements prepared in a manner that presents actual activity against budgeted activity on a monthly and year-to-date basis. It is also helpful if the agency has the ability to compare current year activity against prior year activity. The monitoring of the agency's financial activity must be done in a manner that is as accurate and timely as possible, as the significance of the data representing the agency's current financial activity loses its importance as time passes. If management is to make sound decisions regarding the future of the agency, they must have timely information measuring the results of decisions they have made previously. This can be accomplished by having the financial statements prepared and presented to the agency's governing body on no less than a quarterly and preferably on a monthly basis. The decision and methods for influencing the direction that actual activity has taken would arise from the management's interpretation of the financial statements.

References

National League for Nursing and Council of Home Health Agencies and Community Services. 1979. *Productivity (Home visits per day per employee.)* New York: National League for Nursing.

Serluco, R.J., and Institute of Public and Private Service Trenton State College. 1984. *Innovative financial management and reimbursement strategies for the home care agency.* Trenton: Trenton State College.

Charlotte L. Kohler

Chapter Twenty-Two

Reimbursement

Introduction

Home care costs have traditionally been a small portion of total health care costs (2.6% in 1985 according to the National Association for Home Care). But with the cost of health care continuing to escalate, the home care industry has experienced a rapid growth trend. Some researchers have projected that the market for home health care services will triple by 1990 (Halamandaris 1984,16-17). This has been spurred on, in part, by government (e.g., Medicare) and other insurance carriers seeking alternative ways to hold costs down.

This chapter covers current reimbursement trends for home health care services, as well as some changes that may be foreseen in this reimbursement. Since Medicare still pays for the substantial portion of home care provided (Stewart 1979,96-98; Shaw 1985,8) the chapter will concentrate on the basic aspects of current Medicare reimbursement and address changes that are being proposed by HCFA and the major home care industry organizations.

Medicare Current Reimbursement Trends

The federal government provides home health care or funding for such care under a variety of programs created by the Social Security Act, including Medicare (Social Security Act, Title XVIII), Medicaid (Social Security Act, Title XIX), and the Older Americans Act (PL 89-73, 1965; PL 98-459, 1984), to name a few. These programs provide specific approaches and funding for specific aspects of home care.

Medicare was enacted July 30, 1965, and became effective on what has since become known as "M" Day, July 1, 1966. Medicare is a two-part program commonly referred to as "Part A Medicare" and "Part B Medicare." Under Part A Medicare, beneficiaries receive certain insurance coverage for hospitalization, specifically defined medical care provided in a skilled nursing facility, and specifically defined home health care. In addition to Part A coverage, Medicare beneficiaries may purchase, for a small monthly premium, supplemental insurance for Part B coverage. (Current monthly premium paid by the patient for Part B Medicare is $15.00. This is determined by a formula that sets the rate at 25% of the aggregate amount needed to cover program cost (*1986 Medicare Explained*, Sect. 535).) Physician services provided on an outpatient basis, home health care, pathology services, outpatient hospital services, and others are covered by Part B. As of July 1, 1981, Part A actually pays for home health services to beneficiaries who are covered by both Part A and Part B

Part B (*Home Health and Hospice Manual*, Sect. 208.3). There are currently no deductible or co-insurance amounts charged to the patient for home health services (with the exception of durable medical equipment).

Medicare is an entitlement program with benefits offered to persons who: (1) are at least 65 years of age and eligible for social security retirement benefits; (2) are under age 65 but have been eligible at least two years for social security benefits due to a disability; or (3) have end-stage renal disease (*1986 Medicare Explained*, Sect. 205,8-9).

There are six types of services for which Medicare provides reimbursement under its home care schedule of benefits. They are skilled nursing, home health aide service, physical therapy, occupational therapy, speech therapy, and medical social work.

Skilled nursing is care rendered by a licensed nurse or care provided under her supervision. Observation and assessment, care of wounds, administration of injections, and patient teaching are some of the many services provided as part of skilled nursing. In order for home health agencies (HHAs) to be reimbursed, patients must require skilled care on a part-time (less than one hour per visit with exception of home health aides) or intermittent basis. To be considered "intermittent," care must be for a medically predictable recurring need for which the patient requires skilled nursing at least once every 60 days (*1986 Medicare Explained*, Sect. 420.1, 63). Currently, intermittent skilled nursing visits are allowed on a daily basis for up to eight hours a day for up to three weeks. The interpretation of intermittent care has been the subject of much debate and confusion between HCFA and the HHAs.

Complementing skilled nursing is home health aide service. A home health aide performs many necessary, although nonmedical tasks such as helping patients with personal hygiene, retraining the patient in self-help skills, and certain household services such as changing the bed. The services provided by the home health aide must be determined by a registered nurse and not by the home health aide. Like skilled nursing, home health aide services may be provided only in the patient's home and should conform with the guidelines for intermittent care. Any care provided in a skilled nursing or hospital facility will not come under the home care reimbursement provisions.

Additional types of home health care provided for under Medicare Part A are physical therapy, occupational therapy, and speech therapy. Occupational therapy helps beneficiaries gain the necessary skills to again assume the activities of daily living, while physical therapy helps patients regain physical functional skills such as increased mobility. Speech therapy is provided to help patients overcome speech and language problems related to the physical condition that required home care. For any of these services to be covered by Medicare, there must generally be a restorative potential demonstrated in the treatment of the patient (*Home Health and Hospice Manual*, Sect. 205). Several visits would be allowed to teach a patient how to maintain function if there was no restorative potential. Although physical therapy, occupational therapy, and speech therapy are services that can be rendered either at the patient's home or at a hospital outpatient department, skilled nursing facility, or rehabilitation center, only when the services are actually rendered at a patient's home will they be reimbursed under Medicare's home care provision.

Social work services such as counseling and referral to appropriate community agencies, are covered by Medicare if they are considered necessary to further a patient's medical progress.

To receive any of these home health services, Medicare beneficiaries must meet program requirements. They must, for example, be homebound (*1986 Medicare Explained,* Sect. 420,63). To be considered homebound, patients must have physical impairments making access to outside care difficult. Patients need not be bedridden, however. Lack of readily available transportation does not constitute homebound status. The program also requires that the patient be under the care of a physician (including doctors of medicine, osteopathy, and podiatry) and that the physician submit a Plan of Treatment in writing to the appropriate fiscal intermediary. (The Plan of Treatment is reported on HCFA Form 485 and should be submitted with the initial claim.) (The fiscal intermediary is the third party designated by the Health Care Financing Administration to process claims and payment to Medicare providers.) The Plan of Treatment must be reviewed and signed by the attending physician together with the home health agency at least every two months. If a recertification has not been made and home health services have not been provided in 60 days, then the home health plan is considered by Medicare to be terminated (1986 Medicare Explained, *Sect. 422.3, 66-67).*

Basic Tenets of Medicare Reimbursement

Methods of Reimbursement

Under the Medicare program there are three methods of determining reimbursement to providers: reasonable cost, reasonable charge, and prospective payment. Currently, home health agencies are reimbursed under the "reasonable cost" method; that is, on the basis of the cost deemed necessary to deliver services efficiently to beneficiaries. This method takes into consideration both direct and indirect costs.

In order to determine reimbursable costs, the Health Care Financing Administration (HCFA) carries out a process called "cost finding" that is facilitated by the home health agencies completing the Cost Report (HCFA Form 1728). (The methodology used in the Cost Report is discussed under "Cost Finding.") Cost-based reimbursement must be distinguished from charged-based reimbursement and prospective payment.

Charge-based reimbursement is used under Part B. Medicare uses the amount billed (charges) as the basis for payment. Providers are reimbursed at a percentage of either their customary historical charges, or reasonable charges, whichever are lower. Customary charges are those per-service charges most frequently made by a provider during a given time period. Reasonable charges are the per-service charges used most frequently by similar providers in the same geographical area. Physicians, durable medical suppliers, and hospital outpatient services are reimbursed under this methodology.

The Prospective Payment System (PPS), as the name implies, reimburses hospitals for inpatient services at a predetermined rate. This was enacted as part of the Tax Equity and Fiscal Responsibility Act of 1982 (*1986 Medicare Explained,* Sect. 741,194). A fixed amount is paid to hospitals according to each patient's admitting diagnosis which is categorized into a diagnosis-related grouping (DRG). The hospital receives a fixed per-DRG payment regardless of service intensity, which may vary due to intragroup differences in severity of illness. The hospital must manage its use of resources to provide the required care within the average amounts paid.

Although the amount paid under the Medicare hospice provisions is often called a prospective payment methodology, the significance of the difference between the hospital PPS and hospice payment mechanism becomes apparent when the reward for efficient use of resources is considered. Under Medicare PPS for hospitals, if the hospital incurs less than the payment under that specific DRG-based PPS payment, the difference (or "profit") is kept. If the hospital incurs more than the DRG-based PPS payment, no more is received. On the other hand, if the hospice incurs less than the maximum amount payable under the hospice provision, only that which is incurred is reimbursed by Medicare to the hospice. If the hospice incurs more than the maximum amount payable under the provision, no more is received. The hospice does not have the opportunity to offset "profits" and "losses" for each case; it only is allowed to keep the "losses." In this respect, the hospice provisions are not truly a PPS methodology.

Cost Finding through the Cost Report

Because of the implications of cost-based reimbursement, a working knowledge of the cost-finding process is a basic management skill. Cost-finding is the process of identifying those costs which are to be reimbursed as defined by the Medicare regulations.

> In discussing the overall intent of the Medicare rules of cost finding, we have noted two major goals of the principles of reimbursement as stated in 42 CFR 405.402:
>
> 1. That there be a division of the allowable costs between the beneficiaries of this program and the other patients of the provider that takes account of actual use of services the beneficiaries of the program . . . and
>
> 2. That there should be a recognition of the need for hospitals and other providers to keep pace with growing needs and to make improvements (Booth 1985, 72-73).

To identify appropriate costs, HCFA requires home health agencies and other home health providers to complete a cost report (Form 1728). The cost report is a financial summary which must be submitted at the end of the provider's fiscal year. It contains a variety of schedules which are designed to identify Medicare home health costs (Table 22-1). It is important to realize, that through the use of adjustments required by regulations and nonallowable expenses, Medicare regulations will *reduce* the expenses of the home health agencies to Medicare allowable costs.

Cost reporting involves a three-step process: (1) allocation, (2) cost finding, and (3) cost settlement. The first step in the process is to allocate expenses by Medicare-defined cost centers. A cost center is an administrative unit or subunit, defined by Medicare, that in theory provides a specified service. Cost centers are divided into three different areas: (1) reimbursable services, (2) nonreimbursable services, and (3) general services. Those services included under reimbursable costs are: skilled nurs-

Table 22-1. Home health agency cost report form HCFA-1728

Page 1	*Home health agency cost report* This first page of the report shows the identification name and provider number, as well as details of visits, statistics and the composition of full-time equivalent employees. This cover page is also where the report is signed and certified by the responsible officer of the HHA.
Worksheet A	*Reclassification and adjustment of trial balance of expenses* Worksheet A shows the total expenses per the general ledger trial balance, and the impact of adjustments and reclassifications leading to total costs available for cost allocation on Worksheet B.
Worksheet A-1	*Compensation analysis, salaries, and wages* Worksheet A-1 provides details of total employee compensation.
Worksheet A-2	*Compensation analysis, employee benefits (payroll-related)* Worksheet A-2 provides details of employee fringe benefits.
Worksheet A-3	*Compensation analysis, contracted services/purchased services* Worksheet A-3 provides details of amounts paid for personal services of independent contractors.
Worksheet A-4	*Reclassifications* Worksheet A-4 is used to detail reclassification between cost centers as shown in column 7 of Worksheet A.
Worksheet A-5	*Adjustments to expenses* Worksheet A-5 is used to furnish details of adjustments to general ledger trial balance expenses as shown in column 9 of Worksheet A.
Worksheet A-6	*Statement of costs of services from related organizations* Where Worksheet A includes costs of goods or services purchased from related organizations, the identity of the related parties and the overall cost amounts are detailed in Worksheet A-6.
Worksheet A-7	*Depreciation* Details as to any depreciation expense included on Worksheet A are provided on Worksheet A-7.
Worksheet A-8	*Reasonable cost determination for physical therapy services furnished by outside suppliers* Where independent physical therapists are used to provide patient services, Worksheet A-8 is used to compute the salary and travel Medicare limitations for comparison against actual expenses.

Table 22-1, continued.

Worksheet B | *Cost allocation--general service cost*
The general service cost centers are allocated among the specific service cost centers on Worksheet B.

Worksheet B-1 | *Cost allocation--statistical basis*
The statistical data supporting the allocation of general service cost centers as reflected on Worksheet B are detailed on Worksheet B-1.

Worksheet C | *Apportionment of patient service costs*
Worksheet C shows the computations of actual costs per visit and the cost limitations applicable to each discipline.

Worksheet D | *Calculation of reimbursement settlement*
Worksheet D furnishes the "bottom line" of the cost report, comparing net total allowable costs against interim payments yielding the net overpayment or underpayment of the Medicare program for the HHA.

Worksheet D-1 | *Analysis of payments to providers*
The details of interim payments to the provider during the cost report are furnished on Worksheet D-1.

Worksheet D-2 | *Calculation of reimbursable bad debts*
Where total allowable costs include Medicare bad debts (deductibles and co-payment only), the summary details are provided on Worksheet D-2.

Worksheet D-3 | *Recovery of unreimbursed cost*
The carryover of unreimbursed cost under lesser of cost or charges is shown on Worksheet D-3.

Worksheet F | *Balance sheet*
The balance sheet of the provider, by fund type, is furnished on Worksheet F.

Worksheet F-1 | *Statement of revenue and expenses*
The income statement of the provider is provided on Worksheet F-1.

Worksheet F-2 | *Statement of changes in fund balances*
Changes in the fund balance accounts of the provider, by fund type, are detailed in Worksheet F-2.

Worksheet F-3 | *Return on equity capital of proprietary providers*
This schedule, applicable to proprietary providers, details the computation of allowable return on equity capital includable in allowable costs.

Table 22-1, continued.

HHA-Based Hospices Only

Worksheet K *Cost and data report*
This schedule furnishes Information of a goneral nature regarding the hospice.

Worksheet K-1 *Patient care service utilization analysis*
Worksheet K-1 provides for reporting of visiting service data applicable to the four levels of hospice care.

Worksheet K-2 *Analysis of Direct Costs*
This schedule shows the expense account trial balance for the hospice.

Worksheet K-3 *General service cost allocation statistics*
Worksheet K-3 furnishes the statistical data necessary to compute the allocation of HHA general service cost centers to hospice cost centers.

Worksheet K-4 *Hospice general service cost allocation statistics*
Worksheet K-4 provides the statistical data necessary to alleviate the general service costs of the hospice that are included in the " hospice" cost center.

Worksheet K-5 *Analysis of shared services*
This schedule provides for the identification of shared service data for the HHA and the hospice.

ing, home health aide services, physical therapy, occupational therapy, and the other Medicare-covered services. Nonreimbursable services include non-Medicare-covered services such as home dialysis, homemaker service, private duty nursing, meal services, and health promotion activities. General services include administration, plant operation and maintenance, and depreciation on buildings and fixed equipment. This breakdown is accomplished in Worksheet A on the Cost Report.

Both direct and indirect costs are allocated by cost center. Direct costs are any costs incurred for the benefit of and traceable to a specific cost center. Salaries of employees, such as registered nurses and physical therapists, are direct costs which may be allocated to the specific reimbursable cost center. Indirect costs are those incurred for the benefit of the organization as a whole. The cost of administration, depreciation, and accounting are indirect since they benefit the entire home health agency. Moreover, all other costs under the general service cost center are indirect.

At this point, adjustments are made on Worksheet A. Certain adjustments are required, such as adjustments for insurance and interest. Other adjustments for nonallowable costs must be made before cost finding is started (Table 22-2). The regulations identify the entries to be made. Specific reference is made to those costs that

Table 22-2. Nonallowable Medicare costs for home health agencies

Generally, costs will be allowable for Medicare purposes where they are related to patient care and conform to the prudent buyer concept. Under this concept, costs will be minimized by arm's length bargaining for the best available prices and terms.

Following is a partial listing of costs which have been found to be unallowable for Medicare purposes:

- Federal income and excise taxes
- Net operating losses
- Advertising--for the purpose of increasing patient utilization or for fund-raising purposes
- Research
- Uninsured theft and casualty losses--where insurance was available
- Life insurance premiums--where the provider is a direct or indirect beneficiary of a policy on the life of an owner, key employee, Provider-Based Physician, or officer
- bad debts--unless specifically attributable to unpaid Medicare deductibles or co-insurance
- Charity and courtesy allowances--these are reductions of revenue
- Compensation of owners in excess of a reasonable allowance
- Accelerated depreciation
- Interest expense--to the extent of interest income; any excess over interest income is allowable, however
- Legal fees--incurred in the defense of criminal charges
- Cost of meals sold to visitors
- Cost of drugs sold to persons other than patients, including employees
- Costs of the operation of a gift shop
- Alcoholic beverages for medical staff meetings
- Meals on Wheels
- Political contributions
- Nonvisiting costs--including school visit programs and well baby programs
- Contracted services where the contract term exceeds five years
- Cost of drugs in excess of the maximum allowable cost (MAC) limitation
- Fines and penalties
- Taxes which could have been avoided by a legally available exemption
- Reorganization costs
- Membership dues and costs in social and fraternal organizations
- Malpractice and general liability losses and related expenses where the provider is uninsured
- Costs of influencing employees in respect to proposed unionization

Following are costs which are not allowable in full in the year in which incurred but which are allowable as amortized over a period of years:

- Special water and sewerage assessments--these should be capitalized and depreciated
- Start up costs--amortizable over 60 months
- Issue costs for stocks or bonds--amortizable

Medicare may find excessive, such as excessive compensation of the Executive Director or Administrator.

Once costs have been allocated on Worksheet A, the second step in the process is to separate Medicare and non-Medicare costs. In assigning costs as either Medicare or non-Medicare, providers must carry out a process known as "cost finding" which consists of stepping down indirect costs to reimbursable and nonreimbursable services. This is accomplished on Worksheet B (and B-1). "This method recognizes that services rendered by certain nonrevenue-producing departments or centers are utilized by certain other nonrevenue-producing centers as well as by revenue producing centers." (*Medicare and Medicaid Guide,* Vol. 1, Sect. 2306.1)

The stepping down of costs is performed on a statistical basis. The statistics are developed on Worksheet B-1 using the requirements and guidelines as set forth in the regulations (Table 22-3). Total indirect costs, such as those for administration, are divided by a unit multiplier set by the provider. Transportation costs, for example, are distributed on the basis of mileage, while depreciation of buildings, fixtures, and plant operation and maintenance are divided by square footage. Depreciation costs for movable equipment are distributed by square footage or dollar value and administrative and general costs by accumulated costs. Changes in the statistical basis can have a dramatic effect on the Medicare reimbursement received. Careful planning is necessary to avoid an unfavorable effect on Medicare reimbursement.

"Cost finding" calls for the distribution of these indirect costs on a per-discipline basis. That is, indirect costs are distributed to skilled nursing, speech therapy, occupational therapy, medical social work, and the other types of covered and noncovered services. The allocated, indirect costs for each of these areas are added to the net expense derived from the original direct cost allocation of expenses by cost center. The sum represents the total by Medicare reimbursable and nonreimbursable cost center.

The next step in the cost-finding process is identifying the per-visit cost. This is done on Worksheet C. This is simply the total per-discipline costs divided by the number of visits. For example, if the results of the allocation and step down indicated that cost for skilled nursing was $528,398 for 10,125 visits, then the cost per visit would be $52.19. Medicare reimburses providers on the basis of per-discipline visit costs subject to certain upper limits. (Current reasonable cost provisions are discussed under "Cost Limits.")

The final step in the cost-reporting process is the calculation of the reimbursement settlement. On Worksheet D the provider's reimbursable costs are applied against a variety of payment adjustments including payments already made under the periodic interim payment (PIP) program. (See "Periodic Interim Payment.") If there ha been an excess of reimbursement to the provider, the provider must remit the amount due to Medicare with the Cost Report. If there has been an underpayment to the provider, the provider will be reimbursed the deficit following a review of the cost report by the Intermediary. The Cost Report is due three months after the end of the agency's fiscal year. The remainder of the cost report consists of financial statements including a balance sheet and statement of revenue and expenses, and certain other required disclosures.

Table 22-3. Statistical basis required for cost allocation on Worksheet B-1

A Home Health Agency must allocate general service cost centers in the order prescribed by regulation using the required statistical allocation basis. If permission is obtained from the Intermediary, the allocation may be done in a different order or using some other statistical basis, otherwise the order and statistical basis as listed below must be used.

Depreciation--Building and Fixtures
This cost center includes not only depreciation but also other expenses pertaining thereto, including insurance, interest, rent, and real property taxes. Costs should be allocated to each cost center based upon the proportion of square feet occupied by that cost center to total square feet.

Depreciation--Movable Equipment
This cost center includes expenses closely related to movable equipment such as interest and personal property taxes, in addition to depreciation on such equipment. Costs should be allocated according to square feet, similar to the allocation done for building and fixtures.

Transportation
The Transportation cost center includes the cost of vehicles owned or rented. Costs should generally be allocated on the basis of miles per cost center. As an alternative to this statistical allocation basis, weighted trips may be elected upon request.

Administrative and General
Administrative and general expenses should be allocated on the basis of net costs per cost center after reclassification, adjustments, and the allocation of other general service cost centers.

Where a given cost center has a negative balance immediately prior to the allocation of administrative and general expenses, such cost center should not be included in the allocation base.

Cost Limits

Cost limits are the predetermined maximums placed on per-visit reimbursable costs, by discipline, to assure the efficient delivery of care. Section 223 of the Social Security Amendments of 1972 granted the authority for limits to be set on the costs Medicare would recognize as reasonable for the overall efficient delivery of health services. Cost limits are developed using labor and nonlabor costs as separate costs. Prior to June 5, 1985, the per-discipline limits were established by type of service and compared to the per-discipline costs in the aggregate, based on the number of visits for each type of service. The aggregate was used to determine whether the home health agency was above the limit. Starting July 1, 1985, the limit was issued, and impact calculated, by the individual discipline (*1986 Medicare Explained*, Sect. 749.5,228). This means that an agency can be over the skilled nurse limit by $25,000 and under the home health aide by $25,000, with the result of the loss of reimbursement of $25,000 due to the skilled nursing costs exceeding the limit.

Federal Register 19734 (May 30, 1986) sets forth a new schedule of limits on home health agency costs for cost-reporting periods beginning on July 1, 1986, but before July 1, 1987. "This schedule is an update of the limits," previously set forth in July 1985, "to take into account the effects of inflation on home health agencies' operating costs, and was developed using the HCFA wage index." (*Medicare and Medicaid Guide,* Vol. 4, Sect. 35,406)

In setting limits, HCFA first pulls information on cost per visit from the cost report. Cost limits developed for July 1986 were based on cost report information from 1982. Since there is a lag between the cost-reporting periods and the time when limits are set, the cost data are adjusted. The Health Care Financing Administration updates cost information using a special home health agency price index (Table 22-4). It is a market basket of the goods and services used by the home health industry. The home health agency price index is monitored by HCFA in an effort to minimize the difference between the estimated market basket rate and the actual rate.

The second step used by Medicare in setting per-visit limits is to divide each cost limit into the labor and nonlabor component of costs so that an adjustment may be made to the labor portion of costs based on location of the home health agency. Referring to the price index, labor costs include employees wages and benefits and a share

Table 22-4. Home health agency input price index--1986

Wages and salaries	66.46
Employee benefits	8.39
Transportation	4.23
Office costs	2.90
Medical nursing supplies and rental equipment	2.47
Rent	1.19
Nonrental space occupancy	1.10
Miscellaneous	6.39
Contract services	6.87
Total	100.00

Source: *Federal Register* 51 (104).

of the contract services (80.37%). The wage portion of costs is adjusted by multiplying it by appropriate SMSA index based on the location of the home health agency.

For example, the calculation of the adjusted Occupational Therapy limit for a freestanding home health agency in Dallas, TX:

Labor component (per May, 1986, final regulation)		$41.37
Wage index (for SMSA location)	x	1.0733
Adjusted labor component		44.40
Nonlabor component (per May 30, 1986, final regulation)		11.36
Adjusted occupational therapy per visit limit		$55.76

It is this adjusted rate that is used to determine the cost limit on Worksheet C of the Medicare Cost Report.

Before HCFA establishes the wage portion of costs, the cost data are screened for outliers. These are costs that are either above or below the mean cost by a predetermined range. To screen for outliers the cost data, are " . . . transformed into their natural logarithms . . . in order to determine the mean cost and standard deviation for each group." (*Medicare and Medicaid Guide,* Sect. 35, 406) All costs not within two standard deviations of the mean are excluded from calculation of the mean. A per-service limit then is determined. Currently, for 1986, the basic service limit is 115% of the mean labor and nonlabor portions of the cost per visit; for 1987 and after, it is scheduled to be reduced to 112% (1986 Medicare Explained, *Sect. 749.5, 228).*

To account for a variety of circumstances, adjustments are made to the service limits. These include an adjustment for hospital-based home health agencies and an adjustment for the fiscal reporting year that is different than those that coincide with the limit's effective date. The first adjustment is designed to account for the higher administrative and general costs related to the Medicare cost allocation requirement for hospitals. The adjustment for the cost-reporting year helps to account for higher prices which home health agencies will be expected to pay after the limits have become effective; in terms of inflation, these adjust for increases relating to inflationary pressures.

"Before the limits are applied at cost settlement, the provider's actual costs will be reduced by the amount of individual items of cost (for example, administrative compensation or contract services) that are found to be excessive under Medicare principles of provider reimbursement." (*Federal Register* 1986, 51:104) In this way, Medicare reduces costs during the cost-finding process before the question of cost limitation is to be addressed.

Under certain circumstances, a new provider can request an exception from the cost report for discipline limits. To qualify, the agency must demonstrate that the limits were exceeded due to the initial set-up to comply with Medicare regulations of participation. HCFA strictly enforces the "new agency" requirements and will not consider a newly certified Medicare agency that preexisted as a non-Medicare agency as a new Medicare agency (DHHS 1985, 405.460(f)).

In addition to limits based on per-discipline costs, there is also a limit based on the lower of costs or charges. This is the only case where charges have a basis for determining the reimbursement under Part A. The theory behind this limitation is that the provider must charge an amount at least equal to (or greater than) cost. Should the provider charge an amount (in the aggregate) less than cost, the amount charged will be the maximum that the provider can receive from Medicare. This is true even if the provider is under the per-discipline limits. Amounts not received due to this limitation can be carried forward until the difference between cost and charges is enough to absorb the carry-forward.

Periodic Interim Payments (PIP)

Home health agencies are reimbursed on the basis of the lower of reasonable costs or customary charges. Reasonable costs are developed through the Medicare cost report and cost-finding process. Customary charges are the aggregate amount billed by the home health agency. There are other limits, as previously discussed, based on a per-discipline amount.

There are three different methods in which payments are made to home health agencies on an interim basis, that is, during the course of the year as services are provided. Of course, as with any cost-based reimbursement procedure, the annual Cost Report will determine the final allowable costs of the provider, and hence, any overpayment or underpayment for the period made to the provider on an interim basis.

Of the three Medicare payment methods, the per-visit method is the most basic. Under the per-visit method, estimated total Medicare costs of the provider based on the prior year cost report are divided by total estimated Medicare visits to yield a cost-per-visit amount. As Medicare visits are then billed to the Fiscal Intermediary (FI), reimbursement will be made at the predetermined cost-per-visit amount.

Another method used by Medicare intermediaries to pay providers is based upon a percentage of charges. Under this method, an estimate is made of expected total Medicare costs and total Medicare charges for the period. From dividing the charges by the costs, a rate is determined for the reimbursement of the provider. As an example, assume a provider with anticipated total costs of $800,000 and anticipated total charges of $1,000,000; the costs expressed as a percentage of charges would be 80%. For each Medicare visit billed by this provider to the FI, the provider would be reimbursed for 80% of the charges billed. Medicare found that the providers could manipulate reimbursement by increasing charges. Although notification by the provider to the FI is required, the FIs were not always adjusting the percentage to compensate. To establish better reporting and payment control, and to provide an even, expectable payment from Medicare to health care providers, the Periodic Interim Payment (PIP) method was developed (*Medicare and Medicaid Guide,* Vol. 2, Sect. 7281).

The PIP method is the third and most popular method of Medicare payment. Under this method, total estimated Medicare costs are reimbursed to the provider evenly at regular intervals. The interval used is usually every two weeks, but can be from once weekly to once monthly at the agreement of the provider and the intermediary. The interval is generally established to coincide with home health agency payroll requirements.

Reimbursement under PIP is available to qualified providers upon election of that provider in a formal written request to the fiscal intermediary. The request for PIP reimbursement is reviewed by the Fiscal Intermediary, which results in a recommendation to HCFA to allow or disallow the election.

To be eligible for PIP reimbursement, a provider must meet certain qualifications. The home health agency must have a total Medicare reimbursement of at least $25,000 for the year or an estimated Medicare reimbursement equal to at least 50% of total allowable costs. In addition, the agency must have already filed at least one acceptable cost report, thus providing the intermediary with a basis for making an accurate estimation of payments to be made. This requirement generally restricts use of the PIP reimbursement method to providers who have been in operation for at least one year. Most importantly, the provider must possess the capability to maintain accurate and timely data regarding costs, charges, and statistics, in order to properly monitor the status of PIP payments against actual costs. As an additional requirement, a provider who commences PIP reimbursement must first make arrangements to repay any overpayment due to the intermediary under the reimbursement in effect prior to the conversion to PIP.

Once a PIP reimbursement amount is determined, it will be paid to the provider on a regular basis until modified. Modifications to the PIP reimbursement amount result from any of several different factors. HCFA requires the Fiscal Intermediary to monitor the PIP status on at least a quarterly basis. The provider is required to furnish a quarterly report of such items as total costs, adjustments to costs, the number of total visits, the number of Medicare visits, total charges for the quarter, and whatever other information the Intermediary may need in order to perform the review and adjustment function. Upon review of the quarterly report, the Intermediary may adjust the PIP reimbursement amount accordingly. In some cases, the results of the review of the quarterly report will show that the provider is in an underpayment situation. In these cases, the provider may receive a lump sum adjustment (payment) simultaneous with the adjustment of future PIP payments in order to compensate for the underpayments.

The Intermediary is also required to review the PIP reimbursement amount and adjust as necessary upon their completion of the desk review of the annual Medicare Cost Report.

On its own, the provider may act to adjust PIP reimbursement amounts whenever it has reason to believe that costs of the provider have decreased significantly. Similarly, the Intermediary may act to protect the financial interest of Medicare whenever a provider is found to be in a situation of impending bankruptcy or insolvency. Here, as in all cases, the fundamental objective of the Intermediary is to attempt to assure that periodic payments made to the provider exactly match the allowable costs, thus avoiding underpayment and overpayment situations.

The Intermediary may terminate the PIP status of a provider based upon the provider's failure to comply with certain standards. Such termination is generally not automatic, and the standards are used more as general guidelines. If the provider's cost reports show an overpayment situation on a consistent basis (within prescribed parameters), the Intermediary may terminate PIP status on the basis of "abuse." Other potential reasons for termination include failure to file accurate cost and quarterly reports in a timely manner, failure to notify the Intermediary of a significant decrease of Medicare service levels (volume) and failure to notify the Intermediary in cases of significant overpayments where the provider either knew of the overpayment or should have known.

In the case of a new provider, not eligible for PIP as discussed above, reimbursement for Medicare visits is made under special conditions and results in a percentage of charges payment or a cost-per-discipline payment method. Since there is no actual historical cost data to rely on, the Intermediary will first attempt to base the reimbursement upon that made to a similar provider. In cases where the Intermediary can find no "similar provider" on which to base the comparison, the budgeted costs of the new provider will be used as a reimbursement basis. After the first quarterly report is reviewed, the Intermediary will adjust the reimbursement rate as appropriate to take into account the actual cost experience of the new provider.

During the last year, HCFA has made significant effort to eliminate the use of PIP for home health agencies. However, the use of PIP is effective until one year after the transition to the ten intermediaries for freestanding home health agencies. (*1986 Medicare Explained*, Sect. 828.6, 270).

Denials and Waiver of Liability

The findings of a National Association for Home Care (NAHC) study during October to December 1985 found that the "Department of Health and Human Services has instituted a wide panoply of administrative cutbacks in the Medicare home health care benefits." (Halamandaris 1986,5) In this study of 5,300 home health agencies of which 2,100 home health agencies responded, NAHC found that the use of "denied" visits was the main method used to accomplish the cutbacks.

The term "technical denial" was created by HCFA to label a denial of a visit when the Intermediary believed that the home health agency should have known that the patient's condition would not qualify for Medicare reimbursement. In the use of "technical denials," HCFA is distinguishing between a situation where a particular visit to a patient is determined unskilled care, and a situation where *all* visits are denied because the patient's condition does not warrant medical coverage. These include denials for patients who are "too sick" for intermittent care, those "not sick enough," and those determined not to be homebound. Currently, technical denials are not subject to waiver of liability (as defined below) and are appealable only by the beneficiary, without assistance from the provider. On June 24, 1986, the Health Subcommittee of the House Ways and Means Committee introduced legislation under HR 4638 which would allow providers to appeal certain "technical denials." HR 4638 would also allow the provider to assist beneficiaries in their appeals and would extend waiver of liability to the "technical denials."

About 49% of the agencies surveyed in the NAHC study indicated significant increases in technical denials (Halamandaris 1986,5). Part of this increase resulted from some intermediaries increasingly using a standard of "bedbound" instead of "homebound."

Through increased reviews, HCFA has increased denials and consequently decreased payment. "The introduction of the new Medical Review Forms (Form 485-488) is having the intended effect of increasing the denial rate, but is also slowing down the claims-payment process. The national denial rate is up from 3.5 percent in FY 1985 to 5.2 percent in the second quarter of FY 1986. There has also been an increase in nonmedical or technical denials in the second quarter of FY 1986." (HCFA Research Paper 1986)

The result of these denied or rejected claims is significant on the Medicare Cost Report and the fiscal viability of the home health care agency. This stems from:

1. Services rendered which are deemed to be technical denials are not paid by Medicare and are considered due from the patient. However, the patient generally does not understand why Medicare will not pay, and therefore, the payment for the visit is generally not received by the home health agency.

2. Since services were rendered, they are counted in the total visits by discipline for the home health agency. When the Medicare Cost Report is prepared, costs are allocated to the denied visits and away from the Medicare program. This reduces Medicare costs and reimbursement.

Through this analysis, the home health agency may never be paid for the services determined to be "technical denials."

The "waiver of liability" principle was created by Section 213 (a) of the Social Security Amendments of 1972. The purpose of the waiver principle is to "hold harmless" a beneficiary or provider who acted in good faith in accepting or providing services later determined to be noncovered because they were either not reasonable or necessary, or custodial in nature. Specifically, the program will make payments in those instances where the provider and beneficiary "did not know, and could not reasonably have been expected to know, that payment would not be made for such items or services . . . " (*1986 Medicare Explained,* Sect. 828.6, 269-270)

"Because of the many claims that providers submit to Medicare, a system of presumptions was devised to avoid case-by-case review of liability waivers for providers. Under this system, if a provider's denied claims for a year fell below certain pre-established percentages, the provider would be presumed to be capable of making accurate Medicare coverage decisions (this is called a favorable waiver presumption), and therefore would be entitled to a waiver of liability for the few cases where a wrong coverage decision was made." (*1986 Medicare Explained,* Sect. 828.6, 269-270) A favorable waiver presumption is granted to home health agencies with claim denial rates under 2.5%. The denial rate is calculated by dividing the number of visits for which the Intermediary denies coverage by the number of covered visits billed by the home health agency. Under presumptive favorable waiver, payments are made and then the paperwork supporting the visit is reviewed. When the waiver is eliminated, all paperwork is reviewed by the Intermediary before payment is processed.

Regulations enacted in February 1986 eliminated the favorable presumption waiver, thus requiring review of denied claims on a case-by-case basis. (HCFA estimated in the *Federal Register* (February 12, 1985) that elimination of the favorable presumption waiver would save Medicare $93 million in FY 1987, $22 million of which would have been reimbursed to home health agencies.) However, the Consolidated Omnibus Budget Reconciliation Act, passed on April 7, 1986, restored the favorable presumption waiver (except for denial for custodial care grounds) at the 2.5% rate. "Technical denials" do not become part of this calculation. This will be in effect until twelve months after the ten regional Intermediary system has begun operations (*1986 Medicare Explained,* Sect. 828.6,270).

Appeals on Medicare Cost Reports

There are certain appeal rights granted to the home health agencies through Section 1878 of the Social Security Act and the implementing Medicare Regulation (DHHS 1985, Sect. 405.1801 et seq.). The procedures for appeals are specifically stated in the regulations including the time limit in which such an appeal must be made.

In general, the amount of reimbursement in dispute (as a result of the Medicare Cost Report), must be $10,000 or more to qualify for review by the Provider Reimbursement Review Board (PRRB). For amounts over $1,000 but less than $10,000, a Medicare Administrative Law Judge (ALJ) will review the dispute at the request of the provider. This is called an "Intermediary hearing." Although the route is generally not taken, the provider has the right to seek judicial review (in District Court) of a final decision by the PRRB or any action by the Administrative Law Judge involving a question of law. Civil action must be commenced within 60 days after notification of determination is received.

The Provider Reimbursement Review Board is composed of five members, knowledgeable in the field of health care reimbursement, appointed by the Secretary. At least one member of the Board must be a certified public accountant. As required under Section 1878(h) of the Social Security Act, the Secretary selects two of the members from qualified and acceptable nominees of the providers. The Provider Reimbursement Review Board is authorized to make rules and establish procedures necessary to its operation, in accordance with regulations established by the Secretary.

The general requirement for a PRRB appeal is as follows:

- The provider must have filed a timely cost report.
- The adverse final decision of the Fiscal Intermediary must result in a disputed amount of reimbursement of $10,000 or more. (Note: any cost to be disputed must have been originally filed in a cost report or on an acceptable supplemental filing in order to come under these regulations.)
- The appeal must be filed within 100 days after the Fiscal Intermediary renders its final determination.
- Group appeal must be filed by providers under common ownership and amount at issue must aggregate $50,000 or more.

The home health agency has rights as to notice (of time and place) of hearing, representation by counsel, and introduction of reasonable and pertinent evidence to supplement or contradict the evidence considered by the Fiscal Intermediary. All decisions by the PRRB must be made based on the record from this hearing, which can include evidence submitted by the Secretary.

The positions of the PRRB and Administrative Law Judge are unusual in the American judicial system. Both come under the jurisdiction (and are employees of) of the government unit upon which they are ruling and can be reversed, affirmed, or modified (Social Security Act, Sect. 1878(f)(1)) by the Secretary or Assistant Secretary (on behalf of the Secretary). In other words, they are reviewing the work of their "boss."

General Discussion of Increasing Reimbursement

Discrete Costing. The home health agency cost report reflects the three different types of cost centers found within a home health agency. General service cost centers are those for divisions or departments operated for the benefit of the provider as a whole. Reimbursable cost centers are those for which Medicare will reimburse the provider on a reasonable cost basis. Nonreimbursable cost centers are those relating to services not covered by the Medicare program. The nonreimbursable and reimbursable cost centers are also known as "specific" service cost centers, in contrast to the general service cost centers which represent overhead costs.

The objective of cost finding in the context of preparing the cost report is to allocate the general service costs among the various reimbursable and nonreimbursable cost centers.

Until recently, home health agencies were required by regulation to allocate general service costs using the step-down method of cost finding. Under this method, the general service cost center costs were allocated among the other cost centers (both reimbursable and nonreimbursable) on the basis of prescribed statistical basis. For example, depreciation expense is allocated to the specific service cost centers on the basis of square footage. Accordingly, a specific service cost center occupying 10% of the total provider floor space would be allocated 10% of the depreciation expense.

A similar allocation is made for administrative and general costs. This is a sort of "catch all" cost center which tends to accumulate all of those costs which cannot be specifically assigned elsewhere. In the case of administrative and general costs, allocation is made to the specific service cost centers based upon total accumulated costs. This includes not only those costs specifically attributable but also those allocated from the other general service cost centers, all of which are allocated prior to the administrative and general cost center.

The step-down method of cost finding was not considered satisfactory by many home health agencies who felt that the prescribed statistical allocation basis did not fairly allocate general service overhead costs between the reimbursable and nonreimbursable cost centers. A specific example of the impact of cost finding on non-Medicare reimbursable centers is found in home health agencies who contract with HMOs. The accounting and administrative costs are allocated based on the accumulated costs in this cost center even though there is very little accounting and administrative time required. The portion of these expenses that are allocated to the HMO contracts would share on a direct percentage with the Medicare cost centers even though it is not reflective of actual costs incurred. In response, many providers initiated corporate reorganization designed to legally segregate the reimbursable and nonreimbursable activities, and the related general and administrative costs.

In response to the trend toward reorganization, HCFA had prepared a new position memorandum on discrete costing by home health agencies (Booth 1985) which resulted in the revision of Chapter 23 of the Medicare Provider Reimbursement Manual (HCFA Publication 15-1) in early 1986.

Discrete costing involves the direct assignment of general service costs to specific service cost centers based upon measurements of actual usage, instead of the prescribed statistical allocation basis per the step-down method. The advantage of discrete costing is that overhead costs can now be assigned to specific service cost centers before the step-down process, resulting in what is presumably a more equitable cost finding.

Although the new cost-finding methodology allows the provider relative flexibility in the establishing of cost centers within what was previously the administrative and general "catch all" category, there are other very specific requirements which must be met.

In order to take advantage of discrete costing, the entities within the provider must be kept physically distinct. In addition, they must be operated and supervised separately, and maintain separate records and accounting data contemporaneously.

Also, the provider must request permission from the Fiscal Intermediary to use discrete cost finding in advance of the start of the fiscal year for which it is to be adopted. To obtain this, the provider must satisfy the FI that the cost-finding changes proposed by the home health agency represent an improvement to the step-down method and will result in greater accuracy in cost finding. This claim is, of course, subject to audit verification. Cost reports prepared and filed using the new discrete cost-finding methodology must be accompanied by supporting schedules detailing the cost allocations reflected in the report.

Shared overhead cost centers must be directly costed between the reimbursable nd nonreimbursable cost centers; the total portion attributable to reimbursable cost centers will then be allocated to specific reimbursable cost centers using the step-down method.

There are two critical factors to be considered in the decision to use discrete cost finding in lieu of the traditional step-down method. The first is the need to establish and maintain wholly separate records and accounting. Where this is not or cannot be done, the step-down method remains mandatory. The second is that although HCFA has published revision to the Medicare Provider Reimbursement Manual, specific instructions were not given to the FI, only guidelines. There is concern in the industry that since each Intermediary approves the discrete costing methodology for their specific home health agencies, this will provide too much discretion at the FI level in the application of these regulations (Thomas 1986,131).

The Impact of the Restructured Agency on Medicare Reimbursement. After reviewing the methodology behind Medicare cost reporting and cost finding, it is often fiscally and physically possible to separate noncovered Medicare activities from the Medicare-covered services. Medicare will review such reorganization very carefully, but as long as the organizational structure and operations actually conform to the new corporate organization, these attacks can be mitigated. The use of the corporate structure that includes a parent foundation and subsidiaries for the different services requires the use of a "Home Office" cost report, but does provide for the most defensible structure (Table 22-5).

The reimbursement impact of providing non-Medicare services in a Medicare agency is that the costs will be allocated to all cost centers (Medicare and non-Medicare) based on the allocated costs (and other statistics). This generally results in

Table 22-5. Sample corporate structure

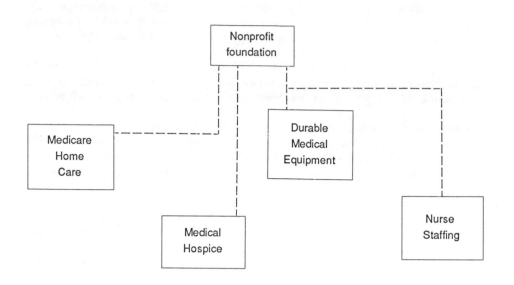

the costs of Medicare billing and compliance (plan of treatment, documentation, audit, etc.) being shared by non-Medicare cost centers, and thereby not being paid by Medicare through traditional cost finding. Since non-Medicare services are generally lower costing services, there is not enough gross margin in these services to cover their own direct and indirect costs, plus the allocated costs from Medicare.

Experienced legal and accounting counsel should be obtained to determine the impact to the agency (reimbursement, legal, functional) and the many options available to meet the objectives of restructuring.

Medicare Future Reimbursement Trends

What HCFA will develop for home care will probably result from the hospital reimbursement changes. Based on the lead of hospital reimbursement, the home health agency should expect some form of a Prospective Payment System (PPS) (Lorenz 1984,27). It is hoped that such a system might promote efficiency and help to contain costs among home health providers. One major problem is that the diagnosis-related groupings in use for hospital prospective payment systems are not applicable to home health care. In addition, the availability of appropriate rating methods for a home health care PPS are in the infancy of development.

In December 1983, HCFA awarded a contract to Abt Associates to conduct a five-year Prospective Payment Demonstration utilizing 120 home health agencies in ten states to test alternative methods of paying for home health care services. There were three payment methods being considered: (1) rates per visit by type of service (e.g., skilled nursing); (2) rates per patient month; and (3) rates per episode of care (Williams and Spencer 1984, 24-25; Rak 1985).

The proposed "per-visit" method would set a rate per visit for each agency, one for each of the six visit types. A separate rate per patient would be set to cover overhead and would be paid by lump sum. This method would not allow for year-end adjustments.

The "per-patient-month" method would establish three different rates for the first three months of care, with the highest rate paid for the first month and the lowest for the third month. After 180 days, payment would switch to the per-visit method. These rates would be predetermined and would not change, regardless of the severity of the patient's illness. This method would include a year-end case-mix adjustment.

Last, the "per-episode" method would involve a single, flat payment for each episode of care up to 180 days. After 180 days, payment would again revert to the per-visit method. This method is ideologically similar to the prospective system of diagnosis-related groupings (DRGs) utilized for hospital payments. This method would also include a year-end case-mix adjustment.

Other proposals have been made for a "PPS" type of system. These proposals have come from the home care trade organizations for consideration by HCFA and Congress. None of these proposals have been adopted as of this writing.

Reimbursement under a home health PPS would allow home health administrators to make business decisions, knowing the amount that will be paid, without the "second guessing" that results from the end of year cost report/cost-finding calculation. With the increased possibility for gain, the badly managed agencies will not be able to stand behind the shield of the cost-based reimbursements. Dynamic and positive managers will be needed to respond to a prospective payment systems environment.

In the meantime, reimbursement for home health care will continue to be squeezed. The Balanced Budget and Emergency Control Act of 1985 (also known as the Gramm-Rudman-Hollings Act) reduced reimbursement to home health agencies by 1% starting March 1, 1986. This was a reduction from reimbursements, not limits, which may again threaten the longevity of many home health agencies who have high Medicare utilization. In addition, the cost limits are to be decreased to 112% of the mean starting in 1987. Medicare has also developed more standards to calculate excess costs by specific categories, such as administrator's salaries and fringes.

The result of these Medicare reductions in reimbursement may be that many reluctant home health agency mangers may look forward to a known prospective payment system method of reimbursement.

Other Payment Sources

Home health care benefits are available from sources other than Medicare. Sources include private commercial insurance companies, Medicaid, Blue Cross, and prepaid plans such as health maintenance and preferred provider organizations. Increasingly, insurance carriers are being pressured into including home care as a health insurance benefit; however, home health agencies often experience difficulty in collecting reimbursement from these carriers. This is due in part to a lack of uniformity among these carriers concerning home care benefits and to a certain lack of experience by home health agencies in working with the insurance companies.

Commercial insurance carriers write benefits differently for each contract. As a result, each client's benefits are different. A home health agency has a responsibility to determine coverage by dealing directly with the insurance company. Like Medicare, commercial insurance companies limit coverage for home health care. Limits include: cost caps, "total benefits available" amounts, and deductible and co-insurance amounts due from the patient. There are also time limits imposed and "medical necessity" determinations to be made. Commercial insurance companies usually pay on the basis of reasonable and customary charges. Unlike Medicare, the patient is responsible for any amount not covered by the insurance.

Under the Medicaid program, each state administers its own home health care service program and acts as a third-party insurer to reimburse home care agencies. Therefore, the extent of home care benefits varies from state to state, although each state is required to offer certain nursing and home health aide benefits. As with Medicare, there must be a written treatment plan submitted by a physician. Unlike Medicare, regulations are not as stringent as to "skilled" nursing and restorative potential. Unfortunately, home health care services have generally been poorly utilized under the Medicaid program because reimbursement is low, often lower than actual costs. Medicaid reimbursement may differ from the Medicare reimbursement tenet of lower of cost or charges. In some states, Medicaid pays at a flat rate per visit, regardless of the cost of that visit.

Blue Cross-Blue Shield offers benefits for home health care under Blue Cross, with some pharmaceuticals and supplies covered under the major medical portion of the plan. There are 79 autonomous Blue Cross organizations in operation nationwide, with greater than 90% offering home health benefits. Each Blue Cross organization negotiates its own contracts with participating home health providers and thus there are variations in the type of benefits offered and in the method of reimbursement utilized. Generally, home health benefits are offered in lieu of a hospital stay and a prior hospitalization is required. The core of covered services includes: physician visits, skilled nursing, physical, occupational, and speech therapy, home health aide service, medical social services, and respiratory therapy. The majority of Blue Cross plans reimburse providers based on customary and reasonable charges. Some reimburse on a cost basis similar to Medicare, and require submission of a cost report. A few have implemented a prospective payment system for home health or hospice care.

The Veteran's Administration has made a commitment to home health care. Veterans in need of home health care following hospitalization receive services from either a VA hospital-based home care program or from a community home health agency selected by the VA. Some of the services available include: physician care, professional nursing, home health aide, rehabilitation therapy, dietetic and social work services. In addition, there are special home care units for veterans with spinal cord injuries offering services similar to those of the hospital-based home care programs.

Prepaid health plans, such as HMOs and PPOs, "are and will continue to be important users of and customers for home care products and services." (Louden and Leavenworth 1986,4-6) Due to the inherent financial nature of such health plans, HMOs and PPOs are driven to keep health care costs down and are, therefore, dependent on home health care as an effective alternative to hospitalization. The results of a recent survey of HMOs and PPOs revealed that only 1 to 3% of total enrollee health care expenditures were spent on home health care, but the forecast is for expenditures to increase to 5 to 10% within the next five years (Louden and Leavenworth 1986,4-6). Further, HMOs are now enrolling Medicare-eligible patients on a prepaid basis, with HMOs entitled to keep 100% of any cost savings they are able to attain. As a result, some HMOs are now actively going after Medicare beneficiaries. The services offered by most HMOs and PPOs vary from plan to plan, but generally seem to be patterned after Medicare. However, HMOs seem to cover more services than Medicare. Some of the terms of coverage are: caps on number of days and visits allowed, copayment and deductible amounts charged to the patient, required purchase of plan rider, physician prescription for services, and per-case evaluations.

As HCFA continues to try to tighten the purse strings of the Medicare program, home health care providers will need to explore new opportunities for growth and will need to generate more revenue from the private insurance sector. Given the dramatic growth of HMOs and PPOs and future trends in the health care system, home health care providers will need to look toward developing relationships with such prepaid plans to ensure survival.

Postscript

On October 17, 1986, the Omnibus Budget Reconciliation Act of 1986 (OBRA) was passed by both the House and the Senate. The significant features of OBRA include:

1. Cost limits are returned to the aggregate for reimbursement for cost-reporting periods beginning on or after July 1, 1986.

2. Cost limits established for cost-reporting periods beginning on or after July 1, 1986, must be set by the Department of Health and Human Services (HHS) based on the most recent data available, but no earlier than for cost-reporting periods October 1, 1983, and must account for increased costs due to requirements of billing and data collection imposed by HHS.

3. Congress requires a General Accounting Office (GAO) report by February 1, 1988, regarding the impact on Medicare beneficiaries of applying per-visit limitations on a discipline-specific basis and the overall appropriateness of percentage limits established by regulation.

4. Provider representation of beneficiary Part A and Part B appeals is now allowed. However, only the cost of successful appeals will be considered a reasonable cost. In addition, providers can not charge beneficiaries for the ser-

vice. Under Part B, an administrative judge hearing is provided for amounts of $500 to $999; and a judicial review is provided for amounts over $1,000.

5. Prompt payment of 95% of all "clean claims" are required within 30 days beginning October 1, 1986; 26 days, as of October 1, 1987; 25 days, as of October 1988; and 24 days beginning October 1, 1989, and thereafter. Interest will be paid for the period on the day that the payment should have been made until the day the payment is actually made. The definition of "clean claim" is embodied in the Act as a claim having "no defect or impropriety (including any lack of required substantiating documentation) or particular circumstances requiring special treatment that prevents timely payment from being made." Claims received on or after November 1, 1986, are affected by this provision.

6. The Peer Review Organization (PRO) is now to assure quality of care in home health agencies as of October 1, 1987. In addition HHS must report to Congress by two years from the date of enactment based on a study in the development of a quality review and assurance strategy. As part of this report, Congress is requiring HHS to develop uniform needs assessment instruments that can be used by discharge planners, hospitals, nursing facilities, other health care providers in evaluating the need for posthospital services covering any extended services such as home health services on long-term care. In addition, the intermediaries will be required to use the same standards.

7. In conjunction with the quality of care issues, Congress has established a "demonstration program: of at least four projects on *prior and concurrent authorization* for posthospital home health services and extended care under Part A or Part B. These projects must be started by January 1, 1987. Specific requirements for this project and the advisory board are in the legislation.

8. Congress has established a demonstration project for Alzheimer's Disease.

9. The 2.5% favorable presumptive waiver of liability has been extended to coverage denials based on "technical denials" (homebound or intermittent care requirement issues) effective for denials occurring on or after July 1, 1987, until September 30, 1989. This timeframe allows for the report required from HHS to Congress in March 1987 and 1988 on denials: type, frequency, rates of reversals, and "other information as may be appropriate to evaluate the appropriateness of any percentage standards established for the granting of favorable presumptions with respect to such denials."

10. Occupational Therapy Services are now a covered Part B service in the therapist's office or in the beneficiary's home after July 1, 1987.

Health Care Financing Administration has issued regulations to comply with the Deficit Reduction Act of 1984 (DEFRA) and also to eliminate the carryover of amount not reimbursed under the lower of cost or charges (LCC) principle. The effective date of the LCC elimination will be determined when the final rule is issued. The changes required by DEFRA are effective for cost-reporting periods beginning October 1, 1984, and cover:

- Elimination of the aggregating Part A and Part B costs and charges for LCC comparisons

- Home health agency durable medical equipment (DME) reimbursement at the lesser of cost or charges (not to exceed 80% of cost)

- Changes to the "nominal charge" provisions

HCFA has now released the new Medicare Cost report (Form HCFA-1728-86). This cost report incorporates the cost-per-discipline limitations and some changes in format on the schedules. The 1728-86 is required for all cost-reporting periods beginning on or after July 1, 1985.

References

Booth, C. 1985. Cost finding for HHA's. Memo March 5, 1985. *Caring* July 1985.

Department of Health and Human Services. 1985. Code of Federal Regulations (Title 42): Section 405.1801 et seq. Washington, DC: Government Printing Office.

Federal Register. 1986. Volume 51, Number 104. Washington, DC: Government Printing Office.

Halamandaris, V. 1984. Home health care market trends. *Caring* June 1984.

Halamandaris, V. 1986. Medicare: The broken promise. *Caring* March 1986.

Home Health & Hospice Manual. 1985. Owings Mills, MD: Rynd Communications, Inc.

Have HCFA initiatives impacted too heavily on home health agencies (HHA's)? 1986. HCFA Research Paper, Bureau of Program Operations.

Lorenz, B. 1984. Prospective reimbursement in health care; Related problems and opportunities for home health agencies. *Caring* February 1984.

Louden, T. L., and E. R. Leavenworth. 1986. HMO/PPO perspectives on home care: A national survey. *Caring* May 1986.

Medicare and Medicaid Guide. Chicago: Commerce Clearing House, Inc.

1986 Medicare Explained. 1986. Chicago: Commerce Clearing House, Inc.

Rak, K. 1985. Home Health Line Vol. X (March 11, 1985).

Shaw, S. 1985. The changing marketplace. *Caring* July 1985.

Stewart, J. E. 1979. *Home health care.* St. Louis: C. V. Mosby Co.

Thomas, J. 1986. HCFA considers a new Medicare costing fix, but will it work for home health? *Home Health Line.*

Williams, J. L., and S. E. W. Spencer. 1984. Home health agency prospective payment demonstration. *Caring* October 1984.

Chapter Twenty-Three

Management Information Systems

Charlotte L. Kohler

What is MIS?

By analyzing the words "Management Information System" it is easy to see that computerization is not part of it. Any systematic information-gathering and recordkeeping method that allows accurate, timely, and useful information to the management of a business is a Management Information System (MIS).

MIS has become closely aligned with the concepts and theories of computerization, where the words "data processing" imply the need to process a large volume of small data elements to provide the needed information to management.

In our experience, we have audited some health agencies that have maintained a very timely and efficient manual billing and accounts receivable systems. Until recently (1984), we determined that there was no need to go to a computerized system. However, the manual system did not provide the home health agency management important information needed to assess the demographics of their patient population and evaluate growth trends.

The use of manual systems, often called "one-write or pegboard" systems, will provide a method to analyze and summarize data. However, when a home health agency has a large number of individual items that must be analyzed and summarized, the time and personnel time requirements will become burdensome. As a result, in a manual system, the amount of analysis will be reduced to a level justified by the cost and the time available.

The benefit of computerization is that after the data are entered, the billing is prepared, data can be summarized, analyzed, and reported. If a data base software package is used, the management reports available to management are generally unlimited. Analysis of data may be current, by comparisons to prior months or years, or by the analysis of data elements at any time they become important in the management of the home health agency.

A good example of how data elements can change in their relative importance to a home health agency is the analysis we performed to determine the financial implications to a home health agency which was considering a prospective payment methodology based on episodes of illness. This methodology also included additional payment for outliers. With the data base in the computer system, we were able to sort on data elements for which the home health agency had no managerial reason to analyze and compare before this prospective payment alternative had required such an analysis. This database was available as a by-product of patient registration and daily charge input. The management of these agencies developed a clear understanding of the impact and how they should respond to the proposal.

The movement toward some prospective payment mechanism for home care reinforces the need for management information systems with managers that effectively utilize the information available to them.

A new concept in MIS for home care has been introduced as "Medical Information System" by J. H. Muellin (1986), in response to changes in PPS for hospital reimbursements. Dr. Muellin believes that the use of computers will move HHAs toward the gathering of clinical data; they will not be limited to the financial data. The use of Medical Information Systems will provide both administrative information and procedure. The availability and use of these data will assist the home health agency in becoming a strong provider of those services not found in the traditional home health agency. Portable data acquisition devices (DADS) will obtain clinical data (from EKGs, for example) which will be transferred to the computer system for clinical analysis. Although it may take the computer and medical industry some time to catch up with the idea, the home health care agency, through the use of more sophisticated MIS, "has effectively leveraged its only assets: cost-effective and timely access to patients at home." (Muellin 1986, 36)

The Marvelous World of Computers!

To see the computer circus in action just visit any of a dozen major computer shows. You'll experience dazzling bewilderment: giant bananas, jumping frogs, flashing lights, models in bikinis, blaring music, free gifts, popcorn and cotton candy. You'll see a lot, you'll also miss a lot. And the systems will come from all sides—big screens, little screens; big prices—little prices; big promises—empty claims; RAMS and ROMS, bytes and bits, Winchesters and floppies. (Tolos and Moody 1986)

In selecting and evaluating a computer system for the home health agency, it is possible to feel like a part of the circus, not just the audience. Carl Knauer, CPA, believes that prospective microcomputer purchasers can fall into two extremes (Knauer 1984).

"Extinct by Instinct"—this is the impulsive decision maker who is easily persuaded by the flashy demonstration and dazzling display.
"Paralysis by Analysis"—the mystery of computers causes these managers to ponder all avenues waiting for better prices, technology, or new products. No decision is ever made.
It is time to stop, and proceed slowly but diligently.

A commitment of effort and time is required before a manager can be comfortable with a computer system selection. Your mission is to evaluate your needs and select a computer system that will do exactly what the home health agency needs and wants. You are committing the future of the home health agency to whichever computer system you select. It is one of the most important financial decisions that a home health agency makes.

As difficult as this decision may be, and even in this period of constant changes in both hardware and software, you should consider the substantial benefit of computerization and move forward.

The increased complexity in home health care billing and reporting increases the need that management has for a sophisticated computer and MIS system. The use and selection of an automated system must be made systematically to obtain the desired results. Otherwise, the home health agency may find out what the first theorem of computers really is: GIGO (garbage in garbage out).

The needs will be determined by performing a detailed analysis of the computer system specifications. This will require a significant amount of time from the home health agency administrator and staff, in addition to, proper use of outside consultants. Outside consultants can either help or hinder the process. At the present time, unfortunately, there is no certification process to identify a consultant with bona fide training and experience in computer applications related to home health care organizations. The contract must be specific and is generally established on an hourly fee arrangement. Although it may seem easier to have one of the vendors perform this function, the vendor can hardly be in a position to provide you with an independent analysis of which system would be best for your HHA.

What to Look for in Automation and MIS

Computerization or automation is available to the home health agency on several levels. These range from batch processing, to home health agency terminal entry (batch processing, or on-line) to an in-house microcomputer-based system and finally to mainframe home health agency software applications.

The choice of which type of processing depends on the internal application needed by the home health agency, the available staffing and capabilities, and the initial and ongoing costs (Exhibit 23-1). These costs are measured by including the costs of software, hardware, on-line processing costs, personnel, office space needs, paper, insurance and any other directly related cost associated with each option.

In making the decision to computerize, software is selected first, then the compatible hardware is selected. The most common mistake for first time buyers is to select hardware first. You may select an excellent machine but you need the programs to run on it. The software programs should be specifically designed to help you perform your tasks. The modules, or application programs, commonly available are:

- Billing, statistical reporting, and accounts receivable
- General ledger
- Accounts payable
- Payroll
- Sick and vacation (accrual and taken)
- Fixed asset reporting
- Inventory/DME control

Exhibit 23-1. Comparison of Data Processing Levels

Type	Considerations
Batch processing	• Low front end dollar commitment
	• Monthly processing costs directly related to volume
	• Little control over processing time
	• Balancing with service bureau may be difficult
	• Little management reporting above basic (standard) level
	• Reporting to management at specified time (monthly)
Batch processing with home health agency terminal input	• Moderate front end dollar commitment
	• Monthly processing costs increase over batch processing but are generally directly related to volume; include data transmission costs
	• More control over processing
	• More personnel costs due to input requirements.
	• Balancing done by home health agency staff at time of entry
	• Generally, reports have the same level of sophistication as batch processing
On-line processing (service bureau)	• Front end dollar commitment covers terminals and printers
	• Monthly costs are a combination of volume related processing costs and fixed payments relating to equipment
	• Balancing and processing performed at home health agency (some service bureau may perform certain tasks, such as mailing bills or statements from the service bureau location)
	• More control over processing
	• Reporting may be more responsive and flexible by allowing home health agency to run its own specialized reports
In-house system	• Front end costs can be significant in both hardware and conversion
	• Monthly costs tend to be at a fixed level regardless of volume
	• All processing performed internally with schedule established by home health agency based on their needs
	• May include customizing of software for home health agency
	• Responsibility for data backups left to home health agency

- Plan of treatment (and Form 485-488)
- Word processing
- Spreadsheet program (for modeling, end of year planning, etc.)
- Cost reporting
- Electronic bill transmission
- Scheduling

The terms "bundled," "unbundled," or "turnkey" are often used in the sales presentation on in-house systems. Bundled or turnkey systems are substantially the same in concept: the vendor combines hardware and software into a "package" to be sold as one unit. Unbundled software allows you the choice of several hardware vendors with which the software is compatible.

In choosing a turnkey or bundled system, the vendor is responsible for any problem with both software and hardware. In choosing an unbundled computer package, the home health agency must coordinate activities and problems between the software vendor and the hardware vendor. In some cases, the unbundled system is the better choice if:

- The software vendor's location is far from you and faster service could be provided from a local hardware vendor (down time is more often caused by hardware problems than by software problems).

- You can negotiate a better price for hardware from local vendors (however, this "savings" must be offset against the future coordination time between hardware and software vendors).

- You already have compatible hardware in your home health agency.

In addition, the home health agency must decide whether to choose "multiuser" (at multiple branch locations, as well) or "multitasking." Multiuser is the ability of the system to accept and process from several terminals at a time. Multitasking permits several users, all doing different things. For example, the accounting department could process general ledger and payroll, at the same time that new patients are being entered and scheduling is being revised by someone else at the HHA.

After the software is selected, the hardware needs are determined. The pertinent areas to be considered are:

1. Processor size — This equates with the speed required for the number of unique data elements and the volume of visits (or data elements) to be processed.

2. Memory size — This is a result of determining the storage capacity needs, based on size of home health agency, software file structure, and level of multiuser, multitasking sophistication.

3. CRTs and printers — The number of each must be determined based on function, staff, and layout of office (or branches).

4. Communication lines — These are used for electronic billing and also for communication between different locations. In considering modem communications, the cost/benefit of this method of data transfer must be investigated.

In all these areas, the experienced systems analyst from your selected software vendor must assist you. It is prudent to have a guarantee by your vendor for upgrade requirements above those recommended for the first year. This is because you may incur substantial additional costs if the hardware or software requirements have been undersized in an effort to make the sale. However, to do this, the vendor must have realistic volume projections from the home health agency to estimate the input/output specifications.

There are other concerns that are often overlooked in computerizing: freight, supplies, sales tax, installation, training (cost and location), conversion (costs and timing), hardware and software support, computer consulting, legal review of contracts, adequacy of air-conditioning, special carpeting, and costs of laying cables.

Therefore, in determining what the expectations should be for automation, your steps are to: (1) select the applications needed; (2) determine the hardware requirements; (3) determine the total costs to computerize; and (4) evaluate the contract provisions and guarantees.

Why Should We Computerize?

Sometimes the feeling starts as an uncomfortable choking experience. This normally happens as the mounds of paper swell and management and staff are overwhelmed. It is difficult to make decisions based on data, trends, or projections.

Although the reasons to computerize may be more subtle, the basis for automation should be evaluated considering the future needs of the home health agency.

Mary Lou Pritichard (Executive Director, Buckeye Home Health Service, Inc., Logan, OH) had to consider resources within her rural home health agency and determined that "one of the hallmarks of her plan was to implement computing capabilities which were financially feasible and for the agency management to have control of the system. She emphasized that the lack of capital resources made it important to place a priority on having the financial system in excellent condition and then plan for clinical systems when the technology she believes is appropriate is technically available and financially affordable." (McIlvane 1986, 50)

On the other hand, David Baker (Director of St. Mary's Home Health Hospice Center, Knoxville, IN) (1980, 21-26) addressed the needs of a hospital-based agency with rapid growth. Baker was concerned about the transition from having the hospital perform the billings and statistical reporting to a computer system that the home health agency could use itself to perform these functions. He also believed that increased and more sophisticated reporting from the home health MIS system was required for good management. This industry-specific data gathering and analysis was not normally available from a hospital system.

Although these two home health agency directors were analyzing the needs of agencies substantially different in growth, size, and corporate structure, their concerns were similar. General concerns which will develop into a "should we computerize" are:

1. More efficient managing. Detailed reports can be generated weekly, daily, or immediately. The computer can handle many routine decisions that often tie up home health agency management. Management, in addition to analyzing historic business and patient care patterns and trends, can initiate realistic projections and forecast techniques.

2. Reduced costs. The system can reduce costs by reducing the level of paper-work and clerical activity.

3. Increased profit potential. The system can increase profit potential by generating all insurance and third party invoices quickly and by following up on over-due accounts. Comprehensive reports provide current information on patient and third party payments and balances.

4. Becoming more competitive in the marketplace. Increasing productivity, improving efficiency, and raising the level of patient service enables a home health agency to become more competitive. The financial impact of a capitated or prospective payment system can be evaluated, and the home health agency can be with the leaders in home health care.

Before choosing to computerize, each home health agency must analyze why computerization is a correct decision. "Keeping up with the Jones" is not a good reason unless the Jones' home health agency is becoming a stronger home health agency due to better management, better marketing, and better fiscal planning resulting from their MIS.

When Should A Home Health Agency Computerize?

It would be simple if there was a home health agency industry standard based on the number of patients or visit which would say, "A home health agency should always automate when they reach 12,000 visits per year." Fortunately, or unfortunately, there is no simple and fixed rule. The reasons for computerizing will provide guidance to the right time to computerize.

Philip Elam (the former director of MAS for Dohm & Wolf, a Dallas CPA firm), President of Business Computer Solutions, provides the advice that the "when" is generally as soon as possible. He uses several indicators to gauge the need for automation.

- Disappointing revenue growth. Because of the past, the economy, the competition, or Medicare reduction in coverage, business growth is not matching predictions.

- Disturbing profit trends. Compared with previous performance in the industry, profits are down.

- Various financial and statistical indications of suboptimal operation. These include factors such as lengthening of the average age of receivables; increases in bad debt losses; excessive employee overtime; reduction in the ratio of reimbursement to revenue-generated equity or other assets; and reduced revenue dollars per patient.

- A chaotic work environment. Employees rush frantically from problem to problem.

- Lack of information. The frustration of knowing too little about what is happening reduces productivity and reimbursement.

- Lack of uniformity. Records are not updated with any degree of standardization, procedures are not followed in every situation, and decisions are not always made on a uniform basis.

After determining that it is time to computerize, there will be some normal hesitation as to what the concept of "change" can bring. Additional hesitation is a natural response in realizing the high level of effort required to computerize. When still in doubt "that now is the time" to purchase the computer system, Mr. Elam indicates that four additional points should be considered:

- If a small business computer would save money or make money for the home health agency *now,* then the HHA is *losing* money by not having it.

- Peripherals (i.e., printers, hard disks, etc.) and software will be useful even if the computer becomes obsolete. The computer itself is usually the least expensive component of all and can be used for other, noncritical processing.

- The features of today's computers probably are more than a home health agency needs, but this means that the computer bought today should continue to meet the needs as the home health agency grows.

- By owning a computer now, a home health agency can obtain the benefits of automation while learning. If the need arises to upgrade to a larger, more powerful system, it will be easier.

Additionally, while Medicare reimburses using cost finding, many of these costs for computer conversion will be covered by Medicare. A prospective payment methodology will not generally provide additional payments to the HHA to automate.

The Durable Medical Equipment (DME) companies discuss standards of 75 to 100 patients per month (Liska 1986, 139) as the optional point in their industry, at which time the DME supplier should start shopping for a computer. DME companies have been generally more aggressive in automation and are outspoken as to the consequences of not automating. Per James Liska on DME companies:

"After the dust settles I think you will find out the strong [DME] dealers will survive, the weak will not. The strong ones will appreciate the value of a computer to keep them managed and expand their business and to pinpoint marketing effort." (Liska 1986,138)

These comments are appropriate for the home health agencies, as well. The home health agency that has strong data processing and management reporting systems, early in its development, will manage its growth with effectiveness and efficiency.

Developing Your Own Computerized Software

By using existing software products that meet your specifications, the home health agency will save time and money. However, one disadvantage of using standard, or "canned" packages is that the user will often have to make some compromises in its specifications or in the way in which they have traditionally processed their paperwork or coding. Nonetheless, it is better to have a compromise system that works and does most of what a home health agency wants (and needs) than to insist on a "perfect" system that never is achieved.

After hiring an experienced systems analyst (with home health care experience), the development of a home health care billing, statistical reporting, and accounts receivable package can require 18 months for programming and testing, development of documentation and the users manual, and the creation of support services; add to this time factor several hundreds of thousands of dollars. (Robert Robertson, President, CareData System, Indianapolis, IN, June 1986)

One of the prime risks of using customized software is that it can contain bugs or errors which, surprisingly, can exist undetected for months or even years before making a sudden and very unwelcome appearance. Existing software packages, on the other hand, allow users to examine their performance. Even if a package has been on the market for only a few months, it probably has the equivalent of many years of usage. This extensive usage tends to minimize the risk of bugs or errors.

In an industry that must adapt quickly to new Medicare requirements, the vendors with existing software are ready for these changes. The home health agency needs software that is specifically developed for home care, that can accommodate changes in a timely manner, and that is at the forefront of improving management and the medical information system.

Are There Any Guarantees?

Warranties are a source of continuing and troublesome questions. Generally, existing software is provided "as is" without any warranties. Unlike many other products, software is subject to so many variables in use, and its evaluation is so subjective that vendors, as a practical matter, could not charge enough for mass-marketed software to cover their exposure to warranty problems. *This means that the home health agency assumes all risk for the operation and suitability of the selected package.* Thus, the home health agency must be aware of the strengths and weaknesses of a given package before selecting it.

A home health agency who contracts for custom software may be able to obtain a warranty that the product will substantially conform to the agreed specifications for some period of time. This is why clearly defined and written specifications are crucial to any determination as to whether a warranty has been breached. Even these warranties, however, will not protect you from missing requirements in your specifications.

For existing or "canned" packages, use the following steps to test the software package:

1. Use the package itself for testing, not the demonstration model. Try a section of the program *yourself.*

2. Determine if the software is "user-friendly" by determining how the help screens, menus, and on-line tutorials assist you.

3. Test your requirements against the features included in the package.

4. Review the documentation (instruction manual) to determine that it is clearly written, understandable, and helpful.

Even though a contract disclaims all warranties, vendors will generally attempt to limit their liability for damages usually to the cost of the package, if they are found liable for breach of contract.

Acceptance Testing for Custom Software

Since software in intangible, there is always the question of whether a package (written or modified to the home health agency's specifications) is performing in accordance with such specifications. Consequently, an acceptance test should be incorporated into a software development contract to provide an objective measure of whether the software corresponds to the specifications, using data supplied by the home health agency. This test should be performed on the vendor's premises to the satisfaction of the user before the software is installed in the home health agency's place of business and before any final payment is made.

Final Thoughts

Custom software is the most expensive option in software selection. It will require the greatest expenditure as well as the greatest effort from your staff. You will generally need to hire an experienced systems analyst or developer to assist you in negotiating with the software development house. During the time of development, the home health agency must have another system to handle the ongoing billing and reporting. It is a decision to be made with a great deal of forethought and foreboding.

In contract negotiations, be sure that the *source* code and all documentation will be property of the home health agency. In this way, if the home health agency and the software development company choose to take different paths, the home health agency is safeguarded by having all its programs which can be maintained and modified by some other software house. For "canned" software, the source code should be maintained by some third party (banker, lawyer, trade association) so that the HHA would be protected should the software vendor go out of business.

In your software and hardware maintenance agreement be sure that the response time is stated and that there is a clear description of costs and timing of software upgrades.

Minimize the Risk of Buying Inadequate Software

The bad story: Software often turns out to be unsuitable or unworkable. A great deal of time and money can be devoted to software that does not perform as expected. The ultimate costs of poorly performing software can far exceed the direct costs paid for the packages.

To minimize the risk in the software purchase, the unexpected problems should be avoided. To avoid these problems, the five major reasons why users encounter software problems and the appropriate response should be understood and are listed below.

1. Software cannot be examined. Only the results of using it can be examined. The home health agency staff will purchase the software but may fail to test all functions of a given piece of software. As a result, inadequate capabilities — such as insufficient report-generation capacity, or ability to retain month-to-month data for comparison or update purposes may go unnoticed.

2. There are no objective home health agency industry standards for comparing the capabilities of various software packages. (Each package is, to a great extent, unique.) To a certain degree, this difficulty can be surmounted by the use of standardized tests, called benchmarks. Although, these are time-consuming and expensive to develop, the home health agency is often left to develop them on their own based on what may be limited exposure to software selection requirements.

3. Many users, surprisingly, do not really understand their business operations. This problem is often compounded by the unrealistic assumption that a few hours of discussion will allow a software vendor to understand both the home health agency's business operations and the home health agency's data processing needs.

4. Many prospective computer users do not have a clear understanding of the capabilities and inherent limitations of computerization.

5. Users and vendors have substantially different expectations as to the transaction. Users (home health agencies) expect to obtain a program that will make a continuing contribution to their business operations, while vendors are interested in concluding the sale and moving on to the next one.

Before you are in a position to evaluate software, you have to define your needs. This is not only a time-consuming process, but it is also one of the biggest stumbling blocks for first time users. This critical, multifaceted review of current and futureoperations will impact on selection, implementation, and results.

To ensure a good system selection, there are five steps a user can take to minimize risk in a new software acquisition (although they do not guarantee a trouble-free installation):

1. Obtain the services of a home health care or computer consultant to assist you in the next four steps. These steps should be left to the consultant. The consultant should work in a objective capacity.

2. Define, as specifically as possible, the organization's goals and objectives. These have nothing to do directly with any particular software or hardware: rather, they define what is to be accomplished. Typical goals are improved information on how the home health agency is functioning and improved internal operations. More specific goals, for example, can include improving skilled nursing productivity (by installing a word processing system), providing better management control (by requiring an automated plan of treatment, or development of a medical order expiration notification system), and improving cash flow (by having weekly billing for self-pay and commercial insurers and electronic filing for Medicare).

3. Specify the functional requirements that must be met to reach the defined goals and objectives. Typical functional requirements are (a) the generation of various accounting or staff productivity reports to provide improved information to management, and (b) the ability to input a given number of documents per day to improve internal operations. More specific functional requirements might include generating invoices in a specific format on existing forms, the use of UB-82, state Medicaid forms, HMO billing formats, using a predetermined and alterable charge schedule to calculate prices, and being able to call up accounts receivable on an aged basis and in a predetermined format.

4. Develop a list of what feature, or benchmark, will be used to evaluate the vendors (see Exhibit 23-2). Determine the relative weight of each feature. For example, the staff of the home health agency would like the new system to print labels for every physician who has written orders during the last 12 months. Although it would be a nice feature, it would not significantly prejudice the ultimate selection. Therefore, on a scale of 1 to 10, it would rate a "1". On the other hand, the printing of UB-82 is very important and would rate a "10".

5. Prepare written, functional, solution-oriented specifications, often called a Request for Proposal (RFP), for the software package based on the goals and functional requirements. These specifications could include:

   - The types and quantity of input to be supplied and the related video screen formats.

   - The types of processing to be carried out on the information.

   - The amount of information to be stored and processed and the time intervals for this storage and processing.

Exhibit 23-2. Software selection criteria (sample).

		Rating	
Feature benchmark	Relative weight	Vendor A	Vendor B
Must prepare UB-82	10	10	10
Productivity at five levels	10	10	8
Able to post late charges	10	3	8
Interface charges for hours directly to payroll	8	10	8
Prepare dunning notices	10	10	10
Prepare HMO listing	5	4	0
Prepare daily census	10	10	9
Prepare mailing labels	2	0	10
Total points	65	530	534
Relative weight		8.15	8.22
			selected due to higher index

- The output required, including the types of reports and their contents, the types of video screen displays, and how often each type of output is to be produced.

Mail the RFP to all selected vendors.

After reviewing the responses from vendors based on your RFP, the ultimate test is "checking out" the package. When evaluating software products, you should take the following steps:

1. Review the literature and documentation for the packages being considered.

2. Obtain references for other users and contact them. If possible, speak with them about their experiences, watch as they run their versions of the software and get copies of their input and output data to compare with your specifications.

3. Use the software yourself with samples of your input and generate typical samples of your expected output on hardware that is similar to what you intend to use. The results of these test runs will provide benchmarks you can use for meaningful comparisons of the various packages.

4. Determine the effect, if any, that having or not having various input/output devices, disk drives, or memory capacity will have on the performance and the useability of the software.

5. Be skeptical of everything unless you are able to verify it yourself or it comes from an independent and reliable source.

The last caution: after making the initial evaluation of available software, review the top two or three vendors again. The second look at these vendors will provide a better decision since the home health agency evaluation team will be more aware of the negatives and positives of many software packages when it is time for the second review, and the making of the final decision.

Selecting the computer system and negotiating a good sales contract are not the ends to this process. Your concerns must now turn to the actual installation and implementation. This requires careful planning between your staff and the software vendor. The planning for installation are covered in the following steps:

1. Define responsibility. Who will handle the actual delivery of the hardware, putting it in place and verifying that it works satisfactorily? The vendor will usually assume this task, but it should be agreed upon in advance—and even specified in the sales contract. Determine if there is a separate installation charge.

2. Training of personnel. All the employees in your office who will use any aspect of the system should be encouraged and perhaps required to attend the vendor's regular training sessions. Will that number of people and the desired training dates fit into the vendor's schedules? Determine if there will be an extra charge for the amount of training your staff may demand, and how additional training will be arranged and billed. Determine how future training is handled.

3. Running parallel. No matter how well your new system has performed elsewhere, you must operate it for several months in parallel with your existing system—even if a manual one. This involves a duplication of effort and careful cross-checking of each system's outputs against the other. Are your office employees properly instructed as to this phase, including which items must be checked? Who among the vendor's personnel will be available to handle the inevitable "bugs" which the parallel runs turn up?

Installation can be a frustrating and difficult time. Knowing the duties and responsibilities of each party will help. Keeping the outlined time schedule for conversion and implementation are a requirement to maintaining the future sanity of the HHA by "getting back to normal" operation as quickly as possible.

The final step in computerization is the evaluation of performance. This should be done at least once a year to determine that all systems are functioning satisfactorily. It should become part of your annual budgeting process to evaluate the needs of your HHA with regards to upgrades of or expansions in data processing.

Description of One Home Health Care Computer System
Clay Figard, Jr.

Computer systems designed to meet the unique needs of home health agencies became available in the early nineteen seventies. The original systems were very basic, providing minimal statistical data, billings, and accounts receivable information. Today, with the availability of very comprehensive management information systems, home health agencies have access to the sophisticated data they need. Comprehensive automated systems consist of many modules which address specific functions within a recordkeeping system. Various modules included within a total system are general ledger, accounts payable, payroll, admission/referrals, scheduling, plan of treatment, and home health. A home health module was developed by Delta Computer Systems Inc. (of Altoona, PA), pioneers and leaders in the software development for home care agencies.

The collection of information centers around a few specially designed input forms. Patient information is recorded on a patient master update form (Exhibit 23-3) and a patient master II update form (Exhibit 23-4). Employee activity is recorded on the daily report (Exhibit 23-5). The cash receipt and adjustment form (Exhibit 23-6) is used to record cash and adjustments. A year-to-date visit correction form (Exhibit 23-7) provides for correcting any incorrect visit or non-visit time entries. Each form was designed for ease of use; many areas require only marking a check in a box for accuracy.

Patient Master Update Forms

The patient update forms are used for each new patient and all subsequent update information. Each patient is assigned a patient number upon admission into the system. The patient number and the first two characters of the patient's last name become the patient identifier. The patient form is completed and then entered into the computer. All patient statistical data (i.e., name and address) are obtained from this master file. The patient name and address are the first areas to be completed on the patient master update form. A team number may be assigned to each patient. The patient is assigned to a substation which will identify where the statistical data for this patient will appear. A substation may represent an office or a program within an office. Utilizing the substation concept the same data may be reported in many different ways. For example, an agency with three distinct programs providing service from five offices would have 15 substations. However, this agency provided service in six different counties and needed to report services by county. In the reporting process, the standard 15 substations are replaced with county codes and the county reporting requirement is met. Patient billing information, which includes pay source and Medicare, Medicaid, and private insurance data, is entered. The patient update form provides a space for an effective date which is used in conjunction with pay source changes. At the end of the month, the system will use this date to retroactively correct visits being billed to the prior funding source. This feature saves time and eliminates incorrect bill preparation. Start of care date, plan established date, and recertification date are entered for the patient. Hospitals and physicians are assigned identifying numbers

Exhibit 23-3.

PRINT ONLY   DATE MAILED

PATIENT NUMBER ☐☐☐☐☐☐   ACTION CODE   3 ☐ NEW PATIENT   5 ☐ CHANGE

                                                                SUBSTATION ☐0☐1

☐ A. NAME _____   _____   ____   TEAM   ☐☐
        LAST   FIRST   M.I.

                                                                READMISSION ☐ Y

☐ B. ADDRESS _____   _____   _____   _____
        STREET   CITY   STATE   ZIP

☐ C. STATUS   DISCHARGE REASON   ☐☐-☐☐-☐☐
     1 ☐ ELIG. REQUEST NEEDED   1 ☐ DIED   5 ☐ MOVED   DISCHARGE DATE
     2 ☐ WAITING APPROVAL   2 ☐ PATIENT REFUSED SERVICE 6 ☐ OTHER
     3 ☐ ACTIVE   3 ☐ NON ACCEPTANCE 7 ☐ NURSING HOME   ☐☐-☐☐-☐☐-☐☐
     4 ☐ DISCHARGED   4 ☐ HOSPITAL   SERVICE CODES

☐ D. BILLING   PRIMARY   SECONDARY
     10 ☐ MEDICARE A   41 ☐ SELF PAY   A ☐ SELF   ☐☐☐☐☐☐☐☐☐☐☐
     20 ☐ MEDICARE B   42 ☐ V.A.   B ☐ PRIVATE INS.   MEDICARE NUMBER
     30 ☐ MEDICAID   43 ☐ PRIVATE INSURANCE C ☐ BC & BS
     37 ☐ CHHC   44 ☐ OTHER AGENCIES/HMO D ☐ EMPLOYER   ☐☐-☐☐☐-☐☐-☐☐☐
     38 ☐ BLUE CROSS   45 ☐ AMERICAN CANCER SOCIETY E ☐ PUBLIC AGENCY   MEDICAID NUMBER
     39 ☐ BOARD OF HEALTH   F ☐ OTHER
                                                                ☐☐-☐☐-☐☐
     PAY STATUS 1 ☐ NO FEE   PAYOR CHANGE EFFECTIVE DATE
                 2 ☐ PART FEE   INSURANCE DESCRIPTION |_|_|_|_|_|_|_|_|_|_|_|_|_|_|_|_|_|_|_|
                 3 ☐ FULL FEE

☐ E. DOCTOR _____ NO. ☐☐☐☐ START CARE ☐☐-☐☐-☐☐ PLAN ☐☐-☐☐-☐☐

     HOSPITAL _____ NO. ☐☐☐ STAY FROM ☐☐-☐☐-☐☐ TO ☐☐-☐☐-☐☐

     HOSPITAL _____ NO. ☐☐☐ STAY FROM ☐☐-☐☐-☐☐ TO ☐☐-☐☐-☐☐

     RE-CERTIFIED DATE ☐☐-☐☐-☐☐

☐ F. ILLNESS ☐☐☐.☐☐ DIAGNOSIS |_|_|_|_|_|_|_|_|_|_|_|_|_|_|_|_|_|_|_|_|_| EMPLOYMENT RELATED
             ☐☐☐.☐☐ DIAGNOSIS |_|_|_|_|_|_|_|_|_|_|_|_|_|_|_|_|_|_|_|_|_| Y ☐   N ☐
             ☐☐☐.☐☐ DIAGNOSIS |_|_|_|_|_|_|_|_|_|_|_|_|_|_|_|_|_|_|_|_|_|

☐ G. PATIENT   REFERRAL 1 ☐ HOSPITAL   5 ☐ STAFF   RACE 1 ☐ CAU   SEX
     INFORMATION   2 ☐ DOCTOR   6 ☐ COMM. AGENCIES   2 ☐ BLACK   M ☐
                                3 ☐ FAMILY, FRIEND/SELF 7 ☐ NSG. HOMES   3 ☐ OTHER   F ☐
                                4 ☐ OTHER   4 ☐ SPANISH
                                                                        5 ☐ ORIENTAL

        TOWN _____ ☐☐   LIVES ALONE   01 ☐

☐ H. SELF PAY CHARGES   LIVES WITH OTHERS 01 ☐

     A — ☐☐-☐☐ F — ☐☐-☐☐   DATE OF BIRTH ☐☐☐☐☐☐☐   MARITAL STATUS
     B — ☐☐-☐☐ I — ☐☐-☐☐   MO. DAY YEAR   1 ☐ SINGLE
     C — ☐☐-☐☐ N — ☐☐-☐☐   PHONE ☐6☐1☐7 ☐☐☐☐☐☐☐   2 ☐ MARRIED
     D — ☐☐-☐☐ O — ☐☐-☐☐   AREA   NUMBER   3 ☐ WIDOWED
     E — ☐☐-☐☐ S — ☐☐-☐☐   4 ☐ OTHER
                                VISITS TO BE MADE EVERY ☐0☐6☐0 DAYS

FORM 958 BELM
7/84

Exhibit 23-4.

PRINT ONLY
PRESS FIRMLY USING
A RED BALL POINT PEN

AGENCY NAME
PATIENT MASTER UPDATE II

DATE   / /

PATIENT NUMBER [ ] [ ] [ ] [ ] [ ]   PATIENT NAME _____

VISIT REASON		ICD9	START OF CARE	DISCHARGE DATE	NUMBER OF VISITS	LAST VISIT DATE	DIAGNOSIS
A	1						
B	2						
C	3						
D	4						
E	5						
F	6						
G	7						
I	8						
J	9						
K	10						
L	11						
N	12						
O	13						
S	14						

FORM 722   PREPARED BY:_____

which are recorded for each patient. Hospital dates, diagnosis, and ICD9 codes are also entered into the system. The ICD9 codes are referenced when visits are recorded so visits may be distributed by illness. The patient master II input form provides for ICD9 codes by different types of service; this feature enables an agency to obtain more accurate statistical data instead of all services defaulting to the primary illness. Additional information which helps profile patients includes race, sex, age, locality, marital status, and living status. Each patient may have up to four service codes which enable special studies based on the patient database. Agencies have used these special study codes to analyze the patient's care and level of achievement at discharge. If an agency renders service to self-pay patients at reduced rates, the sliding scale may be entered for each type of service. The patient master II form is used to enter start of care dates and discharge dates by individual service types. As the information is entered into the computer from the patient update forms, all conceivable validation is done to preserve the integrity of the database. For example, if a patient's funding source is being changed, an effective date must be entered. The system will not allow the operator to proceed to the next patient update until all errors have been eliminated in the current entry.

Exhibit 23-5.

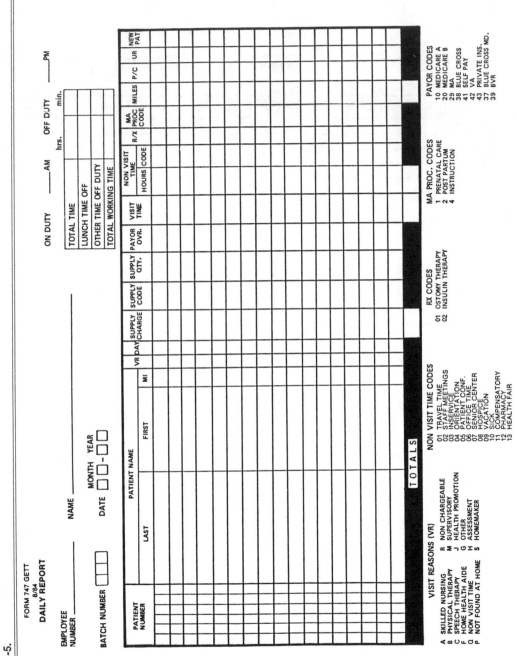

Exhibit 23-6.

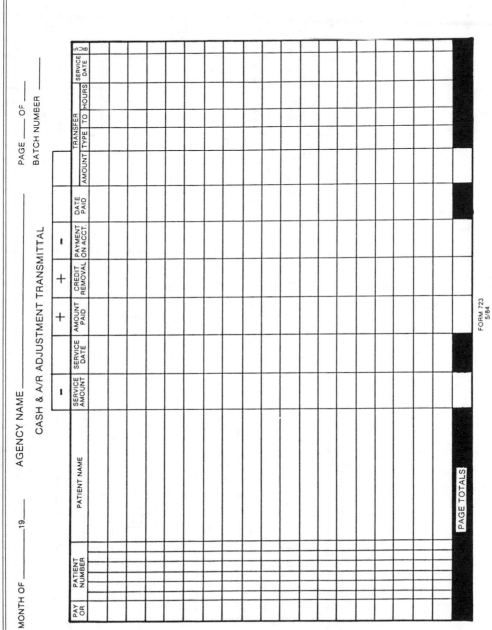

Exhibit 23-7.

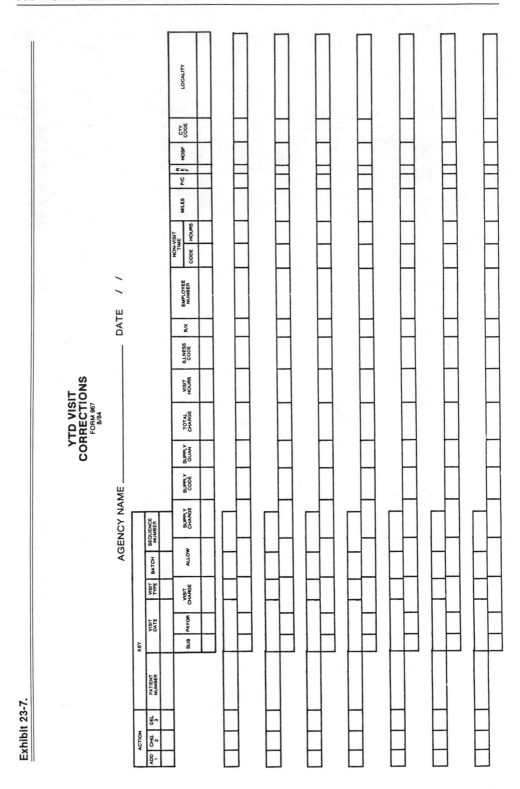

Daily Report Form

Each caregiver completes the daily report form which is used to capture payroll information and to record patient service data. An employee records his unique number and name at the top of the form. Each visit is entered by recording patient number and name, visit reason, day of visit, and visit time (actual time spent with the patient). All supplies are assigned a supply code and price. If supplies are to be charged, the supply code and quantity would be recorded. The computer would automatically price the supplies and add them to the visit charge. If the patient's normal payor is not going to pay for this visit, a pay source override may be entered. Any time not involved in direct patient care is recorded under the non-visit time and each non-visit activity is assigned a code which is entered with the non-visit time. Many agencies are interested in obtaining statistical data on high-tech type visits or hospice visits and may accomplish this by using RX codes. A group of daily activity forms are combined to create a batch; batch numbers are assigned and counts on the number of records and hours are accumulated. Such controls ensure the accuracy of the information being entered into the system by the terminal operator. If a visit were missed or inadvertently entered twice, the batch controls would detect a problem. Entry into the computer begins with entering the batch number and batch counts. This is the external count that will be compared against the totals being accumulated by the computer based on the terminal operators entries. Now the detail visit and non-visit time entries are entered. Patient number and first two characters of the patient's last name are entered. The computer looks at the patient file, verifying the number and first two characters of the last name, and displays the patient's full name on the screen. Visit reason is entered and the computer checks to see whether this particular employee may render the service type. This check avoids keying errors made by the terminal operator. The computer then displays either the patient's normal pay source or a message relating to the patient's specific billing considerations. An alternate pay source may be entered over the normal pay source by the terminal operator at this time. Visit hours are entered into the system. Now the computer may automatically price the visit based on payor, substation, visit reason, and visit hours. Non-visit codes and hours are now entered. Miles driven by each employee are entered into the computer. As visits are accepted by the computer, locality codes, referral information, age of patient, illness code, and substation are extracted from the patient database and stored with the visit. Visit information, in turn, updates the patient file with the number of visits by discipline and last visit date by discipline. After all visits for the batch have been entered into the computer, a batch balance listing may be printed, displaying all entries in the exact sequence as they were entered. Visit registers may be produced in a variety of sequences, the most common being by pay source, patient, or employee. If an agency detects an error while reviewing the visit register, the terminal operator may reopen the batch and correct the error prior to statement preparation. The computer system maintains a batch control file which monitors each batch as to revenue figures, if the batch has been printed, and if the batch is in balance.

At the end of the month, after all visits have been entered into the computer, a procedure called automatic payor change is executed. This reviews every visit that was entered for the month, ensuring that the proper funding source and the correct amount are being charged for the service. If a patient's pay source was changed at the end of the month, but was retroactive to the fifth of the month, all visits from the fifth on would be automatically updated with the correct payor and billing amounts. Also, if an agency had a rate change for a particular service, but did not have approval until the middle of the month, all visits processed under the old rate would automatically be updated to the new rate. This feature saves considerable employee time and results in more accurate and timely statement preparation.

Accounts Receivable File

Applying cash to open accounts receivable is accomplished by completing the cash and accounts receivable adjustment form, or by directly applying cash receipts from Medicare or Medicaid transmittal forms. The accounts receivable file is maintained in the computer as the cash receipts are expected. In the case of Medicare, the open receivables are maintained just as the UB-82 billing form is produced. Thus, multiple treatment plans would create multiple open accounts receivable items. Since receivables match bills submitted, this greatly simplifies the cash application process. The key to the accounts receivable record is the pay source and service date. All cash transactions being recorded on the forms and, in turn, entered into the computer, must be in balance for the computer will not accept a transaction if it is out of balance. Transfers are entered when adjustments are to be made to the accounts receivables. The transfer of bad debts, income adjustments, Medicare contractual allowances, and receivables from one funding source to another are all entered through the transfer columns. For instance, the transfer column is used when an insurance company pays 80 percent of the charges. The insurance company's obligation is satisfied upon its payment of 80 percent and the remaining 20 percent is transferred to self-pay. Statements will be produced reflecting the transfers entered into the computer. As cash transactions and visits are accepted by the computer, the accounts receivable file is updated so each account is current.

Correction Form

Each visit and non-visit time record is stored in a year-to-date file. By maintaining each visit, greater flexibility is obtained for reporting purposes. If statistical data are needed at the end of the year that were not planned for, the information is available by accessing this data file. The year-to-date correction form is used to add, delete, or correct visit or non-visit time entries. All fields within the records may be changed so all reports displaying year-to-date information will be accurate.

"Just Ask" Feature

Information is stored by the computer on magnetic disks. This information is referred to as the database from which all reporting is extracted. The computer system has an ad hoc reporting feature, which is called "Just Ask." Using Just Ask, an agency has the ability to interrogate the database for information without having a specific program written. Just Ask does not completely eliminate the need for customized programming, but is ideal for generating simple extract and list functions. If an agency wanted a list of patients living in a particular locality, receiving care due to a specific illness, the Just Ask procedure would be used.

Financial Management Reports

The system encompasses an extensive variety of management reports which address all the financial and statistical requirements of an agency. From an accounting perspective, the system provides audit trails of information which have entered the system with appropriate external controls. If the information is changed by the system as in the automatic payor change, a report displaying what information was in the computer and what it has been changed to is printed. Regardless of how detailed an agency's general ledger is, the system produces reports which provide the information for posting. The visit summary by discipline is produced in substation (office or program), payor, and discipline sequence. The gross charge, supplies, allowance, and net charge figures are displayed. Revenue and accounts receivable figures for posting are obtained from this report. Many accountants want to see detail supporting the numbers being posted into the general ledger. Visit registers which display each visit and charges may be printed in substation and pay source sequence. A cash journal is printed by the computer which displays in patient sequence all cash receipts and adjustments. Those transactions are summarized and printed on the cash journal summary. Numbers are obtained from this report to post general ledger figures to cash, accounts receivable, income, bad debts, and allowance accounts. If an agency keeps its general ledger by discipline within payor, an additional report is provided which displays all adjustments so the proper accounting entries can be made. These accounting entries can interface with the automated general ledger which means the home health module automatically transfers information to the general ledger system. This interface function reduces the manual effort and potential errors, resulting in faster financial reporting. After all visits and cash entries have been processed by the computer, the system produces statements for Medicare, Medicaid, and third-party pay sources. As in all businesses, good cash flow enables an agency to meet payroll and pay vendors for materials and services. Timely statement preparation is essential—the computer system facilitates this process. Once statements have been produced and forwarded to the funding sources, it is imperative to collect the money as quickly as possible. The monitoring of money owed to the agency is accomplished by using the accounts receivable schedule, which is an aging analysis of all money owed the agency. By combining timely statement preparation and effective monitoring of their receivables, agencies have reduced average receivable days from 120 to 55. Accurate and timely financial reporting enables agency administration to respond quickly to changing trends.

Employee Activity Reports

Employee salaries represent the largest single expenditure for a home health agency. Monitoring employee activity is essential and the system includes a number of appropriate reports. The monthly caseload summary displays each employee in employee number sequence. Employee numbers may be assigned so the first three positions of the number represent a group. When the group number changes, a summary of all employees in the group is printed. Totals by discipline or by certain individuals within a discipline may be obtained by using the group numbers. This report displays the number of visits by type, hours of service, average visit length, and the number of visits per day for each employee. The number of miles driven and the number of different patients seen are also on this report. A recap of all non-visit time is displayed for each employee; this makes feasible a complete analysis of each employee's monthly activities. Standards may be established for all employees of the agency and may be quickly and easily monitored by using the monthly caseload summary report. Detailed employee activity is available on the employee register by day report. Patient number, name, date of service, visit reason, charge, supplies, allowance, net charge, visit time, patient illness, and RX code are displayed on this report. Visit patterns for each employee can be seen by analyzing this report. The same report is available sequenced by employee and then patient and will make possible the comparison of visit patterns to patients from one employee to another as well as total revenues generated by each employee for the month. From a management perspective, the monthly reports reflect current trends providing the tools to react quickly to problem areas. The year-to-date visits by employee report displays the number of visits and hours of actual service by type of service, funding source, major illness classification, and patient's age. It is an invaluable tool in assessing year-to-date revenues generated by each employee.

Clinical and Quality Assurance Related Reports

Management reports which eliminate the need for tickler files and the necessity to do extensive chart reviewing are a natural byproduct of the computer system. Patients are required to have doctors' orders renewed every 60 days, and a report, displaying the patient's and the doctor's name and address whose orders are due, simplifies this process. When a patient is added to the master file, the longest elapsed time between visits is entered. The system keeps track of the last visit date and if the number of days between the last visit date and the end of the current month exceeds the visit interval, the system displays the patient on a patient not seen report. If a patient appears on the not seen report, either the patient has not been discharged in a timely manner, or a visit was not made, or a visit was not recorded in the system. Since Medicare is considered a patient's primary pay source, it is important for community-based agencies to move a sliding scale self-pay patient to Medicare when a patient reaches the age of 65. A report which displays patients who will turn 65 next month and are not Medicare patients alerts the agency to the needed funding source review. Agencies performing quality assurance functions have had problems in the patient selection process. The system generates a monthly report displaying random patients that the quality assurance personnel may review. The automated selection process will not consider a patient selected in the past six months and will give greater consideration to the patients receiving multiple services. Each month 3.33% of the agency caseload will appear on the quality assurance report with one-third of the patients being admissions, discharged patients, and carryovers. These computer-generated management reports are more reliable than those accumulated manually and save valuable employee time.

Statistical Reports

Statistical reports generated by the system are provided using the same database from which the accounting and other management reports are extracted. The service statistics report is printed by substation (offices or program within office) and displays monthly visit totals and hours in service by discipline, fee source, major illness, locality (up to 40), and age. Patient statistics as to the number of patients served, admitted, and discharged are also displayed. All information for each substation is displayed on one page which permits easy comparison between substations. This report is excellent for board reporting for community-based agencies. A year-to-date visits by locality report displays visits and hours by service, fee source, major illness classification, referral, and age. All information for each locality is on one page. The number of individual localities which may be included on this report is unlimited. For community-based agencies, the fee analysis section includes the allowance figure written off for sliding scale patients. Agencies may go to townships and municipalities to request revenue sharing money to offset the write offs supported by this report. Some agencies have detected high occurrences of certain illnesses within a specific locality using the locality report. Reports which reflect patient data are produced by the system and allow agency management to monitor admissions, discharges, and patients receiving service. The reports are printed by substation and display patients by discipline, referral source, race, sex, age, locality, fee source, living status, and major illness classification. These reports also display service codes used by agencies for their own studies. One agency compiles discharge information as to patient, goals, and level of achievement.

Statistics by major illness classification provide some useful information. But most agencies are interested in a finer breakdown of illnesses served. The system allows each agency to define ranges of illness that it wants to evaluate; using this concept, details on specific types of cancers may be retrieved. The diagnosis statistics by discipline and the discharge summary report are two reports which use the dynamic illness file. The diagnosis statistic by discipline report is printed in diagnosis sequence as defined by the agency. Under each diagnosis, the different types of services are listed, displaying the number of patients, number of visits, hours, average hours per patient, and average visit length. All numbers are displayed for the current month, and year to date. This report is an excellent analytical tool in evaluating the impact different illnesses have on agency personnel resources. A variation of this report is to print the same figures within each pay source. Surprisingly, the average number of visits and time vary significantly, depending on the funding source. This could be attributed to the age of the patient which usually has a direct correlation to funding sources. The discharge summary report is also defined by the agency. Under each diagnosis the different types of services are listed and are broken down into length of stays. The different length of stay categories are 1-Day, 2 to 30 days, 31 to 90 days, 91 to 180 days, and 181 and up. Within each category, the report displays number of patients, visits, hours (for visits billed by hour), case revenue at current rates, average visits, hours per patient, median length of service, and median revenue per day. The database consists of patient discharges over the past three years. This report enables an agency to project the resources required and cost when a patient is admitted with a particular illness based on agency history.

The home care industry has undergone dramatic changes over the past few years and the environment will continue to change over the years to come. Effective and professional management of an agency in these times requires accurate, reliable, and timely information, which can only be obtained through a comprehensive automated system designed to meet the unique needs of home health agencies.

References

Baker, D. March 1980. Managing a hospital based home health information system. *Computers in Healthcare*

Knauer, C. 1984. The microcomputer in hardware purchaser decision from the user's viewpoint. *Healthcare Financial Management* August 1984.

Liska, J. 1986. *Home Health Line*

McIlvane, M. E. 1986. *Computers in Healthcare* March 1986.

Muellin, J. H. 1986. Strategic importance of MIS for home healthcare. *Computers in Healthcare* June 1986.

Tolos, P. C., and D. Moody. 1986. *Choosing and using the right medical office computer.* Oradell, NJ: Medical Economics Books.

Glossary

Application program	Program written to accomplish a specific purpose.
Application software	Series of programs written for a specific purpose.
ASCII (pronounced "AS-KEY")	American Standard Code for Information Interchange character code is used for representing information by most non-IBM equipment.
Audit trail	Records of every transaction together with a record of the source of the entry; a means of tracing errors.
Backup	Duplicate of a file made to protect information.
Batch processing	Method by which data are handled by an outside organization and the results sent to the submitting office; see OFF-LINE.
Baud	Speed of communications between devices. (300 baud is 30 characters a second)
Benchmark	Tests of computers against performance standards.
Billing and statements	
Contract billing	Bills sent out for a set amount per month as agreed to under a contract and not for services as they are rendered (such as HMO).
Cycle billing	Statements sent out at specific times for part of the accounts (A to L on the 15th and M to Z on the 30th).
Monthly statements	Sent to all patients when a balance is owed.
Statement	Notification of the status of an account, even though balance may be zero.

Third-party billing	Bills sent to insurance companies or other guarantors, such as UB-82.
Bit	Contraction of Binary Digit; operating unit of a computer; essentially an on/off switch.
Board	Thin, flat component that serves as the base for one or more layers of electronic circuits.
Boot	Starting up a computer.
Buffer	Memory that holds data prior to transactions being performed on it in order to speed up processing.
Bug	Error or anomaly in a software program.
Byte	Usually 8 bits, the unit of symbolic transfer, that is, every character, alphabetic or numeric, is one byte.
Cartridge disk	Removable disk (5 or more Megabytes) in a convenient cartridge form.
Central Processing Unit (CPU)	Part of a computer where data are processed and manipulated; contains the main memory, operating system chip, RAM and ROM, controller for the entire system.
Character	Numbers, letters, or symbols represented to the computer by a unique pattern of bits; see ASCII.
Characters Per Second (CPS)	Number of characters printed per second; a measure of printer speed.
Chip	Integrated circuit, the building board of a computer.
Circuit board	Systematic arrangement of circuits that can be easily inserted or removed; electronic building blocks of a computer.
COBOL	Common Business Oriented Language

Compatible	Ability of hardware and software components to work synergistically.
Configure	To design the components of a computer to perform assigned functions in a particular manner.
Console	Terminal that has the most control in the system or may sometimes be used to refer to any terminal or CRT.
Continuous form	Fan-folded, pin-fed paper.
Controller	Device to control peripherals.
Conversion	Entry of manual records into a computer.
Coprocessor	A second CPU in a single device.
Core or core memory	Central or main memory.
CPU	Central Processing Unit; the heart of a computer system.
Custom program	Software written especially for an individual application that has limited use outside that application.
Data	All information processed by the computer.
Database	Organized information available for access by a computer, e.g., names and addresses, diseases and their symptoms, a bibliography, etc.
DBMS	DataBase Management System.
Debug	To identify and eliminate errors and anomalies on the software program.
Disk	Any flat, circular, magnetic storage medium which is continuously rotated when in use.
Disk crash	Destruction of information on a disk by a mechanical malfunction in the disk drives.

Disk file	File residing on a disk.
Diskette	Another term for a floppy disk.
Documentation	Written instructions for operating hardware or software.
DOS	Disk Operating System.
Downloading	Sending information or programs from one system (generally larger) to another (generally smaller) through a modem.
Downtime	Time when a computer is not operational.
EBCDIC	Like ASCII, a means of assigning binary codes to character sets on IBM computers.
Edit	To edit (correct) and maintain text.
Field	A database space reserved for specific information.
File	Collection of records in the same type and in the same format, such sa patient demographic information.
Fixed disk	Hard disk that is permanently attached in a computer.
Flag	Indicator associated with a special condition (an insurance flag would indicate a patient has insurance).
Flow chart	Symbolic representation of a program sequence.
GIGO	Garbage In, Garbage Out.
Hard copy	Printed copy or microform output.
Hard Disk	Peripheral memory storage unit in a rigid format.
Hardware	Electronic data processing equipment.
Head crash	Head failure that damages the disk.

Index	Shortcut means of locating specific data on a file, a key for accessing data.
Interactive	Equipment that responds directly to your input.
Interface	A. Boundary, meeting, or connection between components.
	B. Ability of components to work synergistically.
	C. Human/machine interaction.
Internal memory	Memory of the central processing unit.
LAN	Local Area Network; a means of interconnecting microcomputers in a facility.
Line surge	Sharp change in voltage that can cause equipment damage.
Load	Transfer data or a program to execute it.
LPS	Lines per second; speed of a line printer.
Mainframe	Large central computer.
Main memory	High-speed, readily addressable memory.
Memory	Data held in storage.
Menu	Listing of options in functions or programs.
Merge	To combine two or more records or files into one.
Microcomputer	Small computer system usually costing under $40,000.
Microprocessor	The CPU of a microcomputer.
Modem	Communications device that allows the computer to use telephone lines to access other devices.

Module	Pertaining to software, any part of software program that performs a specific function, i.e., billing, patient/staff scheduling, recertifications, and so on.
Monitor	CRT for displaying computer information.
Motherboard	Essential electronic board in a computer to which daughter boards may be connected to extend functions.
MS/DOS	MicroSoft Disk Operating System; IBM PC operating language.
Multiplexor	Device to tie in several modems.
Multitasking	Performs more than one task simultaneously.
Multiuser	System which allows multiple terminals to be used simultaneously.
Network	System of interrelated computers.
Object code	Output code readable by the computer.
Off-line	A. A processing operation completed separately from the mainframe, e.g., BATCH.
	B. Storing mass memory in a removable disk format.
On-line	A. Direct processing between a satellite or peripheral equipment and the host computer.
	B. Having data or information available to call immediately into use.
Operating system	Internal language to control hardware.
Output	Information delivered by the system after processing.
Overhead	Amount of disk space or main memory consumed by system requirements including keys, indexes, programs, and instructions.

Parallel	Simultaneous performing of tasks.
Parameters	Descriptions of limitations or control levels.
Password	User identification to allow access.
Peripherals	Devices attached to the computer, adding to its value and the functions it can perform.
Power surge	Flow of current exceeding 110 to 120 volts that may damage the data set, programs, or computer.
Program	Logical sequence of instructions.
Purge	To clean or eliminate data.
RAM	Random Access Memory; portion of core dedicated to the storage and manipulation of data.
Random	Not sequential, accessible at any point.
Record	Data arranged in sequence to make up a file.
Record length	Limit to the amount of information on a file.
Response time	The method of timing different computer operations, a measure of speed and efficiency.
RFP	Request for Proposal; formal document used to gather consistent information from a vendor for making a decision.
Save	Reading information from temporary storage into permanent storage.
Sort	To sequence data according to specified parameters.
Source code	Original program code which is translated to object code for the computer to use.

Spool	Allows an action, like printing, to occur while the computer can still be used for other work.
Standalone	System complete in itself.
Streaming tape	Quick backup system for a hard disk.
Surge protector	A device used to prevent line surges from damaging data or equipment.
Systems analysis	Determination of the detailed components that make up a system and the development of specifications.
Systems design	Plans drawn up to achieve the specifications, tasks, and objectives of a system.
Systems integrator	Vendor who puts together hardware and software from different manufacturers and sells it as a system. (Also called a value-added resaler.)
Terminal	Input/output device.
Throughput	Speed at which processes occur.
Time sharing	Multiple users on one system.
Turnkey system	A computer system completely assembled, installed, and ready-to-use.
Unbundled	When software, hardware, and other components are sold and priced separately.
Upgrade	To improve a system by trading up.
UPS	Uninterruptible power supply; a device to maintain a constant current flow preventing power surges or brownouts.
User friendly	Computer jargon defining a system which is designed to be easy to learn and use.
Utilities	Programs used to accomplish normal data processing tasks (e.g., SORT).

Volatile storage	Storage device, such as RAM, which loses data when the current is turned off.
Winchester disk	Sealed high-density hard disk.
Windows	Ability to look at and process information on a second file or record while the screen continues to show the original record.
Write	Process of entering or changing data.
Write-protect	Process or code that prevents overwriting of data or programs.

Part VII

Legal, Ethical and Political Issues

Chapter Twenty-Four

Risk Management and Home Health Care: The Time is Now

James Tehan and Sharyn L. Colegrove

Over the last five years, the number of Medicare-certified home health agencies has more than doubled, from 2,858 in 1980 to 5,825 toward the end of 1985. There has been a corresponding surge in the number of non-Medicare-certified agencies providing health services at home; recent estimates suggest that Medicare-certified agencies represent only 50% of the industry. Many factors have influenced this remarkable growth in home health care. A prominent perception exists that the very survival of new entrants depends on their capturing patients in a system of care that ensures "cradle to grave" loyalty.

Among home health care providers, there is a consensus that governmental health policy, technological advances, and changing consumer health care attitudes have combined to make the industry one of the fastest growing segments of the health care system. Although payments to home health agencies make up only about 2% of Medicare expenditures, home health services represent the fastest growing component of Medicare outlays. Similarly, home health care accounted for 1.7% of the nation's total 1983 health expenditures. Clearly, the home health care industry has grown up, almost overnight.

Rationale for Risk Management

The development of risk management in the hospital industry was fueled by the medical malpractice crisis of 1973 to 1975 and the accompanying withdrawal of the insurance industry in the face of escalating claims. In the home health care industry, increasingly complex patient care procedures have increased risk exposure. Insurance coverage is much more difficult for agencies to obtain, and the increase in premiums has had a significant impact on many home health agencies. Carriers willing to write policies for home health agencies are beginning to closely evaluate specific policies, procedures, and mechanisms for reporting unexpected outcomes or adverse patient reactions. In many cases, carriers require comprehensive risk management audits for agencies lacking a formal reporting system.

Risk management for home health agencies involves developing a well-coordinated process that identifies, evaluates, and addresses potential and actual risks. The primary purpose is to safeguard agency assets through monitoring mechanisms designed to reduce risk once a decision has been made that a particular program, ser-

Reprinted from QRB 12 (6): 179-186. May 1986. Reprinted with permission.

vice, or product involves a risk worth taking, within the context of the agency's mission and goals.

Not all risk can be eliminated. As more complex procedures become possible in the home, administrative and clinical staff must determine when it is reasonable to provide a program or service that is associated with increased risk. For example, the addition of a chemotherapy program introduces the possibilities of extravasation, anaphylaxis, and increased susceptibility to infection. A home health agency that accepts referrals from a cancer center or medical center with a large oncology section has a responsibility to develop policies and procedures that will ensure the patient's safety. In addition to staff in-service training to ensure technical competency, it may also be necessary to make evening or unscheduled visits, provide 24-hour availability of registered nurses, and develop understandable patient care manuals.

When all this has been accomplished, the home health care provider will undoubtedly be approached by a cancer hospital or tertiary treatment facility asking the agency to accept patients receiving investigational drugs. Again, the agency must evaluate the risks, ask researchers and pharmacists about the safety of specific drugs, and develop procedures that reasonably permit safe administration in the home.

The focus of the traditional Medicare-certified home health agency is on providing high quality services, either directly or under contract. At the same time, since its inception, the Medicare program has restricted the range of reimbursable services. Respected national organizations have urged more comprehensive coverage, including greater emphasis on supportive and custodial care. The simple reality is the Medicare law and regulations dominate the scope of the home health care industry mostly because of the lack of national standards of care. (In December 1985 the Board of Commissioners of the Joint Commission on Accreditation of Hospitals approved a two-year development project to develop standards for community-based and hospital-based home health agencies; the project will examine Medicare-certified agencies, high-technology programs, durable medical equipment, and use of homemakers. See "JCAH Forum: The JCAH Home Care project," page 191 in this issue. [*QRB* 12(6): 179-186.]

All Medicare-certified home health agencies must continuously meet Medicare's ten Conditions of Participation. These regulations govern day-to-day operations and constitute the industry's only nationally accepted standards. Still, they are only minimum standards, and no incentives currently exist to implement higher operating standards. The burden lies with the industry's leaders to formulate a comprehensive, systematic, and practical approach to risk management that is tailored to the special needs of home health agencies. In the absence of accepted national standards for quality of care, this approach encourages organizational behavior consistent with general legal principles related to negligence that govern the standard of care.

Home health care is undergoing great change with the introduction of competition models and prospective payment systems. At the same time, agencies are being asked to care for sicker patients, under increasingly restrictive guidelines, for essentially the same amount of real dollars that were made available prior to the introduction of prospective payment. (Home health agencies also face rising insurance costs. Although agencies must consider these costs in risk management decisions, risk financing is beyond the scope of this article.) Home health care providers are responding to this changed environment with a variety of innovative strategies, but the message is clear that the scope of Medicare benefits will not significantly expand in the immediate future.

This article examines the major areas of risk exposure for Medicare-certified home health agencies, with particular emphasis on patient care issues. Although the non-Medicare portion (private insurance, prepaid health plans, and self-pay) of the industry has steadily increasing influence, Medicare reimbursement remains the dominant payment source for home health services; it is beyond the scope of this article to address these additional variables.

For the remainder of this century, home health agencies face three areas of significant risk:

- Patient care services, including the selection, orientation, and ongoing in-service education of field staff;

- The role of the primary caregiver; and

- Employee health and safety.

New forms of business relationships pose a significant risk to the long-term viability of home health agencies, but again this is beyond this article's scope. Finally, this article proposes a workable structure for a risk management program.

Patient Care Services

From a risk management perspective, agency survival depends on professional staff precisely understanding Medicare coverage and then searching for ways to provide greater support to primary caregivers. By Medicare's definition, home health benefits are part-time, intermittent skilled services that are medically necessary and ordered by a physician for homebound patients. Without documentation that all of these criteria are met, Medicare will not reimburse for services rendered.

For a home health agency that provides comprehensive services, most day-to-day operations involved routine nursing functions such as wound care, medication instruction, physical assessment, Foley catheter insertion, and management of diabetes. All nursing functions involve varying degrees of risk; the appropriate focus is how best to reduce that risk. The recent introduction of intravenous therapy programs represents a small but significant portion of the home health care market and an area of nursing practice that carries the highest levels of risk.

Increasingly, technology has brought portable, simplified machines into the home, permitting earlier hospital discharge. While technology and governmental health policy have combined to slow the growth of health expenditures by decreasing in-patient length of stay, home health agencies and primary caregivers have shouldered the bulk of these changes. Medicare's prospective payment system has altered hospital incentives, and more seriously ill patients with multiple nursing, rehabilitation therapy, and personal care needs are now commonplace home health care referrals. Several years ago, an oncology patient might have required only symptom control; today that same patient frequently requires chemotherapy administration, intravenous pain killers, and central venous line care. Consequently, the caregiver must become proficient in more nursing tasks. (Owing to its limited scope, this article will not discuss the essential role of the home health aide. To contain costs, agencies in the future will rely more and more on such aides, as well as substituting lower-cost nursing personnel for registered nurses. This will impose greater training expense and expose agencies to higher risk.)

Whether services are for basic or specialty home health care, they carry significant and increasing risks that involve procedures performed at home, machines that support patient care, and home environments that are not subject to institutional control. Each of these risks is substantial in and of itself; in combination they can provide the planting ground for a lawsuit.

Risk management in day-to-day operations. The risks now associated with home health care have substantially increased insurance premiums in a segment of the health care system that, until recently, had minimal claims activity. Advances in home clinical practice require measures to control and prevent loss. Three prevention measures must be used: selection, orientation, and in-service training of staff; documentation that clinical practice and administrative functions are carried out in accordance with established policies and procedures; and a centralized reporting system that identifies, evaluates, and resolves patient care problems in a timely fashion.

Perhaps the most important area of responsibility and potential liability for home health agencies is that of staff selection, orientation, and ongoing in-service education and training. Field staff selection is the essential first step for agencies in maintaining a focus that eliminates poor quality care. With registered nurses, this means verifying current licensure, checking employment references, and assessing skills thoroughly. Nurses should demonstrate the ability to make decisions, to request assistance or backup when necessary, and to pay attention to detail. Most often, home health agencies must evaluate whether a nurse with hospital experience will adapt successfully to the demands of home health care.

Home health agencies must also choose contractors carefully. The industry has traditionally relied on independent contractors for rehabilitation services (physical, occupational, and speech therapy) and, to a lesser extent, nursing services. A home health agency facing a lawsuit involving an independent contractor generally will be required to defend against the allegation that the agency hired the contractor negligently.

Orientation for new professional staff generally results in one to three months of reduced productivity expectations, depending on the field assignment and the worker's home health care experience. The registered nurse new to home health care must become familiar with agency policies and procedures and documentation standards, and he or she must obtain certification to perform specialized procedures such as chemotherapy or intravenous medication.

Government regulations influence the duration of staff orientation by forcing home health agencies to cut indirect expenses such as in-service training and development of patient care manuals. Certainly, agencies with extensive orientation programs (including supervised home visits, reduced initial productivity expectations, and extensive documentation review) can trim the intensity or duration of orientation. However, every resource reduction ultimately works against risk reduction. Health care providers, as well as policymakers, must remind themselves that the licensed home health care professional must conduct a thorough assessment to keep the physician fully informed and, therefore, must be competent to perform a wide range of basic and specialty functions without immediate backup medical response. For this, training is necessary.

Complicated home nursing procedures such as chemotherapy, intravenous medications, and parenteral nutrition are increasingly becoming standard practice for home health care. At the same time, new legislation in many states has enlarged the scope of nursing practice. However, expanded nursing practice statutes are a double-edged sword for nurses and their employers: the result is a continuously rising standard of care that requires more training, which is often expensive, time-consuming, and in need of continuing revision. (See Exhibit 24-1.)

In California, the Nurse Practice Act allows for the development of standardized procedures in areas of overlap between nursing and medicine. A standardized procedure is a written document defining and summarizing the parameters and circumstances under which certified nursing staff may act. Procedures such as chemotherapy or intravenous morphine sulfate administration are examples of standardized procedures

Exhibit 24-1. Development of Specialized Programs

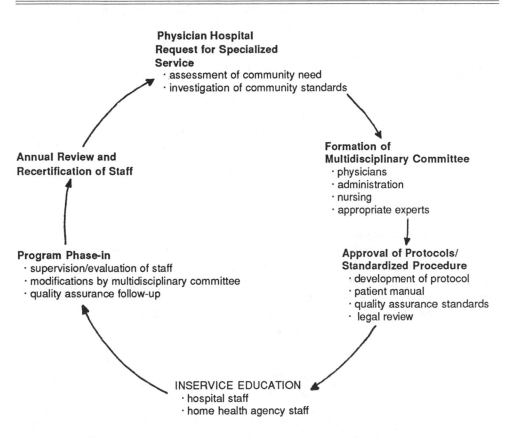

Physician Hospital Request for Specialized Service
· assessment of community need
· investigation of community standards

Formation of Multidisciplinary Committee
· physicians
· administration
· nursing
· appropriate experts

Approval of Protocols/ Standardized Procedure
· development of protocol
· patient manual
· quality assurance standards
· legal review

INSERVICE EDUCATION
· hospital staff
· home health agency staff

Program Phase-in
· supervision/evaluation of staff
· modifications by multidisciplinary committee
· quality assurance follow-up

Annual Review and Recertification of Staff

currently in use at Hospital Home Health Care Agency of California. The nurse makes judgments about patient care in response to changes in the patient's condition, within the parameters of the standardized procedure. For example, the intravenous morphine sulfate standardized procedure in use at Hospital Home Health Care Agency of California gives the nurse discretion to titrate medication after assessing the patient's pain.

Development of standardized procedures involves collaboration among nursing staff, administration, and at least one physician. The document should be detailed and comprehensive and should clearly establish specific circumstances under which the nurse will operate. Since the nurse authorized to perform procedures will be performing functions that overlap with medical practice, it is essential that the in-service training, policies and procedures, and documentation requirements be clearly delineated. Furthermore, the nurse must be taught to recognize situations that indicate alternative interventions, as well as when he or she should notify the attending physician. Finally, complete, comprehensive documentation of the nurse's actions is essential for evaluating the patient's condition and the quality of care received.

Documentation is the lifeblood of home health agencies. Unlike hospitals, where a variety of inputs are reviewed by intermediaries, home health agencies rely almost exclusively on the quality of the treatment plan, progress notes, and discharge summary to support their billing. The importance of appropriate documentation by field staff requires thorough training and ongoing reinforcement of their documentation skills. A precise understanding of changing Medicare definitions is critical to providing quality patient care as well as simultaneously ensuring the organization's viability.

From a risk management perspective, the medical record is the best indicator of the patient's status, and it is the most reliable source of communication among members of the home health care team. In addition, the medical record ultimately serves as the data base for the quality assurance program. Concurrent and retrospective reviews rely on the written record for decision making; an incomplete record will result in a financial impact as well as the untimely withdrawal of services from a patient. This scenario has obvious potential for claims exposure and emphasizes the importance of thorough and completed documentation.

Centralized patient care reporting system. In addition to policies and procedures that govern day-to-day operations, home health agencies must evaluate trends that indicate the need to alter methods of delivering patient care. Recurring errors, patient complaints, or documentation gaps are signals that an alternative approach to the status quo may be necessary. Apart from monitoring documentation of day-to-day visits, the best way to evaluate risk exposure is through incident reports. An incident report records an event that is inconsistent with the routine care and treatment for the patient's admitting or working diagnosis. Incident reports should be developed with specific reporting criteria based on exposures that are apparent after reviewing the agency's services. Consideration must be given to whether paraprofessionals, such as home health aides, report incidents directly or through their registered nurse supervisors.

An incident report should document the type of event, the effect it has on the patient's physical or mental functioning, and the severity of the effect on the patient. For example, the attending physician might order one unit of insulin twice each day.

The nurse who mistakenly administers ten units has clearly become involved in an event inconsistent with the physician's orders. The nurse's first responsibility is to monitor the patient for an immediate or delayed reaction. If the patient experiences a hypoglycemic reaction, then the nurse must administer sugar by mouth. If the patient does not respond the nurse should summon the paramedics. Depending on the patient's reaction, the nurse must also document the severity of the reaction.

The risks of malpractice by registered nurses or rehabilitation therapists are obvious to experienced clinicians. These risks can be controlled through carefully selecting, training, and monitoring agency staff. Another type of risk is the necessary reliance on less than ideal caregivers, where reimbursement constraints make treatment choices and alternative placements increasingly difficult. The potential exists for a *Darling*-type decision that would expand corporate liability to home health agencies for inadequately assessing the competency of the primary caregiver or family member. Over the years, the judicial system has clearly established that custom does not necessarily determine whether the standard of care has been met. Inadequate reimbursement or the lack of clear standards is unlikely to convince a court that the home health agency should not be held responsible for injury caused by a caregiver found to be incompetent.

Role of the Primary Caregiver

The nature of intermittent home health services generally requires the assistance of a spouse, family member, or close friend to assist the patient's return to maximal functioning. Particularly for the Medicare patient, the caregiver is usually an elderly spouse, often with functional limitations of his or her own. Such limitations affect how the caregiver handles patient services, necessitating careful assessment by the primary nurse in developing a plan of care.

In the absence of recognized national standards, agency resources must be allocated to 24-hour on-call capability, patient and caregiver manuals, and written instructions for specific procedures. These patient and caregiver supports are reasonably easy to develop and are designed to identify and resolve areas of foreseeable risk for seriously ill patients or those with special needs or circumstances.

For example, the intravenous care manual issued by Hospital Home Health Care Agency of California provides step-by-step instructions for preparing medication, managing the cannula site, heparinizing the cannula, infusing medication or fluids, and removing the cannula. For particularly complex or potentially confusing tasks, illustrations, graphs, or record-keeping charts are included. Such manuals remind the caregiver to follow certain steps in a particular order, and allow for easy reference while he or she infuses medication. This approach guards against the risk of a caregiver with limited knowledge not following tested techniques that ensure the patient's safety.

A 24-hour on-call nurse provides a source of backup information and expertise to the caregiver who may be confused or unsure about specific procedures. Furthermore, caregivers often have questions during the first few days after the patient has returned home, usually before a routine has been established. When an on-call nurse can give assurance or walk the caregiver through a procedure, it will go a long way toward reducing patient injuries, particularly for procedures involving pumps or other machinery.

Of particular ambiguity and concern is the agency's liability for the caregiver who appears competent at the outset but who becomes physically or emotionally worn out later during the patient's illness or recovery. This situation is difficult because frequently it is the sign of a family unit trying to avoid institutionalizing the patient. The primary nurse must carefully evaluate changing conditions and determine whether additional services can stabilize the situation.

The most important factor to assess is the caregiver's potential to injure the patient if he or she does not perform a procedure as taught. Additional resources may be available through the home health agency or other community agencies, but if the level of risk is such that the environment becomes unsafe, then either a new caregiver must be found or the patient must be institutionalized.

For example, if the physician has ordered the administration of insulin for a newly diagnosed diabetic with poor eyesight, and the primary nurse reports significant fluctuations in the patient's blood glucose levels, a potentially unsafe situation clearly exists. If the caregiver is unable to comply with the medication regime because of lack of understanding or inability to remember prescribed dosages or time of administration, then nursing visits should be increased until another person can be identified and trained to administer the medication. On the other hand, if a reliable person cannot be found, and the patient has hypoglycemic reactions and/or the caregiver administers incorrect dosages, then the patient will have to be institutionalized. Again, manuals specific to the patient can be invaluable in assisting motivated caregivers who may forget specific details or need the reassurance of written instructions. Printed materials for patient use require easy-to-read, concise instructions. On-call and field staff must be completely familiar with the content of these materials so that patient and caregiver reinforcement will be consistent.

Employee Health and Safety

The preventive nature of a centralized reporting system, discussed under patient care services, should also be applied for the protection of employee health and safety. A variety of work-related accidents, security concerns, and employee illnesses or injuries related to patient care must be identified. A centralized reporting system will identify these risk exposures and develop appropriate policies and procedures to reduce or eliminate unnecessary risk.

Many patient care activities cause employee injury just as in a hospital. Back injuries are the most frequent, with more than one-half of hospital nurses experiencing back pain associated with lifting patients in bed and transferring patients. Home health personnel, when caring for sicker patients, must lift and transfer patients many times with little assistance available.

In addition, treatment procedures now performed in the home involve the same risks as in the hospital, but without the institutional controls. For example, there is no assurance that the area where medication is prepared is clean and that the caregiver uses sterile technique. The registered nurse must assess these environmental factors and determine that care can be provided safely.

The development of specialized services requires careful planning and development of procedures to ensure employee safety in the uncontrolled home environment. Infection control techniques, employee training, and program protocols must include the many variables encountered by an employee who works independently.

Another employee health and safety concern related specifically to home health care is security. Agency personnel travel into various communities, often at night, and encounter an assortment of neighbors and family members. Alone, the staff must deal with issues in family dynamics that can be threatening. Often, the patient most in need of care resides in an unsafe neighborhood. It is critical to address security issues through policies and employee education. Measures such as defined procedures for nighttime visits are essential. Furthermore, in those areas known to be unsafe, the agency should consider using security guards to accompany the nurse.

Risk control and prevention may also require use of emergency telephone procedures and/or pages. Safety and security policies must clearly define management's expectations for employee conduct, especially for such issues as the use of security guard services. The personnel manual must clearly define safety and security activities and their relationship to the risk management program. It is important to establish immediate notice of accidents, injuries, and all incidents related to employee health and safety.

Risk Management Program

The development of a comprehensive, practical risk management program for a home health agency must address the exposures identified in the discussions of patient care services, the role of the caregiver, and employee health and safety. Existing programs and reporting procedures, as well as information on losses experienced in the past, can provide a basis to develop the program's structure. The obvious goal is a coordinated process that identifies, evaluates, and addresses potential and actual risks of agency operations; constantly monitoring all factors will permit the agency to continuously refine its programs and to eliminate or reduce unnecessary risk.

An effective risk management program begins with an agency corporate policy that states the commitment to safe and efficient delivery of services and allocation of resources to ensure that the risk management effort succeeds. A formal policy statement from top management lets all employees know that the commitment to safe delivery of quality patient services is the primary operating philosophy. An effective risk management program involves interaction with all levels of employees, often crossing department lines, and requires the cooperation of all agency personnel. It is critical to avoid the association of risk management activities with punitive results; the emphasis must be on preventing incidents, solving problems, and upgrading skill levels.

The corporate policy also establishes the authority and responsibility for the risk management function. Risk managers agree that the responsible person must be one with sufficient authority to initiate appropriate changes in response to identified problems. Furthermore, the individual must be sufficiently removed from supervising field staff to avoid punitive overtones. Centralizing this function will facilitate the reasonably standardized treatment of loss exposures among the departments involved in developing and delivering patient care services. Once the program policy and authority are established, the agency must evaluate its current operations as they re-late to the goals of services provided. The following steps should help to develop and implement an effective risk management program.

- *Identify exposures to loss in existing programs and services.* An assessment checklist can facilitate this process (see Exhibit 24-2 for an example). Reviewing current services and practice will provide information needed to develop future programs.

- *Establish a formalized communication network with management, clinical supervisors, and physician consultants.* A team conference on risk management issues will provide a forum to discuss and resolve identified problems. The risk management reporting system should be separate from the operations chain of responsibility so that employees clearly understand that this communication network exists to protect the organization and the employees.

- *Develop a reporting mechanism to identify problems experienced in delivering services and provide timely intervention.* The home health care incident report should be structured to take into account the major identified risks particular to home health care. This would include risks typical to hospital care such as burns, medication errors, and falls. Caregiver competency, physician communication, and adequate assessment involve the potential for major risks specific to home health care. It is useful to apply reporting mechanisms and information sources that are already part of agency operations. Established information sources include internal quality assurance mechanisms, patient grievances and complaints, infection control activities, employee injury reports, recent patient care audits, and patient satisfaction questionnaires.

- *Educate all personnel on risk management policies, procedures, and reporting requirements.* All agency personnel need to know about the plan established to identify and resolve problems and why their participation is important to the agency.

- *Provide a feedback mechanism on problems identified.* Data obtained through established reporting mechanisms provide useful trend analysis for quality assurance activities. In addition, personnel are encouraged and motivated when included in the problem-solving process.

- *Evaluate the results.* As with management activities, it is important to measure progress and allow for review of established goals and objectives. Risk management is a dynamic process. There is so much growth and change in home health agency operations that it is necessary to remain flexible and allow for change and growth of the risk management program.

Conclusion

The explosive growth of the home health care industry in recent years has been fueled by a variety of economic, political, and social factors, and most experts believe that it

Exhibit 24-2. Checklist for assessing risk associated with intravenous antibiotic administration program.

Risk Assessment for Intravenous Antibiotic Administration Program

1. Classes of Patients and Clients Served
    - Diagnosis of controlled infectious disease.
    - Patient with adequate venous access.
    - Primary caregiver (family member) competent, if applicable.

2. Risk and Responsibility of Registered Nurse
    - Successful completion of in-service education.
    - Administration of medication.
    - Establishment of peripheral line.
    - Obtaining of laboratory specimen.
    - Monitoring of patient response to treatment.
    - Communication with physician.
    - Instruction of patient/caregiver.
        Performing procedure.
        Observing patient response.
        Recording and reporting patient response.
    - Documentation.

3. Operating Procedures
    - Collaborative definition of scope of procedure.
    - Certification and recertification of agency staff.
    - Clinical risks:
        Anaphylaxis.
        Nerve, tissue, and/or vascular damage.
        Toxic reaction to drugs.
        Assessment of patient/caregiver competency to perform procedure and monitor patient.

4. Medical Equipment and Supplies
    - Preparation of medication.
    - Intravenous start-up kit, including tubing and cannulas.
    - Intravenous pumps, including pole and cassette.

5. Regulations
    - State law regulating nursing practice.
    - Medicare rules.

6. Social and Economic Considerations
    - Cleanliness of home environment.
    - Cost of medication.
    - Preauthorization requirements (MediCal/Medicaid, health maintenance organizations, preferred provider organizations).

7. Corporate Assets
    - 24-hour on-call coverage and communication.
    - Computer services.

will continue as the elderly population continues to expand. At the same time, home health agencies are caught in a financial vise because of pressures exerted by governmental and private payers. In the absence of accepted national standards of care, the temptation is strong to reduce commitments to quality patient care even as patient acuity levels and the need for specialized care increase.

The scope of the typical home health agency's services and products has similarly expanded in recent years, and increasingly the diversity of programs demands a formal risk management system to reduce the attendant exposure to risk. Certainly, the most important area on which to focus is the delivery of clinical services in the home. This includes not only monitoring high technology programs such as intravenous medication, chemotherapy, and parenteral nutrition but also documenting that basic nursing procedures related to catheter care, diabetes management, and wound care are conducted according to defined policies and procedures.

In addition, the use of incident reports and follow-up study helps identify the potential for risk exposure before a serious problem in patient care or employee safety can occur. Close monitoring of incidents that have actually occurred promotes the likelihood that potential claims will be eliminated or better controlled.

An effective risk management program also addresses the issue of caregiver competency, undoubtedly the murkiest area of liability for home health agencies. In the area of governance, organization, and operation of a home health agency, Medicare rules define minimum standards of operation; responsibility for caregiver actions, however, has not been defined. As a result, home health agencies need to carefully assess caregiver competency throughout their involvement in a case. In situations where a significant question arises regarding the caregiver's proficiency to perform a particular procedure, other alternatives must be investigated, even if the end result is placement of the patient outside the home. Of greater practical importance is the need for the home health agency to prevent injury in the many cases where the caregiver's ability to function is generally consistent. Patient/caregiver manuals, extended hours of operation, 24-hour on-call nurses, and the ability to provide unscheduled visits are all practical interventions designed to prevent patient injury and ensure high quality patient services. Finally, there are a number of related operations areas that must be monitored by risk management staff, including staff selection, orientation, and in-service education and training, as well as established policies to ensure employee health and safety. Taken together, all these factors truly point to the reality that a centralized risk management program is a necessity for the long-term survival of the Medicare-certified home health agency.

References

Bureau of Data Management and Statistics: *Medicare Data,* Oct 1985.

Williams J, et al: *Home Health Services: An Industry in Transition.* Cambridge, Mass: ABT Associates Inc, 1984.

Note: Home health care for the elderly: Programs, problems, and potential. *Harvard Journal on Legislation* 22:193, 200, Winter 1985.

Orlikoff JE, et al. *Malpractice Prevention and Liability Control for Hospitals.* Chicago: American Hospital Association, 1981, pp 22-24.

Stewart JE: *Home Health Care.* St. Louis: CV Mosby, 1979, pp 1-4.

42 C.F.R. §4051220-.1229 (1984).

CAL. BUS. & PROF. CODE §2625 (West 1985).

Darling v Charleston Community Memorial Hospital, 33 Ill.2d 326 (1965).

Harber P, et al: Occupational low back pain in hospital nurses. *J Occup Med* 27:518-524, Jul 1985.

Chapter Twenty-Five

Ethical Issues

Charmaine McMaster Fitzig

Introduction

According to Bandman and Bandman (1985, 4), "Ethics . . . is concerned with doing good and avoiding harm . . . possibilities of good or harm depend partly on knowledge and partly on values. Both must be consciously and critically evaluated for their potential of good or harm to human beings, well or sick." The practice of nursing is concerned with doing good and, in attempting to define what is good, one could begin with a review of several different pledges or codes which have defined the practice of nursing over time. The following is one of the statements in the Florence Nightingale Pledge, written in 1893 by Lystra Gretter (Kalisch and Kalisch 1978, 141-142):

> . . . I will abstain from whatever is deleterious and mischievous and will not take or knowingly administer any harmful drug. . . .

The International Council of Nurses Code of Ethics begins with the statement: "The fundamental responsibility of the nurse is fourfold: to promote health, to prevent illness, to restore health and to alleviate suffering. . . . (Kelly 1985, 209)

The code which is probably best known and cited most often, because of the seeming increase in ethical dilemmas due to several court cases which have had extensive media coverage (*Doe versus Bolton* 410 U.S. 179; *Roe versus Wade* 410 U.S. 113), is the American Nurses' Association Code for Nurses. Only 2 of 11 provisions are cited here:

> The nurse provides services with respect for human dignity and the uniqueness of the client unrestricted by considerations of social or economic status, personal attributes, or the nature of the health problem (ANA 1976, 4).
> The nurse assumes responsibility and accountability for individual nursing judgements and actions (ANA 1976, 9).

The early philosophers like Socrates, Plato, and Aristotle attempted to define the meaning of good, the role of the individual, and the role of the state. But today, after centuries of debates and hundreds of treatises, we are no closer at deciding absolutely what "good" is or what an individual or state should do. The final decisions must be based on several factors, among them, but not limited to time, knowledge and technological advances, the culture and values of a people, the available resources, and ultimately, the cost. Given the uncertainty of the decision-making process, however, several positions or theories have been developed over the years which could serve as guidelines for action in the health care delivery system. Bandman and Bandman (1985,

40-41) have developed an interesting and graphic representation of what they call "models of morality in nursing practice." (See Exhibit 25-1.) They state:

> As one studies ethics, one finds no single science of moral values. One, instead, finds alternative models of morality and dialogue between these. Alternative models of morality orient the role of nursing in the care of patients. These models

Exhibit 25-1. Models of morality in nursing practice.

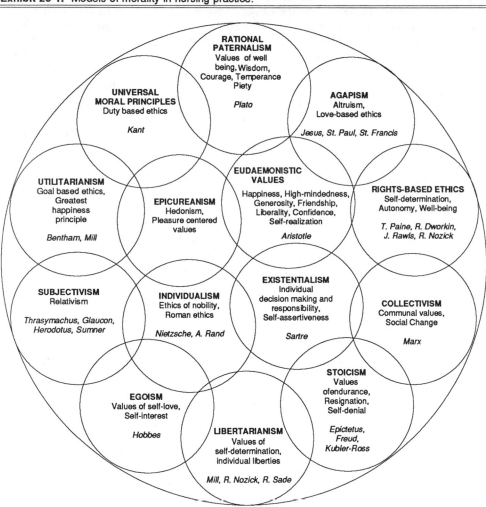

Reprinted with permission. Elsie L. Bandman and Bertram Bandman, 1985. "Models of Morality in Nursing Practice," Figure 4.1, *Nursing ethics in the life span*, p. 41. Norwalk, CT: Appleton-Century-Crofts.

of moral values are like overlapping circles. Each model sets out its values along with an attempted justification to some decision-making aspect of nursing.

Ethics, also called moral philosophy, is generally divided into three major subdisciplines; metaethics, normative ethics, and applied or bioethics. Metaethics deals with questions related to the nature of moral concepts and judgments. Normative ethics is concerned with establishing standards or norms for conduct, and is commonly associated with general theories about how one ought to live. Applied or bioethics is the application of normative theories to practical moral problems such as human rights, the quality of life, and the ethical implications of various developments in medicine and the biological sciences such as *in vitro* fertilization and the operation and use of sperm banks or gene manipulation, etc. (*New Encyclopaedia Britannica*, s.v. "egoism").

It has been postulated that ethics began with the introduction of the first moral codes, and examples of ancient codes or laws would certainly include the Ten Commandments and the code of Hammurabi. . . .

Ancient Beginnings

A description of selected positions or theories is presented after a brief historical review of the ancient beginnings of western ethical thinking, starting with the classical period of Greek ethics.

Socrates (470-399 B.C.), considered one of the seminal thinkers of Greek Philosophy, operated under two assumptions (*New Encyclopaedia Britannica*, s.v. "history of western philosophy").

1. The principle never to do wrong nor to participate, even indirectly, in any wrongdoing; and

2. The conviction that nobody who really knows what is good and right could act against it.

Plato (428-347 B.C.), the most important disciple of Socrates, is best known for his "Theory of Ideas," one of which was the ideal of good which he described as "beyond being and knowledge" (*New Encyclopaedia Britannica*, s.v. "history of western philosophy"). Aristotle (384-322 B.C.), a younger contemporary of Plato, believed in the doctrine of purposiveness. He felt that all human activities are directed toward the end of a good and satisfactory life (*New Encyclopaedia Britannica* s.v. "history of western philosophy").

The latter period of Greek and Roman ethics included the Stoics and Epicureans who presented very different positions as to how one ought to live. The Stoics felt that all human beings share the capacity to reason, and that what is important is the pursuit of wisdom and virtue. They rejected passion as a basis for deciding what is good or bad. Suicide, as a means of avoiding inescapable pain, was acceptable to the Stoics (*New Encyclopaedia Britannica*, s.v. "ethics"). The Epicureans regarded pleasure as the sole ultimate good, and pain as the sole evil. The founder of this philosophy, Epicurus, taught that the greatest pleasure obtainable was the pleasure of tranquility which is to be obtained by the removal of unsatisfied wants. (*New Encyclopaedia Britannica,* s.v. "ethics").

Selected Ethical Theories

Egoism

From the Latin *ego,* I, egoism is an ethical theory holding that the good is based on the pursuit of self-interest. The egoist sees perfection sought through the furthering of a man's own welfare and profit (*New Encyclopaedia Britannica,* s.v. "egoism").

Utilitarianism

The fundamental principle of utilitarianism, a tradition in ethics stemming from the late eighteenth and nineteenth century English philosophers and economists Jeremy Bentham and John Stuart Mill, is that an action is right if it tends to promote happiness and wrong if it tends to provide the reverse of happiness—not just the happiness of the performer of the action but that of everyone affected by it. This theory is in opposition to egoism (*New Encyclopaedia Britannica,* s.v. "utilitarianism").

Altruism

Ethics governed more by man's social aspects, which stresses the importance of the community rather than the individual (*New Encyclopaedia Britannica,* s.v. "altruism").

Deontology

A theory that judges actions by their conformance to some formal rule or principle, such as the ethical system of the German philosopher Immanuel Kant who felt that our actions possess moral worth only when we do our duty for its own sake (*New Encyclopaedia Britannica,* s.v. "ethics").

The Theory of Justice

Put forth by John Rawls, the "theory of justice" was a welcome alternative to utilitarianism. His theory had two principles. The first stated that each person should have the maximum amount of liberty. The second principle required that wealth be distributed so as to equalize the resources and afford the greatest benefit to the least advantaged (Rawls 1971, 257-258).

Theory of Obligation

William Frankena, a modern philosopher, in 1973 published his work *Ethics* in which he described his "Theory of Obligation" which contained two basic principles. The first principle of beneficence included four "oughts" — not to inflict harm or evil, to prevent harm, to remove evil, and to do or promote good. The second principle was one of justice as equal treatment — the equal or comparative treatment of individuals, dealing with people according to their merits (Frankena 1973, 47).

Two other modern-day philosophers have written on the rights of individuals and the role of the state. Robert Noziak (a deontologist), in his 1974 book, *Anarchy, State and Utopia,* presented the ideal that life, liberty, and legitimately acquired property are absolute and that no act can be justified if it violates them. He further indicated that no one, not even the state, had a right to assist people in the preservation of their rights (Noziak 1974, ix). Although Ronald Dworkin agreed with Noziak's theory of individual rights, his ideas were much broader. In his work *Taking Rights Seriously,* he indicated that respect for others might require us to assist them and not leave individuals to fend for themselves. In addition, Dworkin felt that the state had an obligation to intervene in areas where it was necessary to ensure the preservation of individual rights (Dworkin 1977, xi).

Characteristics of Ethical Issues

The five criteria proposed by Rawls (1971) for looking at the rightness of any ethical principle can serve as a guide in the identification and analysis of all ethical issues or dilemmas:

1. Universality — the same principles must hold for everyone.

2. Generality — reference must not be made to specific people or situations.

3. Publicity — the situation or issue must be known and recognized by all involved.

4. Ordering — conflicting claims must be ordered without resorting to force.

5. Finality — the issue may override the demands of law and custom.

The health care delivery system is replete with instances where ethical dilemmas have had to be resolved through the convening of ethics committees or through the courts. In the early days of kidney dialysis (prior to 1972 when Public Law 92-603 was enacted and made dialysis procedures financially available to all), many hospitals initiated interdisciplinary teams to define the criteria for deciding who was put on the machine. Many of these teams were later called ethics committees and were involved in decisions regarding more than the kidney machines. A practice which is fairly common within many hospitals, and known to few outsiders, is sometimes placing in pencil the initials DNR (Do Not Resuscitate) on selected patients' charts. This custom was discussed at length by Dr. Korein who testified in the Karen Ann Quinlan case about the unwritten and unspoken standards of medical practice (*In the Matter of Karen Quinlan* 1976, 655).

... cancer, metastatic cancer, involving the lungs, the liver, the brain, multiple involvements, the physician may or may not write DNR . . . it could be said to the nurse: if this man stops breathing don't resuscitate him. . . . No physician that I know personally is going to resuscitate a man riddled with cancer and in agony and he stops breathing. They are not going to put him on a respirator. . . . I think that would be the height of misuse of technology.

Several other important issues have been tried in the courts. Among them are the following interesting cases which have implications for public health nursing practice.

Individual Rights and Abortion

In *Roe versus Wade* (41.0 U.S. 113 [1973]) and *Doe versus Bolton* (410 U.S. 179 [1973]), the right of every woman to have a legal abortion was established.

Quality of Life and Right to Die were issues addressed in the Karen Ann Quinlan case. Her father, as her guardian, won the right to obtain a physician who would agree that the respirator should not be used, based on the medical decision that there could be no reasonable possibility of Karen's returning to a cognitive state (*In the Matter of Karen Quinlan* 1976, 671).

The Right to Life issue resulted in a national debate after a six-day-old infant, "Baby Doe," born with Down's Syndrome and an incomplete esophagus, died from lack of food and water. The courts in Illinois supported the parents' decision to refuse surgical intervention (*New York Times* April 20, 1982). In response to the public outcry, the United States Department of Health and Human Services Office of Civil Rights issued the now infamous "Notice to Health Care Providers" which directed anyone with knowledge of the denial of food or customary medical care to immediately contact the Department's handicapped infant hotline or the State's child protection services. These notices were to be placed in conspicuous places. This directive was later found to be invalid by the United States District judge.

Unfortunately, many nurses and hospital administrators failed to take advantage of the furor caused by the Baby Doe case to initiate permanent ethics committees. In addition, few hospitals have realized the need for ongoing continuing education or training programs on decision making relative to clinical issues dealing with ethical dilemmas.

Ethical Issues in the Administrative and Clinical Areas of Home Health Care

In general, although the types of ethical issues and dilemmas encountered in home health care are, by and large, no different from those encountered within the whole spectrum of the health care delivery system, there are several issues which are unique to home health care. The following issues will be addressed:

1. Case finding.

2. Documenting for reimbursement.

3. Public health nursing and complex care in the community; are they compatible?

4. The quality of life.

5. The role of the home health aide and supervision within the home.

Case Finding

Two decades ago, when I was a student and later a staff nurse in a public health nursing agency, one of the criteria which was used to evaluate my effectiveness was my case-finding ability. In those days, we had the luxury of actively seeking out individuals and families who were potential users of health services. They were the other family members or neighbors who were present when actual home visits were made (the pregnant teenager, the elderly diabetic, etc.). These new cases were contacted and cared for without the reimbursement limitations. Today, even though, theoretically, case finding is still considered a "good public health practice," it is not pursued as vigorously as was done in the fifties or sixties. The general feeling is, "Why look for cases to increase your caseload when the majority may not be reimbursed?" Of course, there are some public health nurses and supervisors within the public health agencies (voluntary and public) who still do some case finding, and who have budgeted a small percent of their funds for case finding. Many, however, have developed strict criteria in deciding which types of cases to go after.

Documentation for Reimbursement

The importance of recording accurate data is stressed in nursing schools; nurses' notes have played prominently in several malpractice suits. Many examples of court cases lost or won have been reviewed in classrooms during discussions of the legal aspects of documentation. Hospitals and home health agencies have recognized the importance of accurate recording not only to serve as evidence of good patient care, but as safeguards in some future malpractice suits. Many hospitals have also hired individuals, known as risk managers, to evaluate, monitor, and modify practices which can have deleterious effects on patient care and safety.

Continuation programs stressing the legal aspects of nursing, and especially the issue of documentation, have been very popular among nursing audiences. In a 1974 survey on ethics done by *Nursing '74*, four questions out of seventy-three dealt with recording information. The survey results were interesting and confirmed the fact that almost all nurses (96%) — at least among those who responded — would not record inaccurate data. The questions and their responses were as follows (*Nursing '74* 1974, 56-65).

In making notes have you ever done the following?

N - 11,681

Q. 50.	Added information by writing between lines?	48%
Q. 51.	Erased or altered information?	11%
Q. 52.	Purposely omitted information because it might make you look bad?	9%
Q.53.	Recorded inaccurate information because of a delicate situation?	4%

Contrary to these data, Mary Mundinger (1983), in her book *Home Care Controversy: Too Little, Too Late, Too Costly,* found several instances where nurses omitted or "adjusted" data in order to maintain nursing services which the clients needed. The nurses ignored the Medicare restrictions and recorded whatever data were necessary to conform to the rules. In order to comply with these rules, three important criteria had to be met:

1. The patient must require skilled care.

2. The patient must have a doctor's plan of care.

3. The patient must be homebound.

Mundinger's study involved 50 home visits in which she compared the care given to the Medicare eligibility criteria as noted earlier. At the time of the visits, 16 (or 32%) of the clients did not meet the requirements for skilled care (Mundinger 1983, 58), only 25 (or 50%) of the doctors' plans of care were judged to be adequate (Mundinger 1983, 88), and only 15 (or 30%) of the patients were actually homebound (Mundinger 1983, 85). Mundinger notes, "Nurses learn how to document cases to assure reimbursement. Fabrication is rare but adjustment of the data probably is frequent." (Mundinger 1983, 66) Mundinger does not indicate how many nurses she observed in her study of 50 home visits.

Although the *Nursing '74* survey did not include the place of work of the nurses who responded, one can safely assume that the majority worked in hospitals and there were no indications that public health nurses responded. It would be interesting to conduct a similar study among public health nurses. Invariably, the question of recording to meet the reimbursement criteria would be an important issue. It would be enlightening to know how common this practice is in public health nursing.

Another author, Shirley Hoeman (1984), in her unpublished doctoral dissertation, describes how nurses record data to ensure the maximum benefits for clients. She notes that the restrictions of the reimbursement procedures make it difficult for nurses to "give care in a curing system."

Milar Aroskar in "Ethics in the Nursing Curriculum" describes a survey which was based on questionnaires sent to the deans or curriculum coordinators of some 209 accredited baccalaureate nursing programs in the United States. Eighty-six schools (or 80%) responded. Two-thirds of the respondents said that ethical aspects were integrated throughout the nursing courses (Aroskar 1977, 260-264)

Public Health Nursing and Complex Care Within the Community—Are They Compatible?

Many nurses working in public health or community health nursing agencies are graduates of baccalaureate nursing programs. Many of them forego experience in the hospital and go directly into community nursing. The community agencies usually welcome these new graduates since many of them would have completed their clinical experiences at the agencies involved. Many agencies require one or two years hospital experience for the nonbaccalaureate-prepared nurse. As a result of many cost-containment strategies, hospitals have responded by discharging patients sooner and sicker. The needs of these patients are complex and include administration of peripheral and central intravenous therapy, passage of nasogastric tubes for feeding, ventilators, chemotherapy, etc. In order to respond adequately to the increasing referrals of patients in need of complex care, many of the voluntary community home health nursing agencies have modified their services to offer 24-hour nursing and support services (Bowyer 1986, 24-29; *American Journal of Nursing* 1984, 341-342). In addition, these agencies have identified the learning needs of their staff nurses and have, in cooperation with many hospitals and equipment companies, developed in-depth, in-service education programs for their nurses and support staffs.

Many proprietary home health nursing agencies and equipment manufacturers have recognized the financial rewards of establishing specialized, clinical nursing teams who make home visits and care for clients in need of high-technology nursing services. Many of these nurses are recruited from the intensive care and medical-surgical units of hospitals. The majority are registered nurses without public health preparation, experience, or orientation. Consequently, they are unable to function as public health nurses. Their purpose in the home is to complete a special task. The functions of public health nursing, which include health education, health promotion, and risk reduction, are usually not addressed. We have these mini-medical-surgical teams operating in the home and the practice of public health nursing is nonexistent.

Fortunately, a few of these commercial agencies do have supervisors or staff nurses who are public health practitioners and who recognize the importance of obtaining individual and family assessment data on each referral. These nurses become the coordinators and work closely with the 'high-tech' specialized nurse in the development of appropriate comprehensive care plans.

Quality of Life

Webster defines quality as a "peculiar and essential character" and as a "degree of excellence." (*Webster's New Universal Unabridged Dictionary,* s.v. "quality"). Obviously, each person who is capable of reasoning will determine what constitutes quality of life or "degree of excellence" for himself or herself. The final decision as to what "degree of excellence" the individual is willing to accept will, to a large extent, be influenced by several factors, among them: state of health, ability to function independently (financially and personally), adequate housing or living conditions, meaningful family or significant other relationships, changes in lifestyle, etc.

Quality-of-life issues have gained importance with the increase in technological advances. Although no age group has escaped quality-of-life considerations, for certain groups of people the quality-of-life issue is a daily experience in decisions and choices. These groups or populations at risk include the handicapped or disabled, the poor, the minorities, the chronically ill, and the elderly. There have been several situations dealing with quality-of-life issues among the chronically ill which have had extensive media coverage. The following court cases all have implications for public health nursing.

Elizabeth Bouvia, a 25-year-old quadriplegic cerebral palsy victim, in 1983 filed suit against the hospital because she wanted to starve to death. At the time, she contended that her pain-ridden body was useless and that her physical disabilities prevented her from taking her own life. The judge refused her request (*New York Times* January 22, 1986). In January 1986, she filed suit against a second hospital—where she was hospitalized—because, against her wishes, the doctors had inserted a feeding tube through her nose and she was fed by force. Ms. Bouvia later stated: "I didn't want to ever depend on others in an institution. I'm caught in a legal bind because other people can't realize I'm not living, I'm existing . . . " (*New York Times* February 13, 1986)

In April 1986, a state appeals court panel declared that "the right to refuse medical treatment is basic and fundamental" and ruled that Ms. Bouvia has the right to refuse to be force-fed (Chambers 1986, 5-6).

Another equally dramatic case involved a 30-year-old woman. In March 1980, Nancy Jobes, who was four-and-a-half months pregnant, was injured in a car crash and the fetus was killed. During surgery to remove the fetus, she had a cardiac arrest from an anesthesia accident. This resulted in severe brain damage and coma. Several months later she was transferred from the hospital to a nursing home. Nearly five years later her husband and family petitioned the courts to allow her to die by removing the artificial feeding tube since she had been in an irreversible vegetative state since the cardiac arrest. The State Superior Court Judge ruled that the artificial feeding tube could be removed (Sullivan 1986, 1-4).

The third case deals with an individual who was maintained at home on a respirator. Ms. Farrell was 37-years-old and suffered from amyotrophic lateral sclerosis. She was paralyzed except for the muscles controlling her eyes and lips. Ms. Farrell and her husband petitioned the court to allow the respirator to be disconnected because she did not wish to live. The judge approved saying that "it would be cruel to sustain a life so wracked with pain." The decision by Judge Wiley of Superior Court in Toms River was the first in New Jersey to allow the withdrawal of life support from a person who was being cared for at home (Sullivan 1986, 6).

It is interesting to note that the majority of the cases involving quality-of-life issues were initiated by, or on behalf of, patients who were either in hospitals or other institutions at the time the suits were initiated. One might speculate that, for the patient receiving nursing services at home, the public health nurse would have obtained vital information (through an adequate initial and periodic assessment of the patient) prior to any need for emergency treatments. This would then necessitate a plan of care, with the patient's involvement, that would allow the patient's wishes to be followed. Many terminally ill patients and nurses working in oncology units have enthusiastically welcomed the expanding hospice movements.

The proportion of the population 65 years and older is growing at a faster rate than of other age groups, and the 85 years and older group is growing very rapidly. Recent data indicate that although 60 percent of the two million users of home health services are less than 65 years of age, the most intensive users are the elderly who average 22.3 home health visits annually. The data show that 78 percent of all home health visits are received by Americans older than 65 years of age even though they account for only 43 percent of the user population (National Center for Health Services Research 1985, I).

That the elderly are at risk for institutionalization was confirmed by a National Center for Health Statistics survey, which indicated that almost half the elderly report some degree of limitation of activity resulting from chronic disease or impairment (DHHS 1983, 67-70). These same data indicated that an estimated 4.7 million adults in the civilian noninstitutionalized population needed functional assistance from another person for selected personal care or home management activities. More than half (2.7 million) were 65 years of age and over, 1.3 million were 44 to 64 years of age. Less than one million were between 18 and 44 years of age. The percentage of the noninstitutionalized population needing another person's help increased with age. Functional assistance was needed by only one percent of young adults but by 12 percent of the elderly. As expected, the proportion of the population needing help continued to increase with age among those 65 years of age and older. Those needing help varied from 7 percent for those 65 to 74 years, 16 percent for those 75 to 84 years, to 39 percent for those 85 years and older (DHHS 1983).

The ability to maintain independent living is dependent on a number of factors which include the following: extent of disability and functional impairment; sociodemographic characteristics of the individual (sex, age, and living arrangements); availability of another person to provide needed assistance; and the availability of community services and their accessibility to people who need them (DHHS 1983).

For the elderly person receiving public health nursing services at home, the countdown begins when he or she begins to have difficulty in personal care and home management skills. As his or her abilities decrease, decisions about living arrangements have to be made. As living arrangements change—whether by moving to a relative's home or to an institution, or staying at home with the assistance of a home health aide—the quality of life is compromised.

The Role of the Home Health Aide and Supervision within the Home

Among the benefits of the Medicaid and Medicare legislation of the 1960s was the increased availability of home health aide services. The primary function of a home health aide is to give or assist a patient in personal care. The public health nurse, who is a registered nurse and the patient's primary nurse, supervises the services of the aide. The primary nurse assigns the home health aide to a particular patient based on a written plan of care initiated by the physician who certifies the patient's need for personal care, in addition to other services which may be needed (speech, physical or occupational therapy, or skilled nursing care). The training of home health aides varies by agency even within the same geographic area. The length of training can be as short as five days and as long as twenty days. The goal of care for the patient is to maintain or increase the patient's ability to function independently. The level of assistance from the home health aide depends on many factors, among them: the patient's functional ability as defined by the primary nurse; the patient's motivation and willingness in engaging in a therapeutic relationship; the skill of the home health aide in developing and maintaining a supportive environment; and the skill of the primary nurse in initiating and nurturing the supervisory process.

Personal care duties which may be performed by the home health aide include: assistance getting in and out of bed, in bathing, and in eating; grooming, to include mouth care; an exercise program, in and out of braces; meal preparation, to include special diets; and facilitating the prescribed medications which are ordinarily self-administered.

All the duties assigned to a home health aide are written with space for the aide to check off daily at the completion of each task. Although the primary nurse would have instructed the aide and would have observed her in the completion of selected tasks, the aide is very much on her own in between the supervisory visits. The quality of the work and the fulfillment of the duties, to a large extent, is dependent on the integrity and level of sensitivity and ability of the aide.

The intricate balance between the primary nurse, patient, and aide is strained or broken when there is a change of assignments for either the nurse or aide. Another factor, over which the nurse has no control, is the level of preparation of the aide. The agency supplying the aides is usually not from the same public health nursing service from which the nurse is assigned.

In an ideal situation, the same aide will remain with the patient for the duration of the period specified for skilled nursing. Over time, this aide may know more about the patient than the nurse or other health professionals who visit. With limited education (many of them have not completed high school education) and with a patient population which is getting older, and returning from hospitals sooner and sicker, the aide is at a distinct disadvantage.

It takes a well-prepared public health nurse who is patient and plans her supervision visit so that she can assess the aide's ability to follow instructions "to the letter." Her gentle probing of the aide by way of asking "What else do you do for Ms. A to help her with her arthritis?" may elicit the response, "I put warm packs on her knees." The nurse then has to remind the aide that even though Ms. A directed her to apply the warm packs, they were not prescribed. . . . What about assisting the patient in taking medications? How many nurses really know the extent of this assistance? How many nurses would routinely ask a patient to open a medication bottle and observe the kind of assistance Ms. A needs before writing down on the instruction sheet "assist with medications." The aide can assist Ms. A by loosening the medication bottle cap, or even taking the pills out, but she may not pick up a pill and hand it to Ms. A. To do that would be dispensing medications and that is illegal. What happens if Ms. A's arthritis makes her unable to bend her fingers to pick up the pill and then transfer it safely to her mouth? What happens if Ms. A has no "significant other?" How much of this sort of activity is recorded, much less discussed. Of course the nurse says to the aide, "You may not give her the pills . . . you may help by loosening the bottle cover."

But the nurse and the aide both know the extent of the assistance will be more than loosening the bottle cap—a sort of gentlewomen's unspoken agreement.

Strategies

Case Finding

Agency administrators need to decide if case finding and preventive care is an important function and, if so, to include these services with the necessary criteria for eligibility. The policy should be clear and shared openly with agency staff. One way to determine the importance of case finding through the seeking out of at-risk population groups would be to compare the agency's caseload with the community's mortality and morbidity database obtained through complete and current population and community assessments.

Documentation

Accurate and timely recording can facilitate change. Policy decisions need hard data in order to support the need. Agency personnel and administrators need to discuss the problems openly. Nurses have to accept the responsibility of recording all data even if it means that a service visit would not be reimbursed. The agency then would have to assume a larger deficit until the reimbursement regulations are changed. If all the agencies coordinated their efforts and lobbied for changes based on the data which are recorded and not omitted, that would be, in the long run, a more professional and ethical posture to take.

Quality of Life

A problem which is virtually ignored is the increasing number of elderly persons committing suicide. Statistics indicate that more than any other age group, the elderly are more prone to commit suicide. According to Dr. Nancy Osgood, an assistant professor of Gerontology and Sociology at Virginia Commonwealth University in Richmond, seven out of ten elderly persons who attempt suicide succeed. In addition, she indicated that 25 percent of the country's elderly population commits suicide. The population at risk for suicide includes the isolated lower class, elderly males in urban areas, and the widowed male who may have suffered multiple losses including physical, mental, financial, and social. According to Dr. Osgood, all these factors increase the likelihood of depression and, ultimately for many, suicide (Bugman 1985, 91). Public health nurses can increase the degree of the quality of life for each patient by consistently obtaining and recording assessment data of individuals and their families. By analyzing the data, the nurse identifies those individuals at risk and develops appropriate short-term and long-term goals with the individual's and the family's participation. Within the first visit, the nurse should be aware of the patient's preference to die at home, for example, and would—with the patient's permission—engage the "significant other" in the plan of action for the time when the patient's condition would necessitate decisions being made.

It is disheartening that, at this point in time, we do not have recreational or occupational programs geared to the homebound in any systematic fashion. Even though the meals-on-wheels programs are limited in their scope, at least a fair number of elderly can get one meal per day for five days per week. How many crafts-on-wheels programs are there? We keep our elderly alive only to die of boredom or suicide.

Many industries have begun to implement pre-retirement programs to help their employees adjust to retirement. Many senior citizen centers have outreach and friendly visitor's programs, but they are not organized and not widespread enough. Recreational programs should be an essential home health service. These programs would certainly add to the quality of life among our elderly population.

Home Health Aides and Supervision

One of the most important factors in this relationship is the initial complete physical and mental assessment of the individual and identification of concerned and available family members or other "significant others."

Nurses must take the necessary time to instruct, to demonstrate important tasks, and to have the aide return the demonstration; all of this "instruction-demonstration-return demonstration" must be recorded.

It may be time for public health nursing agencies to consider adding the risk manager to the supervisory team. This person would review records on a regular basis, or, through planned discussions with supervisory personnel and staff nurses, identify situations which are unsafe or which have the potential for future litigation. These reviews would encourage nurses and their supervisors to discuss problems early so that they can be corrected before harm is done.

The quality of the supervision process must be strengthened. Many beginning staff nurses have not had experience with supervising aides. Many of the agency supervisors are not prepared at the master's level and may not even have had supervisory or administrative preparation. Administrators of public health nursing agencies need to be more aggressive and either require master's preparation for supervisory personnel or develop on-site instruction prior to, and at least during the first six months of a new supervisor's position. The supervisor's role is one which is demanding, creative, and interesting; she must be adequately prepared to handle such an important and awesome task.

Summary

Nurses in community health are involved in many decisions and, increasingly, these decisions deal more with patients' choices. The community nurse is truly a guest in the patient's home and, as such, needs to recognize the patient's right to direct his or her own care. Community nurses need an awareness of the ethical and legal principles which are involved in, or which have implications for, practice. Both staff and supervisory personnel need to discuss issues which are sensitive and potentially explosive —

the quality of the supervision of home health aides and the closing of cases due to non-reimbursement capability are obvious examples.

Ethical Concerns of Home Health Administration: The Day to Day Issues

Catherine H. Pignatello, Patricia Moulton, and Maureen A. Eng

The purpose of this section is to illustrate how home health agencies experience ethical dilemmas. Ethical issues identified as significant to administrators and staff of New Jersey home health agencies are presented, along with specific case examples. Recommendations are then made as to how agencies can establish processes for addressing these issues.

Significant Issues

Home health administrators are faced with a wide variety of ethical concerns, ranging from those related to maintaining agency solvency to ensuring employee safety on the job. In recognition of this fact, and in an attempt to address the ethical concerns of administrators, the Home Health Agency Assembly of New Jersey formed an ethics committee in December, 1985. (The Home Health Agency Assembly of New Jersey is a voluntary nonprofit state association representing the home health industry.) One of the first tasks of this newly formed committee was to elicit from agency administrators and staff what they perceived to be the most pressing issues. Questionnaires, round table discussions, and informal telephone interviews were utilized. As a result, the following problem areas were identified:

1. Trying to maintain agency solvency while at the same time trying to meet even minimum basic home health care needs of patients and families.

2. Ensuring employee safety without compromising patient care.

3. Maintaining an agency standard of productivity while still meeting increasingly complex care needs of patients and families in a qualified manner.

4. Addressing treatment decisions and truth telling issues in the care of the terminally or incurably ill.

5. Dealing with patient abuse or neglect involving both children and vulnerable adults.

6. Meeting patients' needs and demands as well as those of caregivers when such needs or demands conflict.

7. Resolving conflicts with physicians when physician intervention or lack of intervention is determined to be not in patients' best interest.

Case Examples

In order to give the reader a better understanding of the above issues, specific case examples will be given and each issue elaborated upon.

Agency Solvency. A major concern of home health administrators in this era of federal budget cuts and increased scrutiny of the health care industry is insufficient or nonexistent third-party reimbursement for home health services—services that are often needed just to provide minimum care. Many nonprofit agencies rely on grants, donations, or funding through programs such as the United Way to provide "free" services to those patients and families that cannot afford to pay. Yet these monies are limited and priorities must be set. The following case illustrates this dilemma.

"Mrs. A"

Mrs. A was a 91-year-old widow with diagnoses of severe degenerative arthritis, peripheral vascular disease, and mild dementia. She was bedbound secondary to bilateral contractures of the knees. Her daughter, age 58 and a widow, was Mrs. A's only living relative. The daughter worked from nine to five daily and was financially unable to cease working to care for her mother.

Mrs. A's condition had deteriorated to the point where she was totally dependent in all activities of daily living. Maximum assistance was required to transfer her out of bed. Although she had received home care services under Medicare for several weeks, the services had been terminated when Mrs. A's care reached the custodial level. Most importantly, this meant the withdrawal of home health aide services.

The agency's social worker met with the daughter and Mrs. A to discuss alternatives for care. Mrs. A's income exceeded the eligibility level of all available programs except for Medicaid nursing home. Both Mrs. A and her daughter refused to consider nursing home placement. At the same time, Mrs. A's daughter indicated that she would not consider purchasing home health aide services on a private-pay basis. As a result, Mrs. A was referred for home health aide assistance through a Medicaid waiver program. Because of this program's waiting list, Mrs. A would not receive any assistance for several months. In the interim, Mrs. A was given bath service twice weekly using funds provided to the agency by the local United Way.

Although bath service was the only recourse available to Mrs. A, it could hardly be considered adequate in meeting her complex care needs. The Agency, however, received only limited funding through the United Way for the bath service program and was responsible for making the program available to all agency clients in need.

There are several ethical issues relevant to Mrs. A's case. First, what criteria should the agency use in allocating limited funds and who will make the ultimate decision?

Second, what is the responsibility of the agency in providing service when the family is less than willing to care for the patient? It is easy to say that the family bears the ultimate responsibility, but what is the responsibility of the agency from a humanistic point of view?

And third, as the elderly increase in number, so will the demand for home care services. Who will bear the burden of paying for these services? How will home care agencies meet the needs of the chronically ill elderly and still maintain solvency?

Employee Safety. Home health administrators have a certain obligation to ensure the safety of their staff while that staff is carrying out job duties and responsibilities. Patients and families must also be expected to provide a reasonably safe environment for staff if they are able or if this is within their control. The question arises as to how far the administrator must go to fulfill this obligation and whether needed patient and family care should be compromised in order to protect agency staff. Here is an illustration.

"Mr. J"

Mr. J, age 72, lived with his wife in a large apartment building located in a low income urban area. Mr. J had intractable congestive heart failure and was being maintained at home with regular injections of IV Lasix. A twice weekly nursing visit for assessment of Mr. J's cardiopulmonary status, report to the physician, and administration of Lasix was required. His heart failure had responded favorably to the Lasix, allowing Mr. J to be out of bed for brief periods during the day. Mrs. J. was supportive and cooperative in her husband's care. Both Mr. and Mrs. J were determined to avoid rehospitalization at any cost.

The problems in this case arose because of the environment in which the family lived. The nurses had been warned of active drug dealing in the streets surrounding the J's building and in the building itself. The nurses believed that their safety was in jeopardy when they visited the J's, and the supervisory staff concurred.

Although the agency had its own escort program, this program was fraught with many problems. Escorts were frequently not available when needed by the nursing staff. Their character and reliability were often questionable, and in several instances, the escorts failed to meet nurses for scheduled visits. The agency was attempting to improve the escort program. At this time, however, reliable escort service was not available to the nurses when visiting the J's.

From an ethical perspective, how does an agency ensure the safety of its employees in this type of situation and still provide a needed service? How should the agency deal with the nurse who refuses to visit the patient because she believes her safety is jeopardized? Is it ethical to deny the patient home care services because of the environment in which he lives?

The issue of employee safety might also apply to the care of AIDS patients. Jonsen et al. (1986) in their article on "AIDS and Ethics" note that:

Despite evidence that health care workers are not at great risk, the undertone of fear remains. The maximal incubation period for AIDS may be as long as five years. Lack of definitive information engenders a climate of uncertainty, and uncertainty in turn promotes fear.

Many suburban and rural home health agencies are just beginning to get requests for home care of AIDS patients and thus just beginning to address the fear and uncertainty described above. An example follows.

"Mr. C"

An agency serving a suburban, primarily middle class population received their first AIDS referral. Mr. C was 37-years-old. He had an open, draining abdominal wound as a result of an intestinal fistula and subsequent surgery. He also had a Hickman catheter in place for the administration of antibiotics and chemotherapy. Mr. C was quite weak and required assistance with dressing changes, intravenous administration of medications, personal care, ADL, and meals. He lived with a male friend who worked and was out of the home from 7 a.m. to 7 p.m. No other family or significant others were involved in his care.

Despite the fact that Mr. C was the agency's first AIDS patient, they had infection control procedures in place in anticipation of just such a referral. However, there had not been an all out effort to educate and inform agency staff about AIDS and home care because of the lack of such patients. A nurse who had previously cared for AIDS patients in the hospital was assigned to the case and willingly accepted. Nevertheless, it was clear that other professional staff (nurses, social workers) would not be so willing. They expressed fear and concern when it was thought that they too might be assigned to Mr. C. Also, the agency was unable to secure a home health aide, either from their own staff or from five contracting aide agencies, who would take the case.

What can and should an administrator do to prevent such situations from arising? Is employee safety even an issue here or should all staff be expected to care for AIDS patients? What if the proper infection control procedures cannot be maintained in the home? What recourse does the administrator have if staff refuse to accept AIDS patients? Will education, information, and support to staff be enough to resolve the issue?

Productivity. Staff productivity is a significant factor in the determination of agency cost per visit, a factor that cannot be ignored. Most agencies require their salaried nursing staff to make a standard number of visits per day. On the other hand, with the advent of DRGs, patients are experiencing much shorter hospital stays or are not being admitted to the hospital at all. Home health care providers are picking up the slack, caring for much sicker patients and providing more high-tech care such as IV therapy, chemotherapy, and care of ventilator-dependent patients. Also staff is often faced with complex psychosocial factors that must be dealt with in order to ensure the safe home management of patients. All of this care takes time. This can be illustrated in the following case.

"Mrs. H"

Fifty-two-year-old Mrs. H had complete intestinal obstruction secondary to metastatic ovarian cancer. She was discharged from the hospital to her daughter's home with a double lumen Hickman catheter for administration of parenteral nutrition (TPN) and continuous Morphine Sulfate drip. She also had a nasogastric tube attached to suction.

Intense coordination by the primary nurse was required. Vendors providing equipment and supplies, a laboratory, three different physicians, the clinical nurse specialist, on-call nurses, social worker, physical therapist, and home health aides were all involved in the patient's care. The daughter required instruction and supervision in complex procedures and the nurses visiting had to be skilled and knowledgeable in these procedures and the use of equipment. Moreover, the psychological and emotional needs of the patient and her family needed to be identified and addressed. Mrs. H was still talking about a cure.

Should the nursing staff be allotted extra time for such cases or should they be expected to meet the agency productivity standard despite the complexity of their caseloads? If a certain productivity standard is an expectation, is there potential for quality of care to be compromised? Or can ways be found to provide quality care in complex cases in a more efficient, less time-consuming manner?

Treatment Decisions. Caring for the terminally ill at home probably presents some of the most challenging, confusing, and difficult cases to the staff of home health agencies.

In very few other situations does the complexity of issues surface, as patients, families, and staff confront head-on the inevitable issue of death, bringing with them their fears, experiences, religious and cultural beliefs. Whether agencies have a hospice program or not, caring for the dying, or the irreversibly chronically ill involves decisions regarding the refusal, withdrawal, and direction of treatment. Truth telling versus withholding of information from patients regarding their prognosis and diagnosis are continuous issues.

While end-of-life decision-making must be addressed as each concern surfaces in the patient and family situation, there are common themes that surface in many cases. The following cases might help to illustrate these points.

"Mr. E"

Mr. E was a 45-year-old man with the progressively degenerative disease of Amyotrophic Lateral Sclerosis. He had been cared for by his wife and children at home. Over the past five years, for every major decision about the direction of his care, he and his family discussed the implications, possibilities, and probabilities. It became increasingly difficult for him to swallow much more than soups, custards, and water. Mr. E, who could barely speak, and was no longer able to move his extremities, decided that he did not wish to have the feeding tube, which his physician recommended, inserted. The home health agency staff wanted to continue to care for Mr. E and were supportive of his decision, but found it increasingly difficult to work with the physician.

"Mrs. A"

Mrs. A was a 60-year-old woman with advanced metastatic carcinoma. Although she did not speak with the nurse about her prognosis, in spite of repeated attempts, Mr. A spoke to the staff about the many conversations he and Mrs. A had had about her diagnosis and prognosis.

Mrs. A's condition had slowly deteriorated since early September. Even so, in November she was anxiously awaiting the birth of her grandchild, due the next month.

Mrs. A became obstructed, and after outpatient tests, it was determined that tumor growth had caused the small bowel obstruction. The BUN was also rising, and while not confused, she became increasingly lethargic and unable to participate in any decision making. The surgeon recommended surgery to relieve the obstruction. Mr. A was unable to decide what course of action to take. He knew that his wife did not want any invasive or extraordinary means used to prolong her life. Yet he also knew how many times she spoke about the expected grandchild.

"Cheryl"

Mrs. T recently called the hospice program requesting care for her eight-year-old daughter, Cheryl. She had been diagnosed with a brain tumor one year ago, and the physicians told the parents that they had no further treatment modalities available to them. After heart-wrenching discussions, she and her husband requested hospice care.

Unfortunately, relatives and neighbors could not accept the direction of treatment that the family accepted. They became nonsupportive and hostile. Not only was the family dealing with losing a child, but also losing their support systems.

The questions raised here include some very basic ones. Who has the right to make decisions regarding health care treatment when the patient is competent or when the patient is incompetent? What is the role of the home health staff and the physician in these cases? Are they responsible for deciding what treatment should be given and what should be withheld? Rather, shouldn't the health professionals be the ones to facilitate decision making by the patient and family
through the giving of information and support? What does the home health agency staff do when the physician is contributing to the dilemma by recommending treatment that will only serve to prolong death? Who should inform the patient that they are going to die—the physician, the nurse, or the family? How does the staff handle a case in which the family feels they must protect the patient and thus deny the patient any opportunity to express theirs fears and anxieties? Or what if the family is in denial and thus unable to provide the support that the dying patient needs?

Patient Abuse and Neglect. Home health agency staff are in a unique position in regard to observing and evaluating the presence of patient abuse and neglect. Because they are perceived as helpers, they are accepted into patients' homes and given the opportunity to witness first-hand patients' environments and how patients are cared for. When abuse or neglect is seen, however, the role and responsibility of the home health staff and the agency may be unclear. Here are some examples.

"Mrs. M"

Mrs. M, 52-years-old, had a 30-year history of multiple sclerosis and 10-year history of insulin-dependent diabetes mellitus. She was referred to the local home health agency by concerned neighbors. Confined to a wheelchair, Mrs. M was also losing the dexterity in her fingers. Although still able to transfer herself to the bed and commode, she had been falling repeatedly during the transfers. She lived with her husband who was an executive for a local insurance company. There were no children.

Mrs. M was home alone from early morning to early evening and occasionally overnight when Mr. M was away on business. She was unable to safely prepare her own food and self-administration of her insulin was questionable. Mr. M kept food supplies in the home but did not prepare meals in advance. He would assist with drawing up the insulin but refused to administer the injections.

Mrs. M did not show any signs of direct physical abuse. The nurse's assessment, however, revealed obvious neglect of Mrs. M's needs. When the nurse attempted to discuss this with Mrs. M, Mrs. M accused the nurse of meddling and suggested that she would not allow the nurse to return if she pursued the subject any further.

"Michael T."

Michael T. was born at eight months gestation with severe anoxia and an apgar score of 1-3-3. He was diagnosed with Hirschsprung's disease and a colostomy was performed during the first week of life. Tube feedings via gastrostomy were instituted.

Michael was the child of a 22-year-old unwed mother who was on welfare and had two other children aged three and five.

At six months of age Michael was discharged from the hospital. Teaching the mother about Michael's care was begun before his discharge, but hospital staff members were concerned because the mother rarely visited. Referrals were therefore made to the child protective services and the visiting nurse agency for follow-up.

Michael was brought home to live with his mother and two sisters in a crowded, cluttered one-room apartment. Although the room itself was clean, the kitchen and bathroom facilities shared with the owner of the house were not. The house itself was in bad need of repair.

According to the visiting nurse, Michael's mother was capable of colostomy care and tube feedings and appeared to love Michael. Michael's supervision and safety, however, were a concern. He was left alone on the bed and his three-year-old sister was allowed to "play" with him unsupervised. Moreover, there was no follow-through with developmental stimulation and many clinic appointments were missed. Michael was hospitalized twice during the three months after his first discharge—the first time for fever and diarrhea and the second time for a displaced fracture of the arm.

The hospital staff demanded that Michael be removed from the home. The child protective services worker stated that home care was safe and adequate.

The M's situation presents several ethical questions. What is the agency's responsibility to Mrs. M? Should measures be implemented to protect Mrs. M from a hazardous situation? Should local protective services for the vulnerable adult be notified? If they are not notified and Mrs. M sustains harm, what is the agency's responsibility? What if there are no local protective services for adults? Finally, should the nurse attempt to discuss the problem with Mr. M against the expressed wishes of Mrs. M? Can this breach of confidentiality between the nurse and patient be justified? Might Mr. M retaliate by further neglecting or harming his wife?

The case of Michael T. presents some further questions. The nurse's assessment of the child's care may influence the decision as to whether Michael should be removed from the home. What should the nurse recommend? What is to be done when it is apparent that the mother loves the child but is overwhelmed with the care and the circumstances of her environment? Would a foster home be any better? Would the child be guaranteed the love, physical care, safety, and stimulation that he needs in a foster home?

Patient Needs versus Caregiver Needs. Home health agencies should provide holistic care. They cannot treat a patient in isolation. Often the caregiver in the home (a family member, significant other, etc.) will need as much or more support than the patient. Also, the needs of the caregiver may conflict with those of the patient. Thereby the home health care staff, and thus the agency, is caught in the middle. For example:

"Mr. B"

Mr. B was a 65-year-old man with a diagnosis of advanced cancer of the lungs with metastases to the bone. His prognosis suggested a two- to three-month life expectancy. Mr. B lived with his 69-year-old wife and 29-year-old daughter. They understood that his condition was terminal. Because he wished to die at home, Mr. B was being followed by the agency's hospice program.

Mrs. B had several physical limitations related to cardiac disease and was visually impaired secondary to diabetic retinopathy. The daughter, who had recently returned to live with her parents, had been hospitalized three times during the past five years for a schizo-affective personality disorder. The hospice nurse was able to work with the B's to establish and implement a reasonable home care program. Nevertheless, Mr. B was reluctant to accept assistance in personal care from anyone other than his wife or daughter. He refused both home health aide and volunteer assistance.

The family did well for three weeks when Mr. B's condition deteriorated to the point where he was bedbound and totally dependent in his physical care needs. Mrs. B was then hospitalized with an exacerbation of her congestive heart failure and subsequently suffered a myocardial infarction. A home health aide to assist the daughter with Mr. B's care was assigned with much resistance from Mr. B. The daughter became increasingly distraught and was unable to provide for any of her father's needs. She would refuse to let the home health aide into the home and was also unreliable in administering pain medication. Throughout this period,

Mr. B remained mentally alert and demanded that he stay at home. The hospice nurse was seriously concerned about the care Mr. B was receiving and his safety, but she was also concerned about the wife's impending discharge from the hospital and the daughter's mental and emotional health.

Here is a situation whereby the patient's exercise of his autonomous rights are jeopardizing the emotional and physical health of his family. This problem is compounded by the fact that the patient chooses to remain in what the nurse perceives as an unsafe situation. To whom is the nurse an advocate first, the patient or the family? Should the agency honor the patient's wish to die at home at any cost? What right does the agency have to "force" patients to accept help or to be institutionalized? If family members or patients refuse to cooperate, should the agency withdraw its services? What if the involved individuals are mentally or physically incapable of cooperating? If the agency continues to provide service, is the agency guilty of perpetuating a dangerous situation and legally responsible if harm results to those involved?

Conflicts with Physicians. In order for home health agencies to provide a medical regimen of care to patients, they must operate under the direction of the patients' physicians. Occasionally, physician orders are, in the determination of the agency, in conflict with agency policies or accepted standards of practice. Here is an example.

"Mrs. L"

Mrs. L was 80-years-old. She was a diabetic who was treated with NPH Insulin during her last hospital stay but was discharged on Diabinese p.o. and a 1500-calorie ADA diet. Her blood glucose levels were not controlled at home even with diet compliance and the maximum recommended dose of Diabinese. The physician continued to increase the dose of Diabinese up to 250 mgm five times per day, far beyond the recommended maximum therapeutic dose of 750 mgm daily. Mrs. L's blood glucose remained uncontrolled. The physician would not prescribe insulin because the patient lived alone, she was occasionally forgetful and had poor vision. He did not feel that she could safely self-administer the insulin. The visiting nurse advised the physician that with adequate instruction, weekly visits by the family to prefill syringes, periodic monitoring of her blood sugar, and a daily phone call through the phone alert system, Mrs. L should be able to follow a daily insulin regime. The physician still persisted in keeping the patient on 1250 mgm of Diabinese per day.

Consider in this and in similar cases to what extent an agency should go in order to act as advocate for the patient. Is informing the patient of the potential adverse effects of the physician's treatment enough? Is pulling out of such cases in the best interest of the patient? Where does the agency's legal and ethical responsibility stop and the patient and family's responsibility start when the patient and family have been adequately informed by agency personnel? What leverage do agencies have, particularly nonhospital-based agencies, when trying to resolve such conflicts?

Addressing the Issues

As was intended, the cases presented raise a number of ethical issues. But to offer a solution for each case is not the purpose of this chapter. On the other hand, it is proposed that home health administrators can establish certain practices within their agencies which will assist in resolving some of the issues. These practices include education and development of staff, development of policies and procedures that address ethical issues and are consistent with ethical principles, and the collaboration and networking with other home health agencies and health care institutions.

Before going into the specifics of these practices it is appropriate to note here that one very basic assumption about the agencies to which this chapter is addressed must be made. It is assumed that these agencies, no matter what their structure or form (for-profit, not-for-profit, voluntary, public, freestanding, hospital-based, etc.) are committed to the delivery of high quality services in a manner that is consistent with high ethical and moral standards. Without this commitment from agency boards of directors, owners and administrators, the agencies, and thus their staffs, will not be free to act ethically and morally. Yarling and McElmurry (1986) in their article, "The Moral Foundation of Nursing" refer to hospitals' responsibility to be moral. This concept can be applied to home health agencies as well.

When social institutions are so construed that they systematically create overwhelming disincentives to responsible action, they must be held responsible for the suppression of the moral impulse in everyday life. In a word, nurses are not free to be moral because they are deprived of moral agency by the repressive character of the hospitals in which they practice.

Home health administrators must be willing to take a close look at agency organization, policies, and practices in order to identify barriers in the system which prevent their staff from acting ethically and morally.

Education and Development of Staff. The importance of providing educational opportunities for home health administrative and direct care staff in order for them to become more knowledgeable in regard to the ethical issues in home health care cannot be overemphasized. Educational programs could include, but not be limited to, topics such as ethical concepts and principles, identification and evaluation of an ethical dilemma, decision-making processes, legal aspects, values clarification, communication skills, and family dynamics. Case conferences, in-service programs, and out-of-office educational programs may be arranged.

Ongoing staff support is also essential. Resource persons within agencies who have an understanding of ethical concepts and principles and are familiar with agency policies should be identified. For example, clinical nurse specialists and social workers are professionals to whom staff can refer to and consult with when problem cases arise.

Policy Development. In those cases in which an ethical issue exists, there is usually more than one way to deal with the issue and more than one "right" answer. How a case is handled will be dependent on the characteristics and resources of the agency and its personnel, the resources within the community, and case-specific characteristics such as staff-patient relationship, time constraints, patient-family characteristics, and more. Nevertheless, agencies should be prepared, as much as possible, in advance to handle the issues. A proactive versus a reactive approach can be utilized by having in place certain processes in the form of policies and procedures to be followed when such situations arise. For example, a process for resolving conflicts with physicians can be developed whereby the first step recommended is to have the staff nurse try to work out the problem with a telephone call. Following steps may include encouraging more patient and family communication with the physician, involvement of agency administrative staff, and finally, if all else fails, a referral of the case to the agency professional advisory committee.

The home health administrator should have in place a system for the development of such policies drawing upon resources within and outside of the agency. A system such as that depicted in Exhibit 25-2 might be developed whereby an interdisciplinary agency policies committee is formed. This committee would consist of both staff and management level professionals to ensure that those professionals who are familiar with the day-to-day problems and who must carry out the policies and procedures have input into their development. (An agency policies committee might include but not be limited to: a nursing administrator, a nursing supervisor, one or two staff nurses, a clinical nurse specialist, a social worker, and a physical therapist.) The committee can both draft new policies as well as review and, if necessary, revise policies al-

Exhibit 25-2. Developing a Policy

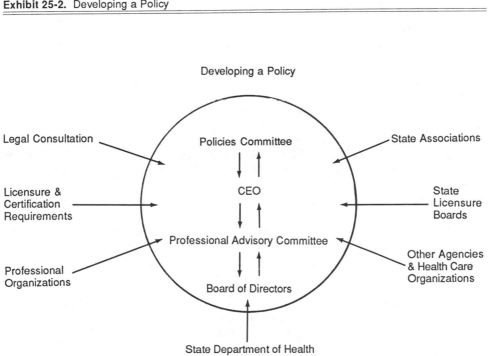

Developing a Policy

ready in place, always taking into consideration whether the policies are consistent with ethical principles. Of course, this committee need not confine itself to the development of policies related to ethical issues; it should be prepared to address the need for policies in other areas as well.

The committee may seek advice and consultation before or after it drafts a policy, depending on its nature. For instance, in New Jersey a child abuse policy must follow the guidelines of the state department of health; or the committee may want legal advice before drafting a policy on informed consent.

After a policy is drafted by the policies committee and has the appropriate administrative approval, it should be brought to the agency's professional advisory committee. The professional advisory committee may at this time advise legal consultation particularly in regard to ethical matters. In some agencies a lawyer who is knowledgeable about health law may sit on this committee and can provide the necessary consultation when the policy is presented. Finally, when applicable, important policies should be brought to the governing board of the agency.

Types of policies that may be developed in this manner include policies for the care of AIDS patients in the home, acceptance of patients, termination of services, provisions for uncompensated care, and conflict resolution procedures when conflicts regarding patient care occur between agency and patient and family or agency and patient's physician.

Other sources of consultation for policy development can include professional organizations, state licensing boards, etc. See Exhibit 25-2.

Collaboration among Home Health Agencies and Other Health Care Organizations. Each home health agency need not and should not work in isolation when attempting to find ways to resolve the more complex ethical issues. The ethics committee for the Home Health Agency Assembly of New Jersey has found that home health administrators share similar concerns and face similar problems. Thus, collaboration and networking among agencies is essential.

In some instances, an agency may have developed a policy that effectively deals with an ethical issue and may be willing to informally "share" this policy with other agencies. What may be more ethically and legally appropriate however, is that highly controversial issues such as the withdrawal of treatment for the incompetent patient or the lack of reimbursement for custodial care be dealt with on a more formal collaborative basis. * In fact, this is one of the main reasons why the Ethics Committee for the Home Health Agency Assembly of New Jersey was formed. This committee is comprised of representatives from nursing, medicine, clergy, law, social work, ethics, and the community. It plans to serve in an advisory capacity to assembly membership throughout the state. See Exhibit 25-3.

The committee also recognizes that collaborative relationships need not be confined to relationships among home health agencies. Hospitals, nursing homes, and other health care organizations are facing the same or similar issues. In addition, the

---

* Two cases have been decided by the New Jersey Supreme Court. In both, the withdrawal of treatment was allowed—a respirator in the case of Karen Ann Quinlan and artificial feeding in the Claire Conroy case. A third case involving a woman, Kathleen Farrel, at home on a respirator is scheduled for a hearing in the spring of 1986. See In re Quinlan, 355 A. 2d 647 (NJ, 1976) and In re Conroy, 486 A. 2d 1209 (NJ, 1985).

Exhibit 25-3. Assumptions, Purpose, and Goals of the Ethics Committee of the Home Health
Agency Assembly of New Jersey

I. Assumptions

The following assumptions shall serve as a basis for the purpose and activities of Home Health
Agency Assembly of New Jersey Ethics Committee.

A. All persons possess intellectual, moral, spiritual, physical, legal, and social rights including
the right to make decisions regarding their health care.

B. Human life at every stage of development and in every condition should be respected.

C. All persons should be treated in accordance with universal principles of social justice.

D. All health care professionals have the right to make patient care decisions based on their
professional code of ethics.

E. The Home Health Agency Assembly of New Jersey acts according to the highest ethical
and professional standards in carrying out its mission of leadership and planning for the
future.

II. Mission and purpose

The mission of the Ethics Committee of the Home Health Agency Assembly of New Jersey is to
provide a mechanism whereby Home Health Agency Assembly members can examine ethical
and legal issues related to home health care and find effective ways to deal with these issues.

III. Goals

A. To educate and inform home health agency administrators and staff of issues concerning
ethical and legal dimensions of health care.

B. To develop guidelines which will assist home health agencies in their development of
policies regarding ethical and legal decisions.

C. To develop position statements on ethical issues which are of importance to home health
agencies and their clients.

D. To collaborate and consult with individuals, groups, and organizations who are engaged in
research and examination of ethical issues in the delivery of health care services.

E. To monitor legislative activities and seek legislative support in areas concerning ethics in
health care.

Reprinted by permission of the Ethics Committee of the Home Health Agency Assembly of N.J., Inc.

policies and practices of these organizations, their discharge-planning processes, for
example, may significantly exacerbate the ethical problems of home health agencies.
Therefore, home health agencies must explore ways in which they can work with not
only themselves, but also other health care organizations to address the issues.

Conclusion

Ethical issues in health care are not confined to institutional settings. Home health agencies have historically been faced with ethical dilemmas—although the problems are now exacerbated with both the push toward out-of-hospital care and the insufficient reimbursement for home care.

Agency boards, owners, and administrators must be aware of the nature of such issues in home health and develop ways to address them, recognizing that some issues may be too controversial or too broad for each agency to deal with individually. Moreover, agency commitment to provide quality care consistent with ethical principles is essential. Without this commitment, attempting to resolve the issues is futile.

References

American Nurses' Association. 1976. *Code for nurses with interpretive statements.* Kansas City, MO: The Association.

Aroskar, M. April 1977. Ethics in the nursing curriculum. *Nursing Outlook* 25:260-264.

Bandman, E. L., and B. Bandman. 1985. *Nursing ethics in the life span.* Norwalk, CT: Appleton-Century-Crofts.

Bowyer, C. 1986. The complex care team: Meeting the needs of high-technology nursing. *Home Health Care Nurse* 4(1):24-29.

Bugman, C. October 27, 1985. Suicide among elderly virtually ignored despite highest rate of any age group. *Star Ledger* I:91.

Chambers, M. April 17, 1986. Appeals panel says quadriplegic has right to end forced feeding. *New York Times* I(28):5-6.

Department of Health and Human Services. Public Health Service National Center for Health Statistics. 1983. *Health United States,* pp. 67-70. Washington, DC: Government Printing Office.

Dworkin, R. 1977. *Taking rights seriously.* Cambridge, MA: Harvard University Press.

Frankena, W. 1973. *Ethics,* 2nd ed. Englewood Cliffs, NJ: Prentice Hall.

Hoeman, S. Unpublished Ph.D. dissertation. 1984. *Counting whatever counts--An ethnography of a hospital-based home health agency.* New Brunswick, NJ: Graduate School, Rutgers, The State University.

Home care today--An interview. April 1984. *American Journal of Nursing.*

In the matter of Karen Quinlan. 1976. 355 A2d.

Kalisch, P., and B. Kalisch. 1978. *The advance of American nursing,* 1st ed. Boston: Little, Brown and Company.

Jonsen, A. R., M. Cooke, and B. A. Koenig. 1986. Aids and ethics. *Issues in Science and Technology* Winter: 56-65.

Kelly, L. Y. 1985. The International Council of Nurses Code of Ethics (1973). In *Dimensions of professional nursing,* 5th ed. New York: MacMillan Publishing Company.

Mundinger, M. 1983. *Home care controversy: too little, too late, too costly.* Rockville, MD: Aspen Systems Corporation.

National Center for Health Services Research and Health Care Technology Assessment. October 1985. *Research Activities.* 78:I.

The new encyclopaedia britannica, micropaedia, 15th ed, s.v. "altruism."

New encyclopaedia britannica, micropaedia, 15th ed, s.v. "egoism."

New encyclopaedia britannica, micropaedia, 15th ed, s.v. "ethics."

New encyclopaedia britannica, macropaedia, 15th ed, s.v. "ethics."

The new encyclopaedia britannica, macropaedia, 15th ed, s.v. "utilitarianism."

Noziak, R. 1974. *Anarchy, state and utopia.* New York: Basic Books.

Nursing '74. Nursing ethics: The admirable professional standards of nurses: A survey report. October 1974: 56-65.

Patient finds just existing is not living. February 13, 1986. *New York Times* I(15):1.

Rawls, J. 1971. *A theory of justice.* Cambridge, MA: Harvard University Press.

Sullivan, R. April 24, 1986. Judge sanctions end of feeding in a coma case. *New York Times* B(3):1-4.

Sullivan, R. June 24, 1986. Dying woman wins Jersey ruling to end life-sustaining care. *New York Times* B(I):6.

The prosecutor closes case in death of Indiana baby. April 20, 1982. *New York Times.*

New encyclopaedia britannica, macropaedia, 15th ed, s.v. "history of western philosophy."

The International Council of Nurses Code of Ethics (1973). In L. Y. Kelly. 1985. *Dimensions of professional nursing,* 5th ed. New York: MacMillan Publishing Company.

Webster's new universal unabridged dictionary, 2nd ed. 1983. New York: New World Dictionaries

Simon and Schuster.

Woman who sought to starve sues hospital. January 22, 1986. *New York Times* I(15):1.

Yarling, R. R., and B. J. McElmurry. 1986. The moral foundation of nursing. *Advances in Nursing Science.* January 1986: 63 73.

Chapter Twenty-Six

Political Issues

Understanding the Political Process
Kathleen A. Carlson and Elizabeth Z. Cathcart

Many federal, state, and local laws and regulations impact directly on the ability of a home health agency to provide care. It is important that home health administrators develop an awareness of the many issues that affect their agencies. It is also important to develop positive relationships with political leaders at all levels of government and to be familiar with the legislative and regulatory processes. This chapter will provide information on how to develop relationships with political leaders and an overview of the legislative and regulatory processes.

Building Relationships

Health care delivery and the regulation of health care are changing rapidly and have become increasingly complex. Thus, when a legislative crisis at local, state, or federal levels is imminent, there is no time to search out political allies. Home health administrators, therefore, should develop active networks of support.

One of your first tasks, as either a newcomer to the state or to your agency's service area, is to register to vote. If your state has mail registration, applications can be found in post offices and state agency buildings. If, however, you must register at the courthouse, take advantage of the opportunity to gather as much data as possible about your elected officials and the demographics of your voting district.

The administrator can ascertain if a community is politically conservative or liberal in its posture toward health and social issues by networking with other community agencies. This can be accomplished with a local Health and Welfare Council or the Chamber of Commerce. Both groups have deep community roots and an astute awareness of the political and business climate. Most chambers have regular meetings with local elected officials which vary from informal gatherings to formal meetings.

Local politics form the base from which state and federal politics evolve. In some areas, you will find there are "friendly" political rivalries; in others, members of opposing parties seldom will be seen together at the same functions. At any function where elected officials are present, make every effort to be introduced by someone who is known to the elected official. This contact becomes a bridge for later communications with the officials.

The home health administrator should strive to develop a good relationship with at least one or two key political figures in the community. However, it is important to communicate with other officials periodically since at some time you may need their help as well. Board members are an asset in identifying these key political players.

They have usually been associated with many of these individuals through past community activities.

A representative of your agency should be present at major political fundraisers to create an awareness of the agency's interest in the community's political process. Sometimes it is important who attends, but that the agency is represented. At other times, who represents the agency carries more weight. At the same time the administrator is developing a working relationship with elected officials, liaisons should be forged with other agencies sharing similar concerns.

Local coordinating groups synthesize information from multiple sources. This coordination broadens the approach to resolving a problem impacting on the delivery of services. Group information gathering is valuable in developing strategies and in coordinating materials to be shared with elected officials. Through memberships in national and state associations, the administrator can keep on top of issues affecting home health care at those levels.

As an administrator, you should only be involved with legislative issues relevant to your organization. It is not effective to support or oppose every health care issue. While legislative proposals frequently receive the most attention, changing regulations may have a greater impact on the day-to-day operation of your agency and should not be ignored.

Local Government

The second step in the development of political and legislative awareness is to assess your county and local forms of government. By now you know their general political posture but you also need to evaluate their positions regarding your primary interest, health care. For example, when an agency serves more than one county, you might find the county with its own health department being reluctant to provide financial support to an outside visiting nurse association. On the other hand, another county may find it less costly to support community agencies delivering health care services and as a result provide funding for specific programs.

Political subdivisions such as townships or wards are concerned about accessibility of public buildings by the handicapped, and about low income housing or transportation of the elderly. Whatever the subject, involvement with groups studying broader issues identifies the home health administrator as a citizen concerned for the total health of the community. All of these issues bear a direct relationship to the problems faced by the clientele served by home health agencies.

While health systems agencies are still intact in many communities, their degree of influence on health care delivery systems varies. Involvement with any local planning group, however, gives the agency director visibility in the health care community as well as an opportunity to be on the forefront of evolving changes within the health care delivery system. Some health systems agencies have been leaders in identifying gaps in health care delivery as well as providing leadership in solving the problem. At meetings such as these, the administrator collaborates not only with politically appointed individuals, but also with influential citizens in the community. The major goal is to maximize your visibility as an agency administrator whose interest includes not only his own organization but also the general health of the community.

Increasingly, county officials are responsible for the direct provision of health care. Therefore, attendance at county commissioners meetings concerning special health care issues provides an opportunity for the administrator to present public testimony. A well-developed presentation with emphasis on the problem from the home health administrator's perspective has impact. You need to focus on the benefits or deficiencies of the plan under consideration rather than highlight the implications for your organization.

Another approach to increasing your visibility has been to host or sponsor joint luncheons or affairs for county commissioners and state legislators. Although emphasis may be on national issues or state issues, their local impact is of great importance. County officials frequently take advantage of this forum to raise pertinent questions on your behalf. Additionally, this is a good opportunity to provide legislators who sponsor health care proposals with the opportunity to update the group. This reinforces the legislators' involvement and support of health care issues. The legislator not only provides the public with information but is also viewed by his colleagues as a knowledgeable resource on health care.

It should be apparent, however, after interacting with elected officials for a short time that your issues and their issues are seldom the same. The home health administrator needs to investigate an elected official's special concerns in order to develop a creative approach to gain attention. For example, if an elected official is concerned about a segment of the population, place emphasis on how proposed legislation will impact on that group. By arranging to have your elected official accompany you on a home visit, you may create a graphic impression of the legislation's impact.

How often you or your agency are asked to participate in county-appointed task forces or study groups is a gauge in evaluating your effectiveness in your community's political process. You will be one of the first invited, if you have been accepted as a knowledgeable and politically astute individual in your field.

Legislative Process

All 50 states have an established process for creating laws. In Pennsylvania, the constitution of the state outlines the specific steps required to introduce, consider, and pass legislation. Each state has its own distinct system of checks and balances to protect the individual rights of its citizens. You can usually obtain pamphlets outlining your state's system from your elected state officials. Although it is not necessary to learn all of the intricate maneuvers, it is very important to understand the varying time elements involved in passing legislation.

In any given legislative session, more proposals are developed than any one person or special interest group can follow. For example, in 1985, the Pennsylvania House of Representatives introduced 1,999 bills and the Senate introduced 1,282 bills. These bills addressed many subject areas such as taxes, appropriations, licensing laws, health care cost containment, sunset of government agencies, and insurance changes. When issues arise which affect your special interest, administrators should take time to communicate their views to their legislators. Most of the information you need about a particular piece of legislation can usually be obtained from a professional or trade association.

Your role in the legislative process as a member of an organization is to follow through with association directives for legislative action. Your role as the director of an agency is to seek ways to protect or further your agency's interest. Occasionally, an association position does not exactly meet your agency's needs. When this situation occurs, contact your professional or trade association to make sure you understand their position. Associations frequently evaluate legislation based on the broadest application of a proposal to its entire membership. If, in your judgment, you cannot support the association's position, do not take any action unless the position specifically jeopardizes your agency. It is imperative that you work through your association, not your legislator, to resolve any differences.

Whatever your sources of information it is helpful in communicating with your legislator to include the following: 1) bill number; (2) committee or subcommittee the bill has been assigned to; 3) your position; 4) rationale or supporting examples; and 5) specific request for support or opposition.

Public hearings may be part of your state's process to give proposed legislation as much exposure as possible. Differences can be aired and, as a result of the hearing, negotiated compromises may be achieved. Input at this stage is critical. If you have never testified before a legislative committee, it is advisable to learn the committee members' position on the issue prior to the hearing. Legislators on opposing sides of an issue can become aggressive in their questioning, particularly when an audience is present. It is important to remember that the hearing's purpose is to address the issue, not the position of an individual legislator.

Personal visits to your legislator lend emphasis to a critical issue. Even though your legislator may not serve on the committee considering the bill, his influence in caucus may strengthen your position. Thus, while initially communications should be with the legislators serving on the committee reviewing the bill, you should keep your own legislator apprised of your actions.

Once a bill has progressed to final passage and a vote is imminent, the home health administrator may not have sufficient time for the U.S. Postal Service to deliver a letter. Mailgrams are appropriate for action occurring during the next 48 hours. If action is to occur within 24 hours, telephone contacts are more appropriate.

It is appropriate to follow through after action has occurred. A thank you to officials who supported your position is always appreciated. If the legislator voted in opposition to your position, you have several options in your communication: (1) ask for the legislator's rationale; or (2) agree to disagree, restating your position. This follow-up correspondence keeps the lines of communication open between you and the legislator. The goal is to maintain a working relationship with the official. Remember all legislation is a compromise!

The following is a list of essential items to include when writing a letter to a legislator.

1. Use the proper address.

   (Frequently letters never reach their intended destination because of incorrect addresses.)

2. Use proper salutation.

(Although "The Honorable" is appropriate for the address, it is not appropriate within the letter. Dear Senator/Representative/Assemblyman is correct.)

3. Include the bill numbers when referring to legislation.

4. Include a generalization of what the bill proposes.

5. State your position.

6. Give your rationale.

7. Use specific examples of how the legislation/regulations/policies affect you and the delivery of client services in the legislator's district.

8. Include the action you wish the individual to take.

9. Be clear, concise, and credible.

10. Make sure your address is included within the letter itself, not just on the envelope.

Regulatory Process

Most laws, once enacted, have implementation and enforcement provisions vested in a state authority. Rules and regulations are subsequently promulgated to outline how the government will implement the laws. State governments have various methods for proposing these rules. Some follow an orderly process; others have no specific requirements. In some states, regulations are merely guidelines but in others they carry legal implications. This determination could affect your next course of action. Whether you take further action or not, you need to understand the process required. Regulations may affect the delivery of home health services to a greater extent than the original law.

Frequently, the regulatory process provides for public input. If so, this is an excellent opportunity for you as a provider to influence the health care delivery system.

Once again, start with statewide organizations if you are affiliated with one that regularly follows legislative and regulatory activities. Significant groundwork and the legal opinions may have already been obtained. If on the other hand you find that little or no work has been accomplished, volunteer to serve on a committee that was established to address the regulatory issue. Offer to serve as a resource with expertise in the area being regulated. If public comments are requested, respond and send copies to your legislators. By sending copies of your correspondence to your national or state organizations, you assist the associations in monitoring how much membership activity is taking place.

Perhaps you are not affiliated with an organization, or your issue is not a priority for them. By networking with other organizations who share your concerns, a quality document can be produced in response to requests for public input. While it is usually beneficial for each administrator to respond as an individual, there are also times when a group effort has greater impact.

The same strategy used by national and state associations can be applied by you as an individual. Contact the government agency or individual within the agency by expressing your interest in the development of the regulations. Some agencies prefer no outside involvement until an initial draft has been prepared. However, written recommendations with rationale may be appreciated. You should request a copy of the draft document if it is to be disseminated to special interest groups. When and if public input is sought, you should respond with documentation supporting your position.

Political Action

For educational purposes, it helps to look at political action separately from the legislative process. Political action is people-oriented rather than issue-oriented. Legislative action, sometimes referred to as lobbying, focuses on the direct efforts of an individual or group to influence the outcome of laws, regulations, and policies of state government. In some states this is a regulated activity. Political action deals with the direct efforts of an individual or group to affect the outcome of an election to public office. There is a natural flow between the two processes. Most often, political action efforts are translated into raising and expending financial contributions to run political campaigns. In addition to dollars, anything of value such as personal services, loan of property, or gifts of stationery can be considered in the definition of "effort to affect the outcome of an election." State laws vary on the amount of control they impose on campaign financing.

Since the purpose of political action is to affect the outcome of an election, before you make personal financial contributions you must carefully evaluate the potential consequences for you and your agency. As an agency administrator, you must be clear on both state and federal laws before your direct involvement in any political activities. However, you as an individual are probably not restricted from engaging in political action, including financial contributions to a candidate's campaign. (Federal employees are regulated by the Hatch Act; state employees may be restricted by specific state laws.) In most states, campaign records are open to public scrutiny. As an administrator, you need to weigh carefully the value of having your name appear in these records.

The neophyte is advised to work through organized groups such as the political action committees (PACs) of state and national organizations. If you have worked with a legislator for longer than six months, you are in a position to evaluate how that legislator responds to you and the issues affecting your agency. Your input can assist these PACs in their evaluations of candidates, since PACs use information from many sources.

Involvement with a PAC does not negate your opportunity to work with a specific legislator or elected official. However, if you are clearly identified in the community as an agency director and are very active in personal party politics, then you should consider ways to identify yourself as a private citizen to offset any potential community backlash for your agency.

As a rule of thumb, PACs consider seniority, committee chairmanships, party position, committee membership, and financial need. It follows then that the majority of financial contributions are given to incumbent candidates. Frequently, legislators who don't serve on health care committees or who don't hold party seniority are overlooked by small health-related PACs. Nevertheless, you can usually request a review of your particular legislator with accompanying documentation of how he has supported your issues. The big question is how well does an incumbent interact with constituents and can this official generate support for your special interest initiatives.

As a private citizen, you may always make an assessment of a candidate's commitment and make a personal contribution to the campaign fund. Agency donations may be restricted by state or federal campaign laws. In particular, a nonprofit agency's tax status can be jeopardized by direct political contributions.

General fundraisers for political parties provide an opportunity for the administrator to participate in political action without endorsing specific individuals. When attending political functions, make certain that the candidates know you are there. A follow-up letter commenting on the success of the event gives you yet another opportunity to point out your participation.

In political action, the name of the game is access to people rather than access to information as it is in the legislative and regulatory processes.

Conclusion

Many federal, state, and local laws and regulations impact directly on the ability of a home health agency to provide care. Changes in any program which decrease the availability of state and local funding may be obscured by larger issues but can create serious service delivery problems. An agency therefore needs many information resources to keep abreast of the constant changes.

Sometimes issues being considered are so crucial that the staff and board members of an agency should take the initiative to contact their legislators. To assist these individuals, who are not involved in governmental issues on a day-to-day basis, it might be necessary to circulate a legislative fact sheet stating the problem, the alternatives, and the expected outcomes. Agency directors should understand lobbying restrictions placed on tax-exempt organizations before they embark on any assertive campaign.

While it should be obvious that there are many nuances in dealing with the players of the legislative-regulatory arena, the final impact is related to your ability to communicate. Individual letters are far more effective in influencing lawmakers than are petitions or form letters. At key times, telephone contacts are even more effective. Whatever the mode of communication, it should be clear, concise, and credible. There should be no doubt about your position on the issue. When it is necessary to communicate with federal legislators, the same communication techniques are appropriate; however, you should send a copy to your state officials. This creates the potential to generate a chain of support for your position. As you get more involved in the process, information sharing between you and your elected official should be mutual.

The best communication tool for all citizens and yet the most frequently ignored is the power of the vote. Voting is your final evaluation of the overall effectiveness of an elected official in responding to you as a concerned citizen with a special interest. Although no one can expect an elected official to support his positions 100% of the time, you nevertheless have the right to expect a knowledgeable response to your inquires as well as the official's rationale.

Home health administrators have known for years how to generate community support. Since communications and networking are common activities for any agency director, it is not difficult to expand this activity to include the politicians and key elected officials to your community. Be aware that they too have a role to play in the future of your organization.

Political Issues in Home Health Care: A National Perspective

Margaret J. Cushman

The host of political issues of interest to home care providers today spans a broad range: from the quality and availability of health care for the nation's elderly, poor, and infirm,; to more mundane concerns about reimbursement for services rendered under federal entitlement programs. By far, the dominant focus of home care political activity in the mid-1980s is centered on Title XVIII of the Social Security Act, better known as the Medicare program. Because of its centrality, the Medicare home care benefit and related issues will be the primary topic of this chapter.

The History of the Medicare Home Care Benefit

The Medicare program was enacted in 1965, through amendment to the Social Security Act. The Medicare home care benefit was a minor part of the legislation which was geared to coverage of medical and inpatient care of individuals over age 65. Chief proponent of the home care benefit was Senator Frank E. Moss, of Utah, who was then chairman of the Subcommittee of Health and Long-Term Care of the U.S. Senate Special Committee on Aging. Moss and his colleagues in the Senate Special Committee on Aging, having conducted a series of hearings exposing fraud and abuse in nursing homes, determined that home health care should be made available as an alternative to nursing home placement.

The original home care benefit was quite circumscribed, partially because national policymakers had little knowledge about this rather small sector of health care. Covered services included:

- Part-time nursing, physical or speech therapy on an intermittent basis, as primary services.

- Occupational therapy and medical social work on an intermittent basis if a primary service was also needed.

- Homemaker-home health aide services for the purpose of assisting the patient with personal care related to activities of daily living. Home health aide services were required to be under the supervision of a registered nurse, physical or speech therapist (Social Security Act 1965a).

To be eligible for Medicare home care services, the patient had to be considered homebound. All services had to be ordered by a physician and be considered medically necessary and reasonable. The statute also defined the need for nursing care to be "skilled," which in essence required hands on application of a medical treatment or procedure. Assessment, counseling, and teaching were not considered skilled, and were not covered unless provided in conjunction with other hands-on care (Social Security Act 1965b).

The original legislation also required three days of prior hospitalization for coverage under Part A of Medicare. A patient could be covered under Medicare Part B after meeting an annual deductible requirement and paying a 20% coinsurance. The number of visits was limited to 100 under Part A and an additional 100 under Part B. Investor-owned agencies were barred from participation in the program unless licensed. At the time of passage, however, few states offered licensure and no proprietary agencies were in existence.

In 1967, the first full year of the Medicare benefit, $46 million worth of home care services were provided. One year later, the amount of service reimbursed grew 46% to $67 million, as existing providers geared up to meet Medicare conditions of participation. The growth continued more modestly in 1969, equalling another 16%. Then, due to a series of regulatory reinterpretations of coverage, providers were hit with massive retroactive denials for services rendered in prior periods. These retroactive denials resulted in a real dollar decline in reimbursement for services through 1972.

Despite repeated expressions of congressional interest in expanding the home care benefit, home health expenditures represented only 1% of the total Medicare outlay in 1971, and 1.5% in 1975. After several years of explosive growth, home care reimbursement still accounted for only 2% of total Medicare expenditures in 1981 and 3% in 1985 (U.S. Bureau of the Census 1984, 29, 371, 374).

The growth in Medicare home care in the 1980s has been largely due to amendments to the Medicare statute. The Omnibus Reconciliation Act of 1980, removed the requirement for three days prior hospitalization as well as the 100-visit limitation. The requirement for proprietary agencies to be licensed to qualify for participation was also removed, paving the way for many additional agencies to enter the federally reimbursed home care market. But, perhaps the greatest influence on the recent growth of home care services has been the passage in 1983, of the prospective payment system for hospitals, which brings us to the political climate of today.

The Current Home Care Political Climate

Fueled by these legislative changes, expenditures for home health care increased from approximately $1 billion in 1980 to an estimated $2 billion in 1986, making it the fastest growing part of the Medicare system. At the same time, the number of agencies has increased from about 3,000 in 1980 to nearly 6,000 in 1986, virtually all due to the addition of proprietary and hospital-related agencies.

Viewing these increases, the Health Care Financing Administration (HCFA), the arm of the Department of Health and Human Services responsible for administering Medicare, has concluded that home health care is out of control and must be stopped. Based upon internal departmental studies, HCFA believes that the growth in home care reflects provision of unnecessary service, despite analyses of the contrary (*The Attempted Dismantling of the Medicare Home Health Benefit* 1986, 38).

Acting on its belief that home care must be curtailed, the Administration has introduced more than 35 initiatives against home care since 1983. To quote Val Halamandaris, President of the National Association for Home Care (*Attempted Dismantling* 1986, 7):

... home health care paradoxically has been the most regulated of American industries. At a time when the airlines, the trucking industry, hospitals and nursing
homes are being deregulated, the Department of Health and Human Services has
promulgated an oppressive series of requirements applicable to home health
agencies.

Using the original Medicare statute as a tool of restriction, HCFA has issued
restrictive interpretations of the terms "intermittent," "skilled," and "homebound."
These have been used to deny care, often inconsistently, and when overturned, denials
frequently crop up on the same case on the basis of lack of "medical necessity." A new
form of denial has been instituted: the technical denial. Selective billing has been implemented in cases where beneficiaries choose to purchase more medically necessary
care than the intermediary has deemed Medicare-coverable. Compliance audits have
been implemented, and revised to be more restrictive. The appeal rights of beneficiaries and providers have been challenged, administrative costs disallowed, the cost
limit methodology changed, and waiver of liability eliminated, by regulation.

A comprehensive review of the consistent attack on the home care benefit has
been compiled by the National Association for Home Care. *The Attempted Dismantling of the Medicare Home Health Benefit: A Report to Congress* attracted enough attention to be reproduced as a government document. The American Nurses' Association, concerned over the continuous efforts to erode home health care coverage,
passed a resolution at the 1986 biennial convention to work aggressively to stop the
destruction of home health care.

Home health care today is caught in the midst of a federal government working at
cross-purposes: a Congress supportive of expanding home care services in the interest
of cost containment and consumer preference and an administration run amok with
intent to curtail the same benefit because of that very growth. Yet, of even greater
political importance is the dilemma of the Medicare beneficiary, caught in the tangle
of institutional cost containment and the lack of available alternatives.

What we are witnessing today is an increasing trend for the gap in unmet health
care needs to widen because the pressures of health care cost containment are
reducing access and entry to institutional care without a corresponding adjustment in coverage policies for home care and other non-institutional care to cover
services which were either previously covered in institutions or never covered at
all. (*Toward a National Home Care Policy* 1986, 11)

Preserving the Medicare Home Care Benefit

The first line of political interest in home care is to preserve the Medicare benefit as
interpreted upon enactment. The three key terms that are subject to restrictive and inconsistent interpretation are "intermittent," "skilled," "homebound."

Intermittent is a term originally understood to convey less than full-time or 24-
hour-a-day care. In more recent guidelines, the term has been interpreted to allow
daily visits for a maximum of three weeks. Continuation of daily visits may be permitted with documentation of unusual circumstances. In some instances, the
guidelines have been used to deny visits by more than one discipline in the same day

and twice-daily visits by the same discipline. Daily has also been interpreted by creative fiscal intermediaries (FIs) to mean five days a week. To limit inappropriate restrictions on daily care, especially in the face of earlier hospital discharges, legislation was introduced in the House of Representatives in 1985 by Henry Waxman of California, and in the Senate by John Heinz of Pennsylvania. Senator Patrick Leahy, Vermont, again introduced legislation aimed at the intermittent issue in 1986, as part of the Better Health Care Act.

"Skilled" nursing has been one of the most protested definitions since the inception of the Medicare statute. Home care providers, dominated by the nursing profession, have fought to have the term rescinded on the grounds that all care provided by professional nurses ought to be covered, not just that limited to carrying out medically ordered treatments. However, in the recent administrative cutbacks, the term skilled has been interpreted even more stringently. Some intermediaries have denied care as too skilled for home care if more than one visit a day is needed. These patients have been deemed "too skilled," then because care is more than intermittent.

On the other extreme, coverage has been denied as not skilled enough to instances where a family member can be instructed to assume the care. This has occurred even when the nurse's plan of care is to provide just such instruction in order to speed the transition of independent care management. No legislation currently exists to correct the problems of "skilled" care, but as can be seen from the examples above, denials on the grounds of skilled care and intermittency are interwoven. When agencies and beneficiaries have successfully overturned denials for one reason, care is often denied for the other or as not medically necessary.

Likewise, the "homebound" requirement is receiving increasingly strict interpretation. The current guideline allows a homebound patient to leave the home infrequently, for short durations for medical treatment and "occasional non-medical purposes." In 1983, HCFA proposed a new guideline which would have required patients to be nearly bedbound to meet the definition. Thanks in part to congressional concern, the proposal was never implemented.

Unfortunately, select intermediaries have enforced more stringent interpretations. There have been instances where friends and family have, with extraordinary assistance, enabled a patient to attend a special function such as a wedding, or a last fishing trip—only to have Medicare coverage denied as no longer homebound. In one instance, an American Indian was denied coverage because custom dictated he be moved outside his swelling just before death. In Colorado, between May and July of 1986, providers resubmitted 412 cases involving homebound denials to their intermediary. The intermediary conceded that 190, or 46%, of these denials were erroneous. Another 93 cases were overturned on the basis of homebound and subsequently denied as not "medically reasonable and necessary." (*NAHC Report* No. 172, 4-5)

Elimination of the homebound requirement is a key issue in home care. In the interim, the industry remains vigilant against these more restrictive interpretations, contesting them on a case-by-case basis.

Closely allied with the core requirements of the original Medicare statute is another form of administrative curtailment of coverage. Some intermediaries, acting with the sanction of HCFA, have informed home health agencies that if a patient is receiving any medically reasonable and necessary care beyond the amount which Medicare will cover, all home care coverage will be denied. For example, if an acutely ill patient, recently discharged from the hospital, receives a shift of private duty nursing to allow family caregivers to rest, intermittent care may be denied during the day. Medicare may refuse to pay for any of the care, even if the additional care needed is purchased by the family or another payor. Ironically, former HCFA chief Carolyn Davis did clarify that if the additional care is not medically necessary or reasonable, its purchase will not affect Medicare coverage. This practice has been dubbed selective billing. What the Medicare program is doing in these cases is prescribing the maximum plan of care it will cover regardless of need, and then seeking to act as second payor. Limitations of coverage on these grounds are particularly onerous given the dramatic increase in earlier discharges to home from acute care settings.

As the reader will recall, the original home care benefit was subject to a 20% copayment under Medicare Part B. This copayment requirement was rescinded by the 1980 Omnibus Reconciliation legislation. The Reagan administration has proposed reinstituting copayment for home care in the 1985, 1986, and 1987 fiscal year budget proposals. This provisions has been rejected by Congress each year, but will probably remain an issue throughout the Reagan administration. Copayment presents an impediment to beneficiaries seeking needed care, since they are already subjected to significant out-of-pocket expenses for their medical needs. As opposed to saving program costs, the expense of billing beneficiaries for the copayment coupled with the bad debt from those who could not pay, would actually cost Medicare more in administrative expenses.

Issues Surrounding Coverage Denials and Appeals

Over the past few years, home health agencies have experienced a dramatic increase in the numbers of denials for coverage. Some agencies who had never received a denial since the inception of the Medicare program, receive denials daily on care that was formerly considered covered. Partial denials are also being issued — arbitrarily reducing the amount of care that will be covered in a week, despite physician orders. Denials of coverage are frequently stated in vague terms, not detailing what the reason is for the determination. Intermediaries often use pro forma language to describe the general grounds for denial. Denials usually do not specify which visits are not covered, or why some visits are covered and others not. This lack of specificity makes it nearly impossible for providers and beneficiaries to anticipate what care will be paid for.

The Medicare program has provided a safeguard for providers who, acting in good faith, did not know that services furnished to an individual patient would not be coverable. This safeguard, known as waiver of liability, allows payment to providers under such circumstances, so long as claims paid under waiver are equal to less than 2.5% of the total claims submitted during that period. In the midst of changing interpretations of coverage, the Health Care Financing Administration issued regulations in 1985, to eliminate waiver of liability for all providers. Senior and consumer groups joined in a coalition with providers to lobby Congress to preserve waiver for home care. As a result, Congress included a provision to temporarily extend waiver of liability as part of the 1986 budget reconciliation package.

In order to circumvent payment under waiver and limit the ability to appeal denials, the Health Care Financing Administration has begun administering a new form of denial. The "technical denial" is one which the fiscal intermediary determines does not meet a statutory or regulatory requirement other than medical necessity. In simple terms, denials for reasons of skilled, intermittent, and homebound are considered technical. This form of denial is not provided for under either the current statute or regulations.

Legislation introduced by House Aging Committee Chairman Edward Roybal, of California, would replace the waiver of liability provision with a system of prior and concurrent authorization for home health agency and nursing home claims. The legislation would also require that all claims, including technical denials, be appealable. The Medicare Quality Protection Act of 1986, authorized by Senator John Heinz, Chairman of the Health Subcommittee of the Senate Finance Committee, and Representative Fortney Stark, Chairman of the Health Subcommittee of the Ways and Means Committee, would also address concerns about waiver and technical denials.

The Health Care Financing Administration has also projected denials of claims based upon a sample of claims reviewed. The Region VI office of HCFA conducted a fraud and abuse audit on the Visiting Nurse Service (VNS) of Albuquerque in 1983. Finding no basis for concern, the audit was treated as a compliance review audit on a nonrandom selection of the agency's billing records. The denials rendered on these records (the majority of which were reversed on reconsideration) were then used to project denials on the entire universe of the VNS's Medicare claims for fiscal year 1983. Not only was the sample procedure statistically invalid, the use of sampling for projection of denials abrogates the appeal right of the beneficiaries and agencies because the cases and claims being denied are not identified.

The same sampling approach was used on a second New Mexico agency shortly thereafter. Given the gravity of this circumvention of the normal denial process, the two agencies and the New Mexico Association of Home Health Agencies brought action against the Department in a lawsuit sponsored by the National Association for Home Care. At the first level of contest, the Administrative Law Judge hearing the preliminary argument for VNS of Albuquerque ruled that there was "no statutory or regulatory validity to the statistical sampling and projection." (*Toward a National Home Care Policy* 43) In July 1986, the Appeals Council of the Department of Health and Human Services decided that neither it, nor an Administrative Law Judge had the authority to rule on the issue of whether or not it is legal for overpayment to be calculated and collected based upon a sampling projection. (*NAHC Report* No. 175, 2) The next step in legal action will be taken before federal district court.

As can be seen from the sampling case, the approach of projected claims eliminates the appeal rights of Medicare beneficiaries. The Department has actively discouraged the exercise of appeal rights by issuing a revised manual provisions preventing home health providers from representing the beneficiary in the appeal process. Prior to the revision, this practice was quite common, given the difficulty of the appeals process and the infirmity of the beneficiaries.

In the case *In Home Health Services et al. versus Heckler: U.S. District Court for the District of Columbia Civil Action No. 84-0957: The Right of Medicare Beneficiaries to Select a Home Health Agency as their Representative*, the National Association for Home Care brought suit against the Department. In July 1986, the court ruled that the transmittal went beyond interpretation of existing statutes and regulations. While this ruling does not address the substance of the transmittal, it does represent a victory for home care in requiring that such a change be subject to formal regulatory procedures (*NAHC Report* No. 173, 2-3).

Other Medicare Reimbursement Issues

As part of the Omnibus Deficit Reduction Act of 1984, Congress mandated a change in the system of 47 fiscal intermediaries to a system of 10 or fewer FIs. This was enacted in recognition of the problems of inconsistent interpretation and payment for Medicare claims among different intermediaries. Final regulations for implementation of the 10-FI system were published by the Department of Health and Human Services in the summer of 1986, for beginning implementation in October of the same year.

The change to the new intermediary system is of concern to home health providers. In the process of transition, agencies are concerned about the status of claims review, waiver status, and cash flow. There is also concern that the improved consistency in interpretations will be at the most stringent common denominator. The transition to new intermediaries is to be complete by July 1987.

Legislation enacted in 1972 allowed the application of cost caps to home health agency reimbursement. First implemented in 1979, cost caps limited the reasonable cost for Medicare services to the 75th percentile of all agencies' costs. The cost limits were applied in the aggregate. What aggregation meant was that if a home health agency's cost was over the limit for one discipline and under for others, it could average the differences and be reimbursed accordingly.

New regulations promulgated in July 1985, and applied immediately, implemented major change in the method of calculation and eliminated the ability to aggregate costs against he new limits. The new method was calculated using 120% of the mean of all agencies' visit costs per discipline in the first year. The regulations provided that the limits be decreased to 115% of the mean the second year, and 112% in the third year. In the preamble to the regulations, then Secretary of Health and Human Services Margaret Heckler acknowledged that the majority of all home health agencies would be adversely affected by the regulations.

Legislation was introduced in 1985 to enact a one-year moratorium on implementation of the new cost limits. Although that legislation was not acted upon, provisions were included in the 1986 Budget Reconciliation package to prohibit the removal of aggregation and to require a study on the effects of the regulation. Although it appeared sure to pass, the cost limit provision was removed from the Reconciliation package because it was an issue designated by the Administration as grounds for vetoing the entire package. Cost limit relief has been attached to the 1987 Budget Reconciliation package, and introduced independently.

In the meantime, the new limits have been in effect and have caused significant losses for agencies. Especially hard hit are agencies providing high volumes of high-tech care, hospice care, and rural agencies. As the average length of visits has increased due to sicker patients and increased paperwork burdens, more agencies have found the new limits inadequate to cover the costs of care.

Congress enacted the Balanced Budget and Emergency Deficit Control Act, better known as Gramm-Rudman-Hollings, in December of 1985. This legislation requires that the federal budget be balanced by 1991, through annual reductions in the deficit. If the President and Congress are unable to produce a balanced budget, automatic cuts are triggered throughout federal expenditures. By special consideration of Congress, automatic cuts to the Medicare program are limited to 1% in the first year, and 2% in subsequent years,.

The Department of Health and Human Services has determined that the 1% reduction in home care expenditures is to be applied to cost. This means that regardless of efficiency or cost containment, home care providers are subject to reduction in reimbursement: they are receiving 99% of the cost of rendering care. Between the cuts imposed by the new cost limits and the 1% reduction, home care providers have experienced a tremendous increase in unreimbursed expenses under the Medicare program.

The National Association for Home Care has filed a petition with the Provider Reimbursement Review Board seeking expedited review of the legality of the HCFA approach. This action is a first step toward a federal lawsuit on the Gramm-Rudman application to home care.

Beset by so many problems, one might consider the Medicare home care benefit a lost cause. Indeed, Health Care Financing Administration officials have publicly stated that they are aware that patients are sicker and require more care than is being covered. They believe, however, that it is their job to rigidly interpret Medicare coverage with respect to the original legislative language. The administration has thrown the gauntlet to Congress to change the Medicare statute if they desire increased coverage under the home care benefit. If the interests of serving the growing elderly population while containing health costs, Congress is responding.

Congressional Activity Related to Medicare Home Care

During the first nine months of 1986, more than a dozen hearings were held by various committees, and individual senators and representatives, on problems surrounding the Medicare home care benefit. During the same time, 13 pieces of legislation were introduced which would benefit the provision of home care. Three of these legislative proposals were introduced as companion pieces in both the House of Representatives and the Senate (*NAHC Report* No. 180, 3-4). The Medicare Quality Protection Act of 1986, introduced by Heinz and Stark, has numerous provisions of interest to home care. In addition to the previously mentioned provisions addressing technical denials and waiver of liability, this legislation would require hospitals to provide discharge planning; require fiscal intermediaries to expedite claims review; allow providers to represent beneficiaries on appeals; and require Professional Review Organizations (PROs) to include information on the quality of posthospital care in their annual reports on prospective payment (Cushman April 1986; June 1986).

The legislation introduced by Leahy, The Better Health Care Act, likewise covers several items of importance to home care. The bill would define intermittent care as one or more visits per day up to 60 days; allow aggregation of claims; require HCFA to follow the Administrative Procedures Act requirements; replace waiver as previously discussed; and create uniform assessment criteria for claims review. It would also make all claims appealable and allow providers to represent beneficiaries; require hospital discharge planning with prescribed guidelines; and change intermediary performance evaluation, standards to require accuracy as well as costs savings (*NAHC Report* No. 174, 4).

Other bills addressing current problems in the Medicare program including the Medicare Part C Catastrophic Health Insurance Bill, introduced by Claude Pepper of Florida, Chairman of the Subcommittee on Health and Long Term Care of the House

Select Committee on Aging; The Medicare Health Improvement Act, introduced by Senator Bill Bradley of New Jersey; and The Medicare Timely Payment Amendments of 1986, co-introduced by Dave Durenburger, Minnesota, Chairman of the Senate Finance Health Subcommittee, and Congressman Willis Gradison, Ohio.

Prospective Payment for Home Care

For a variety of reasons, it is becoming apparent that the current cost-based system of reimbursement for home care services is outdated. First, the movement of acute care hospitals to prospective payment for Medicare has created interest in doing the same for all providers. Second, the obvious problems with coverage and claims review would be obviated by a well-designed system of prospective payment. Perhaps most important, patients could receive the services they need, in the intensity they need them, without imposition of rigid coverage guidelines.

There are, however, as many pitfalls involved in movement to a prospective payment mode as there are advantages. Design of an effective system is predicated on accurate data. Unfortunately, neither the Department of Health and Human Services, Congress, nor the home care field have been successful in collecting sufficient accurate data on the resource utilization and consumption, or cost of home care services. A demonstration project, awarded to Abt Associates by the Health Care Financing Administration, was to begin study of prospective payment in 1985. The project has been stalled by the government for nearly two years.

Providers, concerned that a system of alternative reimbursement will be imposed with or without appropriate data, have pressed for the National Association to develop models. Likewise, individual agencies have begun small research projects to identify various cost and resource utilization patterns. In response, the National Association for Home Care has identified the attributes necessary in a prospective payment system (*Toward a National Home Care Policy* 14-15) and has commissioned two projects to examine possible models for prospective payment.

The first of these projects involved a task force representing financial, administrative, and clinical experts in home care; and an external consultant, expert in economic and legal aspects of health care financing. The Task Force on Alternative Care Payment Methods, in its report to the Association, recommended development of a two-tiered prospective payment system: one method for payment of care to acutely ill patients, and a second for long-term care clients. The Task Force also recommended pursuit of a system which takes into account severity of illness and functional disability. The task force concurred with the widely expressed opinion that medical diagnosis does not offer a sufficient basis for development of a prospective payment system for home care (NAHC Task Force on Alternative Home Care Payment Methods 1986).

The second project, still underway, involved commissioning the consulting firm Health Policy Alternatives to review the Task Force report and the current Medicare statute. The project is to suggest possible changes in legislation to move toward a sound prospective payment system. In a presentation at the 1986 Annual Meeting of the National Association, Irwin Wolkstein, chief consultant, indicated that they would recommend a major reconstruction of the Medicare law on home care, rather than a simple prospective payment system (Wolkstein 1986). Clearly, a great deal more study is required before recommendations can be made to design a new reimbursement system for home care.

Hospice Issues

The Medicare Hospice benefit was created in 1982 through P.L. 97-248. The new benefit allows individuals in the last six months of their lives to elect palliative hospice services in lieu of the traditional Medicare benefit. The hospice benefit was implemented in November of 1983, and had a three-year sunset provision built into the statute. The 1986 Budget Reconciliation package included language to make the benefit permanent.

Since the law requires 80% of all services to be provided at home, and no more than 20% for episodic inpatient care; the hospice benefit is home care. Hospice care is reimbursed on a per diem basis, with a per patient capitation ceiling. The per diem payment takes three forms: routine home care, continuous home care, or inpatient. In addition to basic home care services, the hospice benefit requires provision of medical care, pastoral care, volunteer services, and bereavement follow-up. The cost of the last three services is nonreimbursable. Other aspects of the law require the hospice to provide interdisciplinary team management of cases, management of inpatient as well as outpatient care, and acceptance of full financial responsibility for the care of the patient until death.

The Hospice statute also designates nursing and social work services as core services. This means that they must be provided directly by the hospice and cannot be subcontracted. While this provision is theoretically laudable to ensure quality, properly coordinated care, it has also served to restrict the availability of the benefit.

By October of 1965, less than 16% of the 1500 known hospices had sought and obtained Medicare certification as a hospice provider. A 1984 survey found that 78% of all home care agencies in the United States currently provide hospice services. Yet, 85% of those agencies had not applied for Medicare certification, and only 4% planned to do so. The reasons provided for avoiding the Medicare program included: inadequate reimbursement, excessive red tape, inability to arrange inpatient service contracts, and the prohibition on subcontracting nursing care (*Toward a National Home Care Policy* 20).

The inability to subcontract has limited community hospices and community coalitions from participating in the hospice program. It has also impeded rural agencies from participation and caused urban hospices to duplicate existing resources in order to participate. The National Hospice Organization, proponent of the original inclusion of the core requirement, insists that it is essential to the integrity of appropriate hospice care. The National Association for Home Care and Hospice Association of America believe the provision should be modified. They support legislative change to allow hospices in rural and medically underserved areas, and agencies providing hospice care before enactment of the Hospice Law, to subcontract under carefully prescribed conditions. Legislation to this effect has been introduced in two sessions of Congress, but has not received widespread interest.

Medicaid Home Care

The Medicaid program, administered on a state-by-state basis, was created at the same time as the Medicare program. The Medicaid program, Title XIX of the Social Security Act, provides medical and health care to the medically indigent. Expenses of the program are shared by the federal and state governments.

In the majority of states, the Medicaid home health benefit is even more limited than the Medicare benefit. The only services required to be offered by statute are nursing, home health aide, and medical supplies and equipment. All therapy services are provided at the discretion of the individual state. This limitation in coverage represents a serious problem in many states. Home care providers are fighting for states to include at least the same benefit as Medicare, nationwide.

Because the Medicaid program is a federal- as well as state-funded social program, it has been subject to federal cost containment efforts. The 1987 Reagan Administration budget package proposes cutbacks in the federal expenditure for this program. Such cutbacks, if successful, will either force states to increase expenditures, or reduce the benefits of the program still further.

Since the majority of Medicaid expenditures goes toward long-term nursing home care there is considerable interest in reducing unnecessary institutionalization of the elderly and chronically disabled. As part of the Omnibus Budget Reconciliation Act of 1981, the "Medicaid Section 2176 Home and Community-Base Waiver Program" was enacted. This program grants the Secretary of the Department of Health and Human Services authority to waive existing statutory limitations and allow states to finance noninstitutional long-term care under Medicaid.

The Section 2176 Waiver Program restricts the noninstitutional long-term care services to Medicaid-eligible individuals who would otherwise require nursing home placement. Services which can be included under the waivers include chore, handyman, homemaking, case management, respite care, adult day care, and transportation. More than 76 waivers have been granted in 44 states. The information from these projects to date indicates that they have been successful in containing the costs of the Medicaid program.

Convinced of the efficacy of such an approach, Senators Orrin Hatch (Utah), Edward Kennedy (Massachusetts), John Heinz, Paula Hawkins (Florida), Bill Bradley, and Robert Stafford (Vermont) introduced the Home and Community-Based Services for the Elderly Act of 1985. This bill would establish a block grant program to provide services similar to those demonstrated under the waiver programs, educate the public and health professionals, and involve family and community groups caring for the elderly.

In a similar measure, Senators Bill Bradley, John Glenn (Ohio), and Lawton Chiles (Florida) introduced the Medicaid Home and Community-Based Services Improvement Act. This bill would eliminate the waiver process and allow states to provide home-based care to prevent institutionalization.

Expanding Home Care Horizons

The home care services covered by the Medicare and Medicaid programs have been targeted to narrow segments of the American population in need of such services.

With the exception of the waiver programs, described above, the programs have focused almost exclusively on care to the acutely ill. Expanding government funding of home care services to the long-term care population scares policymakers. There is a general fear that opening up home care would encourage people to seek care who are currently managing without government support. The majority of long-term care individuals are cared for by family and friends.

Development of mechanisms to help individuals and their informal caregivers afford and manage care, however, is a necessary step in keeping the self-care system viable. The creation of a respite benefit is one such mechanism. Another approach would be to provide tax incentives for families who take care of a dependent individual in their household. Recently, the concept of creating health and long-term care IRAs has gained popularity. Four bills which contained language on such IRAs were introduced during 1986.

Another aspect of home care receiving recent attention is pediatric home care. Senator Orrin Hatch and Senator Edward Kennedy have been the primary proponents of expanding pediatric home care. During the 99th Congress, several hearings were held on the topic. The hearings have emphasized that numerous children can be deinstitutionalized with the support of home care. Through new technology, these children can receive complex treatment at home at far less cost than in institutions. These breakthroughs allow children to live with their families and grow up in a normal environment. As a result, a number of bills have been introduced in Congress to provide payment for certain types of high-tech care for children, especially for the ventilator-dependent.

As medical technology advances, there may be no limit to what care can be safely and cost-effectively provided at home. It is certainly the setting most preferred by children and families . . . and by the elderly. The future of home care will be determined as much by its success in deinstitutionalizing the public policy mind set and purse strings, as by the care it provides.

References

Cushman, M. J. April 1986. Testimony of Margaret J. Cushman before the Health Subcommittee of the Ways and Means Committee, on behalf of the National Association for Home Care.

Cushman, M. J. June 1986. Testimony of Margaret J. Cushman before the Health Subcommittee of the U.S. Senate Finance Committee, on behalf of the National Association for Home Care.

NAHC Report. July 17, 1986. Washington, DC: The National Association for Home Care.

NAHC Task Force on Alternative Home Care Payment Methods. January 29, 1986. *Toward the development of a prospective payment system for home care.* Washington, DC: The National Association for Home Care.

Social Security Act. 1965a. Sec. 1861(m), 42 USC Sec. 1395x(m):42 CFR Secs. 405.235,236 and

Sec. 1814(a)(2)(B), 42 USC Sec. 1395(f).

Social Security Act. 1965b. Sec. 1835(a)(2)(A), 42 USC Sec. 1395x(m), 42 CFR Sec. 405.234.

The attempted dismantling of the Medicare home health benefit: A report to the congress. March 1986. Washington, DC: The National Association for Home Care.

Toward a national home care policy: Blueprint for action. January 1986. Washington, DC: The National Association for Home Care.

U.S. Bureau of the Census. 1984. *Statistical abstract of the United States: 1985,* 105th ed. Washington, DC: Government Printing Office.

Wolkstein, I. 1986. Reform of Medicare law on home care. Presentation before the Annual Meeting of the National Association for Home Care, September 10, 1986.

Part VIII

Strategic Planning, Marketing And Survival Issues

Chapter Twenty-Seven

Strategic Planning

David Barton Smith

Introduction

Strategic planning is difficult, rewarding, and essential for organizations. It shapes the way an organization changes so that: (1) it can better accomplish its goals, and (2) more effectively adapt to environmental pressures. Organizations will change anyway. Even the most effective strategic planning may not always control the way an organization changes. Successful home health agencies, so dependent on third-party payment regulations and referrals from potential competitors, are like the champion downhill skier, a little out of control.

> The Men's Downhill races in the 1976 Winter Olympics changed the strategies of racers. Franz Klammer seemed "out of control" for the entire run. Yet, he won the Olympic Gold Medal. Up until Klammer's run the prevailing thinking among downhill racers was that the winner of a race would be the one who was in the best condition, had the best technique, and skied just this side of the edge of losing control. The thinking changed. To win one now had to ski on the other side of the edge of losing control. In 1976 Klammer was the only one (of truly world class skiers) who skied out of control. Since every other top skier was trying to ski just short of losing control and since Klammer was lucky, he won easily. Now all the top skiers, perhaps fifteen or twenty, are skiing out of control and on any given day it is largely natural selection stemming from factors beyond the skiers control which determines who wins. During any run there are many blind variations in form of ruts, bumps, mistakes, and so forth, which are beyond the control of the skiers at the speed they are now going. The skier who skis most out of control and is luckiest in avoiding falling will win. Since there are so many good skiers skiing out of control the odds are excellent that one of them will always take enough risks and manage enough miraculous recoveries to beat the under-control skier (McKelvey 1982, 447-448.).

The top skiers made a strategic choice. They chose to go for the gold rather than the less risky strategy of good average performance. Organizations can make risky strategic choices that aim for market dominance or more conservative ones that aim for average performance. The rapid technological, regulatory, and competitive changes in the home health care market, however, make almost any strategy a risky one. Strategic planning helps make those choices and control their implementation.

No matter what choices are made, successful strategic planning must move at the speed of the winning downhill skier. Such planning is *not* a special set of procedures, a committee structure, a set of statistical projection techniques, or a document that can be produced by a consultant for the right price. It *does* involve: (1) an understanding of how organizations change, and (2) the use of that knowledge to shape changes in an organization that will, as much as possible, assure its success. The first section describes how organizations change; the second, how strategic planning can help shape those changes; and the final section, how to develop strategic planning capacity.

How Organizations Change

Organizations resist change. It is stressful and disruptive. Exhibit 27-1 summarizes the process by which changes take place in organizations. An organization must adapt effectively to its environment to succeed. When it fails to achieve at least the minimum performance needed for survival, it looks for ways to turn things around. Change involves risk. The larger the change, the greater the cost and disruption and, consequently, the greater the risk. As a result, most organizations will attempt to turn things around by making modest adjustments that involve little change for the organization. If the more modest changes fail, an organization searches for more drastic solutions. That search will progress through four distinct phases.

Phase I. Manipulation of the Environment

Organizations invest effort in getting others to change rather than changing themselves. One tries to change the reimbursement policies, influence the granting of Certificates of Need to restrict competition, or change consumer patterns of utilization. If such efforts are successful, the organization does not have to change at all. Home health agencies and the associations that represent them fight such battles.

The new interest in marketing reflects this concern with reshaping the environment. Predictably, when most such organizations focus on marketing, they focus on developing an advertising campaign to increase their market share rather than changing their own organization or the services they provide to better respond to market demands. As suggested in the next chapter, marketing is, or at least should be, an integral part of the more extensive process of strategic planning and organizational change.

Most providers of health services, however, are beginning to recognize the limits of such environmental manipulation. Acute care hospitals, which have been eminently successful in the past, are now being drastically affected by changes in the payment system. Average length of stay in hospitals dropped by over a day in the first two years of the prospective payment system (PPS), and the proportion of discharges to home care programs doubled (Chesney 1985; Farley 1986). They must search for more drastic solutions that will directly affect the character and structure of their own organizations.

Phase II. Operational Adjustment

If environmental manipulation fails to assure adequate performance, then an organization will attempt to address the immediate operational issues. Revenue

Exhibit 27-1. Organizational Response to Problems in the Environment

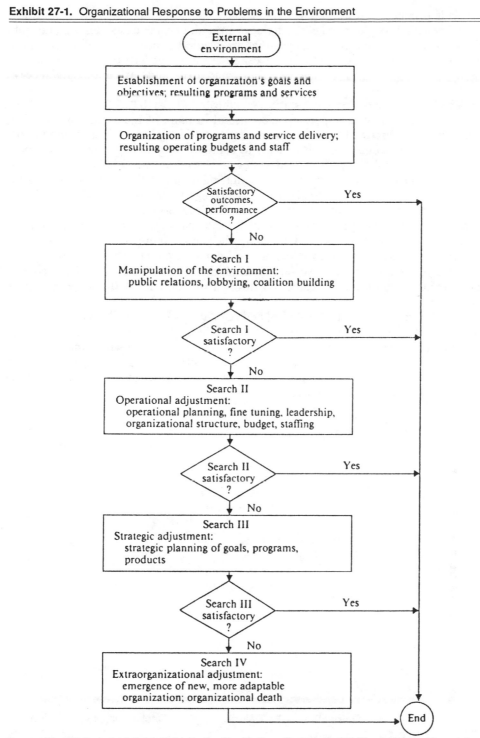

Source: The White Labyrinth: A Guide to the Health Care System, 2nd Edition by D. Smith and A. Kaluzny. (Ann Arbor: Health Administration Press, 1986) p. 116; Reprinted with permission.

shortfalls produce staff and budget reductions. The administrator may be fired and new leadership brought in to help turn things around. In some cases, this is a poor substitute for more fundamental changes that are needed. Operational adjustments can improve efficiency and quality of services. Such efforts absorb most of the time of management. Yet, no matter how well performed, they alone will not assure success, or even survival.

The health care sector is not static. As indicated in Exhibit 27-2, products or services have a life cycle. It is perhaps most useful to think of home care as a market, rather than as a discrete product. That market existed long before the invention of the modern hospital around 1920. It is likely to continue long after its replacement with other organizational forms. The products or services, however, have changed drastically. Some, such as remote monitoring of vital signs, are in the early stages of introduction and rapid growth. Others, such as managed care systems (PPOs, HMOs, capitation case management, etc.) are entering into the more competitive growth stage of the life cycle. Other products, the more familiar packaged array of fee-for-service home health services have reached maturity, where growth in net income is restrained both by competition and restriction of third-party payment. The more traditional private duty nursing services that were in the decline stage of the life cycle, of course, have gained a significant life extension through the shift in Medicare payment for acute care.

Third-party payment, technological and regulatory changes will continue to affect both the actual home health care products delivered and the organizations that provide them. Concentrating on efficiency and quality may not stave off the erosion of its share of health care expenditures in the face of emerging vertically integrated hospital systems of community care or HMOs and other emerging permutations of insurance and service organizations.

Exhibit 27-2. Product Life Cycle

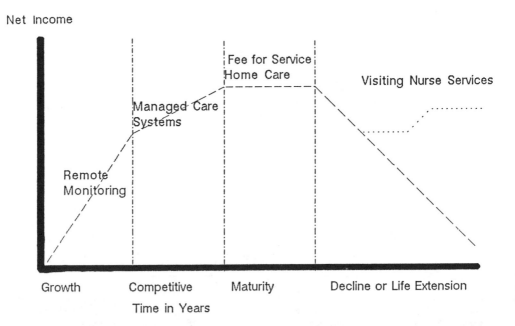

Net Income

Fee for Service Home Care

Visiting Nurse Services

Managed Care Systems

Remote Monitoring

Growth   Competitive   Maturity   Decline or Life Extension

Time in Years

Phase III. Strategic Adjustment

A strategic adjustment involves changing goals, programs, and products to respond better to regulatory or market pressures and to adopt new products in the introduction and growth phase of their life cycle. This is not an easy thing for organizations, particularly with staff having strong professional identifies. Yet, the capacity to engage effectively in such adjustments will determine the ability of an organization to survive. Working effectively at this level, changing products and services to adapt to shifts in the regulatory or market pressures is the acid test of effective strategic planning.

It is often useful to think about "products" as separate and distinct from the medical specialty or allied health occupational group services that form the traditional building blocks of health services organizations. The "product line management" approach attempts to identify a single center of accountability for financial and quality of care issues. This is a logical extension of the matrix-type organizational structure illustrated in Exhibit 27-3. The traditional approach is to divide an organization into major specialty areas. In Exhibit 27-3, these areas are the vertical columns (nursing, billing, etc.). The products are the horizontal rows in Exhibit 27-3. This particular hypothetical home care agency or company has defined four products: a home hospice service, a conventional fee-for-service program, a highly specialized posthospitalization cardiac care program, and a special capitation subcontract with an HMO. While there is a good deal of overlap in the kinds of services offered by each of these "products" (medical consultants, nursing, durable medical equipment rental, etc.), it is often advantageous, particularly in a competitive environment, to manage them separately. That is, organize the home care agency by rows (products) rather than

Exhibit 27-3. Examples of Home Care Product Management

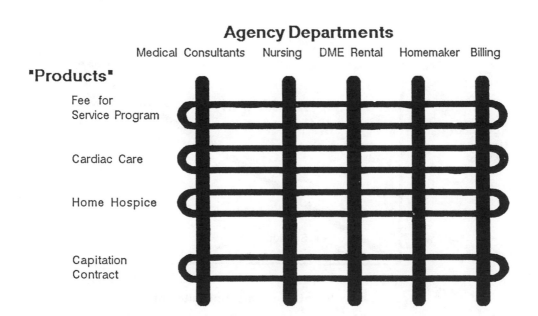

Agency Departments

Medical Consultants   Nursing   DME Rental   Homemaker   Billing

"Products"

Fee for
Service Program

Cardiac Care

Home Hospice

Capitation
Contract

columns. This may assure better cost and quality control and more responsiveness to the needs and demands of a special segment of the market.

Defining the "products" of a home care program may seem like belaboring the obvious. Sometimes, however, it's not that obvious. "Products" may be defined by the geographic boundaries, third-party markets, or medical specialty. There are also three basic additional ways health care "products" or services can be redefined, as illustrated in Exhibit 27-4. First, the time commitment during an illness episode can be either narrowed or widened. One can focus on a narrow time during posthospitalization or view the service or product as one involving a more extensive time commitment. The latter would imply a commitment to serving the chronically ill and providing long-term maintenance and rehabilitative services. Second, the nature of the services can be either restricted to more narrow technical or expanded to include broader social-psychological support services. The broader definition of the product, for example, might involve the development of social and recreational services. The more narrow definition, for example, might simply involve supply on a rental basis of specific pieces of durable medical equipment.

The relative attractiveness of these alternatives, however, depends on how specific services are "bundled" for payment. Arrangements for payment can be negotiated with third parties or the client for each specific service rendered, either by illness episode or admission (a DRG-type payment system) or by person covered (HMO or SHMO). The bundling of services for payment, of course, defines the time commitments and breadth of services that will be provided. The movement from a fee-for-ser-

Exhibit 27-4. Alternative Definitions of "Product"

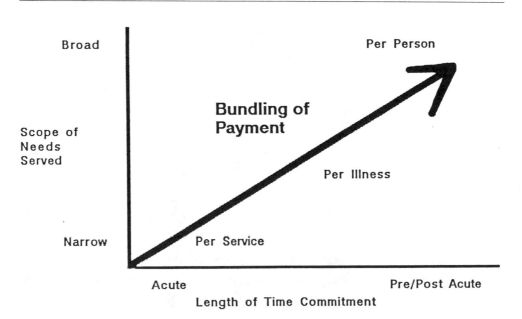

vice payment system, to ones where third parties shift some of the risk onto providers, requires a fundamental change in orientation. A strong financial position for a provider is assured under such payment arrangements not by providing a high volume of relatively costly and complex services, but by reducing the volume of costly services and substituting less costly ones. Health care providers have yet to adjust fully to the shift in bundling of acute care services into payments for illness episodes and are just beginning to adjust to a bundling based on capitation arrangements. The ripple effect of these shifts in financing will force fundamental redefinitions of most products of health services. Both the scope and length of the time commitments will be radically altered by such changes. Home care, as a less costly alternative to acute hospital care and, in some instances, skilled nursing home care, will be directly affected.

Phase IV. Extraorganizational Adjustment

If none of these searches are effective, an organization either dies or is transformed into a completely different entity. In a recent six-year period, for example, 340 hospitals in the United States closed (Mulner 1986). Many others were absorbed, either through horizontal or vertical integration, into another organization that can more effectively control environmental pressures, or it may precipitate such a transformation itself. We are beginning to see a variety of hybrid multi-institutional, multiservice organizations in health care. For-profit hospital chains are merging with HMOs or joining in ventures with insurance companies. Not-for-profit institutions are developing for-profit subsidiaries and developing joint ventures medical groups. Some of these adjustments are acts of desperation, some the result of more thoughtful strategic planning activities, and most are a little out of control. According to one knowledgeable source, half the business of consulting firms involved in corporate restructuring activities in the last several years involve undoing organizational restructuring and joint ventures that have gone sour.

How Strategic Planning Shapes Change in Organizations

Effective strategic planning radically alters the natural process of organizational change. Its focus is on change rather than maintenance of the status quo. It views the stages of organizational change not as places to go only in desperation, but as inevitable steps in an ongoing process of organizational development. It transforms what is essentially a passive, often unconscious, reactive process of organizational change into a self-conscious, proactive one. At each stage in the process of organizational change outlined in Exhibit 27-1, an effective strategic planning process anticipates the questions and develops answers and makes choices. Those choices are based on an assessment of the external environment, a refined sense of the mission and goals of the organization, and a knowledge of the key issues in each of the four phases of organizational development.

Assessment of the External Environment

Intelligence is critical to planning strategy. What do we know, what do we need to know to position ourselves strategically? What trends in payment and regulation of the health care industry will impact on home health care services? What changes in the population and economics will shape demand for home health services? Not just is the population of those over 65 and 75 growing rapidly, but the relative wealth of this population segment appears to be growing as well. For home health services that have suffered from restrictive eligibility requirements and benefits from third parties, this is particularly critical.

Everyone remotely involved in the health sector is engaged in similar types of environmental assessments. The potential of an attractive and growing market invites greater competition. One needs to know what new entrants to the market are likely, and what kind of position existing competitors are likely to take. There is also the threat of potential substitute products or services that will affect the competitive environment; for example, the growth and development of hospice programs, swing-bed and self-care units in hospitals, life care communities, HMOs, and the return of the physician or nonphysician practitioner home visit. Greater competition will in turn increase the bargaining power of customers and produce greater competition for staffing.

Clarifying Goals and Objectives

Goals and objectives have to represent a good deal more than financial ratios and utilization and budget projections. There is a fine line between organizational autism which ignores the environment, and organizational emptiness which ignores any internal vision and is preoccupied with short-run market demand. Either extreme will destroy the organization. One needs to articulate the special vision of the organization that helps to impose order upon the chaotic signals of the environment. It also helps to give a sense of cohesiveness and common purpose to those involved in assuring the success of the organization.

Identifying Strategy in Each Phase of Organizational Change

At each phase of organizational change the question becomes not what action can alleviate the immediate problem, but what can be done to assure the overall effectiveness of the organization's strategy in achieving its vision. Questions such as the following need to be asked and answered.

Phase I.   Environmental Manipulation:
How can we shape our market and influence the regulations that affect us to better assure our success?

Phase II.   Operational Adjustment:
How can we improve what we're currently doing to improve our strategic position?

Phase III.   Strategic Adjustment:
              What choices are available in new goals, products? Where on the
              basis of our own experience do we have the best competitive ad-
              vantage?

Phase IV.   Extraorganizational Adjustment:
              What new organizational forms are possible? Which ones should we
              pursue? Should we compete with others or form coalitions?

Answers to such questions form the framework for the strategic plans of an organization. They link immediate operational issues to efforts for the active creation of
a future for the organization.

Steps in Developing Strategic Planning Capacity

There are many detailed outlines of the specific actions and steps involved in a
strategic planning process (Ackoff 1981; Day 1986; Nutt 1984; Weber and Peters
1983). Others have supplied case studies of strategic planning in health care that help
put some flesh on the abstractions (Reeves 1983; Suver, Kahn, and Clement 1984). In
simplest terms, however, it all boils down to four critical steps.

Commit the resources to do it right

Strategic planning is least likely to be done by those who need it the most. Administrators faced with rapid change in their environment and increasing competition
have difficulty stepping back from the immediate day-to-day crises they face. The most
critical resource that has to be committed is the time it requires of key decision
makers within an organization. This may involve initially several full days to clarify and
get agreement on the process and follow-up sessions to help reinforce and further
clarify it. If effective, this strategic planning process becomes imbedded in the
decision-making routines of the organization and is no longer perceived by executives
as "something else I have to find time for." Outside facilitators can help in these initial
stages of development. There is a need also to build in either the internal staff support
or to contract out for the development of the information base to "feed" the strategic
planning process. The level of effort and cost of these information-gathering activities
will depend on: (1) the size and complexity of the organization; (2) the size and
complexity of the market and regulatory environment it is dealing with; and (3) the
level of detail and degree of certainty that the managers involved determine as necessary to make strategic decisions. Just as with the time commitments of top managers,
the initial cost will be relatively high and, as such information gathering gets built into
the day-to-day operations of the organization, the "maintenance costs" will decline.

Pick the right participants

Strategic planning must be done by the key decision makers in an organization. It is
not something, such as a Certificate of Need application or a required long-range

planning document, that can be delegated to either a staff person or a consultant. The top managers in an organization are responsible not only for strategy formulation but also for making it work. It is thus the responsibility of the chief executive officer to pick the individuals that will be involved in the strategic planning process. These individuals need to have a working knowledge of the organization, and they need to have the intellectual ability to think strategically, rather than parochially or defensively, about their own special concerns. The basic work group should include no less than three and no more than twelve individuals. It need not include all those that hold the key formal organization positions on the board, medical staff, and administration, but should be designed to assure, as much as possible, the support of all those groups needed to implement whatever strategic plans are developed.

Provide an effective link between operational and strategic planning

Strategic planning operates in the gray area between the broad "ends" incorporated in the mission of an organization and the overall direction of its board and the specific "means" incorporated in the operational plans of department heads and middle managers. Those operational plans may include operating budget, staffing, construction and capital equipment, and program and marketing plans. Strategic plans need to be translated into operational ones. This requires the bottom-up participation of those responsible for such operational planning in the creation, implementation, and evaluation of strategy.

Strategic plans that emerge insulated from any understanding of the operational difficulties are doomed to failure. The strategic planning process for one hospital, for example, developed the concept of a multipurpose facility. The construction of the hospital was combined with rental space for shops and physicians' offices. Strategically it was brilliant. Operationally, it almost proved disastrous because of the failure to work out special concessions from third parties in calculating the capital cost payments. (This is done typically by measuring the proportion of floor space allocated to the actual hospital functions and paying that proportion of the overall costs. Because the cost of hospital construction is many times higher than the cost per square foot of office space, the hospital would have had to charge shop owners and physicians three to four times the going rate. It would have been unlikely to attract any tenants and would have had to absorb a substantial loss.) Similar anecdotes of the gaps between strategy and operations abound. They illustrate the need for a regular dialogue between operational and strategic planning.

An effective dialogue between strategic and operational planning can take place through well-designed joint operational and strategic planning sessions. They can also be built into the day-to-day review and consultation process that goes on between top and operational managers. It should provide the opportunity for operational mangers to the shape of strategies as well as its implementation.

Develop an orderly process for accomplishing the tasks

There are many ways that the essential tasks of strategic planning can be accomplished. In whatever way these tasks are accomplished, what is important is that the process is well understood and acceptable to the key participants, and that it proceeds in an orderly manner. This should not exclude the opportunity for more open-ended, chaotic brainstorming and free association, but it should take place within a structure so that the ideas can be subjected to critical appraisal and put to work. These tasks might take place in the following sequence:

Step 1. Assess current situation. Collect information, and evaluate the current strategic position of the organization. Assess potential future opportunities and threats.

Step 2. Revise objectives. Set new objectives based on the assessment in Step 1.

Step 3. Generate and evaluate strategy alternatives. Explore alternatives, in all four phases of organizational change, designed to achieve the desired objectives.

Step 4. Select the best strategies. In the four possible phases of organizational change, make choices. These should have the benefit of review by operational managers and support of the governing body.

Step 5. Develop detailed plans for the selected strategies. Provide opportunities for input from operational mangers or, if this is a new venture for the organization, from outside consultants.

Step 6. Implement the Plans. Delegate responsibility to a manager and those involved in its operation.

Step 7. Monitor performance. Regularly review the success of these implemented plans to see if they accomplish the objectives set for them. Use this to make midcourse corrections and as input into the situation assessment step of the next cycle of strategic planning.

Conclusions

This brief summary may suggest that the process of strategic planning is easy and obvious. It is neither. Some readers, like the individual who discovered one day that he had always been writing prose, may conclude that they are already doing it. That is probably correct. The key question is not whether organizations should do strategic planning, but how well do they do it and how can that process be improved? There are many tools and techniques that can be applied to strategic planning. There is no end to the information that could be collected, analyzed, and utilized in such a process. What improves the process in one setting may be ineffective in another. Strategic planning is a process for bringing about organizational change and growth. Like the process of individual change and growth, it is very personal and individualized; you learn by doing it. Organizations that have the most successful strategic planning are motivated to engage in it not so much by grim survival pressures but by the uniquely human drive to grow, and to become all they are capable of becoming. To paraphrase Rene Dubois's conclusion in his classic work *The Mirage of Health*, "has never been a Garden of Eden but a Valley of Decision where resilience is essential to survival...To grow in the midst of dangers is the fate of the human race, because it is the law of the spirit" (Dubois 1959, 281-282).

References

Ackoff, R.L. 1981. *Creating the corporate future.* New York: J. Wiley and Sons.

Chesney, J.D., and Long, M. 1986. Medicare case-mix complexity and product change: what has happened since prospective payment. Presentation at Association for Health Services Research Third Annual Meeting, 24 June, Boston, Massachusetts.

Day, G.S. 1986. *Analysis of strategic market decisions.* New York: West Publishing Company.

Dubois, R. 1959. *Mirage of health.* New York: Harper and Row.

Farley, D.E., and Rosekamp, J. 1986. Changing patterns of occupancy, length of stay and admissions. Presentation at Association for Health Services Research Third Annual Meeting, 24 June, Boston, Massachusetts.

McKelvey, B. 1982. *Organizational systematics, taxonomy, evolution and classification.* Berkeley: University of California Press.

Mulner, R. 1986. Hospital closures, mergers and consolidations. Presentational Association for Health Services Research Third Annual Meeting, 24 June, Boston, Massachusetts.

Nutt, P.C. 1984. *Planning methods for health related organizations.* New York: J. Wiley and Sons.

Reeves, P.N. 1983. *Strategic planning for hospitals.* Chicago: Foundation of the American College of Hospital Administrators.

Smith, D.B., and Kaluzny, A.R. 1986. *The white labyrinth.* Ann Arbor: Health Administration Press.

Suver, J.D., Kahn, C.N. and Clement, J.P. 1984. *Cases in health care financial management.* Ann Arbor: AUPHA Press.

Weber, J.B., and Peters, J.P. 1983. *Strategic thinking: New frontiers in hospital management.* Chicago: American Hospital Publishing, Inc.

Chapter Twenty-Eight

Marketing: An Overview

Susan C. Nolt

Introduction

The traditional concept and delivery of home health care changed in the mid-sixties with the advent of Medicare. In the late seventies and into the early eighties, the general economic outlook forced further changes in the area of operations and cost efficiency. And as we steam ahead toward the next century, no one can be certain just where or how it will all end. For this reason, it is increasingly important that individual agencies utilize their energies in a well-organized manner to achieve their organizational goals. Marketing, then, becomes an important function in assisting agencies in meeting these unknown challenges of the future.

In the broadest sense of the word, marketing is an exchange process. Although it is a concept that has existed since the days of bartering, it became a recognized profession in the early twentieth century. In spite of this, the health care profession has historically viewed marketing as hard-core selling, an anathema to professional codes of ethics. Today's informed consumer and increased competition are forcing the health care industry to rethink this position. Recognizing this, Philip Kotler, a noted marketing authority, offers the following definition of professional services marketing:

> Professional services marketing consists of organized activities and programs by professional services firms that are designed to retain present clients and attract new clients by sensing, serving, and satisfying their needs through delivery of appropriate services on a paid basis in a manner consistent with creditable professional goals and norms. (Kotler and Cox 1980)

Before proceeding with the formal discussion of the marketing process, a few items need clarification. The approach that was taken in the compilation of this chapter is generic in nature. If marketing concepts are understood, then individual agencies can modify and build upon these concepts as they develop their marketing program. Under the Medicare and Medicaid programs, certain aspects of marketing, i.e., in the area of communications, may not be considered an allowable administrative cost, and therefore, frequent references should be made to provider reimbursement manuals for appropriate guidelines. Traditional marketing frequently deals with a tangible product. Although this may be true for the home health care agency, quite often it is more likely to be a service. Therefore, product and services are used synonymously as are the words patient, consumer, and client.

The Marketing Process

Step 1: The Mission Statement

The first organized activity of the marketing process is the development of a mission statement or a review and update of your current one. Although seemingly the buzz-words in today's corporate world, the mission statement is indeed the focal point of your organization for it defines your business. For instance, you are in the business of providing home health care, home care, or health care? The word home may have some limiting features for your business image, whereas without it, services might be provided in the home, as well as in selected long-term care facilities, or in industry. Whatever is ultimately decided, the development of a mission statement may perhaps be the most difficult and time-consuming task ever undertaken within the agency. Therefore, the end product should have a broad focus with enough flexibility to make changes as indicated by the competitive environment.

The responsibility for the development of this mission statement lies with the governing body working in concert with the agency's top management. Additional input may be obtained from employees, referral sources, other human service organizations, business community, and consumers.

Topics for consideration when developing the mission statement may be, but are not limited to:

1. Agency history and background: Why was the agency originally formed? Who were the referral sources? How have these changed over the years? What type of formal and informal relationships have occurred over the years?

2. Philosophy of the governing body and top management: Each individual brings to the agency specific personal and professional values and beliefs. A conflict between the mission of the agency and the values of the people in charge may act as a detriment to the daily functioning of the agency as well as have a negative impact on the quality of the services rendered.

3. Environment: How has the regulatory and competitive environment changed over the years?

4. Agency resources: What financial and staff resources are available? What are the past, present, and potential competencies of the agency staff?

Once the mission statement is established, two more activities must be completed before moving on to the next step. First, recognizing that this statement provides the agency with a purpose, it must be communicated to all administrative and provider staff. This, then, provides the staff with a sense of unity and allows them to perform their jobs within the appropriate parameters. Second, goals, which will give direction to the agency, can now be established and should be focused in three general areas: financial, growth through retention of current clients and addition of new ones, and diversification.

Step II: The Analysis

The Kotler definition indicates that in order to retain and attract clients, an agency must sense, serve, and satisfy needs. Likewise, to remain viable in today's health care environment, an agency must be aware of its strengths and weaknesses, as well as the opportunities and threats it faces. This awareness and the identification of consumer needs begins with a detailed analysis both inside and outside the agency.

Assessing your own agency provides top management with an opportunity for some organizational introspection. It is time to ask such questions as:

1. What is the historical background of the agency and how has the agency grown over the years? These questions were addressed during the development of the mission statement and can be referred to later on when the marketing plan is developed.

2. What is the detailed financial history of the agency? What percent of the service is reimbursed by third parties, by private pay? Is there an endowment? What is the ratio of reimbursed care versus nonreimbursed care? Are there any problems with the accounts receivable?

3. What are the visit trends? If they are decreasing, has it been due to underutilization of services or greater competition?

4. Who are your current referral sources and how have they changed over the years? Has the advent of hospital-based programs had an impact on referrals? Are patients aware of home health care and the fact that they may still have a choice of agencies for their home care?

5. What is the skill level and attitude of the staff (providers as well as administrators?) Is management attuned to the fine balance between business acumen and the provision of a quality service? Is the provider keeping up with the technologically acute needs of a sicker patient as well as the more routine home care services? Is the administrative staff prepared to deal with computerization and more efficient time management?

6. What is the image of your agency in the community at large? Is the community aware of your existence of the scope of your services? Or are you perceived as an agency for the "poor"?

7. What is the attitude of your past and present patient population toward your agency? Can they differentiate between your agency and your competitor?

Once you have completed the detailed analysis of your agency, there are six areas to be considered in the macroenvironment.

1. Population demographics: Consideration should be given to such factors as age, sex, birth and death rate, income, education, place of residence, and population shifts. Much of this information can be obtained from your state's Office of Planning.

2. Economic situation: Currently much of health care is paid for by third-party reimbursement ranging from private insurance to capitation. In the future, health care costs may be paid for on a private basis. Therefore, an agency must monitor the rate of inflation and keep their prices competitive. What is happening to individual income, and what are the spending and saving patterns of your target population?

3. Technology: Over the last 20 years, health care technology has changed tremendously. These changes are now also affecting the way a home health care agency does business. One can anticipate that this trend will continue, and it therefore becomes imperative that a member of the agency act as a liaison with the medical community to remain current with these advances so that the agency can be prepared to meet the patient's potential needs at discharge.

4. Political: As an agency administrator, you will want to be aware of state and federal regulatory issues which will impact on your ability to do business. These may be related to certificate of need, licensure laws, and changes in government regulation. The state and national associations for home care should serve as a resource for this information.

5. Cultural: Where possible, try to identify the value system of the members of the population you hope to serve. What is their lifestyle? What is the role of the extended family? What are their religious values? What is their attitude toward health care?

6. Competition: It is important to know who is competing with you for the patients and what kinds of services they provide. What are your competitors' strengths, weaknesses, capabilities, and future goals? Who are the members of their staff and what is the skill level of the staff?

This analysis may be completed by an individual member of your staff, through staff brainstorming sessions, by an outside marketing firm, or by a college student as a requirement for a business course. If you choose to perform this assessment by your own staff, the information obtained may be more subjective than objective; consequently, further marketing plans may be biased and ultimately not appropriate. It may also be more difficult to obtain accurate information about your competitors. An assessment by an outside marketing firm may provide you with the best information upon which to build your plan. Depending upon your community, the cost for such a service may be more than $6,000. By tapping into the educational system, the benefits to your agency would be twofold: input from an enthusiastic student who has access to the skills and knowledge of a faculty member.

Having completed the detailed analysis of your agency and the environment in which it functions and having appropriately identified consumer needs, the process continues with the development of a market plan which will meet these needs.

Step III: The Marketing Plan

The marketing plan consists of three phases: a matching phase, an implementation phase, and an evaluation phase. Although separate and distinct steps, they are closely linked, and the following concepts have implications for all three phases.

1. Service: This is your agency's programs which will meet the previously identified market needs and is the core element in the marketing mix. The home health care agency has the unique characteristic of having to please two markets simultaneously: the patient, who may not be fully informed about home health care; and the referral source, who is most likely very aware of the home health industry. For instance, although the concept of "one-stop shopping" is important, it may be more important to the busy referral source than to the patient. This must be kept in mind as the agency modifies existing programs, develops new programs, or becomes specialized. It is equally important that these programs be identified appropriately so it is clear to the consumer exactly what they are purchasing.

2. Price: Price may be governed by third-party reimbursement. With the advent of HMOs, PPOs, and prospective payments, as well as an increased focus on self-pay, pricing must be creative and competitive. To achieve creative pricing, the agency administrator should work with the agency's financial officer to consider such options as discounting, credit programs, prepayment strategies, skim pricing, market-share pricing, etc.

3. Distribution: This essentially applies to where and when the services will be provided. Besides the home, rehabilitation services may be provided at long-term care facilities, whereas health assessments and wellness programs may be provided in industrial settings. Besides service provision during normal work time, it may be essential to offer selected services on holidays, weekends, evenings, and nights.

4. Promotion: This is how you promote your agency to the community at large and specifically to your target markets, but it has often been construed as marketing per se. As members of society, each day we are bombarded with examples of promotion, and it is now time to make them work for your agency. Within promotion, there are certain communication tools; which ones you use may depend on your target market, as well as the purpose of your communication. What are the target market's media habits? What magazines or newspapers do they read? What is their education level? Do you as an agency want to create an awareness or assure referrals? There are four communication tools which are used within promotion. They are:

   - Advertisement: This is use of the spoken or written word through a specific medium (radio, TV, newspaper, brochure) and is basically used to create an awareness about your agency and its services.

   - Publicity: Again, this is the use of media to inform the public about your agency or a new program. The focus may be a human interest story which is less likely to have a negative impact on the audience. Publicity is also used to create awareness. Neither advertisement or publicity allows for clarification to the target market, and consequently, may not be the most efficient way to generate referrals.

- Promotional Activities: Many activities and tangible items are included in promotional activities. Gimmicks, such as personalized agency pens, mugs, etc., and participation in community programs, such as health fairs, are included in this category. Quite often these activities include some dialogue between potential consumers and agency staff, thus creating a greater understanding of your agency and its services, as well as the industry.

- Personal Selling: This is the best but perhaps a more costly way to assure referrals. It encourages direct dialogue between your agency and the target market. It also affords an opportunity to listen to complaints and recommendations, to answer questions immediately, to identify problems, and to assure solutions. Never negate the power of personal contacts and professional friendships.

When developing the market plan, consideration should also be given to the life cycle of the service as it impacts on the previously mentioned concepts and promotional activities. The aspects of a service life cycle are:

- Introductory stage: This is the first time the service is offered and, indeed, may be offered only to a small test market in a specific geographic area. During this stage, a high level of promotional activity as well as a higher price for the service can be anticipated.

- Growth stage: Service utilization begins to increase substantially and your competition may increase. The level of promotional activities should remain the same since services will be expanded to other areas. Price likewise may remain the same or decline slightly since volume is increasing. You will want to continue to pursue the market aggressively.

- Maturity Stage: Utilization of the service may plateau or even slow down. This is perhaps the longest stage of the life cycle. When reached, it is time to take a serious look at your service or the market for evaluation and modification. The decision may be to lower the price or alter your communication with the public or target market.

- Decline Stage: Again the service that is declining must be evaluated as to why—is it the economy, the quality of the service, industry trends, or technological changes? Is it time for management to evaluate the service to see if it is worth saving, to continue it as is, to concentrate on a revitalization of the service, or to phase it out?

The matching phase of the marketing plan should be completed by representatives of the governing body and the agency's top management staff utilizing the data obtained during the analysis process. If marketing specialists were used to perform the analysis, your agency may continue to utilize their expertise throughout the remainder of the marketing plan. Should an agency choose to do so, the additional cost may be more than $5,000.

The implementation phase should be coordinated by one staff member, preferably someone with a marketing background, but is the responsibility of all persons affiliated with your agency. The final market plan should be communicated to the staff since they all play a role in attracting or retaining clients.

The personnel department needs to be aware of the new market plan in order to recruit staff that can provide services in the new market arena.

The provider staff needs to be highly skilled and able to provide a quality service which satisfies the consumer need. They may, indeed, be your agency's sales force either directly or indirectly.

Because new programs or the expansion of existing programs always present a degree of financial risk, the marketing plan should be reviewed thoroughly with the finance department. A member of this department should be responsible for a projected revenue and expense statement, concurrent financial data, and cash flow management.

The general administrative staff should also be aware of the agency's new focus on marketing and how it is applicable to their job. Does the switchboard operator know how to handle inquiries? Are efficient billing and collection systems in place? One frustrating experience by the consumer may send him to another agency for his care.

The final phase of the market plan is the evaluation phase. It is during this stage that the agency will learn if the matching and implementation phases have indeed met the needs of the target market as well as the goals of the agency. The staff member, who coordinated the implementation phase, shall also have the responsibility for coordinating the evaluations. At periodic intervals, the plan should be evaluated for:

- comparison of projected versus real revenues and expenses

- customer satisfaction

- new competition and

- effectiveness of communication tools.

The data received from these periodic evaluations should be reviewed annually and used when planning for the following year.

Summary

The agency which is able to sense, serve, and satisfy the consumer's needs will occupy a strong position in today's competitive home health care environment. The goal of this chapter has been to acquaint the service-oriented administrator with some broad marketing concepts which would be applicable to their agency. There are many details of the marketing process which could not be condensed into this chapter. Although there are relatively few texts on marketing currently available for home health care, a general textbook on marketing in business should be added to every home health care administrator's library.

Marketing: A Case Illustration

Rebecca A. Walker

Introduction

Broadly viewed, marketing tools have been identified by Kotler as price, planning, place, and promotion (Kotler and Cox 1980). They have further identified marketing communicational tools as advertising, sales promotion, publicity, and personal selling. This marketing mix was described earlier in the chapter. This section will describe a program which capitalized on the foregoing marketing theory: the Liaison Nurse Program at The Visiting Nurse Association (VNA) of Baltimore.

The VNA of Baltimore has stated its mission as follows:

> "Health Care is a right, not a privilege, for all members of a community. A Home Care Agency, therefore, is a basic health resource which should be available to all citizens regardless of the ability to pay. Home care is an essential link in the chain of health care services needed by a community to provide the full range of services that constitute a quality health care system. All activities of the Agency are directed toward meeting the health needs of patients and their families at home. Participation in community planning activities for the purpose of extending and coordinating health resources to improve the total health system is, therefore, an important responsibility of professional staff."

Driven by this mission statement and an analysis of the markeplace that demonstrated a lack of information about and consequent underutilization of home health service, the VNA of Baltimore developed a Liaison Nurse Program in concert with Medicare regulations governing "Home Health Coordination (or Home Care Intake Coordination) Costs—General." Part of the planning for this program considered the marketing mix of service and product, price, distribution, promotion, and personal selling. Planning decisions were heavily influenced by marketing communications theory.

Description Of The Program

Over the years (1970-1980), the VNA of Baltimore had tried a variety of approaches to improve relations with hospitals, to enhance coordination and communication around referrals, to improve feedback to referring sources, and to effect joint management of patient care. The assistant director visited area hospitals and met with key members of the discharge planning team; nurses stopped by selected hospitals in their districts for a half-day per week to meet with discharge planners; one nurse was hired, called a "liaison nurse" and assigned to seven area hospitals to carry out this coordination function. None of these efforts had any significant impact on enhanced coordination or improved hospital relations.

In 1980, the agency committed to an expansion of previous efforts that translated into one liaison nurse, in just one or no more than two hospitals, depending on bed size, and placed on-site in the hospitals full- or half-time. A job description was developed that closely followed permissible activities as spelled out in the "Home Health Coordination Costs—General" Section 2113 of the Medicare Provider Reimbursement Manual. (See Appendix A.) The description charged the liaison nurse to coordinate and participate in physician referrals for home health care, and to assist with the development of care plans and identification of services required to achieve optimal effectiveness in the transfer of patients to home health care settings. Cooperative agreements were negotiated with eight area hospitals initiating contact with Departments of Nursing, then continuing discussions with hospital directors, administrators, and Departments of Social Work. (See Appendix B.) Four liaison nurses were placed into these eight hospitals. This effort experienced the success that the three previous attempts had not, and that success was based largely on decisions that were made about our marketing communications mix.

Use Of Marketing Communications In The Program

Decisions about marketing communications were tied into our goals—improved hospital relations through enhanced coordination and communication around referrals, improved feedback to referring sources, and joint management of patient care. Communication was obviously key, both in our task environment (hospitals) and our home environment (agency). Decisions about marketing tools were also tied into these goals. The decision concerning price was to continue to maintain one of the lowest charges in town. Planning took place with and through hospital administrators and Departments of Nursing and Social Work, resulting in important alliances within the hospitals at the outset. Decisions, referring to place, assigned the liaison nurses to work in the hospitals full- or half-time, and these decisions were seen in retrospect as critical to the success of this fourth attempt. With respect to promotion, the decision was to concentrate strictly on service with no gimmicks.

Decisions concerning communicational tools were tied into the stated goals. Kotler has described these as advertising, personal selling, sales promotion, and publicity. Personal selling had the end result of the liaison nurse doing the job, as earlier described, extremely well. Personal selling's distinctive qualities of personal confrontation, cultivation, and response are implicit in the job responsibilities. The liaison nurse works frequently in a one-to-one situation, providing helpful responses immediately, and over time is earning a reputation for competence and trustworthiness, as well as the respect and confidence of the hospital's professional staff. Effective response finally becomes almost automatic.

Factors Influencing Decisions Regarding Communication Process

Decisions regarding use of the communication process were based on the following factors. There was a concern for our target-audiences' perception of our agency's performance both in the past and on an ongoing basis. We assessed the current image of the agency and its service delivery. We listened to complaints regarding deficient areas of performance and did what was necessary to correct these deficiencies as quickly as possible. Desired target response was identified as improved hospital relations through effective communication and coordination. Appropriate message content would hopefully be that good deeds followed our good words. The message was a factual stating of what we could and would do by way of service delivery, and then following through on every promise. In considering efficient media, the liaison nurse was recognized as the media, the channel of communications. A working definition of liaison is "...a person who interpersonally connects two or more groups." Attributes of the message and the messenger were that both had to be highly credible. The liaison nurse had to be seen as the expert, trustworthy and with the necessary authority to accomplish what was planned. Finally, feedback, what would we learn about the success or failure of our liaison nurse efforts; how would we monitor this; how would we assess whether or not agency relations with hospitals had improved; whether coordination and communication around referrals had been enhanced; and whether feedback and joint management of patient care had had a positive impact?

Planning Process

The foregoing decisions led to the following planning process. Our communications objective was "to improve hospital relations through efficient, effective coordination of referrals, timely and effective service delivery, and prompt feedback." Liaison nurses needed to have a thorough understanding of the business, the agency's strengths and weaknesses, and the perception of the agency held by the institutions to which they were assigned. The liaison nurses dealt with a marketing mix of product and personal selling. The product was service to people. The end result of doing their jobs extremely well was a kind of personal selling.

The program has experienced a life cycle that included an introductory phase, a growth phase, a stage of maturity, and presently, at least in relation to hospital sites, a decline. Due to the presence of 12 hospital-based home care programs in the city of Baltimore, there are now three liaison nurses in five hospitals. The order of the day clearly is to look to a revised mix of sites according to shifts in the marketplace.

Outcomes

Improved quality and coordination of referrals and communications between institution and agency resulted in an increase in quality of patient care, as measured by (1) the date of the first nursing visit compared with the date of hospital discharge; (2) the dates on which other services were in place; (3) the dates on which patient goals were met (e.g., discharged to self or caregiver care); and (4) decreased frequency of hospital readmissions. There was an increase in total numbers of referrals received from all hospitals served. (See Appendices C and D.) A significant decrease in monies not billed, due to unsigned physician orders, was realized. There were almost no unsigned orders originating from the institutions served. Finally, new linkages for the VNA based on the performance of the liaison nurses were effected. These linkages were with a community hospital, an institute for handicapped children, and a hospital-based home care program.

Summary

More than ever home health agencies need to recognize the importance of including a major marketing effort in overall operational planning. Our work environment has become fiercely competitive. Agencies have proliferated and patients are moving through inpatient settings so rapidly that discharge-planning efforts, which might have included a referral to a home health care agency, are often not implemented. This chapter has offered a theoretical overview of the essence of marketing, its application to the home health field, and a practical illustration of the way in which one agency put the theory into practice.

Why Market?[*]

Nancy L. Rhodes

Why market? "We've never done that; referral sources know who we are and what we have to offer; it costs a lot of money." These statements had become familiar discussion topics among longstanding home health agencies.

The Visiting Nurse Association of Milwaukee faced competition from 45 other home care agencies. Visiting nurse was becoming a generic term. It referred to *any* nurse who came to the home to provide care, *not* the visiting nurse from the VNA of Milwaukee.

The Visiting Nurse Association of Milwaukee has been a home health care leader since 1906 and has responded to the multiple changes and challenges in home health care. The acceleration occurring in the health care delivery system applies not only to time spent in each link of the system, but also to the complexity of care each link now provides. Rapid growth, multiple agencies, and earlier discharges leave the health care consumer faced with difficult and confusing choices about home health care.

The Visiting Nurse Association's mission is to continue to have a concern and be a voice for those underserved by the health care system; to grow through careful planning in response to identified community needs for home health care and related services; and to develop related services and markets in response to changing community needs. The VNA of Milwaukee welcomed the opportunity to educate the community about home health care and assist consumers in making informed and knowledgeable decisions about their health care. The time had come for the VNA to make its many services known to the public.

Planning Process

What is the best starting point for planning a marketing strategy? How should we begin? A benchmark research study was the answer to our questions. We needed to measure awareness, attitude, and opinion about home health care and the Visiting Nurse Association of Milwaukee. The first challenge was to interview and hire a

* A special thanks to Mary Jane Mayer, President of the Visiting Nurse Corporation-Milwaukee and all my colleagues who lent their support and assistance.

market research firm since we did not have the expertise in-house. Proposals were solicited from four area firms. Bisbing Business Research was selected. The study began in April 1985, and was completed with results and recommendations by mid-May 1985. The study consisted of two sample bases — consumers (the general public) and professionals (physicians, hospitals, HMOs, and insurance companies.) The consumer sample size was 500, with all respondents 40 years of age or older, and the male or female head of household. The sample was drawn from the Milwaukee telephone directory on a systematically random basis to be representative of the total Milwaukee area. The professional sample size was 44 and drawn from the Milwaukee Yellow Pages. The cross-tabulations for consumers were done by age, education, income, sex, and whether anyone in the household ever used the VNA. The results of the study were as follows:

- The VNA has the greatest awareness among home health service agencies.

- The VNA is selected most often as the agency which would be used if the respondent or a family member were in need of the services provided by a home health agency.

- Respondents not selecting the VNA do so because they are not familiar with what the VNA is or what services it provides.

- In some cases respondents are not aware to whom the VNA provides their services. There is some confusion as to whether VNA services are provided free or if there is a charge.

- When choosing a home health agency, people want an agency which provides quality care and is caring and concerned.

In summarizing the professional section of the study, the results were:

- The VNA has the greatest awareness among home health services agencies.

- The VNA is referred to most often.

- The VNA would be recommended most often.

- VNA does a good job keeping in contact with physicians about patients' care.

- VNA staff do an excellent job.

- Some hospitals think VNA has difficulty in providing service promptly.

Competitive analysis was done internally to review the number of agencies, the services they provide, and the area they serve. Although the research results were positive toward the VNA of Milwaukee, the need to maintain and protect current market share and garner new target markets would not allow us to rest on past laurels. Our strong reputation and tradition of quality service were precious assets to protect. The next step in lifting the bushel basket was to retain an advertising and communications firm to help plan an effective promotion program as part of our marketing plan. One idea was to utilize a successful marketing vehicle which a colleague, Rich Roberson, Executive Director of the Kansas City VNA, had shared with us, a Preferred Patient

Card. The card allows past and present VNA patients, and those people who may need home health care in the future, to be preenrolled for VNA home health care when it is needed.

Selecting an agency was a critical factor to ensure a successful campaign. A VNA board member and Dr. Phillip Kotler, Professor of Marketing at the J.K. Kellogg Graduate School of Management, recommended a number of agencies. We gave each agency a hypothetical situation and requested they prepare a short presentation of a marketing plan. Along with that presentation, client references and chemistry in working with that individual closely for an extended time frame were key factors in making our decision. McGlinchey and Associates was chosen. The decision works as effectively one year later as it did at the onset. After a thorough orientation about the VNA of Milwaukee to John Dunn, a principal of the agency, we rolled up our sleeves, sharpened our pencils, and got down to the hard task of creatively designing a communication program to create and maintain marketwide awareness of the VNA and at the same time, use the Preferred Patient Care concept as the communication vehicle.

Objectives and Strategy

What objectives would best build the framework to create and maintain marketwide awareness of the VNA? After much discussion, the following three objectives emerged as the guides in designing an effective marketing plan:

1. To promote and increase public awareness and knowledge of home health care, and to assist consumers in making informed and knowledgeable decisions.

2. To keep the VNA "top of mind" among the centers of referral and continue reinforcement of VNA's image as a leader.

3. To retain VNA's share of the market.

The strategy to meet these objectives was to develop a long-term marketing campaign and use a rifle versus a shotgun communications approach to retain our current patient base. In addition, it was felt that these objectives could best be accomplished through mass media advertising. A series of brochures, direct mail pieces, and public relations supported and supplemented the advertising efforts. Strategies included developing special communications channels to directly reach and influence target audiences; implementing an editorial program utilizing an informational kit and feature stories; pursuing opportunities for presentations or speaking engagements before local community groups, media talk shows, etc., and developing public service announcements for selected radio stations in the four-county area.

Budgetary constraints were in place from the beginning of the plan. A budget of $30,000 was available for 1985 with limited discretionary funds. Once objectives were defined and the budget was delineated, it was time for creativity to emerge in the design, content, production, and implementation of all the components. The Preferred Patient Card and the slogan "Don't Stay Home Without It" became the umbrella theme for all advertising and collateral material.

Creativity and careful planning cannot be hurried. Impatience to see results was the major hurdle to overcome during the development process. Regular progress reports at management and board meetings lessened the impatience of seeing the finished products.

Execution and Evaluation

The Preferred Patient Program began in July 1985, to assist in retaining the current patient base. Each current patient and all new patients received a laminated card (see below) with their name and record number, along with a letter welcoming them as a member of the VNA Preferred Patient Program. Educational and informative materials about health care, changes in the health care system (Medicare, Medicaid, HMOs, etc.), and the VNA newsletter *"The Visitor"* continue to be developed for mailing to preferred patients. (For letter, see Exhibit 28-1.)

Board members wanted cards for identification also, but did not wish to be called preferred patients since they were not ill. As a result, we developed a "Preferred Member Card" for the board and top management. See Exhibit 28-2.

The other components of the program, which is copyrighted, include billboards rotated to new sites every two months, 50 king-sized transit posters on the sides of buses, and newspaper advertising. The newspaper advertising was scheduled for the metro dailies, select suburban weeklies, and the *"Business Journal."* Additional advertising was scheduled for the quarterly editions of the Wisconsin Senior Citizen and special health issues of the *"Catholic Herald"* and the *"Jewish Chronicle."*

Advertising to the target market, initially the general public, began with goals to increase and promote awareness. Primary and secondary target markets were then defined and reached by using the Visiting Nurse Association's Long-Term Care Program as the advertising vehicle. Primary audiences included physicians, discharge planners, and senior groups. Secondary audiences were health care providers such as HMOs, medical clinics, etc., selected clergy members, and major corporate human resource departments.

The official date for advertising began on September 23, 1985, with newspaper ads followed one week later by transit posters and billboards. Collateral materials, a brochure, and an application for the Preferred Patient Card, became available by the end of October. Then came a critical question. How could we evaluate the effectiveness of our marketing efforts? Within two weeks of mailing the Preferred Patient Card, several patients had presented them in hospitals and insisted on returning to the VNA. Field staff reported patients' positive feelings about having the card, and how it assisted them in retaining the same agency. Approximately 15 VNAs throughout the country inquired about the program and intend to utilize it for their patients. The opportunity for other VNAs to benefit is exciting and gratifying.

The initial mailing of cards totaled 2,500. Through May 14, 1986, another 3,214 cards have been sent out, for a total of 5,714. One week after implementation, informational calls increased by 10 per day. Members of the staff, management, and the board were enthusiastic and reported where they had seen the advertising. Community agencies with whom we network and coordinate (including one accounting firm) called to express their enthusiasm and support for the VNA.

Exhibit 28-1.

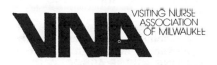

VISITING NURSE
ASSOCIATION
OF MILWAUKEE

VNA-MILWAUKEE'S MOBILE MEALS INTRODUCES "PREFERRED CUSTOMER PROGRAM"

CONGRATULATIONS! YOU ARE NOW A MEMBER OF THE VNA MOBILE MEALS PREFERRED CUSTOMER PROGRAM.

The Visiting Nurse Association of Milwaukee is starting a Mobile Meals "Preferred Customer Program" to ensure that area residents receive the best in home delivered meals. This program will allow past, present, and future VNA Mobile Meals customers to be pre-enrolled for VNA Mobile Meals options when they are needed. There are no enrollment or membership fees for VNA Mobile Meals Preferred Customer Program members.

The Visiting Nurse Association has been a leader in home delivered meal programs for such a long time that Mobile Meals has become almost a generic term for home delivered meals. To receive meals from the Visiting Nurse Association, you must ask for the Visiting Nurse Association of Milwaukee's Mobile Meals Program. The new Mobile Meals Preferred Customer Program will help area residents get the real thing!

HOW THE PROGRAM WORKS

As a Mobile Meals Preferred Customer, <u>anytime</u> you feel you can benefit from VNA Mobile Meals, you can call us to start meal services. We will check with your physician for your current diet order. If you are hospitalized and your physician recommends that you purchase home delivered meals, you can receive VNA Mobile Meals by presenting the membership card and specifically requesting VNA Mobile Meals. A discharge planner, usually a registered nurse or a hospital social worker, will visit with you prior to discharge from the hospital. Together, you both can determine which of the Mobile Meals program options you will need when you return home. The membership card will help make the discharge process easier for you and ensure that you receive the Mobile Meals option best suited for you.

ADDED PROGRAM BENEFITS

Preferred Customer Program members will also realize other important benefits. Your card lists a phone number which is answered 24 hours a day, seven days a week. This number may be used by you to receive answers to any home health care question that you may have. Program members will also receive updated information about the rapid changes in home health care of local, statewide and national interest. Other information may also be sent to you including home health education materials. Along with your Preferred Customer Card is a program identification card with our phone number. We suggest that you keep this card in a prominent place.

KEEP YOUR CARD WITH OTHER IMPORTANT MEDICAL INFORMATION

You will want to keep your card in your wallet or purse, along with your other important health insurance information so it is available at all times. Remember, don't stay home without it.

Exhibit 28-2.

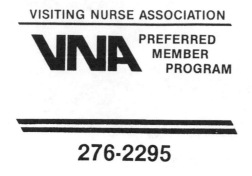

VISITING NURSE ASSOCIATION

**PREFERRED
MEMBER
PROGRAM**

276-2295

VNA PREFERRED MEMBER CARD:

1. **Present this card to your physician or hospital discharge planner and specify that you want home health care from the VISITING NURSE ASSOCIATION.**
2. **One call to the VNA at 276-2295 will ensure you receive the best possible home health care.**

**VISITING NURSE ASSOCIATION
OF MILWAUKEE**

Requests from the community to become preferred patients had not been anticipated, but we were quickly able to establish a mechanism for handling these requests. We now utilize opportunities such as heath fairs and speaking engagements at senior and community groups to promote enrollment in the Preferred Patient Program. All of our board members and staff have been included in the program as preferred members.

Additional opportunities for new referral sources have arisen through increased awareness of the VNA. Another opportunity is the growing awareness of utilizing the VNA as a resource and informational center. This has potential for developing a specific program targeted at assisting the consumer with questions and information.

The mechanisms for evaluating the impact of the awareness program will be long-range. Follow-up research will be done in the future to measure the public's awareness, attitude, and opinion of the Visiting Nurse Association. All informational and referral calls from the patients, their families, and community agencies are being screened to determine how they learned of the VNA. A service representative tativetativetativetativewhose responsibility is to identify service needs and educate referral sources, visits HMOs, physicians' offices, and other referral sources on a regular basis, so feedback can be solicited. Referral data are analyzed monthly as to volume and source. A quarterly report is prepared for the board and regular updates in the employee newsletter serve as ongoing communication.

In April, we received notification of a national recognition for part of our campaign. *Healthcare Marketing Report* chose our outdoor and transit advertising for the gold medal award in that category. Our Preferred Patient concept was really launched!

This is only the beginning of marketing the VNA of Milwaukee. We are truly in exciting times in health care with many challenges and opportunities ahead.

Reference

Kotler, P., and K. Cox, ed. 1980. *Marketing management and strategy: A reader.* Englewood Cliffs, N.J. Prentice-Hall, Inc.

Appendix A

The Visiting Nurse Association
Of Baltimore
Position Description

TITLE: Home Care Liaison Nurse

REPORTS TO: Director of Clinical Development

PRIMARY FUNCTION:

Coordinate and participate in physician referrals for home health care; assist with the development of care plans and identification of services required to achieve optimal effectiveness in the transfer of patients to home health care settings.

RESPONSIBILITIES:

1. Coordinate physician referrals in order to facilitate the transfer of patients from health care facilities to home care environments.
2. Determine the need and arrange for predischarge visits by community health nurses when unfamiliar or non-routine procedures are involved or when special problems related to home care are involved.
3. Participate and assist in the development of appropriate home health care plans. Includes making assessments of the appropriateness of requested services, supplies and equipment.
4. Ascertain that referrals are complete, providing all required medical, nursing and psychosocial data, and that all services required are prepared to respond in a timely and coordinated manner.
5. Assist in and facilitate communication between physicians and home health agency staff to assure uninterrupted and continuing medical care for patients.
6. Assure that physician and other professional staff receive prompt and accurate feedback regarding patients referred.
7. Interpret and communicate agency policies, procedures, and practices to patients and caregivers following referral, and to professional staff.
8. Serve as educational and information resource and consultant to professional staff in matters involving home health services, policies, and practices.
9. Assist the agency in its service delivery evaluations. Maintain qualitative and quantitative records of liaison activities.

QUALIFICATIONS/REQUIREMENTS:

1. BSN and a minimum of two years experience in community health nursing.
2. Licensed as a Registered Nurse in the State of Maryland.

Reprinted by permission of the Visiting Nurse Association of Baltimore, MD.

Appendix B

Cooperative Agreement
Between
The Visiting Nurse Association Of Baltimore
And

_____
(Facility)

THIS AGREEMENT is entered into this _____ day of _____, by and between the Visiting Nurse Association of Baltimore (hereinafter called "the agency") and _____ (hereinafter called "the facility");

WHEREAS, a collaborative relationship between an acute care facility and a community-based home health agency will facilitate a more systematic, comprehensive and consistent approach to provision of home health care services to facility's patients, and,

WHEREAS, both facility and agency desire, by means of this agreement, to insure continuity of care and treatment appropriate to the needs of facility's patients by establishing a coordinated system for home care services,

NOW THEREFORE, in consideration of the mutual agreements and covenants herein set forth, the agency and the facility mutually agree as follows:

ARTICLE I - AGENCY RESPONSIBILITIES

1. The agency shall provide one liaison nurse who will be present in the facility _____(hrs. per wk.) to assist with the development and coordination of care plans and identification of services required to achieve optimal effectiveness in the transfer of patients to home health care settings after the patient has been referred to the agency. The liaison nurse will not perform or replace any of the discharge planning responsibilities of the facility.

2. The agency's liaison nurse shall interpret and communicate agency policies, procedures, and practices to patients and caregivers following referral, and to professional staff of the facility; and shall serve as an educational and information resource and consultant to professional staff of the facility in matters involving home health services, policies and practices.

ARTICLE II - FACILITY RESPONSIBILITIES

1. The facility shall assist with the coordination process by assisting the liaison nurse to become familiar with the facility and to develop relationships with members of the health care team.

2. The facility shall provide opportunities for the liaison nurse to participate in orientation of new staff and in service education programs as they relate to home health issues.

3. The facility shall provide the liaison nurse with a desk and chair, and access to a telephone.

ARTICLE III - TERM AND TERMINATION

1. This agreement shall be in force and effect from _____ through _____.

2. This agreement may be terminated by either party upon giving written notice of such intent to the other party by registered mail at least thirty (30) days prior to such termination.

IN WITNESS WHEREOF, the parties have executed this agreement.

THE VISITING NURSE ASSOCIATION OF BALTIMORE

_____   _____

PRESIDENT   DATE

FACILITY

_____   _____

AUTHORIZED SIGNATURE   DATE

_____

VNA 11/85

Appendix C

THE VISITING NURSE ASSOCIATION
OF BALTIMORE

STATISTICAL SUMMARY OF LIAISON NURSE PROGRAM

Comparison of Admissions for Fiscal Years
1980 through 1985

HOSPITAL A

67% increase FY'81 over FY'80
58% increase FY'82 over FY'80
105% increase FY'83 over FY'80
119% increase FY'84 over FY'80
175% increase FY'85 over FY'80

HOSPITAL B

62% increase FY'81 over FY'80
63% increase FY'82 over FY'80
132% increase FY'83 over FY'80
230% increase FY'84 over FY'80
315% increase FY'85 over FY'80

HOSPITAL C

210% increase FY'83 over FY'82
477% increase FY'84 over FY'82
480% increase FY'85 over FY'82

Abbreviated Version of
Complete Report

Appendix D

THE VISITING NURSE ASSOCIATION
OF BALTIMORE

LIAISON NURSE PROGRAM

COMPARISON OF TOTAL HOSPITAL A, B & C DISCHARGES
WITH TOTAL REFERRALS TO VNA FOR FYs 1984 and 1985

HOSPITAL A

FY'84 Discharges - 11,782 Referrals - 606 5.2% *of Discharges*
FY'85 Discharges - 11,783 Referrals - 763 6.4% *of Discharges*

HOSPITAL B

FY'84 Discharges - 16,058 Referrals-1,136 7.1% *of Discharges*
FY'85 Discharges - 15,994 Referrals-1,428 8.9% *of Discharges*

HOSPITAL C

FY'84 Discharges - 8,646 Referrals - 444 5.1% *of Discharges*
FY'85 Discharges - 5,708 Referrals - 447 7.8% *of Discharges*

Chapter Twenty-Nine

Diversification Issues

Corporate Reorganization
Bernard R. Lorenz

Corporate reorganization is becoming increasingly more attractive to many home health agencies as they strive to expand services, meet new competition, and operate more efficiently. In many instances, Medicare cost reimbursement can be made more accurate and supportable, to the advantage of the agency.

Reorganization also offers the potential to provide a number of in-home services that are not reimbursed by Medicare, but for which there appears to be an increasing need. These include, but are not necessarily limited to:

1. Private duty nursing.

2. Homemakers.

3. Personal care.

4. Home management.

5. Companion services.

6. Chore services.

7. Medical day care.

8. Child care.

9. Hospice and related services.

10. Durable medical equipment.

The decision to reorganize must be based on careful study which includes an analysis of community demographics, the agency's competition, as well as its goals and objectives, the latter of which should be projected for at least five years. The agency's analysis must consist of projections for every service the market will support, anticipated levels of changes, and expected costs. An operating budget must then be prepared to determine the potential profitability of each service and the cash flow that can be realized from it. Projections must be constructed for different volumes of services and changes in costs and charges to determine what effect they will have on profitability.

An ideal organization would meet the needs of long-range goals while providing sufficient flexibility to respond to new opportunities and to meet the competition as it arises. The variety of corporate structures available to approach the ideal is almost unlimited. However, most fall into two general categories: the single corporate entity and the multicorporate entity.

Single Corporate Organizations

Single corporate entities, as their name implies, are the simplest type of organizational arrangement. They are a single legal entity, usually a corporation.

Single corporate entities have several advantages. They are the least expensive to establish, require only one corporation, one management group, and one accounting system, and lines of authority are clear. In addition, issues and problems relate to only one corporation, and additions and deletions of services can be made without creating too many problems.

There also are several disadvantages to single corporate organizations. Those which are Medicare-certified find that all of their operations are affected by governmental control through Medicare and Medicaid regulations. Hence, lines of business that are not covered by government programs cannot be separated from those that are. Consequently, allocations of costs, especially administrative and general costs, using federally prescribed methods, may be disadvantageous; and assignment of costs to various activities may not be as clear or defensible as they would be with a more definitive separation of programmatic entities. While it is true that Medicare does have some provisions for discrete cost finding, it is easier to justify the allocation of costs between different corporations than between different departments within one corporation.

Multicorporate Organizations

The most common and simplistic form of a multicorporate organization consists of a parent corporation with two or more subsidiaries (depending on the size and complexity of the agency). The parent company provides overall management and some centralized administrative services such as human resources, accounting, billing and collections, management information systems, etc. The subsidiary companies provide the different medical and other services. For example, one subsidiary could provide the traditional home health services for Medicare, Medicaid, private insurance, and self-payors, while another could provide services not covered by federal programs. These include private duty nursing, homemaker services, personal services, chore services, etc.

There are several advantages to the multicorporate organization. First, it provides greater flexibility in operations, as each corporation has its own separate legal entity, its own board of directors, its own accounting system, its own assets and liabilities, and its own financial statements.

As more services are provided by the group of entities, more corporations can be added without disturbing the others. Costs can be more accurately charged against the services for which they were incurred, and allocations can be better recognized and defended. Where services are provided by related organizations, charges can be assessed between or among them. Although Medicare will substitute costs for charges for reimbursement purposes, charges are still important. Further, the allocation of general and administrative costs will be clearer and more accurate since usually only the costs of the parent corporation need to be allocated. The administrative costs of each subsidiary remain within it. Finally, costs in the parent corporation that are directly allocated to the subsidiary are directly allocated prior to cost-finding.

Multicorporate organizations are not without their disadvantages. These begin with the costs of organizing the multiple corporations which are much greater since everything that must be done for one must be done for all of them. In relating to one another, the entities must always remember that they are separate as well as related, and accounting and information systems must adhere to that fact.

In the event a provider becomes a different legal entity in the reorganization, a change of ownership occurs. This requires that all things related to change of ownership be done. (This is not usually recommended.) Another problem is that staff, clients, and providers of service to the agency can become confused by the diversification. The accounting for transactions between corporations, for transfers of assets, and for the services provided can become complex and confusing. This can be reduced, however, by decentralizing management to the maximum feasible extent.

If any of the corporations are not-for-profit, great care must be taken to assure that there are no violations of the inurement of benefit requirements for maintaining that status, especially with grants and contracts. Violations could result in loss of the tax-exempt status. Care also must be taken to account for any unrelated business income earned by the tax-exempt organizations.

Conclusion

There is no easy answer for any organization concerning corporate diversification. It is important for the agency to research all the possibilities of corporate reorganization but *not* to copy the ideas of any other organization. The agency must start with their goals and objectives and the best way of achieving them. There are no easy answers and the agency should review this very carefully from a financial, as well as from many other viewpoints. The financial, management, and other benefits of diversification must be clearly seen before embarking on such a large project. Also, the projections generated in the decision process can be used as a management tool in monitoring the progress of the diversified entities.

Joint Ventures

Keith DeVantier

As the rules of health care change, hospitals are grappling with ways to trim institutional costs yet still provide dependable, quality care while positioning themselves before lucrative new markets. One of the most active areas of exploration is the formation of business arrangements between hospitals and medical equipment suppliers to service the growing home care market.

Such agreements can take many forms, including subcontracts, partnerships, or joint ventures. In any case, the primary goal of the hospital should be to increase and retain the number of clients served, for a longer period of time. In addition, hospitals should be concerned with providing a standard quality of patient care by providing services on discharge. They should want to enter this agreement to develop a competitive marketing edge as an attractive benefit to physicians and patients. Also, it is a way to earn additional revenue for the hospital.

An agreement with a medical equipment supplier like Foster Medical Corporation should complement and expand existing services by providing such services as durable medical equipment (DME), respiratory therapy equipment, oxygen, parenteral and enteral nutrition, intravenous drug therapy, apnea monitoring, home phototherapy, continuous passive motion, and the like.

One hospital—in this case, a hospital system—which contracted with Foster Medical is the Sisters of St. Mary Health Care System, based in St. Louis, Missouri. Under the agreement reached with Foster, the system formed a for-profit corporation (the SSM Home Care Corporation) to operate its DME component. The corporation is wholly owned and controlled by the Sisters of St. Mary, but subcontracts with Foster Medical. They chose Foster, according to the Health Care System's Interim President, Sr. Mary Jean Ryan SSM, because "the company is noted for reliable service, tight financial controls and a well-integrated, standardized distribution system throughout its branches. In addition, Foster Medical already ran DME operations in many SSM-served cities, and they guaranteed service provision in all areas requested by the sisters."

Under the arrangement, the Director of Home Care, appointed by the Sisters of St. Mary Health Care System, is responsible for the overall management, discharge planning coordination, equipment ordering, patient care protocols, marketing, and pricing. Foster Medical's responsibilities are equipment purchasing, warehousing and maintenance, delivery and set-up of equipment, patient instruction, and billing and collection.

About 3,700 patients in need of durable medical equipment are discharged annually from hospitals in the Sisters of St. Mary Health Care System.* The corporation competes with other DME companies in all locations, and is mandated to provide excellent equipment services to all patients. The presence of the Sisters of St. Mary Health Care System in the market ideally provides SSM Home Care Corporation with a strategic advantage over similar DME suppliers, but all clients discharged are given a choice of companies, if other options are available. Its market share eventually will have to be expanded outside of the system.

Another hospital with which Foster Medical contracts is Baylor Health Care System, Dallas, Texas. The contract with Baylor is unique in that the system had attempted to operate its own DME component, but in analysis, decided it would be more profitable if they would operate a joint venture with Foster Medical. The resultant company, Baylor/Foster Medical, was formed in June of 1986; Foster Medical purchased Baylor's DME assets and hired its employees to operate the new entity.

Each of these cases has unique aspects, and highlights some questions that every health care provider ponders when entering the DME market: Should we establish our own company? Should we hire a subcontractor? Should we enter into a joint venture?

**The Sisters of St. Mary have 15 hospitals. The 11 based in Missouri are Cardinal Glennon Children's Hospital and St. Mary's Health Center, St. Louis; St. Elizabeth's Hospital, Hannibal; St. Francis Hospital, Marceline; St. Joseph Health Center, St. Charles; St. Mary's Hospital, Kansas City; St. Mary's Hospital of Blue Springs; St. Mary's Health Center, Jefferson City; St. Mary on the Mount, St. Louis and St. Charles; and Arcadia Valley Hospital in Pilot Knob. Other facilities are St. Clare Hospital, Baraboo, Wisconsin; St. Mary's Hospital Medical Center in Madison, Wisconsin; St. Francis Hospital in Blue Island, Illinois; and St. Eugene Community Hospital in Dillon, South Carolina.

Each approach has its drawbacks. (Please refer to our chart, "The DME diversification decision: An evaluation tool," shown in Exhibit 29-1.) Can the hospital or its system generate enough home care patients to support a dealership and its requisite inventory? Do any hospital personnel have DME expertise? Can we afford the acquisition of equipment — and is it worth the gamble? To aid in the decision-making process, we have compiled some key questions which need satisfactory answers if DME diversification is to be successful.

1. *What are your partner's long-term plans?*
   Does your partner have a long-term commitment to the DME industry, or is the company merely putting the proposal together to secure referrals? If your partner is shortsighted and not totally committed, the venture will fail, usually within one to two years. Can the company grow and change as your needs do? Flexibility will be vital as you forge your partnership.

2. *What are your partner's motives in submitting a proposal?*
   It is important to know whether the DME industry is your partner's main business or a sideline, and whether the company only provides equipment to promote its main (and more profitable) supplies product. Is the proposal being submitted out of fear of losing your business? If so, the bid might be unrealistically low to try to wrap the contract this year. But what happens next year? The contract should not favor one party or the other; it must be a "win-win" arrangement or there will be *no* winners.

3. *Look at the partner's fiscal stability.*
   Look at the bottom line; if the company cannot make a profit for itself, how can it make a profit for the partnership?

4. *Evaluate the partner's services and products.*
   Check your partner's references and learn what is thought of your partner: Does the company have a reputation for providing quality products and services? Is it responsive, prompt, and efficient? A good provider will have an established quality assurance program, utilization review, and a clinical program with an adequate number of qualified clinicians. Further, the company should be willing to develop new programs to meet *your* needs.

5. *Is the partner aware of the ever changing regulations?*
   Rent and purchase regulations and oxygen guidelines drastically affected the DME industry in 1985, and industry leaders anticipate even tighter controls in the future. Does your partner know and understand these changes, and can the partner explain them to you? Realize that if federal cutbacks hurt your partner, they will hurt you, too.

6. *What type of sales support can the partner provide?*
   Your contracting partner should have a strong sales and sales support team — a team that is knowledgeable about what type of equipment and services are available in the home. They should be able to act as a resource to you and to explain this new service element to your staff and physicians.

Exhibit 29-1 The DME Diversification Decision: An Evaluation Tool

DECISION: Start your own company

PROS:

Control of the company

Control of quality of care

100% of all profits are yours

Easier access to patients and physicians allows for marketing

CONS:

High initial investment/continuing high capital expenditures

Difficult to show profit in first year

Lack of experience/industry knowledge slows the "learning curve"

Billing would be at the 50th percentile for Medicare patients

Difficult to implement

If done poorly, affects the entire institution's reputation

DECISION: Buy an existing company

PROS:

Buying experience in the business

Control of the company

Control of quality of care

100% of future profits

CONS:

High risk: the company you acquire may have hidden weaknesses

Expensive

Existing referral base will probably drop

Purchase may create personnel changes, unrest, and instability

DECISION: Contract for goods/services

(Set up a for-profit subsidiary and get it a provider number as a DME supplier. Contract for all needed services (i.e., equipment, billing, etc.))

PROS:

Control of the entity

Ability to negotiate spreads between costs and allowables

Relatively easy to implement

Some control over quality of care

Low investment

Good financial returns

CONS:

Billing *may* be at 50th percentile for Medicare patients

Reimbursement rules adversely affect entity like any other DME supplier

Need to overcome existing referral patterns/internal sensitivities

Risk of bad debts

If done poorly, reputation suffers

DECISION: Contract for a joint venture partnership

(Set up a for-profit subsidiary and enter into partnership contract with a DME supplier. Profits of the venture are split on a predetermined basis.)

Exhibit 29-1 continued.

PROS:	CONS:
Como control over quality of care	Shared control of entity/quality
No provider number problems	Not as easy to implement, especially with legal concerns
High financial returns	
Bad debts are shared	Small investment is required
Lower risk, financially and to reputation	Need to overcome existing referral patterns

Source: Foster Medical Corporation, 1986

7. *Involve your staff in the decision-making process.*
   Before deciding to enter the DME market, it would be helpful to know where your patients are going for equipment now, and who handles the arrangements and referrals. Be aware of your referral history and why it was shaped: Are there past relationships (such as a close, former employee moving on to another DME provider), sensitivities, perceptions which will have to be overcome? Without your staff's support, your venture will not succeed.

8. *Have realistic expectations and projections.*
   After you have quantified and qualified your needs, discuss them with your contracting partner to ensure that their proposal is on the right track. Ask for fiscal projections, and then do your own. Be realistic in your expectations.

   Determine what you can expect from your internal coordinator of the program, and provide clear direction. This person should develop, coordinate, and monitor the agreement and the discharge planning referral process. He or she should be able to analyze pricing structures and reimbursement patterns, as well as budget and set rates for the corporation.

9. *Study your contract for legalities.*
   Before you sign the contract, make sure that there is no fraud or abuse, kickbacks, or antitrust in your agreement. Check it out yourself, with your legal counsel.

10. *And finally, communicate.*
    Both you and your contracting partner should each assign one person who is responsible for the administration and the success of the contract. They should be in constant communication with one another, to discuss and resolve problems, services, and any other concerns. Even if the service area is wide, it should be treated as though it were a local company, with corporate caring and sensitivity. Learn to trust your partner, and grow with him to make the business the success you both want it to be.

An Experience in Diversification

Mary Ann Keirans

Interest in diversification has grown tremendously in the last few years. A review of the current literature about home care leads one to believe that diversification is the cure-all for the problems which plague the home health industry. Many agencies are considering diversification without really evaluating what they want to accomplish and studying the methods of fulfilling these goals without diversifying.

This chapter relates the experiences of a voluntary, nonprofit home health agency and its decision to diversify. A brief review of the agency's history is necessary in order to understand why the diversification route was chosen.

The Visiting Nurse Association/Home-Health Services (formerly known as Home-Health Services of Luzerne County) is located in the northeastern part of Pennsylvania. The agency was started in 1908 by a group of local citizens who were concerned about the health and sanitary conditions of the community, especially among the families who had immigrated to the Wyoming Valley area of Pennsylvania in order to work in the local coal mines. The Visiting Nurse Association developed a reputation for excellent services and quickly became a primary caregiver in the health and social services delivery system.

Over the decades, the agency changed in response to community needs. These changes were spontaneous in nature rather than planned occurrences. The Board of Directors was composed of numerous volunteers from the community who, according to ancient board minutes, had as their primary responsibility the financial stability of the organization. The Board of Directors was involved in continuous fundraising campaigns, while the professional staff members concentrated their efforts on the care of the patient under the direction of the superintendent of nurses.

The primary sources of funding for the Visiting Nurse Association (VNA) in the early days were the fees collected from patients for services rendered and funds raised by the Board of Directors or allocated to the agency through the Community Chest, which later became the United Way. The blessing of program flexibility was constantly thwarted by limited financial resources. Despite this difficulty, the Visiting Nurse Association continued to flourish and to respond to the changing health care needs of the people in the community.

In the early 1950s, the first major changes occurred in the Visiting Nurse Association. The original agency merged with another Visiting Nurse Association from a nearby town in order to strengthen and coordinate the work of both agencies. A third Visiting Nurse Association joined the other two in the late 1950s and men began serving on the agency's Board of Directors for the first time in its history.

When the Medicare Program was introduced in Congress in the early 1960s, the Board of Directors actively supported passage of the legislation because Medicare was expected to "take care of paying for services for all the needs of the elderly." If government money could be used for that purpose, the Board of Directors would be able to concentrate their fundraising efforts on the needs of the nonelderly population, and would be assured of a degree of financial stability for their organization.

The Visiting Nurse Association had had limited experiences with third-party reimbursement. Funding from insurance companies, such as the Metropolitan Life or John Hancock programs, had existed but was limited in scope and brief in regulations.

After becoming a Medicare provider, the Board of Directors became interested in expanding the scope of the agency's programs from just nursing and physical therapy into the full gamut of Medicare-allowable services. It was decided that a home health aide program, speech therapy, social work, and eventually occupational therapy, would become a part of the VNA's menu of services. At the same time, the local Welfare Planning Council was encouraging mergers of organizations that had similar purposes. The Visiting Nurse Association and the local Homemaker Services began a dialogue about merging. The agency was also encouraged to merge with the two remaining small visiting nurse associations in the county. In 1971, the first of a series of mergers took place creating the new agency which was known as Home-Health Services of Luzerne County. This new name was chosen to reflect the broad array of services available, and to remind the community that the focus of the agency had changed from an emphasis on nursing care to one which was supposed to meet the total health care needs of the homebound population in the area. Expansion was rapid with new programs added on a regular basis. Geographical territory was increased until a countywide service covering approximately 1,300 square miles was achieved.

With the new structure, most of the professional services were reimbursable under the Medicare program; however, it quickly became evident that the homemaker program, which primarily provided care to the chronically ill, would not be able to be sustained through Medicare funding. The Wyoming Valley area was a victim of flooding following Hurricane Agnes in 1972, and had resources made available to it for service delivery programs that were unique in nature. Unfortunately, these funds were also temporary in nature. As flood recovery dollars were withdrawn, the organization found itself in the unique position of having developed a large chronic care delivery system as a part of its Medicare-certified home health agency. The program was extremely popular among the elderly of the community, but it lacked an adequate funding source to support it.

The skilled services section of the organization had grown in size and complexity, causing the cost of the homemaker program to also increase to a point where chronic care services could not be offered on a private-pay basis at a price which was affordable to the average citizen in need of the services. Therefore, with great reluctance and a significant deficit, the agency discontinued its homemaker program and experienced the first layoffs in its history.

From the mid 1970s until the early 1980s, the VNA concentrated on perfecting its professional health care services to the community. The agency had grown from a staff of less than 20 employees to more than 100 in the period of a decade. Funding which had once been more than 80% United Way allocations reversed to being more than 80% Medicare reimbursement. The caseload changed in composition, from maternal and child health care and care of patients with communicable diseases, to an emphasis on service for the acutely ill, homebound geriatric patient. Even the procedures performed by the nursing staff had changed in intensity, requiring the development of more sophisticated continuing eduction programs. The direction of the agency was no longer provided by a superintendent of nurses but rather by a team of specialists under the direction of an administrator. The qualifications for the administrative function were no longer "an experienced nurse of fine repute" but rather a master's prepared individual with extensive experience in home health administration.

The composition of the board of directors and their responsibilities also changed. The role of fundraiser was traded in for the role of policymaker. Accountability, compliance with regulations, cost analysis, personnel policies, patient's rights, professional liability insurance, and other business topics became the focus of the board's agenda.

In the late 70s, the Board of Directors and administrative staff looked at the agency's past history and realized that growth and program development had occurred through spontaneous reactions to community needs rather than through a process of business planning; therefore, a Long-Range Planning Committee was created to help guide the organization's future development. One of the first documents reviewed by the Long-Range Planning Committee, after a demographic analysis had been completed, was the agency's mission statement. The Long-Range Planning Committee realized that the agency was not fulfilling its commitment to the chronically ill, as stated in the agency's purpose. They recommended to the board of directors that either the organization should change its mission statement or should find a way of serving this unmet need in the community. In response to this recommendation, an ad hoc committee was established to study the issue. An extensive survey of community resources revealed that programs existed for care of the chronically ill who were of a low-income level, and resources existed for the wealthy who could afford to pay the going rate for services from private agencies; however, nothing existed in the community for the population between these two extremes.

After the need had been determined, the Board of Directors and administrative staff had many lengthy discussions regarding the agency's responsibility to fulfill this need. The past experiences with a homemaker program under the auspices of the home health agency and the deficits which resulted from the care of the chronically ill caused the Board of Directors to be extremely cautious when considering the reestablishment of such a program. It was finally decided that the agency did have an obligation to fill the unmet community need if a way could be found to do it in a financially viable fashion.

At this stage in the decision-making process, the Board of Directors hired a consulting firm to advise them on their various options. The board had previously decided that an in-depth marketing study performed by consultants would be too expensive to absorb; therefore, administrative staff were assigned to perform a marketing survey on the feasibility of starting a homemaker program for the chronically ill, using the caseload of the visiting nurse component of the agency as the population to be studied. The role of the consultants hired by the Board of Directors was limited to the legal structures available for consideration and the reimbursement impact of each of these structures on both the existing acute care program and the projected chronic care program.

Four corporate structures were studied in depth with the consultants. The first was the foundation model which was rejected by the Board of Directors, since they did not desire to commit themselves to a specific volume of fundraising annually. The second model studied was the holding company model. This model was also rejected by the Board of Directors, since they had decided that each of the corporations involved in the restructuring would be nonprofit 501(C)(3) agencies; therefore, there would be no stock to be held by a holding company. The third model presented was that of a management corporation. This model satisfied the desires of the Board of Directors in the sense that it provided a logical structure for having two subsidiary corporations controlled by one management company.

The last structure studied was that of creating a chronic care component within the existing home health agency. This model was also rejected by the Board of Directors because of concern that the past history of the organization could be repeated, and that a chronic care program which was not financially viable could have adverse effects on the future of the home health agency. Before rejecting this concept, the methods of discrete cost analysis were carefully explored. The administrative staff members were confident that they could avoid many of the previously encountered financial pitfalls through the use of the sophisticated accounting methods currently available. In the past, the agency had neither the comprehension nor the staff to utilize these tools. However, the administrative staff also recommended that the acute care and chronic care programs be separately organized because the service philosophies of the two programs are different. The VNA services are medically necessary and, therefore, are provided to all in need, regardless of ability to pay for the services. A homemaker program is socially necessary, and in some cases, a luxury service. People may be less comfortable or less independent without the service; however, they can survive without it. Implementing these different philosophies requires different management techniques that are easier to accomplish in separate corporations. In addition, types of employees, training programs, personnel policies, and salary levels can be developed to suit the market of each corporation when separate organizations exist.

Now that the agency knew what it wanted to do and how it wanted to set up the structure, the remaining piece of the plan, how to fund the chronic care portion of the total program, remained to be solved. Since the home health agency was serving a large population of patients, it was felt that surveying current recipients and recently discharged patients or their families would provide the agency with sufficient data to determine whether a homemaker program could be financially viable in our community. The administrative staff developed a brief but concise survey instrument and taught the professional staff how to use it for interviewing current service recipients. The same tool was also mailed to patients or families of individuals discharged from the home health agency during the past six months. A total of 827 surveys were returned and tabulated for presentation to the board of directors. Included in this survey tool were questions regarding the need for services to either supplement the skilled services provided by the home health agency including its home health aide program; questions regarding the need for personal care assistance and homemaking help following discharge from the agency's skilled service component; and questions regarding the volume of services desired on a weekly basis and the fee that the individual would be willing to pay for such a program.

The results confirmed the fact that the population surveyed was highly interested in having homemaker services available as a supplement to the other services provided by the home health agency, and that the clients were desirous of having bathing as well as homemaker services continued after the Medicare-certified agency discharged the patient. The survey, however, also confirmed the fact that most patients desired to pay a fee lower than the one established by a budget projection as necessary to cover the cost of the program.

The survey results were logical and had been anticipated because northeast Pennsylvania has a high percentage of elderly who need help. Most of the elderly in this segment of the state, however, are living on fixed incomes and are not wealthy. Since the Visiting Nurse Association was a United Way Member Agency, it received an allocation for supporting those skilled services which were not reimbursable under third-party payment. It uses a sliding-fee scale, based on ability to pay, for determining the patient's financial obligation for services whenever United Way Funds are needed to supplement the patient's payment. The United Way was asked for support of the homemaker program. A small portion of the Visiting Nurse Association's allocation was being used for care of the chronically ill. The cost of providing this service through the Medicare-certified agency's aide component was considerably higher than that projected for services under the homemaker agency. The United Way, therefore, agreed to shift this portion of the Visiting Nurse Association's allocation to the new program and to help the agency with the start-up expenses. It was decided that the target population would be the individual in the community who was unable to afford private-pay rates and who was not eligible for services through other state-sponsored programs. As a nonprofit agency, the financial goal was to cover costs and to generate cash reserves to sustain the agency for the normal turnover period between billing and receipt of payment. It was estimated that it would take two years for volume to build up to the point where breakeven occurred.

The financial consultants made numerous recommendations to the Board of Directors' committee, regarding the structure of the organization, billing practices to be followed, documentation requirements, and the importance of good customer relations. It was recognized from the start that the philosophy of service delivery in the Homemaker Agency had to be considerably different than that of the Visiting Nurse Association, where all patients are served regardless of ability to pay. The homemaker agency would need to limit its free and part-pay services to the size of the annual United Way allocation. In addition, bad debt situations could not be tolerated.

The Ad Hoc Committee of the Board of Directors presented its findings to the full board approximately two years after the study had been initiated. A number of board meetings were devoted to review the committee's findings and their recommendations. Finally, the Board of Directors voted in favor of diversification using the management corporation model. The legal work then began. It was decided that the Ad Hoc Committee would become the incorporators for the two new organizations — the management company and the homemaker services.

It was decided that the management corporation would be called "Home-Care Management of Luzerne County" with the two subsidiary organizations called "Homemaker Services of Luzerne County" and "Home-Health Services of Luzerne County." The home health program had as its mission statement the provision of skilled services and home health aide services to the acutely ill, homebound members of the community, a responsibility for health education, health screening, and the provision of professional services to other segments of the community. The homemaker agency, on the other hand, was clearly identified in its mission statement to be responsible for provision of homemaker, personal care, and companion services to the chronically ill segment of the community. The management corporation has as its sole purpose providing management services including financial, marketing, and public relations to its two subsidiary corporations and any of the corporations that the Board of Directors may determine are appropriate to add in the future.

Articles of Incorporation for the management corporation and the homemaker agency were filed in the Commonwealth of Pennsylvania. Bylaws were drafted and adopted by the incorporators. They also decided how the Board of Directors was to be divided. The original Board of Directors consisted of 30 individuals; therefore, it was decided that 10 individuals would serve on each of the three corporations, with the officers of the two subsidiary corporations also serving on the management corporation board. Therefore, the subsidiary corporations each had boards composed of 10 people with the management corporation board composed of 18 people. A singular nominating committee for all three corporations exists at the management corporation level, budgets for the subsidiary corporations must be approved by the management corporation's board of directors, and the bylaws of the subsidiary organizations cannot be changed without the approval of the management corporation. Because of the structure desired by the Board of Directors, it was decided that the subsidiary corporations are related parties, and that any services sold by Homemaker Services to the Medicare-certified home health agency would be done at cost. Filings were made with the Internal Revenue Service for all three corporations requesting a continuation of the 501(C)(3) status of the home health agency and establishment of a 501(C)(3) status for the two new corporations. These requests were approved approximately seven months after filing.

On February 1, 1984, the management corporation became functional. Four individuals from the Visiting Nurse Association were terminated in that agency and hired by the Home-Care Management. These four individuals consisted of the Administrator, the Director of Financial Affairs, the Director of Marketing and Public Relations, and the Executive Secretary. It was decided that the salary and benefits of these individuals would be the same as they were in the home health agency, and that the personnel policies of the home health agency would be adopted for the management corporation. Separate groups needed to be established in the home health agency's pension and health plans in order to accommodate the employees of the management corporation.

The following month, Homemaker Services started. A nurse from the home health agency was hired as the manager of the homemaker corporation. She developed a training plan for the homemaker and personal attendants, and interviewed, hired, and trained the first group of part-time workers. The title "Homemaker/Personal Attendants" was chosen to distinguish, because of salary differences, these employees from the "Home Health Aide" employed by the home health agency. Consideration was given to developing contracts between the two subsidiaries for home health aide services, but it was decided not to take that action in the Homemaker's formative stage. Since the subsidiaries are related parties, Homemaker Services would have to charge its cost to Home-Health Services for aides on a contractual basis. This did not offer an economic advantage to either party since the home health agency was well below the Medicare cost cap for aide services and had no need to reduce its aid costs. The Homemaker Services would require more administrative staff if its initial volume was too great; therefore, it would not have a lower cost for its private-pay clients by contracting to provide aide services to the home health agency. In addition, it was felt that the Homemaker Services needed time to develop expertise in its management functions before extensive growth occurred.

Because of these decisions, the initial caseload for the homemaker program consisted of 15 patients transferred from the home health agency to the homemaker agency. All of these individuals had completed their need for skilled services but still required assistance in personal care. They had been taken off of the Medicare program and were personally responsible for paying for their nonskilled care.

Homemaker Services offered three programs: personal care, help with household chores, and companion services. The fee for these services was set at $6.50 per hour. Since this fee was considerably less than that charged by the home health agency for private-paying clients, the patients were either able to save money by being transferred to the homemaker program or to purchase additional hours of services. A sliding-fee scale based upon income is used in order to assure proper utilization of United Way resources and to provide equitable guidelines for adjusting client charges when necessary.

Home-Care Management generates its income by charging the two subsidiary corporations for its services. This means that each employee of the management corporation must maintain an elaborate time record on a daily basis. In the beginning, it was difficult for the management corporation employees to get used to continuous timekeeping, but after a few months the task became routine. Funding for the home health agency did not change with the diversification.

The cost of accomplishing the diversification, excluding administrative staff and board time, was approximately $15,000. In order to provide cash flow for the Homemaker Services from the time of start-up until the point breakeven volume was developed, a line of credit of $25,000 was established at a local bank using the home health agency's resources as collateral. The total of $40,000 was considered to be a reasonable amount to risk on the new venture.

It has been two and one-half years since diversification of our home health agency took place. Frequently, we are asked whether the effort was worth it or not. Our response is always a resounding "Yes!" We feel strongly that diversification was the answer for our agency. We knew what we wanted to do and we knew why we wanted to do it. Diversification was the only way in which our company could accomplish its objectives. Because we chose to establish separate corporations, the management staff of both subsidiaries have been able to concentrate their efforts on development of their programs without being diverted by the external and internal influences that tend to determine daily operational priorities.

The management corporation model is a comfortable one for our structure and provides us with a parent corporation that has a functional purpose which can be expanded in the future. The home health agency, now known as Visiting Nurse Association/Home-Health Services, was not changed by the diversification. Our United Way resources are being used for more people and for more hours of client care. We are in a position to add additional subsidiary corporations with minimal cost and effort, if we desire to take advantage of new opportunities to expand our service line in the future; but, the greatest advantage from diversification is that a previously unmet community need is being filled. Homemaker Services of Luzerne County provided 11,536 hours of help during the first nine months of its operations; 30,402 hours of care were provided in the following calendar year; and 36,000 hours are projected for the current calendar year. More than 600 people received help that would not have been available to them three years ago.

Yes, it was worth it.

An Experience with Mergers

Marilyn Seiler

Home health seemed simpler in the fall of 1981. The doctor gave the referral. The nurse went out to see the patient. The agency got paid for the services that were delivered.

In that spirit of naivete, five RNs and two LPNs met to form their own agency. Each nurse had five or more years of nursing experience and six months to five years of home health experience. They were interested in serving the people of Oklahoma and in offering quality nursing care to their patients.

They had few financial resources among them, so they began searching for capital from their friends and other health agencies in Oklahoma. They discovered an agency, that was involved in supplemental staffing for the hospitals of Oklahoma City, that indicated an interest in starting a home care agency. Watchful Nursing had previously applied for incorporation and had made preliminary steps toward starting a home health agency.* Lack of staff and home health experience, however, prevented further development. When approached by an experienced staff, the agency was willing to put up the capital to start home health care.

The nurses started by writing preliminary policies and procedures and designing chart forms. They began marketing to doctors in the metropolitan area of Oklahoma City. Their marketing efforts failed to pay off at that time. Therefore, the decision was made to move out of Oklahoma City into one of the small rural towns to seek referrals. As a result of that decision, the dream that all the nurses be utilized and become a part of the agency was abolished. I was the only nurse who was able to continue with the agency due to my ability to relocate.

Watchful Nursing was already doing supplemental staffing and consultation for nursing service administration in a hospital in southwest Oklahoma, approximately 120 miles from Oklahoma City. Therefore, that seemed like a good place to start.

I moved to that area for the time that would be required to set up an office. Again, naivete. It was originally thought by the nurses that it would take approximately a month or two to set up the first office. When that office was going well, we planned to use its revenue base to market in the Oklahoma City area. In reality, this did not happen. What did happen follows.

I went to the area to set up the first office. I immediately received two referrals from one of the local physicians. I called the patients, briefly explained the services, and set up appointments for a home visit. These became the first admissions to Loving Home Health. As is typical of many rural areas, there were no social services available in that town. Therefore, any help I could offer was most welcome and appreciated by the families. Besides nursing care, I was able to mobilize some sources in the community, such as churches and neighbors, to meet some of the families' needs.

The next 13 months were spent setting up the operation. By the end of the first month of services, I was making 30 visits per week. This necessitated hiring a second nurse to help make visits. An aide was also hired for part-time work. All aide visits had been previously made by the nurses. Loving Home Health offered skilled nursing and home health aide. Staff was added as needed, with the result that by the end of the first year, seven LPNs had been added as well as two RNs. The LPNs made most of the routine visits, while the RNs made the initial assessments and supervisory visits. Staff was recruited from various small communities surrounding the office, so that a wider geographic area could be reached.

I received financial support from Watchful Nursing, but I relied heavily on former colleagues for the answers to technical home health administration questions. Approximately three months later, an administrative office was established. An ad-

---

* All agency names have been changed.

ministrator was added to the staff full-time. He was on the Board of Directors and a partner of Watchful Nursing.

After six months, a branch office was established in a community 30 miles away to provide more cost-effective care and better follow-up for patients. An RN and three LPNs completed the staff working in the branch office area.

I continued to supervise all nursing activities. I also performed all the office and billing activities for the first eight months, at which time a secretary-billing clerk was hired.

The initial goal for establishing the first office was to move to other areas of the state, especially in the Oklahoma City area. Therefore, I needed a nurse to replace me in Cordell in order to move on to other areas. After nine months of operation, a supervising RN was hired and oriented. After two months, she was trained sufficiently to take over the first office.

Geographical Location and Expansion of Offices

Very early in the history of Loving Home Health, the administrator and I surveyed areas and counties of Oklahoma that were felt to be underserved. Statistics from county offices on population distribution over 65 and lower income levels were studied. Statistics on which county health department had availability of home visits were also used.

Based on these statistics, two possible areas of expansion emerged. They were the far northwestern corner of Oklahoma and the south central area of Oklahoma. The northwest area was chosen first, since there were fewer health departments in that area. The income was moderate in the area, but there were few services available to meet the needs of the elderly. A site was chosen as Loving Home Health's second office.

In December of 1982, I moved to establish the office. Two months prior to my arrival, ads were placed in the local newspapers announcing openings for a supervising RN. Based on previous experience through the Cordell office, I did not feel that I wanted to set up the office and then choose a supervising RN. It was deemed too expensive to continue what had been done for the first office.

In subsequent offices, we interviewed and hired nurses before my move. We met with medical staffs of local hospitals. We also hired nurses from various geographic areas to reach a broader base of physicians. I continued to orient staff in home health procedures, home visits, documentation, and marketing. In the second office, I tried to orient two nurses with no prior home health experience at the same time. That experience was overwhelming. I felt I needed to be in two places at once.

Each nurse was taught to market the doctors with whom she was already familiar. The nurses were from different towns and therefore, knew different doctors and had different experiences. This proved to be very advantageous for drawing patients from a wider geographical area.

The second office grew very rapidly. Staff was added more quickly. I hired a secretary-billing clerk much earlier in the development of the office to allow for smoother office operations and quicker response to phone calls. The office progression proceeded much more smoothly than that of the first office. Prior experience paid off well.

The feasibility study for new offices was used again in May of 1983 to establish an office in south central Oklahoma. The same procedure was used for this office as had been used for the second office.

In June of 1983, an office site was chosen, with a different approach taken this time. Real estate was a good buy at the time, so an office site was purchased instead of being rented. This turned out to be a poor decision, as the agency had to be sold soon after opening.

Growth of Loving Home Health was very rapid in the first two years of operation. With that internal growth, rapid expansion of the industry, and changes in Medicare regulation interpretation, hard times were ahead. November of 1983 brought very slow Medicare reimbursement. We were forced to seek a buyer for the entire agency. Changes had been too drastic to keep up with the monetary needs of the agency.

Unable to adapt quickly enough, the third office was closed at the end of December 1983. Patients were referred to another agency in the area.

No new patients were accepted in either of the first two offices. Most of the nurses were laid off. Only skeleton crews were retained.

A buyer for the agency was located in January of 1984. Better Home Care already had three offices in existence in Oklahoma. A fourth one was ready to be established. Better Home Care was a full service agency. It included all Medicare and non-Medicare services from 24-hour skilled nursing care to homemakers and live-in companions, as well as the various therapies. They also operated supplemental staffing and industrial nursing service. The two agencies joined policy and procedure manuals, philosophies, organizational charts, services, and financial and human resources.

Loving Home Health operated the Medicare-certified arm of the agency, while Better Home Care became the non-Medicare section of the company. The mission and philosophy of the combined agency plays an important role in the decision for geographical location of offices.

It has been the philosophy of both agencies since their inception to place nurses in strategic geographical locations in order to capture referrals from a broader geographical base. This means hiring nurses from several different towns surrounding the actual office. The nurses are responsible for coming into the office one time a week to bring in paperwork and time sheets. The nurses are also responsible for contacting the supervising RN at their base office for direct communication and supervision. This has been found to be a very cost-effective tool of the agency.

Organizational Chart and Its Changes Through Growth

The organizational chart has grown with the agency. It started out very simple (See Exhibit 29-2). As offices were added during the first three years of operation, the administrator remained the same, but each office had its own supervising RN. (See Exhibit 29-3).

As more offices were added, the organizational chart necessarily changed. More responsibilities have been added to the individual offices.

In March of 1984, an administrator was appointed for each office. That person has taken on more of the budgetary, financial planning, and administrative duties (See Exhibit 29-4). The Medicare, non-Medicare, and Quality Assurance Managers directly supervise the offices, and are responsible for a particular area of expertise (e.g.,

Exhibit 29-2

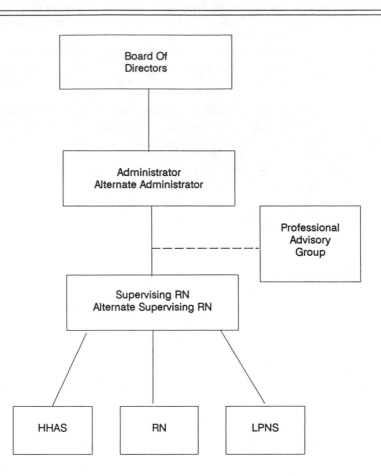

quality control and staff development). A general manager has responsibility for home care supervision, as well as other businesses.

This concept was maintained for approximately one year. Product line supervision and structure has been introduced (see Exhibit 29-5). The administrator of each office continues to care for all administrative, budgetary, financial, and marketing activities. Under the direction of the administrator, the supervising RN supervises all nursing care delivered to patients.

Because the offices are geographically dispersed, each has had to function autonomously and had to be very decentralized. Each office has had responsibility for all of its own billing for Medicare activities. Non-Medicare billing has been centralized at the home office level.

Exhibit 29-3

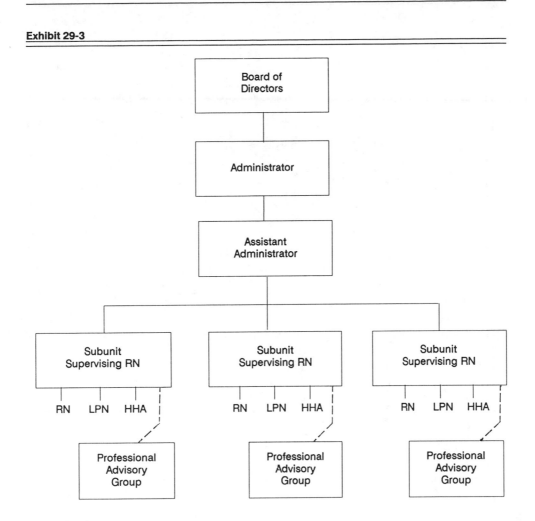

Mission and Philosophy

The mission of the agency has been to serve people of every race, creed, handicap, and age within the financial ability of the agency, which has been limited at times. The agency is proprietary. Resources, however, have always been sought, if the agency was unable to provide the services directly.

Better Home Care has not changed its original philosophy of providing care to underserved areas of Oklahoma, basing all business relationships on honesty, integrity, and mutual trust. They strive to extend health to all areas of wellness: physical, emotional, social, and spiritual well-being. They also believe in a holistic approach to patient care through interdisciplinary means.

Mission and philosophy are a joint effort of the Board of Directors and the management staff. I believe that management is in the best position for implementing the philosophy, and therefore must be part of the development.

Exhibit 29-4

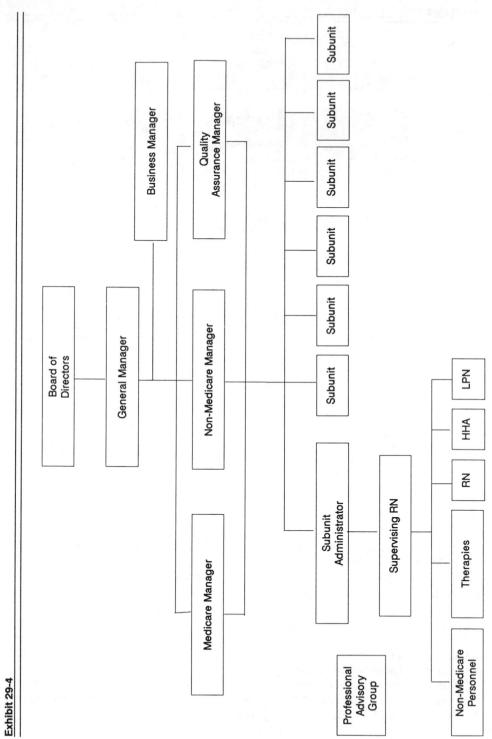

Exhibit 29-5.

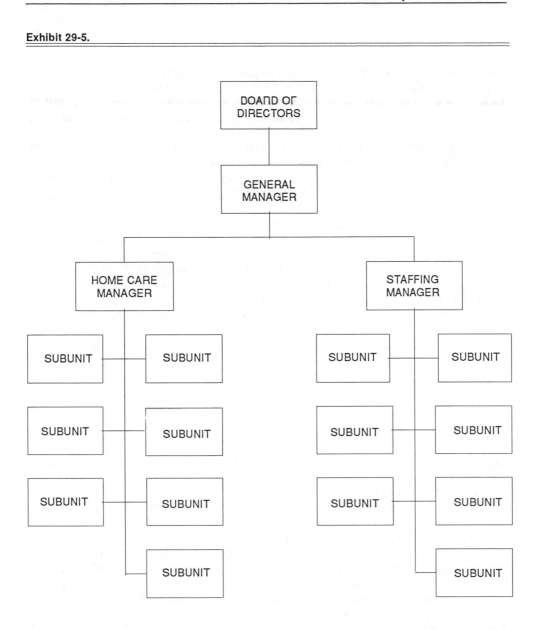

Through the first two years of operation, Loving Home Health's Board of Directors and management staff were the same persons. The administrator and I had very similar personal philosophies. Therefore, the agency mission which was adopted was compatible with our personal lives. In searching for a buyer, an agency with "like minds" was desired and located. The similarity definitely assisted in a smoother merging of the two agencies.

Services and Staffing

Better Home Care has always attempted to provide whatever services a client needs. Depending on the office location, all services are provided: homemakers, live-in companions, skilled care, and therapies. Some locations are able to provide only skilled nursing and unlicensed care, since availability of the therapies in some of the rural areas is nonexistent.

Instead of concentrating almost entirely on Medicare, as was the case early in the history of Loving Home Health, non-Medicare services are offered and marketed on an equal basis in the combined agency. All sources of reimbursement (Medicare, private-pay, and insurance) are utilized so that a broader base of service may be provided.

Staffing standards are provided. Forms have been changed frequently to assist staff persons to provide adequate documentation as expeditiously as possible.

Time utilization is frequently discussed with all staff members and is reviewed often in order to maintain standards and job satisfaction for staff members. Time studies are done on a regular basis to make sure that nurses are staying within the allotted time frames. The primary focus in doing time studies is to document miles per visit and time spent per visit, which includes staff meetings, documentation, visit time, and travel time.

Nurses are primarily hired on a temporary basis. Very few full-time nurses are utilized. Most nurses complete the number of visits or hours mutually decided upon in the desired area.

Policies and Procedures

The policy and procedure manual of November of 1981 consisted of approximately 25 pages. The policy and procedure manual of today fills a three-inch binder. A small agency with one office can get by with very few policies and procedures. Problems are solved on a day-to-day, case-by-case basis.

That is no longer possible as the agency grows. Most of the policies and procedures have grown out of discussions with staff members, and situations that have arisen requiring standards and uniform procedures.

The first manual consisted of job descriptions for approximately five positions. The personnel policies consisted of benefits, hours on duty, dress code, hiring policies, acceptance and discharge policies of patients, and forms. It indeed was very simple.

Today's policy and procedure manual consists of all the above with several additions: new programs, standing orders, and new forms. Billing procedures, general administrative policies, and orientation procedures have been added to the manual. The personnel policies have also been expanded.

The decision to add a new policy or procedure often begins with a staff person who sees a need for a set procedure on a certain situation or topic. That person is then encouraged either to write a preliminary policy and procedure or to offer suggestions for such. It is developed within the administrative group and approved or revised by the General Manager, Home Care Manager, and Staffing Manager. At that point, it is distributed for general policy.

The administrators of each of the subunits meet on a semimonthly basis to discuss new procedures and policies, the need for new procedures and policies, and other administrative concerns, such as the need for new programs and services.

Capital Requirements

Gone are the days when a home health agency can be started on a shoestring or close to a shoestring. Capital requirements are such that a home health agency has to be able to function for approximately six months to a year after inception before full reimbursement for services can be realized on a regular basis. A case mix balance is necessary to maintain solvency.

The home health agency needs to provide for salaries. Medical supplies, office supplies, office equipment, travel expenditures, office expenditures are all major items to be taken into consideration during the first year of operation.

A case mix balance helps assure better reimbursement. For the most part, insurance and private-pay services tend to pay more quickly than do Medicare-reimbursable activities. A good capital base needs to be maintained throughout the life of the agency. There are constant peaks and valleys in both services and reimbursements. Growth can be severely limited if the capital base is not large enough, as we discovered firsthand early in our history.

New Developments, Mergers, Buy Outs, Joint Ventures

It is extremely difficult today to operate a small home health agency. The capital requirements are very large, and the referral base is usually not large enough to support that kind of venture. Hospitals are starting their own agencies. By doing so, they have a fairly secure referral base. Therefore, freestanding agencies need to research the feasibility of contracting with hospitals to secure their own referral base. Another option is linking with other agencies and other referral bases in order to insure their own survival.

Home health is becoming a bigger and much more sophisticated business than when it began. High-tech programs are becoming a very important part of home care. Intravenous therapy, maternal and child programs, phototherapy, ill-child programs, respiratory care, and rehabilitation programs all are taking place in the home. Home care agencies have to update themselves in order to meet the challenges of the future. They must be proficient, not only in the care to be provided to sicker patients, but also in technology and services.

Through flexibility and adaptability, I have grown and learned. The agency has also experienced much growth, both in numbers and experience. It has been very difficult at times, but also very rewarding and challenging. From these beginnings, I believe we are prepared to face the bright future of home care.

Chapter Thirty

Grantsmanship In Home Health

Terrance Keenan

The term "grantsmanship" is often used to denote a set of techniques and talents for persuasion, which in combination constitute a sort of master key to the coffers of institutions engaged in philanthropic giving—government agencies as well as foundations and corporations. Thus, administrators of human service organizations commonly seek people who profess these qualities for their staffs, and in fact an entire profession called "development officers" has arisen to fill what has become a burgeoning job market.

What is unfortunate is not that fundraising is receiving increasing attention from management, for in truth, it warrants the serious and energetic concern of both the administration and the board. The troublesome aspect of fundraising, rather, is that it has tended to become shrouded in a mystique of its own, as if its practice and practitioners embody some magical craft for reaping philanthropic dollars.

The truth is that institutional development officers or external fundraising firms have little direct influence on the decisions of philanthropy. Their influence, although it can be considerable, is only indirect and facilitative, and is wholly dependent upon the strengths of the grant-seeking institution itself, particularly its leadership. Grantsmanship at whatever intensity it is applied—and at whatever cost to the grant-seeking institution—has no magic to generate dollars for a mediocre or marginal organization. Without institutional purpose and leadership, grantsmanship is a hollow exercise.

The Meaning of an Institutional Image

The first step in acquiring the ability to compete successfully for philanthropic dollars is not to hire a development officer but to undertake an honest self-assessment of the institution's precise role in the community. The second step involves a self-audit of the institution's performance with respect to this role and the adoption of prompt management remedies to any shortfalls. Finally, the organization needs to define a mission statement articulating the results of the above steps (role and performance) in a way that is clear and compelling to the public. All of these efforts are preconditions to a successful grant-seeking program, and in combination they shape the institution's image.

Visiting nurse associations and other forms of home health agencies have a serious problem with the first factor relating to their image: mainly, their role and function within our huge, complex, and swiftly changing health care system.

---

*The views expressed in this chapter are those of the author, and no official endorsement by the Robert Wood Johnson Foundation is intended or should be inferred

At an earlier time, when they stood in the vanguard of the settlement house movement, this was not the case. Impoverished immigrant families were in great need of basic nursing care and of advocates to mediate the appalling social misery in which they lived. In rural areas as well, the role of the visiting nurse was abundantly clear. The classic example is the Frontier Nursing Service founded in rural Kentucky in 1925. Visiting nursing services during this period were able to command widespread philanthropic interest both regionally and nationally.

Today, the mission of home health nursing and its governing agencies has somehow lost the conceptual singularity it once possessed. Among other things, home health has shifted part of its base from community ownership to investor-owned chains or to components of investor-owned hospitals. Even where hospitals have remained voluntary, many have unbundled their services in the form of complex corporate structures and established home health as only one component of a multiple product line. For these and other reasons, the traditional identity of the visiting nurse association, whether voluntary or public, has begun to wane as a community service available to all households impaired by injury or sickness.

Ironically, the fading concept of home health as a basic and probably essential community service has occurred at a period when the American household is becoming more vulnerable than at any time in this century. Moreover, the outlook for the future is that it will become increasingly at risk. Single parent families are on the rise among all income groups, including adolescent mothers. Mothers of intact families are entering the job market in record numbers. The frail elderly, people 75 and over, are one of the fastest growing population groups nationwide. Finally, people are being discharged from the hospital so swiftly that the aftercare needs of the general population may reach crisis proportions.

The combination of these forces yields a profile of the American household that is characterized by an alarming state of vulnerability. This is especially the case in a society that is witnessing the demise of the extended family, the breakup of the nuclear family, and hence the rapid erosion of a dependable system of family member caretakers.

These circumstances have clearly increased the need and broadened the opportunity for home health. The household, as in our earlier history, is emerging as a principal locus of care. Home health agencies urgently need to reassert their role as the one institution in the community wholly devoted to meeting the health and personal support requirements of vulnerable families.

As noted earlier, once they have formulated such a role and taken the steps necessary to perform it both fully and well, they need to project to the community at large the image that they are a vital resource that warrants the sustained backing of all of its residents.

Building a Constituency of Supporters

The successful achievement of a meritorious social image, however, does not automatically translate into a flow of financial support. Generating public sector and charitable giving is painstaking work, and it is here that the skilled practice of fundraising or grantsmanship applies. The most valuable commodity any service organization has to market is its reputation. Once this has been guaranteed by its management and board, the organization is in a position to build a constituency of people and groups who will become its advocates. For a home care agency, this would manifestly include its chief referral sources: physicians, hospital social work and discharge offices, local family service, and social welfare agencies. Other important constituents who should be enlisted as advocates would include the community's business, civic, and religious leadership, and beyond this, county, state, and federal offices in such areas as the aging and maternal and child health. While developing a constituency of advocates is, of course, an ongoing task, it is also the foundation of a formal fundraising program, and the program is not likely to do well until this foundation has been laid.

Organizing a Fundraising Program

An effective fundraising program is usually organized around two broad categories of potential givers, and it is important that they be approached with sensitivity to their differences. The first category consists of individuals and groups who are members of the community. The second category consists of institutions which are members of organized philanthropy; namely, foundations and corporations which conduct formal charitable-giving programs.

Contributions from the first category comprise the cornerstone of support for the core budget or ongoing operational expenses of any community agency that depends on voluntary giving to maintain its programs. To reach people and groups within this category, the agency concerned can call upon the constituency of supporters or advocates discussed above—for it should have been made clear at the outset that participation in fundraising would be one of their functions. Members of these constituencies—from the Rotary, the Chamber of Commerce, the hospital board, for example—can be enlisted to serve on annual fundraising committees, or to persuade their organizations to conduct benefits on behalf of the agency. In these and other ways, the agency's local advocates serve as a powerful system for reaching individual community residents.

At the same time, individuals should be approached directly through mailed solicitations. However, these mailings should not be one-shot requests but should arrive at the individual's home as part of periodic informational mailings (for example, a simple newsletter) about the agency's work and its related funding needs.

In sum, generating contributions from individuals and groups in the community requires a constant, year-round effort which is neither routine nor easy. Yet, it is often the level of giving from this source that makes the margin of difference in the local service agency's ability to continue to exist. Moreover, the agency's potential for success in obtaining grants from foundations and corporations will almost always be directly related to its accomplishments in local fundraising. Foundations and corporations will rarely respond favorably to proposals from community agencies that cannot demonstrate a solid record of local funding.

Approaching Foundations and Corporations

The first thing to recognize about foundation and corporate giving, or so-called organized philanthropy, is that it is different from giving by the community membership. The latter can be called upon to help the local service agency complete its operating budget. Foundations and corporations will respond helpfully to requests for this purpose only rarely. Corporations, which have strong local bonds and which are, in fact, part of the civic life of the community, will sometimes make annual general support grants to the community's basic voluntary institutions; but these are the exceptions, and to an increasing degree, the pattern of their philanthropic giving is similar to that of foundations.

If organized philanthropy does not help with operating budgets, what does it do? The answer is that foundations and corporations have a strong preference for developmental funding. They see themselves as the principal source in our society of private investment capital for nurturing new capacity, competence, and ideas in the country's human service enterprise.

For home health agencies, this means that they are a resource for testing and instituting new concepts and ideas to help American families cope with the increasing levels of vulnerability to their independence and integrity.

It is important to emphasize, however, that most foundations and corporations do not have a portfolio of ideas in home health to put out for bid to interested local agencies. From time to time, when there is firm evidence that a particular initiative or approach can serve as a prototype to advance an entire human service area, a foundation or corporation will issue a formal competitive invitation for proposals. In general, however, these institutions depend on the applicant bringing the idea to them.

Ideas in home health might be concerned with such matters as the following: new ways of deploying staff to ensure continuity of care to clients and better communications with physicians; new financing mechanisms, such as prepaid capitation, enabling services to be provided according to clients' needs rather than according to what Medicare or third-party intermediaries will reimburse; new in-service training programs in high-need areas such as geriatrics; new approaches to training family member caregivers in the clinical management of clients: for example, the administration of intravenous solutions.

While in general, organized philanthropy tends to favor proposals for ideas and innovations, some will also participate in capital projects (i.e., buildings and equipment); but this is not common, and requests for this purpose should be sent only to those grant-making institutions with a stated policy of considering capital spending needs.

Identifying Grant-making Prospects

Much of the success in fundraising from organized philanthropy rests in the precision with which prospective grant makers are identified. The most economical and dependable resource for this purpose is the Foundation Center, 79 Fifth Avenue, New York. The center is a nonprofit organization devoted solely to conducting a national documentation and information service on American foundations and their grant-making activities.

The center published the following key directories:

- *National Data Book.* Basic information on all 24,000 U.S. foundations.

- *Foundation Directory.* Concise profiles on the 4,400 foundations with assets of at least $1 million and annual grants of at least $100,000.

- *Source Book Profiles.* Complete summaries of the 1,000 largest independent foundations.

- *Corporate Foundation Profiles.* Similar information on the 230 largest corporate foundations, plus brief summaries of 400 other corporate grant makers.

- *Foundation Grants Index.* Bimonthly and annual compilations of all grants of $5,000 or more by the 500 largest grant makers.

- *Foundations Grants to Individuals.* Foundation and corporate programs providing individual educational opportunities through scholarships, fellowships, and other types of awards.

In addition to its printed directories, the center offers computer printouts of foundation grants across 112 different subject fields. Moreover, it is equipped to conduct customized searches in other areas.

The center's directories and computer services all carry a charge, but the directories are accessible to grant seekers at 160 affiliated sites, largely local libraries, located in every state. (Note: the reader should write the center for a listing of these collections.) Besides the center's directories, each site contains microcard copies of the annual information returns foundations are required to submit to the Internal Revenue Service (IRS).

The microcard information returns lend a good measure of precision to the identification of funding prospects. The directories provide the grant-seeking agency with the names of foundations which make grants within the agency's geographic area and general field of work (e.g., community health services). The information returns list the foundation's actual grants for the IRS reporting year, and thus provide a more exact idea of whether the foundation is interested in the agency's specific field (e.g., home health).

Utilizing the materials produced by the Foundation Center requires a fair measure of practice and skill, and to help grant seekers make the most of these resources the center conducts periodic regional workshops.

Preparing the Proposal

Unlike government, few foundations and corporations have standard application forms or even stated formats or outlines for the preparation of proposals. This does not mean that they are not concerned about content; indeed, they will usually ask for meticulous detail in their study of a proposal and, before they fund it, will commonly require a meeting with the applicant. For the purposes of an initial approach, however, a lengthy application is seldom necessary. Anywhere from five to ten double-spaced pages will suffice and should include the following information:

- Nature of the problem, its size and scope nationally and regionally, and why it is important. This should be documented through a thorough literature search.

- The proposed project or program for dealing with the problem—its conceptual basis as an innovation, whether it has been tried elsewhere, and with what success.

- The anticipated outcome—what will happen as a result of the project, who is likely to adopt the innovation, and how this will help bring the problem under resolution.

- A brief work program for carrying out the project, including time lines for completing its various components.

- A detailed line-item budget by year for completing the work program (personnel, travel, office operations and supplies, consulting costs, etc.). This should include separate line-item columns detailing support from other sources.

- If the proposal is for a new type of institutional service or program, it should explain how the project will be financed after the expiration of the foundation's grant.

- The qualifications of the applicant and the people who will head the project. Include the applicant's size, service load, record of innovation, and the curriculum vitae of the project staff.

Finally, the applicant should include a copy of its ruling from the IRS that it is a tax-exempt entity. In general, voluntary organizations should be exempt under Section 501(c)(3) of the IRS Code.

Foundation indirect cost overhead allowances are modest (5 to 10%). However, foundations will usually pay for institutional costs incurred by the project (space, utilities) when these can be accurately identified. Thus, these costs should usually be incorporated as line items in the budget under some appropriate category such as office operations and supplies. In any event, foundations interested in studying a project will always advise the applicant of their indirect cost policies.

Fundraising and Management

In today's competitive climate, it has become increasingly obsolete to follow the practice of hiring a chief executive officer of any nonprofit organization (home health agency, hospital, etc.) purely on the basis of his or her management expertise, and letting someone else (usually the board) worry about raising the money. Fundraising is a paramount responsibility of the CEO, and agency heads who dislike this function are unlikely to be either happy or successful in their jobs.

On the other hand, the effort to generate external resources, especially when successful, should not deflect the attention of the board from the essential tasks of management to bring expenses under efficient and effective control and, most importantly, to generate service revenue. This means an equitable schedule of sliding-scale fees for uncovered clients and services and prompt billings and collections. It also means an aggressive stance with Medicare and its intermediaries and the state Medicaid office, for if the agency does not protect the entitlements of its clients it is not likely to get clients.

In sum, to complete the basic operating budget and to obtain the developmental funds necessary to enable the organization to expand and improve its service capacity, the heads of home health agencies have to master the strategies of grantsmanship, but neither should this effort be allowed to mask the bottom line responsibility of the chief executive and board to compete for service revenue. It is particularly those agencies which are able to show commendable financial performance while doing their best for the vulnerable families they serve that are most attractive to organized philanthropy.

Part IX

Other Types of Relationships

Chapter Thirty-One

Home Care Volunteer Programs

The Notion of Volunteerism

Carol-Rae Hoffmann

Old sailors know never to volunteer for anything! The implication is that to volunteer places one at risk. To volunteer makes one vulnerable to the experience of injustice, a risk which is prevalent enough in all human interaction but which is intensified by the intrinsic nature of volunteering. To volunteer means to offer one's services out of one's own volition with no guarantee of reciprocity, let alone a guarantee of equal reciprocity. The risk of experienced injustice is high.

To volunteer means to generate a proactive statement of commitment based on faith, belief, and individually felt principle. It is a projection of personal quality, which normally can remain hidden and safe from public perusal, into a concrete act which becomes visible and subject to public judgment. To volunteer is to make an open statement of principle; it makes the individual visible and accountable and consequently binds him by his honor to the fulfillment of his promise. Here again is the potential for felt injustice. The volunteer risks visibility and public judgment by his own volition; he stands alone, in front of the crowd, on his own behalf. He risks exposure and judgment from those who can shout their condemnation from the anonymous safety of the crowd. The volunteer is always vulnerable to the statement, "You offered."

Most of us volunteer with the hope, perhaps even belief, that we will feel the balance of our risk in received appreciation. Sometimes this payback comes through; often, it falls short. The self-perception of one as "volunteer" can easily slip to a self-perception of one as victim."

It is precisely this issue, keeping the volunteer a volunteer and not a felt victim that is the key to a successful volunteer program. The object is to attract qualified, committed individuals who will risk the public statement of volunteering, to stimulate and support these individuals into working at maximum levels of investment and productivity, and finally, to maintain their involvement over an extended period of time. Recruiting quality volunteers, stimulating them to maintain production, and retaining them demands a recognition of the risks incurred by the volunteer and responding to that risk by working toward a reciprocity of justice. A fundamental goal for any successful volunteer program must be mutuality, a mutuality of acted-out commitment, by both volunteer and agency, to a shared justice and fairness which precludes victimization.

Volunteerism: An American Cultural Trait

Volunteerism is a well-established American tradition. The cultural demand to volunteer one's time, energy, and talent seems to be rooted in the American interpretation of the Protestant work ethic. In America, not only are you expected to work hard with every anticipation of financial and spiritual reward, but once your rewards have been recognized, you are expected to "share the wealth"—both material and moral. In America, once the individual is in a position of relative financial stability, he is expected to give over time and talent for the general social good and for the good of individuals who are less fortunate. There is considerable social pressure to share the wealth; individuals who, because of the time restrictions created by their success, cannot give directly of their skills, are expected to surrogate this donation with money! Government supports this practice by making contributions of this sort tax-deductible and in so doing concretely acts out the social sanction of this unique value.

Money is fine, but time is better. Direct action volunteerism has always held cultural esteem in our society. Interestingly, while it has usually been a predominantly female prerogative, volunteerism has consistently been encouraged of men as well as women. Often men volunteer for positions which hold significant social status, volunteer heads of foundations, social and cultural committees, political and economic organizations; while women often volunteer for direct service functions such as the Gray Ladies, institutional fundraising committees, and volunteer service in schools and welfare agencies. All individuals are expected to participate, and if there are inequities in the volunteer system in America, they are inequities reflective of the general social system rather than specific to volunteerism—the culture is consistent.

In summary, volunteerism in America is a well-established cultural trait rooted in moral sanction and perpetuated through significant social pressure. Volunteerism is a collective charge, a cultural norm given to all members of the society with every expectation that the individual will meet the challenge to the best of his or her ability.

Health Care Volunteerism

During the twentieth century, the health care institution in America has gained tremendous esteem. The post-World War II period saw a dramatic rise in social and political power for the health care community, a rise which seemed to reach its peak in the mid-seventies. This rise in power and esteem appears to be rooted in the relatively unique notion, perpetrated in the latter half of the twentieth century, that medical personnel can do more than mitigate pain, they can in fact defeat death. With the "magic" powder of antibiotics tightly in hand, medicine in the post-World War II era came close to gaining theological prestige. Before this period, the power of life and death was pretty much in God's hands; now He seemed to have the assistance of a physician.

The public has done a great deal to increase the prestige of the health care community. It makes sense that if you stand just under God's right hand, or if the public believes that this is your designated position, you acquire a considerable amount of respect, a considerable amount of power. Add to this set of perceptions the popular American image of the "lifesaver" as a romantic hero, and you are well on you way toward sanctification.

The whole notion of a collective cultural fantasy spun around a hero who exercises power over death is an intriguing cultural phenomenon. This fantasy allows the individual to bask in the warm light of public acclaim, of public recognition and esteem, of direct ego gratification at the highest level, through the performance of an act which by its nature is the ultimate in moral behavior. Give back to an individual that which is most morally valued and most ethically weighed, his life, and you earn the right to direct ego gratification. It is a point of curiosity that for many of us in America in order to free ourselves, even in our fantasy, to claim recognition on our own behalf, we must pay the cost of performing an act that comes conceptually close to divine.

It should, therefore, not be surprising that volunteerism in health care settings has been consistently popular in America. To volunteer for service in a hospital or geriatric facility, for example, fulfills the requirement to give back to the society and at the same time allows the individual to gain permitted self-gratification by engaging in "good work." Whether one agrees with the ethical system or not, there is a system operative, and its reality must be recognized and worked within; and truthfully, an ethical system that exhibits through altruism certainly is far better than a system which is non- or antialtrusitic in its expression. Perhaps our motives are a bit bent, but better bent than crooked.

Home Care Volunteerism

Outpatient care is a growing movement in the current health care spectrum. In-home care has always been present, to a greater or lesser degree, in the general health care scene in America. Today, however, because of diagnostic related groups (DRGs) and the payment policies they impose, more and more individuals find themselves at home at stages of more and more acute caretaking need.

In addition, the growth of the hospice movement (which in America involves primarily in-home care) has vastly contributed to the need for trained volunteers for in-home care service.

Home care volunteerism makes good sense. If properly administered, it is cost-efficient and delivers a unique quality of care that can be acquired in no other way. The patient, who is clinically appropriate for in-home care, has the advantage of being in the security of familiar surroundings, in an environment in which he can usually exercise a fair degree of individual control, and in addition, (hopefully!) remains among those who are most significant to him, most trusted by him, and most nurturing in every sense. Well-trained and supervised volunteers through their facilitation can maximize the quality of the in-home care experience, and in many cases, they do more than facilitate the process, for they are essential to its very existence.

In-home care volunteers come in several varieties. They include individuals who volunteer their time and self to provide companionship for the at-home patient, as well as individuals who volunteer their professional services and skills. Without these donations of personal resources provided by volunteers, many patients and their families would not be able to function effectively in the in-home setting; responsibilities would be too demanding, and costs would be too consuming.

In-house care, which incorporates the efficient use of volunteers, has every potential to increase the possibility and quality of good patient care and at the same time stabilize or lower cost. There are some risks, however, which cannot be ignored.

The first issue is the possibility of legal liability. When the volunteer is sent into the patient's home, institutional environmental control is given up and this creates a degree of risk. In addition, in-home volunteers, unlike most volunteers working in institutional settings, usually hold an extraordinary degree of personal responsibility for the patient's well-being. Often, the in-home volunteer is the only individual present and responsible for the patient. This breadth of responsibility demands that the degree of trust and confidence placed in in-home volunteers be extraordinary, and in the extraordinary is risk.

The second issue is the problem of "burn-out." In-home volunteers are giving a great deal of themselves in relatively intense dosages. There is a risk of loosing them or their quality if they are not given some degree of reciprocity and nurturing.

When the effect is balanced against the risk, most in-home care agencies choose in favor of the volunteer's involvement in patient care plans. Volunteers do not need to be present in every case handled by an agency to be perceived as "earning their salt." They need to be present when their presence is critical or appropriate. In addition, they can provide peripheral services such as bookkeeping, secretarial, or library tasks which usually translate into all-around increased quality of service. The bottom line is that volunteers enhance service at every level with a minimal cost in both money and overhead.

The Philosophical Basis for a Successful Volunteer Program

Program Goals

A well-organized volunteer program is designed to meet four basic program goals. These goals are internal and aimed at the creation and preservation of a productive, stable volunteer corps, which in turn will provide quality service both to the service agency and, more importantly, to the public. Well-managed volunteer programs focus on meeting the demands of quality in (1) recruitment; (2) service; (3) retention; and (4) cost effectiveness.

Quality in recruitment demands that the agency knows what it wants and expects from its volunteer corps, and then aims its recruitment campaigns at populations best able to meet the agency's expectations. Targeted recruitment, while it demands a greater effort and time investment up front, pays back with volunteers who bring in skills, and who are more likely to remain in the program because they are wanted; they come to understand that they are wanted and value this recognition.

Another advantage of targeted recruitment is that only individuals appropriate to the function of the agency are approached, thus eliminating the problems which surface when large numbers of individuals who have nonspecific skills are recruited and then the agency must find a use for all of them. Often it is discovered that there are too many individuals who are able to fulfill one task and not enough to fulfill another; consequently, more volunteers need to be recruited, while volunteers already trained must remain idle. This policy is both monetarily inefficient and corrosive to morale.

Quality in service demands that volunteers are well-trained and well-supervised. Individuals recruited into a volunteer corps must be taught and taught clearly what is expected of them and how they are to meet those expectations. Little if anything should be left to chance. It is unfair to assume that the volunteer knows precisely what you want and how you want it done, even if he or she has a professional handle on a given skill. The volunteer must be helped to integrate this skill into the personality and function of the agency. Training is as much a function of integration as it is the communication of information.

Similarly, the function of supervision is more of guidance and development rather than discipline and judgment. Supervision policy and process must encourage the volunteers in the performance of their tasks and assist their growth in both skill and self-assurance.

Quality in retention suggests that skilled and well-functioning volunteers remain in a program not by accident but by design and effort. Since the economic investment in volunteers is primarily their training and only secondarily in their supervision, it makes good fiscal sense to work consciously to maintain the fruits of the initial investment. The longer a volunteer remains productively a part of the corps, the lower the cost to train that volunteer and the lower the cost of the services provided by the volunteer. More importantly the longer the volunteer remains in the corps, the greater their skill and adaptability to work within the process of the agency—they are an incorporated member of the team. It takes time and effort to continually train new people; it takes time, effort, and loss of service to continually integrate new individuals into a team.

The quality of a volunteer program is often measured by its cost effectiveness. While cost considerations need not be the only rationale for a volunteer program, they certainly are important. Any quality program will be designed to achieve the best service for the least amount of money. Volunteer programs have their cost in the staff necessary to train and supervise them. Effective programs which result in a volunteer corps characterized by skill, adaptability, variability, and creativity will be quite cost-efficient. The measure for the cost effectiveness of a volunteer program is not so much what it costs to create and maintain the corps, but how much the corps can provide in both quality and variability of service—what does the corps allow you to offer to the public that could not be offered without it?

Basic Premises Necessary to Attain Goals

The successful attainment of these goals through a system which does not rely on monetary incentive comes just short of being an art form. Volunteerism depends virtually exclusively on an affirmative relational process to attain its specified goals, and this process is a skill under any circumstance; in the context of volunteerism, unbolstered by economic support, it becomes critical.

The relational process necessary to create and maintain a successful volunteer program must flow from a clear, committed philosophical basis. This basis consists of two concomitant sets of premises, the ethical and the relational. The ethical premises, those of integrity, justice, and humanism, are the philosophical foundation for the process; while the relational premises, those of trust, fairness, mutuality, reciprocity, and dialogue, are the actuating behavior of the process. The ethical premises form the essence of the process; the relational premises, the actuality.

The Ethical Premises. The ethical premises form the value system which directs the process of interpersonal relationship. It is commitment to these values which determines the criteria against which behavior is judged, and decisions of policy and procedure are made. Successful volunteer programs are based on policies and procedures which remain committed and faithful to integrity, justice, and humanism.

Integrity is a commitment to reality, consistency, and truthfulness. Integrity demands that individuals and the systems they create recognize the nature of reality and having recognized that nature, work compatibly and affirmatively with that reality. Integrity demands that reality not be denied, mutilated, or distorted, but be honored and credited for its existence and its essence. Integrity demands consistency that actions match spoken words and understood agreements; that policy mirror principle. Integrity demands that truth be honored and continuously respected in thought and deed.

Specific to a volunteer program, integrity demands that administration have a realistic understanding about what is needed and what will be required to meet the need; that these requirements be clearly stated to both the client and the volunteer so that communication is kept open, clear, and appropriate; that what is asked of the volunteer is what is wanted and possible, with no hidden messages, no hidden motives, no hidden circumstances; and that feedback given to the volunteer be inclusive, direct, and always truthful.

Justice is a commitment to fairness, to giving for what is received, to crediting when crediting is due, critiquing when critiquing is deserved. Justice flows from integrity, and while the two are separate in refined essence, they are experienced simultaneously. Justice in a volunteer program demands that all sides be heard and credited, that treatment of the volunteer be fair and equitable in every circumstance, and that there is a recognition of earned trust and reliability as well as open, clear statements of complaints.

Humanism is the capacity to see and respect the other for the honor and dignity they hold by virtue of their status as human. Humanism demands respect, honor, empathy, and judgment that is recognized as individual and subjective, not authoritarian and absolute. Humanism in a volunteer program demands that each individual in the corps be continuously seen, perceived, and responded to with consideration and conscious recognition of his human dignity and needs. Humanism demands that administration relates with constructive process to the volunteer, and that by doing so earns the right for similar consideration from the volunteer.

Relational premises. The relational premises are the modes of behavior which make the abstract principles of ethics concrete. They are the particulars of process which form and maintain relationship; they are the actions and exchanges which engender union and encourage its continuity.

Any relationship which expects to maintain itself and create a constructive history must be founded on trust. Trust building, consequently, becomes a critical dynamic in the relational process. Trust is earned over time and with experience. Trust is generated out of mutual constructive interaction which binds individuals in a common history. Trust cannot be rushed, nor can it be given away, and remain in character. Trust demands mutual disclosure of individual truths; it demands that the individual speak and act with integrity, justice, and humanism. Trust demands appropriate self-disclosure and a corresponding willingness to be held accountable. Trust demands the courage to know one's truth, to say and act one's truth, to hear the other's response to one's truth, and to credit the legitimacy of the other's side.

The creation and maintenance of trust is essential to a successful volunteer program. The trust building must be mutually engaged in by volunteer and agency; it must be mutually earned and felt. The building of trust demands a mutually created history of integrity, honest statements, openly given and carefully adhered to over time.

Fairness encourages trust. Crediting the other's position recognizes his presence and honors his intrinsic value. Fairness encourages reciprocal behavior and works to insure a future in the relationship.

The volunteer must be treated with fairness, fairness based on a commitment to justice. Fairness to the volunteer includes working with him to help make his experience personally enriching. Fairness means openly recognizing his accomplishments and contributions. Fairness requires clearly communicated direction and demands honest criticism delivered with sensitivity and encouragement. Fairness means recognizing that the volunteer is entitled to something back for what he gives.

Reciprocity is the give-and-take necessary to maintain the momentum of relationship. Reciprocity is the interchange within which fairness is experienced, and trust evolves. The balance, which creates reciprocity, actuates in the willingness to give and to receive information, assistance, attitudes, and events. Reciprocity must have the perceived experience of equality but does not need to be tit for tat. It is the recognition of entitlement both in the other and for one's self and the capacity to act on that entitlement.

Reciprocity in the volunteer corps requires that the volunteer be encouraged to share his side, and that when he does share, he is legitimately heard and considered. In turn, the agency also has a right to have its side stated, heard, and worked through to mutual understanding. Reciprocity demands, again, that the volunteer receive from his experience as well as give, and that the agency appreciates and credits what it receives from the volunteer.

Reciprocity requires mutuality. Mutuality is a recognition of relational reality and a willingness to work cooperatively with that reality. Mutuality demands that all parties affected by a given process or decision be consciously, actively included in the evolution of that process or decision. Mutuality precludes authoritarianism and the dictatorial imposition of wants on another. Mutuality demands that all parties involved be given an opportunity to contribute to the processes which will directly affect them, thereby encouraging their sense of inclusion, cooperation, and adaptation. Mutuality forestalls resentment, resistance, and noncooperative reaction; mutuality assists smooth administrative process.

Mutuality with the volunteer corp requires stated recognition of the volunteer's existence and contribution to the process of the organization. It requires that volunteers be included in the development of policy, which will directly affect them as individuals, or which will affect the nature and manner of their work. Throughout the evolution of this process, they must be given legitimate attention and consideration, spoken to with honest, direct statements and heard with openness and sincerity. This willingness to engage in an authentic mutual process does not preclude the legitimate power of the agency to make final policy decisions; in fact, mutuality demands that the volunteer recognize and respect the rights of the agency to exercise its administrative function. The volunteer must credit the administration's side as honorably as the administration credits the volunteer's position.

Trust, fairness, reciprocity, and mutuality are clearly interdependent, each interlocked and supportive of the other in a productive process of human relationship. The key to the actuality of this process is the additional premise of commitment to dialogue. Dialogue, the concrete mutual, reciprocal, fair exchange of each individual's "I" truths, may not guarantee universal positive resolution, but it will generate trust, and consequently lay the foundation for a process which is most often constructive, progressive, and highly productive.

Dialogue not only encourages cooperation and integration but it generates creativity. It is out of dialogue that new perceptions, new insights, and new approaches find their way to consideration and often productive implementation. Dialogue engenders the productiveness of a team model. Dialogue is essential to the team process; an attempt to create and maintain a team approach without dialogue is doomed to fail.

Dialogue, the clear, direct sharing of "I" statements, must be encouraged with and from the volunteer corps. Volunteers must be informed of the agency's position particularly on issues which directly affect them. In turn, their "I" statements must be given the time and place to be voiced and the crediting they warrant. Volunteers must be known, spoken with, and credited. In turn, the agency must also be known, heard, and credited. This requires a system of practices which consciously and deliberately encourages dialogue, support groups, in-service programs, retreats, one-on-one interviews, and reasonable access to volunteer supervisors and agency personnel. The time commitment this requires is reciprocally balanced with a relatively smooth and productive process. It is much easier and much less costly in time and money to proactively forestall personnel problems than to reactively attempt to counter and correct problems after the fact.

Program Design

What has been discussed so far has been a consideration of desires, premises, wants, and beliefs which form the abstract foundations for a successful volunteer program. How to make these principles concrete both in design and execution needs to be addressed next. With concreteness and effectiveness in mind, attention will now be focused on the specifics for a program design.

Director of Volunteers

Any program, no matter how well-designed, is as effective as the individuals involved in its execution. With this postulate in mind, it seems appropriate to begin a discussion of program design with (1) a description of expectations and responsibilities associated with the creation of the position of Director of Volunteers, and (2) a description and recommendation about the nature and capability of the individual hired to serve in this function. Both these points warrant careful consideration, because, realistically, the function given to the position of Director of Volunteers and how that function is executed, greatly determines the success of a volunteer program.

Job Description

The Director of Volunteers is usually responsible for (1) recruitment; (2) selection, (3) placement; (4) supervision; and (5) evaluation. In addition, many programs are designed so that training is included as the director's responsibility, although this can be changed. The advantage, however, of facilitating the entry and bonding of new members into an established corps, is obviously hampered to some degree when training is done by an outside individual.

The Director of Volunteers should hold equal status with other divisional directors in an agency and be directly responsible to the Administrative Director. It must be remembered that the Director of Volunteers will be responsible for the administration of a division which houses a significant number of people; in fact, in many home care agencies, the volunteer corps represents, in gross number of personnel, the largest division in the agency. The degree of responsibility held by the director is measured by the number of functions he is accountable to perform, the number of personnel under his supervision, and the fact that personnel in this division usually have the greatest amount of contact hours with the public which could represent significant risk if mismanaged.

The Director of Volunteers is usually responsible to the executive or managing director of the agency. Occasionally, the position of Director of Volunteers is combined with or responsible to the social service division or, in a few instances, to the pastoral unit. In still other instances, the Director of Volunteers is a volunteer, an arrangement which works well, provided nothing major occurs for which the director might be held accountable. When this position is held on a volunteer basis, it limits the power of the executive administration to hold the division accountable; this is a subtle point but warrants careful consideration before instituting a totally volunteer division.

In addition to administrative and educational responsibilities, the Director of Volunteers should, ideally, perform a counseling function. The capacity to defuse psychodynamic problems as they begin to evolve is invaluable in the administration of a problem-limited agency. The Director of Volunteers, as does any director of any division, needs to be able to keep problems from developing. He must be aggressively proactive in philosophy and policy, so that there is need for a limited amount of reactive administrative decisions. This helps keep the general balance of administrative power and momentum in place, and helps the executive director maintain an effective, assertive leadership role.

In most home care agencies, team work is essential. First, it is the Director of Volunteers' responsibility to inculcate and nurture a cooperative team interaction within the corps itself. Second, the director must function as the chief catalyst to assist the integration of the corps with the general agency team. The director's responsibility is to help the corps remain cognitively, emotionally, and functionally integrated with the agency as a whole. Finally, it is the obligation of the volunteer director to assure that the corps' function meets and matches the general service needs of the agency and its divisions. The director is responsible for seeing that the corps delivers, and delivers with some skill, the services requested by the various divisions of the agency.

Special Skills Required. Ideally, the individual who functions as volunteer director should have administrative, educational, and psychotherapeutic skills. It is difficult to find one individual who has talent, experience, and training in all three of these areas, so often compromises must be made. It must be remembered, however, that the more compromises agreed to, the weaker the structure and the greater the potential for problems. With this in mind, a good rule of thumb would be that any individual hired to act as Director of Volunteers should be skilled in performing at least two of the three ideal functions of the job. In addition, no compromise should be made on administrative capability. Individuals who are skilled in administration and education would be suitable, and the psychodynamic function could be assured by the social service division; or individuals who are skilled in administration and psychotherapy could forfeit the educational function to an outside contract. It is, however, very risky to have as director an individual who has only administrative skills. This creates too weak a structure by dividing responsibility and thereby accountability. It is difficult, virtually impossible, to administrate an integrated division if the majority of responsibilities are farmed out, because this also "farms out" accountability and control.

Background and Credentializing. Individuals who are trained and experienced in administration (particularly health care or social service administration), who have an additional background in teaching or counseling would be very suitable for this position. The individual should be empathetic, perceptive, capable of being supportive to others, have well-developed listening and communication skills, and be relatively charismatic, or at least capable of stimulating bonding, cohesion, and commitment from a group. In addition, the individual should be skilled in evaluation and decision making, capable of exercising his responsibility with decisiveness, strength, and the courage to accept responsibility and be held accountable.

Ideally, the individual should hold at least a master's degree in psychology, sociology, human services, administration, or related fields; and have a minimum of three years experience working with groups or the public. The credentials are important, but the bottom line is the effectiveness of the individual in the job; consequently, exceptions to specific credentials are always possible.

Structure of the Corps

The structure of the corps must be logically and thoughtfully developed. This structuring begins with a careful evaluation of what is expected in performance from the corps; and what they will be doing. Their various functions should be conceptualized in terms that are concrete and specific, e.g., cataloging books for a library, cooking, filling in for personnel shortages in other divisions, such as social service or nursing. Once it is determined what the corps is expected to do, then an educated guess about how many individuals will be needed to fulfill the functions listed must be made. What should be avoided is having too many volunteers who can serve a function for which there is limited use and not enough volunteers to fill functions where there is demand.

Home care volunteer corps should contain individuals who are proficient in general social skills, homemaking, child care, fine arts, and fundraising skills. In addition, a percentage of the corps should have professional skills in nursing, social work, geriatric care, business, law, library science, virtually any area in which the agency sees itself potentially involved. The greater the versatility of the corps, the greater the agency's potential for service and for lowering costs of service. A volunteer corps should be envisioned as a pool of resources, both in the skills contained by the individuals themselves, and the potential these individuals offer through the networking of their contacts. Each individual brings not only himself and his skills into the corps, but he brings his world as well!

All volunteers enlisted in the corps should be required to attend a training program designed by the agency to orient the individuals into the expectations and procedures of the organization. The training program should be structured so that the focus includes orientation and group integration, in addition to factual data. The skills and talents brought into the corps by the volunteers must be recognized and credited; training programs must be flexible enough to enhance and facilitate a variety of volunteer offerings, and never designed to suffocate, mutilate, denigrate, or disregard what the volunteer offers as his own. Training programs must come from a position of respect, reinforcement, and facilitation rather than from a position of haughty authoritarianism and unilateral righteousness.

Program Structure

Recruitment. Appropriate time and consideration given to a recruitment campaign can save a great deal of time, effort, and money later on in the management of a successful volunteers corps. As described before, targeted recruitment is well worth the time and effort it involves, because it guarantees an appropriately populated resource pool and aids morale by assuring that those recruited will be appreciated and used.

In-home care agencies should begin their recruitment programs with a careful examination of the services the agency offers and those which can legitimately be expected from a volunteer corps; what can the corps be expected to do for the agency, and what can they be trained to do for the public served by the agency. The following outline is generally adaptable, and would serve as a base for virtually any in-home care volunteer corps:

Volunteers who have skills most appropriate:

For the agency	*For the public*
Librarians	Nurses
Accountants	Physicians' assistants
Lawyers	Physical therapists
Bookkeepers	Educators
Grant writers	Social workers
Fundraisers	Clergy
Secretaries	Psychotherapists
Computer operators	Homemakers
Publicity personnel	

An attempt should be made to recruit individuals who have specialties within these areas, areas which are concurrent with Physicians' assistants the specialties of the agency. For example, if a particular agency specializes in the care of terminal children, then individuals who are familiar with nursing, psychotherapy, physical therapy, and any other area specific to children, should be sought.

Obviously, familiarity with the structure and service function of the agency is important when choosing a recruitment target, but equally important is a familiarity with the demographic nature of the population served by the agency. A concerted effort must be made to recruit a complementary, representative sample of the service population. Here the issues relevant to the client population which must be considered include:

- Number of males and females in client population

- Age factors

- Racial and ethnic factors

- Educational factors

- Socioeconomic factors

- Religious factors

- And neighborhood ethnocentric factors

Every attempt should be made to recruit volunteers from each demographic group perceived as essential and representative of the client population. Good recruitment policy should result in a corps which has flexibility, adaptability, and enough variety in resources to creatively meet virtually any challenge of service offered by the population. In short, the corps should match in demographic makeup, the makeup of the population served; and it should match in resources the wants and needs of the agency's clients.

Recruits can be gathered from a variety of sources. Individuals with professional and semiprofessional skills can be acquired through tapping into the volunteer programs of business and industry, professional service organizations and clubs, and professional schools, particularly for combined volunteer-internship programs. Contact with these sources should be personal and ongoing, and the director of volunteers must be responsible for the cultivation of a large, solidly woven network of personal contacts in each of these recruitment areas. In addition, volunteers from the existing corps can be trained to speak to church groups, women's organizations, general social service clubs, and special interest groups which might have an interest in the function and services offered by the agency. The development of a speaker's bureau within the corps is an excellent technique. This involves the development of a brochure, listing a variety of topics about which members of the corps are willing and capable to talk, circulating these pamphlets in appropriate places, and following up with phone calls and personal arrangements for bookings.

Publicity is an important factor in the recruitment plan. It's a good idea to begin by seeking out for recruitment an individual who has some degree of skill in creating, developing, and executing publicity campaigns. This individual might be someone who is actually in public relations, but may also be someone familiar with newspaper writing, advertising, etc. Once this individual is in place then they can take the responsibility for designing public relations programs aimed at general recruitment. In addition, remember that every constructively used and credited volunteer in the corps will recruit for the corps through their spoken enthusiasm. Good recruitment demands that you know what you are doing as an agency, and that you have a good idea of where you are going and how you are going to get there. How you are going to get there should include the creation of a corps which has as its goal not only service, but the capacity to be self-generating. When you begin by recruiting individuals who are skilled in recruitment, you are well on your way; simply credit their skill, maintain basic guidance and cohesiveness, and allow your original recruits to do what they do best — recruit.

Evaluation. Evaluation is one of the more difficult functions of the volunteer director. Bad decisions can be costly in many ways; consequently, it is essential that the volunteer director have some basic familiarity with standard evaluation instruments and techniques, but in addition he should have well-developed, well-tested visceral reactions.

Every candidate should be required to have a private initial interview with the director. At this point, the candidate should be evaluated for basic social skills, generally appropriate behavior and expression, and for the identification of any gross problems which would make the candidate inappropriate for recruitment. A conversational interview of 30 to 45 minutes is usually enough time to give a general sense of the individual's personality. If there is a desire to be more clinical, any one of the standard personality tests could be administered at the end of the interview, and then the individual could be told that he will hear from the agency concerning his status.

The guideline for this evaluation must be appropriateness for the program, not whether the director "likes" the individual or not. Evaluations must be kept as fair as possible, and that requires looking at what is needed to do the job and how much the individual being interviewed fits the need.

Once past the initial interview, the candidates should be informed that they will be under ongoing evaluation during the training period. This is one of the reasons it is a good idea to have training periods which extend over a period of time (4 to 6 weeks); it gives the extended opportunity necessary for a fair and accurate evaluation. During the training period, candidates should be evaluated in terms of creativity, insightfulness, cooperativeness, empathetic capacity, adaptability, and capability to work well within the group. In addition, attention should be given to identification of leadership potential and talents. It is an excellent idea to include a practicum period at the conclusion of the training course. This practicum should include at least six hours of on-site observation and supervised participation by the candidate in activities appropriate for the volunteer corps. Candidates should be evaluated by their practicum supervisor, and this evaluation should be reviewed by the volunteer director before the closing interview.

The closing interview should be conducted as a mutual dialogue between the candidate and the volunteer director; both parties should be open and frank in this discussion. If a candidate has been less than appropriate for a particular volunteer program, the individual should be credited for skills they do hold. An explanation should be given for why this particular program is not suitable for them, and constructive suggestions should be given for situations which might prove more mutually fulfilling. Candidates who do appear to be appropriate need to be clearly informed about how their skills will be incorporated into the program and what their rights and responsibilities will be as members of the corps. In all cases, time must be given to hear and discuss a candidate's concerns, questions, and opinions. In addition, candidates should be reminded that they are subject to continuous evaluation, and that there is a mutual right to terminate the relationship at any point if either volunteer or agency finds that necessary. Finally, a contract, stipulating the rights, responsibilities, and terms of the relationship, should be jointly signed and each participant should receive a copy.

Training Program. The goals of a well-developed and well-delivered training program must be focused on: (1) the integration of the recruit into the agency; (2) the inculcation of necessary skills and pertinent information; and (3) the encouragement and direction of pre-existing skills and information brought into the program by the candidate. Training programs should be aimed at enhancement and integration, rather than reformation and visionary indoctrination; and on development and adaptability, rather than reconstruction and remolding.

A syllabus which has proven successful with a variety of training classes includes the following:

Structure: 24 hours of class time, divided into two 2-hour sessions, for six weeks plus six hours of practicum experience, for a total of 30 instructional hours.

Delivery: Appropriate team members with one core instructor to provide continuity and integration as well as group cohesion. Methods should include lecture and discussion, demonstration and guided hands-on experience, and group process.

Content Breakdown

Session 1: The general introduction focuses primarily on structure, function, and general process of the agency, including introduction of personnel and demonstration of procedures.

Session 2: The context presentation focuses on what they will do; where they will do it, and with whom; and how the current program relates to work which they have already done in other areas.

Session 3: The history of the movement involved e.g., if a hospice is involved, a full explanation and differentiation of types, forms, and methods of hospice care is presented along with discussion of the philosophical roots of the program, the notion and practice of confidentiality and professional responsibility.

Session 4: This is the presentation of materials by the social service division including policy and practice and issues of integration and cohesiveness.

Session 5: This is the presentation by the medical division including material on pain control, psychiatry, and other relevant medical issues.

Session 6: This is the presentation and demonstration of material from the nursing division including basic information on lifting the patient, making a bed, etc.

Session 7: This presentation considers basic sociological issues surrounding in-home care, general information and significant demographics in the catchment area served by the agency, and discussion of social and legal issues.

Session 8: This session covers communication skills including nonverbal communication, listening skills and basic evaluation methods — factual, cognitive, and affective levels of evaluation.

Session 9: This session covers communication skills and involves demonstration, practice, and application of methods to various psychological situations.

Session 10: This is a presentation and consideration of issues on family dynamics: variability in family structure and function, what they might find, how they must adjust, and when they need to refer.

Session 11: This session considers religious dynamics and their function and influence on patient and family and includes a chaplain.

Session 12: Discusses ethical issues: suicide, euthanasia, confidentiality, integrity, and responsibility along with a general review and closure.

The case review is a method of engendering thematic cohesiveness throughout the lectures. In addition, it is an excellent method of integrating new members into the ongoing work experience of the agency. A current case seen as didactically appropriate should be chosen, introduced with initial relevant data at the second session, and then in each session thereafter the material being presented that day should be applied summarily to the ongoing case study. The result should be clarity, concreteness, and a growing familarity with the agency process; in addition, there should be a distinct evolution of identification, inclusiveness, and integration, and a feeling of developing familiarity and confidence within the volunteer candidate.

The practicum, as discussed above, gives the agency a unique opportunity for on-site evaluation. In addition, it offers the volunteer candidate a chance to experience concretely what he might have only imagined. Experiencing the reality allows the candidate to discover whether or not he really wants to do this work; it's one thing to imagine a role, but another to live it.

There are two formats which the practicum can follow: (1) accompanying as an observer an in-home care nurse during rounds, and (2) assisting a working volunteer. Ideally, both formats can be included with the nursing observation as the formal practicum experience, and the volunteer assistance as a primary step in actual volunteer function. It is important for the volunteer director to do a debriefing with each candidate as he completes his nursing observation; this gives the candidate a chance to work through any surfaced concerns or anxieties, and at the same time it allows the volunteer director to acquire necessary firsthand feedback from the experience.

It is important that clear recognition and credit be given to the volunteers who successfully complete the training program. This is a factor of both incorporation and morale. Successful candidates should be formally issued certificates of completion at a graduation ceremony. It is not at all inappropriate to schedule an evening event, off-site at a town hall, a church auditorium, etc., with a guest keynote speaker, the distribution of certificates to each recipient, and a reception. Graduation should be seen as a rite of passage and initiation, marking a distinct shift of status, based on the recognition of skill. It is a formal recognition of the candidates as fully functioning members of the corps; it is a statement of welcome, trust, and inclusion.

Retention. The capacity to retain individuals who do their job with skill and dedication is always a goal for volunteer programs. Retention is usually important in any personnel program, because it should guarantee a maintenance of quality in service or product. Consistency, commitment, personal identification and consequent responsibility, loyalty, and increased skill which comes from experience, are all excellent reasons for encouraging retention. In a volunteer program the economic factor makes retention programs essential. The cost of volunteer labor is primarily in recruiting and training. Once the initial investment has been made, the cost of supervision should be significantly lower. Because the largest cost invested in an individual volunteer comes up front and maintenance costs are significantly lower, it stands to reason that the longer the individual remains in active and productive service, the greater the return on the initial cost. The expense of training an individual is clearly and significantly diminished by the length of his service.

The key to a strong retention program is a commitment by the agency to a policy of equitability, mutuality, and fairness. It is essential to remember that while volunteers are not paid, they do need payback! It is essential that individuals get something back for what they give. If this balance of giving and receiving is not maintained, it will not be long before corps members will begin to feel victimized. Volunteers want to feel useful, not used.

Payback is given in recognition, reward, and respect. Recognition demands that volunteers, both collectively and individually, be credited for the nature and quality of what they do. Individuals need to have communicated to them that their immediate supervisor and the agency sees and understands what they are actually producing. The volunteer needs to *know*, by being told, that the director is aware and appreciative of the difficulties involved in the volunteer's performance of responsibilities. Recognition demands that the director be familiar with the person and his performance as a volunteer, and that this understanding be communicated to the volunteer as acknowledgement and praise at regular intervals.

Rituals of reward are part of the paycheck in volunteerism. Open, formal, public rewards for quality of service are necessary for morale and to help maintain retention. Rewards, whatever specific form they take, should always involve some degree of public recognition for the individual or the corps and for the quality of their work.

Authenticity of respect can only be communicated if the director truly does know the volunteer and his work and therefore takes the time and effort to communicate that familiarity. Authenticity of respect demands that the director perform his job responsibilities with a high degree of commitment and involvement. It is the director's responsibility to develop appropriate relationships with each volunteer and within the context of this relationship to understand perceptively the capacity and character of each corps member. Authenticity communicates when it exists; if the goal is to communicate respect, then the director must be committed to behavior which engenders an honest and appropriate knowledge of an appreciation for each individual member of the corps. Basically, the issue here is integrity, an integrity which is quickly recognized by the volunteer and responded to with appreciation, trust, and mutuality.

In an attempt to maintain a high degree of retention, the director must decide how to support the individual members by providing recognition, rewards, and respect. Basically, this goal can be accomplished through structures of interchange which fall into two broad categories: (1) those activities which are the specific personal effort of the director, and (2) those activities which involve the participation of the agency and the corps.

Under the first category, it is essential that the director know the members of the corps. A file containing as much relevant data as can be acquired should be kept on each member. Information which is standard to a resume obviously should be present in this file; but the profile should be broadened to include details of life events, personal traits, unique characteristics and relationships—anything and everything that will help the director to know and understand the volunteer. Obviously, all information should be kept confidential. A complete medical and psychological history enhanced by an appropriate social history should be acquired if possible. Updates of addresses and phone numbers and changes in name, marital status, and jobs are essential. The record should include basic information on the volunteer's mate and family, e.g., names, employment, etc. so that a sense of the volunteer's social context and needs is continuously, accurately maintained.

The director must make every effort to keep the dialogue open with members of the corps. The maintenance of dialogue involves time, relational skill, and commitment to the process.

Approximately twenty-five percent of the director's time should be dedicated to the "cultivation of the garden." This cultivation involves time spent in direct interchange with the volunteers as individuals and as a group. Individual time can be created in a variety of different ways. It is a good idea to have lunch periodically with individual members of the corps at the initiative of the director. The lunches should be informal and conducive to open dialogue. They should occur at least once a year, more frequently if the calendar permits. Individual lunches offer time and opportunity for personal disclosure, needed recognition, mutual evaluation, and for defusing anxiety and receiving affirmation. In addition, they serve to enhance and maintain the bonding and integration of the volunteer with the program and as such are a major tool in retention.

It is important that the director advocate on behalf of volunteers, as individuals and as a group, to the agency. The corps needs someone to speak on its behalf, to exhibit concern for its interests, and to act as a peer representative within the management level of the agency. This can be a delicate balance for the director who is obligated to meet the needs of the agency as well as the corps. Every attempt must be made to keep the corps bonded and integrated with the agency so that goals become reciprocal and mutual. The director must be open and truthful in all communications, both to the corps and to the agency; this includes making statements of the inability to disclose when permission to discuss an issue has not been received from involved parties. Basically, it must be recognized that it is the responsibility of the director to safeguard the fair treatment of corps members and to work to maintain trust, equitability and mutuality.

It is also the responsibility of the director to maintain clear communication between the agency's administration and the corps. Weekly meetings with the executive are quite appropriate when possible. These discussions should center on a mutual exchange of information, interest, and concern in which management is kept informed of the function and character of the corps. The director can then be informed of the management's attitude and insights concerning the corps.

In addition, it is the responsibility of the director to meet with the corps, ideally on a weekly basis. These meetings should function as an open exchange of information and attitudes. They should be conducted as open dialogues directed toward goals of understanding and cohesion. These discussions are clearly an essential tool in maintaining good communication; but in addition, they serve to identify and defuse problems of anxiety, insecurity, rumor, and discontent before they fester into major administrative difficulties.

Mentioned above was the director's responsibility for the organization and facilitation of collective methods to assist retention. These collective tools include operating a weekly support group, conducting recognition events, offering periodic inservice programs, and awarding certification and credentialization when possible.

Support groups are essential in maintaining an effective volunteer program. Ideally, the support group should meet once a week and be open to all volunteers. The group should not exceed 20 participants; if group numbers are consistently higher, a second group should be formed. The group must have a professional facilitator; if the director is not qualified to act in this capacity, someone with appropriate credentials should be enlisted. The presence of a professional is required because the basic function of the group is to be therapeutic rather than "self-help" oriented. The issues which surface from in-home care volunteerism are often heavily ladened psychologically and warrant therapeutic response. A well-conducted support group can forestall numerous problems, even some of a very serious nature, before they have a chance to begin. The group should function therapeutically (defusing emotional or conceptual issues before they evolve into a crisis); educationally (with continued instruction which is relevant to the volunteers' current experiences); and cohesively (members begin to identify with and support each other as a group).

Group sessions should be one and one-half hours in length. This gives enough time for all members to participate if they so choose. It is helpful to have a therapeutic theme for each session. For example, the issue of the volunteer's self-confidence might be chosen. The facilitator then introduces the theme and as the group progresses with discussion of the individual volunteer's experiences and concerns, the facilitator clarifies, interprets, and interconnects individual contributions along the thematic lines. This process serves to educate, to affect therapeutically, and to encourage group identification and cohesion. Alternatively, the thematic line can be extracted by the facilitator from the group process. In this case, the group begins its process immediately, and the facilitator, having paid close and perceptive attention, extracts whatever thematic thread begins to surface, mirrors it back to the group, clarifies, elaborates, and again reinforces the theme as the group process continues. Here again, the same positive effect of education, therapy, and cohesion can be achieved, with a final result of minimal crisis and burn-out within the corps.

Everyone needs to feel a sense of accomplishment and competency, regardless of what it is we have chosen to do; this is especially true for volunteers. For this reason, recognition events are essential to maintain individual involvement in the volunteer corps. Recognition events should include graduation, an awards lunch, a Christmas event, a mate's dinner, and a summer picnic hosted by the agency.

Graduation, as discussed above, should be a special event, held in the evening, off campus, with a guest speaker and the distribution of certificates of completion. A reception following the ritual always is well received and serves to enhance group identity and belonging.

An awards lunch, given by the director usually in the early spring or fall, serves to publicly affirm the director's recognition and appreciation for the corps and its members. The lunch is for the corps, and outside individuals should be invited only at the initiative of the volunteers; this includes invitations extended to other members of the agency. The lunch provides an excellent opportunity for a review of in-house corps business and the highlights of the preceding year of service. In addition, specific awards for contribution and performance can be given. The main theme, however, should be the affirmation of the corps as a unit. An open statement of appreciation for the quality of their performance and commitment should be the central focus of the luncheon.

A mate's dinner is essential for any assertive retention program. In-home care volunteers have a degree of involvement in their work which is rivaled by few paid employees. The work tends to hold the volunteers emotionally and intellectually. It is as though a part of the person is put aside especially for this work, and those who are close to the volunteer are acutely aware of this surrender. Mates may become uneasy, competitive, and in some cases jealous of the volunteer's time and invested concern. Often the mate may experience the volunteer's new commitment as a personal loss, and may subtly or aggressively agitate for their mate to resign from the corps. This agitation can be eased by giving recognition and credit to the mate's position. An off-campus dinner sponsored by the agency and hosted by the corps can be given in February or March. February and March tend to be depressing periods, times when issues that are pieces of sand during the rest of the year become pebbles. It is quite appropriate for all agency administrators to be invited, and the executive administrator as well as the Director of Volunteers, should be asked to address the group. Regardless of the general theme chosen for the evening, it is essential that direct recognition of the mate's position and difficulties be expressed. Statements must be open and discussion direct, not subtle or alluding. The mate's side must be clearly credited, and it is essential that the agency thank these individuals for their support and recognize them as nonrostered members of the team! Again, the goal is cohesion and dissipation of dissatisfaction before it blossoms into crisis; in addition, the dinner serves an advocacy function for the volunteers and consequently directly bolsters their adhesion to the program by increasing their trust in the agency as a concerned personal resource.

Christmas parties and summer picnics are events best sponsored by the agency. The Christmas party can include only agency personnel, while the summer picnic can effectively include family members, mates, and children. Again, the purpose is cohesion, affirmation, recognition, and the nurturing of group identification. In these two events, the stress is on cohesion and identification with the agency, as well as with the corps.

In-service programs provide continuing education for the corps in addition to a psychodynamic function. A full-day, in-service program in the fall, planned and prepared by the volunteers, works very well. A central theme, a guest speaker, and appropriate representation from the agency are the basic ingredients. The day can be broken into a morning and an afternoon session with a luncheon in between; is a good idea to leave plenty of time for group process and participation. What is important is that the volunteers get something and learn something from whatever is offered, that the corps be involved in every aspect of the planning and presentation, that they in fact "own" the day. The goal is to reinforce involvement and commitment and to stimulate the enthusiasm and spirit of the corps with new learning, new insights, and new possibilities.

A feeling of belonging, of being an integral, appreciated part of the team is an essential dynamic in retention. Consequently, it is important that a conscious and consistent effort be made by the agency as a whole to continuously integrate the volunteers into the spirit and function of the agency. This is as much an attitude as it is a mode of behavior, an attitude which must pervade policy and be actively present in the day-to-day interaction of the agency. The bottom line is that volunteers remain present and active if they feel useful, appreciated, rewarded, and a necessary part of the team.

Volunteers who remain with the corps need to feel competent and successful. With this need in mind, the Director of Volunteers should make every effort, when placing the individual volunteer on an assignment, to place the volunteer for success.

Placing a volunteer for success demands that the director know each volunteer, know the particulars of each case, and carefully match the volunteer's skills and personality to the needs demanded in the placement case. It is helpful to envision each case in the context in which the volunteer must function, because the object is to choose an individual who, when placed in the case context, will work productively, for the good of all concerned.

Placement must begin with an evaluation visit to the family by the Director of Volunteers. Evaluation data to be considered should include:

1. Patient's physical and psychosocial needs,

2. Family's physical and psychosocial needs,

3. Family structure and basic dynamics,

4. Relevant demographic data such as socioeconomic levels of family, education, ethnicity, religion, race, etc.

Once this material has been gathered, a general profile of family needs and functions can be created, and a volunteer chosen who is perceived as compatible with the case dynamics. A great deal of this process is procedural, but the director should have an intuitive capacity for match-making. No matter how much data are collected, success often rests on the perceptual ability of the director to match precisely the right volunteer with the right case context. If the match is fundamentally compatible, the success of the case, in terms of resultant positive resolutions, is close to guaranteed barring introduced or unforeseen circumstances.

Once placement has been made, a schedule for supervisory contact must be followed. Ideally, it is good for the director to accompany the volunteers on an introductory visit to the family. This gives the director an on-site opportunity to make sure that there is in fact basic compatibility between the volunteer and the context. On the day when the volunteer actually begins the assignment, a brief visit or phone call from the director is both affirming and supportive. Hereafter, periodic on-site visits for evaluation and morale are appropriate. The frequency of these visits depends on the complexity of the case and its length. Cases which are complicated demand more attention, and cases which extend over lengthy durations demand periodic visits to sustain volunteer morale. In addition, periodic brief meetings in the office for review and suggestion are appropriate.

The volunteer should be present at team meetings and encouraged to participate in the case report. Here again it is the director's responsibility to facilitate this participation and evaluate its content for accuracy, compatibility, and effectiveness. Remembering always that the main objects of supervision include education and development of the volunteer as well as quality service to the client, the director needs to provide feedback privately to the volunteer about his contribution.

There are times when cases do not work out as anticipated, no matter how carefully the preparation work has been done. It is the director's responsibility to initiate and facilitate the exit of a volunteer in these cases. Circumstances which warrant this intervention include situations where the health and safety of the volunteer are at risk, where gross incompatibility of personalities develops, and where the family dynamics are fundamentally dysfunctional and threaten the general procedure of the case.

It is the responsibility of the director to advocate on behalf of the volunteer to the family and to the agency in these circumstances, and in any situation where it is critical that the volunteer's side be heard. In this regard, the director is answerable for the creation and maintenance of an open, constructive dialogue. This demands a degree of diplomatic skill and courage. In the end, however, it takes less courage to deal directly with each crisis as it arrives than to let discontent and antagonism grow to major proportions, and then attempt to deal with them; again, the object is to keep problems from ever developing rather than figuring out how to cope with them after the fact. The object is to be consistently proactive, consistently in control, and thereby minimize the necessity to respond reactively.

Summary

A successful volunteer program demands that the agency in general and the director in particular have a clear, mutual understanding of a relational ethic that is conscientiously and consistently concretized in program design and process. There must be an active commitment to the ethical values of integrity, justice, and humanism. These values must influence policy and decision making at every level, acting as an integrating thread of uniformity and consistency. In addition, there must be an active commitment by all involved parties to the relational premises of trust, fairness, mutuality, reciprocity and dialogue; premises which must be experienced in and through the daily process of the program. The bottom line is that quality recruits, who are appropriately and skillfully trained and supervised are retained and remain productive, thereby increasing the quality of service and cost efficiency of a good volunteer program. Fair treatment and justice for all parties involved pays dividends and insures results on every level in every way, regardless of the currency used, whether it be monetary or relational.

A Cooperative Volunteer Training Program*

How a VNA worked with a hospital to teach volunteers to assist in home and hospital care

Marilyn D. Harris and Bette Groshens

> There's no one left of my friends to visit me. They are all in the same boat. My daughter tries to come once a week, but she has her own life and family. My sight is too poor for me to sew or read anymore. You've no idea how much I would appreciate someone to come over and just visit and spend the afternoon; the days are pretty long. How nice it would be to share an hour with someone.

We will describe a cooperative volunteer training program conceived, planned, and carried out by the Visiting Nurse Association of Eastern Montgomery County (VNA) and Abington Memorial Hospital to prepare volunteers to assist the professional staff with the care of patients at home and in the hospital. This venture also helped to meet an identified need expressed by the patient who wanted someone to "just visit and spend the afternoon."

Background Information. Abington Memorial Hospital is a trustee-operated, nonprofit, short-term community teaching hospital. Since it opened in 1914, it has grown from a 48-bed emergency station erected in the midst of farmland to a 500-bed regional medical center serving a population of 350,000. The hospital is accredited by the Joint Commission of Accreditation of Hospitals and the American Hospital Association. The Volunteer Department of the hospital was formed in 1956 and currently has 450 volunteers (per week) assigned throughout the hospital.

The Home Care Department of the hospital accepted its first patient on July 1, 1980 and is accredited and certified as a hospital-based home health agency. The Department provides home care services to patients who are essentially homebound for medical reasons and who require nursing and therapeutic services on an intermittent basis.

The Visiting Nurse Association (VNA) is a voluntary, accredited, certified home health agency that provides multidisciplinary care to persons who are confined to their homes because of illness or disability. The VNA was established in 1919. The agency started with a staff of one and now employs 75 full-time equivalents. The hospital Home Care Department provides direct service of physical therapy and occupational therapy to selected patients and contracts with the VNA to provide nursing, medical social work, speech pathology and home health aide services to patients in their homes. An excellent working relationship exists between the hospital and the VNA.

Since August of 1980 the Home Care Department has been most fortunate in having very dedicated volunteers. The volunteers perform a number of clerical tasks including statistical summaries, answering telephones, and typing. A hospital volunteer also serves as a member of the Home Care Department's Advisory Committee.

---

* Reprinted with permission of *Home Healthcare Nurse* from a cooperative volunteer training program, Vol. 3, No. 3, pp. 37-40 by Marilyn Harris and Bette Groshens (May/June 1985).

The hospital's Director of Volunteer Services was very interested in initiating a pilot cooperative effort with another community agency. In cooperation with the hospital's Home Care Department and the Department of Volunteer Services, the VNA identified a need for volunteers to work with the professional staff in providing care to persons in their homes.

Support Groups. In October of 1980, the Home Care Department's Advisory Committee supported the concept of volunteers in the home. Although the proposal was approved in 1980, it was not actively pursued until 1982.

Approval for this cooperative arrangement had full support of the Home Care Department's Advisory Committee and the hospital's Board of Trustees. In February of 1982, the Professional Advisory Committee and the Board of Directors of the VNA gave unanimous support to the program.

Why Volunteers? Volunteer services are not new to either the VNA or the hospital. Each facility depends upon volunteers to meet the needs of the facility, including the Board of Directors and Professional Advisory Committee, and the needs of the patients. The hospital has volunteers in most departments. The VNA uses clerical volunteers in several areas, such as Well Baby Clinics, Senior Centers, and in the office. Direct service volunteers are involved in the Hospice Program.

The use of volunteers is essential and beneficial for several reasons:

- Cutbacks in federal, state, and local funding make it imperative that community health administrators make use of resources, both human and physical, within the community so that health care services are available to those in need.

- Volunteers are consumers of services and their direct involvement with the agency and its patients makes for enlightened consumers who are then willing to tell others about the available services and opportunities.

- Volunteers involve community support for an organization.

- Volunteers gain personal satisfaction while being beneficial to patients.

What Tasks Will the Volunteers Perform? Consideration had to be given to developing a mutually agreeable job description (assignment guide) that would be submitted for approval to the Professional Advisory Committees and appropriate committees and boards of both facilities.

As a first step, the hospital's Director of Volunteer Services met with the VNA director and staff nurses to determine the range of services required by the patients in the home. These suggestions were put into an assignment guide that was reviewed with insurance companies for both facilities. The assignment guide included the following:

- major functions;
- duties;
- hours;

- qualifications, and

- training.

The planning phase thus far identified the need for volunteers and their duties. The next step addressed the course content and the instructors. The decision was made to use an outside resource person who was involved in volunteer training programs to teach our first course in cooperation with in-house personnel.

We also explored the possibility of offering this course through the local community college, thereby involving additional community support. The Director of Continuing Education at the college was contacted and the appropriate arrangements were made with an identified resource person.

Course content was most important. To meet the hospital's criteria for volunteers, a person has to be certified by members of the hospital staff for direct patient services, such as feeding, transfer, and ambulation. Because the ability of the volunteer to follow the patient from home to hospital and back for continuity of care was the unique concept, the curriculum included the following:

- psychosocial skills — 24 hours taught by psychologists;

- cardiopulmonary resuscitation — 4 hours taught by hospital personnel;

- transfer, feeding techniques — 2 hours taught by hospital personnel, and

- observation through home visits — 6 hours with the visiting nurse.

The classroom course included an outline of general health care services, description of volunteers, type of services performed, how volunteers function, touching, listening, body language, record-keeping and how to handle specific situations.

Funding. Another consideration was funding. Neither the hospital nor the VNA had funds incorporated into the current budget to cover the cost of this course. Although the amount involved was small in relation to total budgets, it was felt that a local business firm might be interested in underwriting the cost of this course. The VNA's director contacted the gifts chairman of one company requesting money for the cost of the course and books. In a short time, a response was received with a check to cover the cost of the course.

Recruitment of Volunteers. Recruitment and selection of the volunteers was under the supervision of the hospital's Director of Volunteer Services. The director did the initial interview. Applicants interested in this new program who met the criteria had a second interview with the director of the hospital's Home Care Department and the VNA before the final selections were made.

Implementation of Plan. The first course was planned for June of 1982 but was rescheduled for September of 1982 because of vacation schedules of staff and applicants.

Nine applicants were accepted into the program, but only five took the course. One went back to work, one was not interested in a one-on-one encounter in the home, and two others decided not to take the first course. Of the five who completed the program, two of those selected had previous hospital volunteer experience, but three were new to both agencies.

The hospital was able to provide for available space for the scheduled meeting time. Also, arrangements were made for free parking for volunteers during the course and in-hospital service as volunteers.

The five volunteers completed their instruction in November of 1982. A graduation luncheon was held in November, at which time the volunteers were given information on patients who were awaiting volunteer assignment. As of January, 1983, the five volunteers were assigned to patients. It should be noted that the case load and status of patients fluctuates. One of the VNA nursing supervisors is responsible for the coordination of this service at the present time.

Types of Patients. Volunteers have contact with the patient's primary nurse who supported this program so that they can obtain information on the patient and review the Volunteer Care Plan. The nurse may accompany the volunteer on the first home visit.

The following are examples of the patients who can benefit from volunteers in the home:

- Mrs. D., a 73-year old woman, has a long history of depression and lives with her granddaughter and needs socialization.

- Mrs. G., a 70-year old woman who lives alone, would benefit from a visitor. This visit would be particularly helpful at mealtime if the volunteer would bring a bag lunch and eat with her.

- Miss G., a 41-year-old polio victim, is paralyzed from the neck down. She is able to sit in a wheelchair and would enjoy company because it would permit her father a chance to get out of the house.

- Mrs. K., a bedbound patient, lives with an elderly sister who would like to be relieved occasionally for a physician's or hairdresser's appointment.

- Mr. V. lives with his wife. He had recent surgery and is very weak. His wife would appreciate a volunteer to sit with Mr. V. for a few hours periodically so she could go shopping.

Plan of Care. A plan of care for each patient provides background information for the volunteer and identifies those tasks that they may perform for patients.

Volunteers are asked to maintain a log. At this time, information is shared with the nurse on a monthly basis at the scheduled meeting. Volunteers are encouraged to contact the primary nurse or appropriate supervisor if a change in the patient's condition occurs or questions arise.

Evaluation and Followup. Monthly meetings are held in which volunteers, staff nurses, medical social workers and directors of volunteer services and home care services discuss the current case load and new patients who are awaiting assignment. This is also a time of sharing for the volunteers.

Plans are being made for a second training course. Before this course content is finalized, we are continuing to evaluate the first course. The nurses, directors, volunteers, and patients have been asked to identify strengths and weaknesses of the program and make suggestions for future courses.

The following comments have been made by volunteers:

I feel that this new program is invaluable, especially for the elderly. My patient and I have a great relationship and he seems to enjoy my visits as much as I like visiting him.

Matching of a friendly visitor and patient gives a real sense of service. Freedom to reject without guilt is an important part of this program. Benefits are not only to patients, but to the visitor as well. I highly recommend continuation and enlargement of this program.

We have also asked the patients to share their comments with us. The following is one such comment:

I have been under the care of the visiting nurses since 1976 and this new volunteer service is just an extension of the excellent care and compassion we have been receiving. About the same time the visiting nurse spoke to me about this new service, I felt an emptiness because of a friend dying, another friend going back to work, and a relative moving away. Just having a letter written to keep me in touch with family and friends and taking care of small personal needs—these are the services the volunteer provides. It helps relieve Daddy of doing one more thing. Now that he has a health problem, the volunteer services will be appreciated even more. Every household and situation is different, but for me, at this time, this service is fulfilling a need.

As part of our evaluation process we are also meeting with other volunteer agencies in our area who use volunteer services to determine their interest in joining with us in this program. We are also looking at the possibility of offering two separate courses; the original one and an abbreviated version that would limit responsibility of the volunteer to that of a visitor. This may increase the number of persons who would participate in the program.

Summary. The following conclusions can be drawn from this successful, cooperative program:

- Hospital volunteer service departments and VNAs can work together to provide comprehensive services to patients regardless of the setting.

- Cooperative efforts can be made to develop and approve a mutually agreeable assignment guide for volunteers.

- Local industry is interested in funding cooperative ventures in health care.

- Our local community college was able to offer the course at a reduced rate.

- Interested volunteers can become vital members of the health care team.

- To date, volunteers have initiated their visits in the home setting rather than the hospital. But, the mechanism is in place to allow for flexibility when the need arises.

This cooperative effort has benefited the hospital, VNA, volunteers, and patients. An expansion of this program will increase the benefits to the community.

Chapter Thirty-Two

Student Programs

Student Placements in Home Health Care Agencies: Boost or Barrier to Quality Patient Care?

Ida M. Androwich and Pamela A. Andresen

The placement of students in a home health care agency has the potential to both help or hinder the work of the agency. In this section, these boosts and barriers to quality patient care are addressed by two community health nursing faculty members who have taught clinical courses using a home health care agency as their clinical site (Androwich and Andresen 1986). One faculty member was formerly director of a Medicare-certified home health care agency involved with student placements.

A major benefit of student placements is the collaboration or "marriage" between education and service. Motivators for this union include the need for home care for the sick and the desire for faculty-student-shared clinical practice. Opportunities for sharing of information and expertise between these disciplines are great. Nurse educators offer clinical expertise, research skills, the desire to test new models of nursing practice, and students who can make reimbursable home visits. Nursing service brings to the marriage an available clinical site with qualified nursing personnel and support services.

A second benefit to the agency is increased staff support. A typical group of 8 to 10 students is able to visit at least that number of patients during a clinical day. Not only can this produce revenue for the agency (see Cost-Benefit Analysis), but it also allows staff to pursue other endeavors. For example, students making visits may permit staff to complete paperwork or attend continuing education programs without an accompanying drop in the agency's productivity. The agency may find that student clinical experiences in their agency serve as a recruiting mechanism, with the best and most enthusiastic of the students returning as employees after graduation.

Depending on the type or level of student (e.g., AD, BSN, or graduate student) and the length of the clinical program, creative use of students can provide assistance to the agency in many other ways besides making visits. Harris (1984) describes two outcomes of student experiences that have the advantage of being mutually beneficial to both learner and service agency. Graduate students can provide assistance with several types of administrative projects, such as completing needs assessments and quality review audits, developing management information systems, and planning future programs and evaluating existing programs. Graduate students in clinical specialty programs can also assist with staff in-services and serve as consultants to the staff.

Staff usually benefits from student placements. Staff members are given an opportunity to serve as role models for students and are typically rewarded with gratitude and admiration from those students. Students are impressed by the independent judgment and high degree of professionalism demonstrated by the community health nurse. Staff may be renewed by exposure to student enthusiasm.

The nursing care plan for a patient cared for by a student is developed by the student in conjunction with the primary nurse and the instructor, a master's or doctorally prepared expert in community health nursing. The patient then receives the benefit of staff, faculty, and student input. Therefore, the resulting plan of care can be expected to be comprehensive.

Productivity, in terms of the number of patients students visit per day, is typically not a priority of nursing education. Therefore, a student who visits only one or two patients per day has much more time to spend preparing for the visit, as well as actual visit time, than the staff nurse visiting five or more patients on the same day. This is another benefit to the client and can be particularly helpful with cases requiring lengthy teaching, such as new diabetics.

Yet there are drawbacks to student placements. Although the strengths of nursing education and service complement one another, they can also create conflict. For example, a faculty member may wish to use the agency as a site for testing a new model for nursing practice. The time required to orient staff to assist with the research may conflict with the administrator's need for the nurses to maintain a certain level of productivity. At the student level, a faculty member may request that students chart in depth on a family's psychosocial status. This may lead Medicare reviewers to believe that the patient is being primarily followed for nonreimbursable psychological problems versus an unstable physical condition. As was previously mentioned, student visits do generate revenue for the agency. If visits are not documented correctly, however, denials for Medicare reimbursement may follow.

Communications may be another pitfall. Community health nurses have long valued team conferences as a means for receiving input when managing caseloads. Students are continuously in a team environment which includes their instructor and other students. A student seeking advice from diverse sources may find it difficult to develop one comprehensive nursing care plan with clear long-term goals for the patient. Also, instead of communication concerning client status flowing from primary nurse to physician, it may go from the student (who actually made the visit and assessed the client) to faculty to agency coordinator to primary nurse to physician, with each step increasing the opportunity for misinterpretation or miscommunication.

A quality of care concern is discontinuity. A student bringing much time and energy to a case may also create discontinuity as the patient wonders what has happened to her "regular" nurse whom she knows and trusts. Patient visits must also fit into the student's schedule since students are rarely in an agency five days per week. Students are in an agency for a limited number of weeks. A student may have just established a good working relationship with the family when it is time to move on to the next clinical experience. Discontinuity may also occur when students are not present in the agency on days when support staff, such as the rehab team, are available.

Environmental or space problems may be a minor but constant irritant. It is obviously not cost-effective for an agency to maintain more space than needed; so when a team of 10 to 11 students and their instructor are added to a space meant to house 11 fewer people, crowding occurs.

From the above advantages and disadvantages, a set of recommendations has been developed. First, faculty needs to be oriented to the agency prior to the student experience. It is recommended that faculty not only be acquainted with the organizational structure, policies, and documentation, but that they also be given the opportunity to make joint home visits with a staff nurse. The administrator and educator should develop a plan for training students in these areas with each party's role in the orientation clearly spelled out. Some agencies may use faculty in practice roles, or to serve on various agency committees, such as the audit committee or the Professional Advisory Committee. Faculty members, who have knowledge of the mechanics of operations and reimbursement, can only help the agency by providing improved student guidance and decreasing the amount of time staff needs to spend with students and faculty.

Orientation is only one area for which accountability must be determined. Accountability for documentation other than progress notes, Medicare form completion, communication with support services and the physician, and case finding are just a few of the many points to be addressed. From the start, a plan should be developed for evaluation of the experience including feedback from students, faculty, nursing staff, and administration.

Planning for the student experience must begin far in advance of its starting date. It is standard practice within universities to solidify contractual arrangements during the spring semester, preceding a fall semester experience. During the summer months, faculty should meet with administrators to discuss the needs of each party in terms of case finding, space, the orientation process, etc.

It is to each party's advantage to have responsibilities clearly delineated in the form of a contract or letter of agreement. In many cases, this will be initiated by the university. Typically, this is negotiated to outline each party's areas of accountability; the agency assumes primary responsibility for the quality of patient care, and education assumes primary accountability for student supervision. In *Bottorf vs. Waltz*, the Pennsylvania Superior Court ruled that teachers have three main areas of responsibility to their students:

1. To provide adequate supervision.

2. To exercise good judgment.

3. To provide proper instruction, especially when potentially hazardous conditions exist. (Van Biervliet and Sheldon-Wildgen 1981)

Implications of this ruling include the need for agency staff to assist faculty to meet its responsibilities in this area. Often agency staff members are in a better position to evaluate clients' needs and characteristics and can guide faculty in the selection of appropriate clients for the student's level of skill.

Even with extensive planning, unanticipated problems are certain to occur. Communication must not only be open, but the channels of communication must be determined in advance. One thing to consider is whether or not students should communicate patient problems directly to the staff nurse or to their instructor first. The second route may prevent the constant bombardment of staff with diverse student questions. An end-of-the-day report should be developed for both students and faculty. Faculty should be advised of agency policy and preferences for reporting problems and communicating concerns.

Finally, assume that students will create a space problem to some degree. Even with unlimited space, students are often perceived as invading the staff's territory. During planning sessions, the administrator and educator should designate which space and telephones are available for student use.

Cost-Benefit Analysis

The following is a cost-benefit analysis of one agency's experience with student placements. It must be noted that it is extremely difficult to generalize cost-benefit analysis from agency to agency as there are so many variables, which are unique to a given agency, yet must be considered in an assessment of costs.

The first of these is the organizational structure and environment of the agency. At what stage of development is the agency? The stress of accommodating student placements in a new agency may prove to be overwhelming because systems have not become smooth. How adequate is staffing? Is there an individual with primary responsibility for coordinating student-faculty communications? An individual designated in this role can assist the integration of students into the agency routine. Can provisions for alternate staff activities be made while students are in the agency? Unless the agency is seriously understaffed (which is not a desirable situation in which to place students), staff will receive the same salary regardless of the number of student visits, and the total agency visits will not increase. Time can be maximized, if staff can be scheduled for continuing education/staff development, to use the time as a breather and to catch up on documentation, or to assist with program/policy and procedure development or record audit in the agency. The amount of documentation which is expected of students will also influence the time staff spend with student cases.

A second major consideration is the type of faculty and students. Generic, RN-BSN completion, or graduate students may make a difference in the reimbursement. Medicare will reimburse for all nursing student visits, but other third-party payors may require RN licensure for reimbursement; thus only RN or graduate students would be reimbursed for visits. The faculty supervisor's familiarity with the agency, its clients, and general proficiency and experience in home care will influence the time required by the agency in orientation and assistance with documentation and care planning. Faculty members, who can assume the bulk of the student's orientation and oversee charting and client care services, will reduce the amount of time spent by agency personnel in these activities.

Case Study Assumptions

This case study examines one agency's experiences with three student teams for a semester. Each of these teams is made up of RN-BSN completion students and is supervised by a faculty member familiar with home care and the agency involved. No additional costs for insurance are included. For purposes of calculation, it is assumed that the agency will receive no denials for any of the student visits. Quality of visits is also not addressed. Students and faculty provide their own transportation and are not reimbursed for mileage by the agency. It is also assumed that there is no negative effect on the volume of other therapies and services provided by the agency.

Staff salaries will vary. Estimates used for computation are: Director, $20 per hour; patient care coordinator, $17.50 per hour; PHN, $14.50 per hour; and clerical staff, $7.50 per hour. (This includes 15% benefit allowance.) Staff members are reimbursed for mileage at 21 cents per mile with an average of 12.5 miles per visit. Agency charges per nursing visit equal $75.

The agency made 1,756 nursing visits in the 11-week time period covered. Students made 179 visits or approximately 10% of the nursing visits. This accounted for a total revenue of $13,425. It must be remembered that these visits would have been made regardless of the student experience, thus the revenue does not represent additional income to the agency unless (a) visits are made that would not have been made if the students were not present, or (b) staff members are able to actually decrease hours. The three faculties estimated the amount of time spent by and with various agency personnel during their clinical time.

Team 1. Three RN-BSN students in a weekend program at the agency every other Saturday and Sunday for three weekends. They made a total of 20 visits. During this time, the agency had a PHN on-call, but the students' provision of services decreased agency costs because the PHN was not needed for visits and thus was paid not hourly, but on an on-call basis.

Analysis

Revenue: 20 visits @ $75. = $1,500.

Costs:	(Communication-reporting)	
	Director — 1 hour	20.00
	Coordinator — 1 1/2 hour x 3	78.75
	PHN — 1/2 hour x 3 x 3 PHNs	$ 65.25
	Clerical — 1/2 hour x 3	11.25
		$175.25

$1,500.00
− 175.25

$1,324.75 plus mileage savings of 20 x 12.5 x 21 = $52.50

Team 1 — Net $1,377.25 or $68.86 per visit

Team 2. A total of 18 students over an 11-week period — 10 students for 6 weeks and 8 students for the last 5 weeks — making 119 visits. Students in agency 4 hours each day on Tuesday and Thursday.

Analysis

Revenue: 119 visits @ $75.00 = $8,925.

Costs:	Director — 4 hours	$ 80.00
	Coordinator — 2 hours/day x 22	770.00
	PHN — 1/2 hour x 4 PHN x 22	638.00

Clerical — 1/2 hour x 22   82.50

                                                          $1,570.50

$ 8,925.00
− 1,570.50

$7,354.50 plus mileage savings of 119 x 12.5 x 21 $312.38

Team 2 — Net $7,666.88 or $64.43 per visit.

Team 3. Eleven students for 5 weeks made 40 visits. Students were in agency concurrently with the last 5 weeks of Team 2, and difficulty was experienced finding an adequate number of cases for these 11 students plus the eight from Team 2, thus the numbers of potential visits had reached a ceiling.

                                Analysis

Revenue: 40 visits @ $75./visit $3,000.

Costs:	Director — 4 hours	$ 80.00
	Coordinator — 2 hours/10 days	350.00
	PHN — 1/2 hr x 4 PHN's x 10 days	290.00
	Clerical — 1/2 x 10	37.50

                                                          $757.50

$3,000.00
− 757.50

$2,242.50 plus mileage savings of 40 x 12.5 x 21 105.

Team 3 — Net $2,347.50 or $58.69 per visit.

Summary

In the case study, Team 1 had the best cost/benefit (C/B) ratio. This was because Team 1 was using the agency at a time when staff were not normally present and salaried. Team 2 did better than Team 3, because they were alone in the agency for six weeks. When both Team 2 and 3 were together, the number of visits decreased because the agency caseload could not accommodate two teams of students.

Each agency will need to examine its individual situation relative to the variables cited. The ratio of the number of students using the agency and the caseload, as well as the timing of student experiences, will affect the C/B ratio.

Requests for one-day observational experiences often come from diploma and associate degree nursing programs that do not offer full community health nursing experiences. An agency, whose mission statement stresses a perceived responsibility for the education of future health professionals, might wish to accommodate these students regardless of cost effectiveness. A proprietary agency, without such a mission statement, would more closely examine the costs of such arrangements (Androwich 1986).

Student Programs Benefit Nursing Service Agencies[*]
Marilyn D. Harris

The community health nurse has the opportunity to promote health education and reinforce this teaching by providing materials that can be reviewed at a later time.

Community health nursing agencies often have active student programs in affiliation with colleges and universities. One way to maximize this relationship is to have students develop educational materials for the agency, to meet an identified need while allowing the students to meet course requirements.

The series of brochures, "Watching Your Baby Grow," is the product of one such program.

Background

The Visiting Nurse Association of Eastern Montgomery County is a voluntary, certified, accredited home health agency that provides service in 18 municipalities. In addition to providing a variety of health care services, such as a Home Care Program, a Maternal and Child Health Program, and an Adult Health Promotion Program, a variety of patient teaching activities are offered throughout the community.

Teaching is done on a one-to-one basis or in a group setting. Printed materials are provided in order to reinforce the teaching. The materials, which can be taken home and reviewed at a later date, may range from an easy-to-read brochure for adults to a coloring book for the young child.[1]

Student Programs

The VNA also has an active student program with several hospitals, colleges and universities. Eighty-six students affiliated with the program during 1983. The student experiences may vary for each academic institution and with the clinical experience of the student.

The student program is an important component of the student's total experience. It provides a broader prospective of the health care system and an opportunity for

---

* Reprinted with permission of *Home Healthcare Nurse* from student programs benefit nursing service agencies *Home Home Healthcare Nurse* by Marilyn Harris (November/December 1984) vol. 2, no. 5, pp.34-35.

practical application of the theory gained through an academic program. It also serves as an information exchange.

One way to maximize the benefits of this relationship between nursing service and nursing education is to assist students as they develop materials to meet course requirements.

Benefits of Student Program

The VNA conducts ten well child clinics each month. These clinics are staffed by registered nurses and certified nurse practitioners, as well as several physicians.

Based on the physical setting and the number of people who attend, both the quality and quantity of time spent with each mother are important considerations.

One example of student participation in the educational program in the clinical setting is the study conducted by K. Kishi.[2,3] The results of the study are detailed in her dissertation entitled, "Communication Patterns Between Health Care Providers and Clients and Recall of Health Information." Kishi examined the verbal communication patterns that take place between health care providers and clients in well baby clinics and then investigated how these patterns related to recall.

During Kishi's study of 68 health care provider interactions with mothers, encounter times ranged from 5 to 38 minutes, yielding an average visit time of 12 minutes. Although Kishi found that initial recall of instructions received was high, averaging 81% of items taught, the recall ratio tended to decline in longer sessions in which more items were taught. Even though the mothers did not have a problem with the clinical setting or the time frame, the nurses felt that additional take-home materials would be beneficial.

A second example of the benefit of student involvement relates to a series of brochures developed to fill the needs identified by Kishi.

In 1982 and 1983, two of the master's students on affiliation with the VNA were interested in pediatric nursing and worked under the supervision of the certified pediatric nurse practitioners (CPNP). One of the needs identified was for a brochure that mothers could take home and use as a reference between visits to the clinic. As a result of the combination of an identified nursing need and the available resource of the student nurses, the first in a series of four brochures titled "Watching Your Baby Grow" was developed.

Each brochure is divided into age categories and contains the following information: How and what should I feed my baby? How long will my baby sleep? How can I protect my baby? What should my baby be doing? When do I bring my baby for immunizations? The back page carries information such as: common reactions to immunization, food recommendations, and how to choose shoes, car seats and toys.

The Student Design Group at the Art Institute of Philadelphia designed the brochure and prepared mechanicals for the printer as part of a service they offer to non-profit groups.

As each brochure was completed by the students, drafts were reviewed by the Professional Advisory Committee (PAC) of the VNA which approves all policies, procedures, standing orders and standardized information that is distributed by the Agency. The student attended the PAC meeting when a specific brochure was reviewed, thus allowing the student and the committee to agree on mutually acceptable instructions.

Three of the brochures are completed and the fourth will be developed soon.[*] The completed ones are: "Watching Your Baby Grow: The First Six Months," and "Watching Your Baby Grow: The Second Six Months," prepared by Mary T. Folkerth, RN, BSN; and "Watching Your Baby Grow: The Second Year of Life," prepared by Susan Burke, RN, BSN.

In summary, though student placements present valid concerns for administrators, the next time the local educational institution calls to explore the possibility of placing students in your nursing agency for clinical experience, consider the opportunities and benefits of such an experience to the patients, staff and students.

Endnotes

1. Harris, M. One Way to Promote Nursing. *The American Journal of Maternal Child Nursing,* 6(5): 307-310, 1981.

2. Kishi, K. Communication Patterns Between Health Care Providers and Clients and Recall of Health Information. A Dissertation in the School of Nursing, University of Pennsylvania, 1981.

3. Kishi, K. Communication Patterns of Health Teaching and Information Recall. *Nursing Research,* 32(4): 230-235, 1983.

A Student Program in One Home Health Agency

Marilyn D. Harris

The Visiting Nurse Association (VNA) of Eastern Montgomery County has an active student program. Each year 8 to 10 educational facilities use the VNA for observational or practical experience. An average of 125 students affiliate with the agency for varying periods of time each year.

The VNA offers educational opportunities for diploma, baccalaureate, graduate, and doctoral student nurses, physical therapy and medical students, and medical residents. The VNA has developed manuals that include a statement of philosophy and objectives for the overall program (Exhibit 32-1) and for each individual program (Exhibits 32-2 and 32-3). The institutions are also asked to submit program objectives and curriculum outlines to the agency. Exhibit 32-4 is an example of one outline.

* The author acknowledges the valuable contribution of the following individuals to the success of the "Watching Your Baby Grow" brochures: Susan Burke, RN, MSN; Louise Harmer, RN, CPNP, VNA staff; Mary T. Folkerth, RN, MSN; and The Student Design Group—The Art Institute of Philadelphia.

Exhibit 32-1.

Student Program

Philosophy

We, the Visiting Nurse Association of Eastern Montgomery County, believe that our student program is a vital component and is mutually beneficial to both the student and our agency. Further, we believe that it is a valuable experience, because it provides the student with a broader and unique perspective of the health care system by incorporating the community health component. It also provides an opportunity for practical application of the theory gained through an academic program. Finally, we value highly the information exchange which occurs as a result of our experiences with the students.

Purpose

The primary purpose of the program is to provide the student with an opportunity to augment his perspective of the health needs of the aggregate population, as well as the client and family in the community setting. The program also allows the student an opportunity to gain a better understanding of the role of a community nursing organization in meeting these health needs.

Objectives

The individual student experiences are based upon and consistent with the course objectives of the various academic institutions that participate in our program.

Contracts have been approved and signed by both the VNA and the school. These are reviewed and renewed on an annual basis. Sample contracts for diploma (Exhibit 32-5), graduate (Exhibit 32-6) and medical residents (Exhibit 32-7) are included in this chapter with the permission of the educational facilities. The contracts list the responsibilities of both organizations, the number of students to be assigned to the agency at any one time, and other pertinent terms of the affiliation.

In some instances, "Guidelines for Cooperative Relationships Between Clinical Setting and Graduate Program" (Exhibit 32-8) are shared and approved. These guidelines include information related to agency selection, qualifications of the preceptor, functions of agency preceptor, expectations of the graduate students, responsibilities of the faculty preceptor, and the placement process.

The contractual relationships are the responsibility of the administrator at the VNA. The determination of the number of educational institutions and students that will affiliate at the VNA each year is the responsibility of the nursing supervisor in charge of education. This decision is based on consultation with the Director of Professional Services and the clinical supervisors. The educational supervisor is responsible for orientation of the faculty and students to the VNA each semester.

Evaluation of the student placements is an integral part of the total annual evaluation process at the VNA. As part of the evaluation process, students complete, and the

Exhibit 32-2.

Student Nursing Program
Diploma School

I. *Philosophy*

To enhance the student's learning with an experience in a community setting which offers an opportunity to observe the application of nursing principles and adaptations of techniques in accordance with environmental needs.

II. *Objectives*

To identify the functions of a Visiting Nurse Agency and observe methods of providing health services to meet the need of community members by:

1. Introduction to the organization's structure, philosophy, and funding.
2. Description of the community service area and the common needs of its members.
3. Explanation of the role of a community nurse as a team member assisting in meeting the total health needs of the patient, his family, and the community.
4. Identification of various resources utilized to aid in meeting the total health needs of community members.
5. Introduction to methods of referral employed to support a coordinated effort to meet required health needs of community members.
6. Observation of selected individuals and family units receiving health care and guidance including:
   a. Physical environment and nursing care of the patient in the home.
   b. Teaching and supervision of responsible individuals in interim care.
   c. Family-centered care.
   d. Accountability for hospital discharge planning.
   e. Family participation in planning and supporting patient care.

Exhibit 32-3.

Visiting Nurse Association of Eastern Montgomery County, Inc.

Baccalaureate Student Clinical Experience
Objectives

1. To identify the structural and functional differences of voluntary, official, and combined agencies.

2. To identify the changing pattern in community nursing functions which have evolved in response to current needs.

3. To acquire skill in the assessment and provision for required health needs of individual and families in the home.

4. To encourage participation of responsible individuals in planning for and providing care for the patient.

5. To actively participate in the provision of skilled nursing care to selected individuals/families which portray an average agency caseload.

6. To adapt nursing knowledge and techniques to patient/family care in the home environment.

7. To become aware of and arrange for other available community health resources which will support more comprehensive care.

8. To acquire an appreciation and understanding of the effect of chronic or long-term illness upon the patient/family, including its economic and psychosocial impact.

Exhibit 32-4.

Villanova University
College of Nursing—Graduate Program

Title: NUR 8922 - Practicum in Clinical Nursing

Credits: 3

Overview:

The practicum will provide students with an opportunity to operationalize concepts in clinical nursing through intervention modalities. Students will select a clinical specialty setting that provides regular opportunities to plan, implement, and evaluate nursing goals for health promotion, maintenance, and restoration.

Major Purpose:

To study and practice advanced clinical nursing concepts.

Objectives:

1)   To generate a series of individual objectives which reflect the specific scope and purpose of the practicum.

2)   To collaborate with faculty advisor in selection of an appropriate clinical site for practicum.

3)   To collaborate with the agency preceptor in planning a learning experience which will meet the individual student's objectives for the practicum.

4)   To prepare a process log of each learning experience.

5)   To augment the learning experience with readings pertinent to the experience.

6)   To analyze the practicum experience in relation to the individual student's objectives.

7)   To participate in bimonthly seminars.

Requirements:

1)   Participate in the selection of a clinical setting, development of objectives, and evaluation of practicum.

2)   Participate in a two-hour weekly seminar.

3)   Plan, implement, and evaluate nursing intervention modalities.

4)   Submit a written report of practicum.

Exhibit 32-4, continued.

Villanova University
College of Nursing—Graduate Program

Evaluation:

Criteria based on practicum objectives:

1) Seminar participation - 30%

2) Weekly Logs   - 50%

3) Synthesis Paper   - 20%

Reprinted by permission.

schools forward to the VNA evaluations of the experience. These evaluations are shared with the staff. In general, the students, patients, and staff indicate that student affiliations are a valuable aspect of the total VNA service.

Considerations

Productivity. The changing health care climate presents several areas of consideration for the home health agency administrator in relationship to student programs. Current home care services are reimbursed on a per visit basis. Students do have an impact on the productivity of staff. Even though a representative from the educational institution is on site, staff members are involved in the orientation of students to both agency and patients. Having someone accompany the nurse on home visits on a regular basis slows the nurse down. This could result in fewer visits per day which, under the current per visit reimbursement schedule, would result in less income for the agency.

The Medicare regulations allow for student nurses to provide billable service under a general supervision provision. Physical therapy students must work under the direct supervision of the licensed therapist. Once again, this requires the time of the licensed therapist in the home and office.

Documentation. Documentation is another area of consideration. Documentation must be reviewed to determine whether it meets with both agency standards (use of patient classification system, nursing diagnoses) and reimbursements standards. Agencies cannot afford to have visits denied on a medical or technical basis. Therefore, additional supervisory time and expenses are incurred to review and verify that all student documentation meets established criteria.

Exhibit 32-5.

1986-1987 AGREEMENT OF OBSERVATION
BETWEEN

VISITING NURSE ASSOCIATION OF EASTERN MONTGOMERY COUNTY, INC.
ABINGTON, PENNSYLVANIA
AND
ABINGTON MEMORIAL HOSPITAL SCHOOL OF NURSING
ABINGTON, PENNSYLVANIA

It is hereby mutually agreed that the *Visiting Nurse Association of Eastern Montgomery County*, herein referred to as *Agency*, shall provide and *Abington Memorial Hospital School of Nursing*, herein referred to as *School*, shall receive for its students, a clinical facility for observation of the skills necessary for the nursing of clients in the home. The above-described observational experience shall be limited to two days per students and subject to conditions hereby given for the school year 1986-1987.

Conditions

1. The number of students sent to the *Agency* by the *School* shall not exceed 3 or 4 on any one day. Affiliation dates from September to December 1986 and from January to May 1987.

2. The *Agency* will provide each student with orientation and observation under the direction of a registered nurse.

3. The *School* will provide the *Agency* with a master schedule listing names of student nurses and dates of the planned experience prior to beginning of observation. In the event of any change in schedules, either party may notify the other of the change in writing.

4. The *School* agrees to have its students:

   a. abide by general policies of the *Agency* when visiting patients by direction of registered nurse with whom students are observing.
   b. keep confidential all knowledge and records of patients.

5. The *Agency* will make available to students and faculty all pertinent educational material during period of observation.

6. *Abington Memorial Hospital* students will provide individual malpractice insurance coverage.

7. In the event of accident, injury, or illness of student on observation experience, *Agency* will notify *School* and plans for student's return to *School* will be made on an individual basis depending on the situation. The *School* shall assume responsibility for care and emergency transportation of student.

Exhibit 32-5, continued.

8. The faculty of the *School* agrees to present the terminal evaluation of the observation experience to the Executive Director of the *Agency* within 30 days of its completion.

9. The Agreement shall be reviewed and evaluated annually.

10. Renewal of Agreement will be negotiable on application of *School* to *Agency* at least 30 days prior to first date scheduled for observation experience.

SIGNATURES OF AGREEMENT

FIRST PARTY   *SECOND PARTY*

Visiting Nurse Association   *Abington Memorial Hospital*
                of
Eastern Montgomery County

_____
Executive Director

_____
President

_____
Date   Aug. 4, 1986

_____
Chairman, School of Nursing

_____
Executive Vice-President and
Administrator

_____
Date   7-30-86

Reprinted by permission.

Exhibit 32-6.

THIS AGREEMENT, made this 10th day of June 1986, By and Between VILLANOVA UNIVERSITY, of VIllanova, Pennsylvania, a corporation organized and existing under the laws of the Commonwealth of Pennsylvania, (hereinafter referred to as UNIVERSITY) and EASTERN MONTGOMERY COUNTY V.N.A., a corporation organized and existing under the laws of the Commonwealth of Pennsylvania, (hereinafter referred to as AGENCY).

WITNESSETH

WHEREAS, it is of mutual interest and advantage to the parties hereto that the students enrolled in the VILLANOVA UNIVERSITY, College of Nursing, be given the opportunity and the benefit of the clinical facilities for experience in the practice of nursing.

NOW, THEREFORE, it is mutually agreed by the parties hereto, each of them intending to be legally bound hereby, that in consideration of the good and valuable considerations each to the other provided for thereunder, the parties agree as follows:

1. AGENCY agrees to provide clinical facilities for nursing experience for students covering the academic year 1986-87 for such number of students as mutually agreed upon for such period.
2. The said groups of students will receive their instructions and supervision from UNIVERSITY instructors.

Undergraduate

Fall   *Spring*

Health Promotion

Graduate Practica

3. UNIVERSITY agrees to abide by the regulations of AGENCY concerning chest X-rays, physical examinations, and other tests required by AGENCY.
4. The UNIVERSITY agrees to have its students abide by the general policies of the AGENCY regarding patient care.
5. AGENCY will supply, to the best of its ability, to said students and faculty, the prompt referral to the nearest medical facility in any emergency requiring medical attention.
6. Malpractice Liability coverage is supplied by the UNIVERSITY.
7. AGENCY will provide, to the best of its ability, space for conferences for such students and faculty when required.
8. UNIVERSITY will send to AGENCY only students adequately prepared for the stipulated nursing experience and will assume the responsibility for the education of the students in the specified clinical areas as described in paragraph 1 herein. Ultimate responsibility for patient care remains with AGENCY staff.

Exhibit 32-6, continued.

9. UNIVERSITY will withdraw upon recommendation of AGENCY any student who shall fail to abide by the regulations respecting student personnel or who otherwise fails to fulfill the personnel and/or professional requirements of AGENCY.

10. It is understood and agreed by the parties hereto that this Agreement will be reviewed not later than May 30 and provision may at that time be made, at the option of the parties hereto, that UNIVERSITY at that time will notify AGENCY of number of students in succeeding groups and the time when the students will report.

11. The parties hereto further agree to form a coordinating committee of UNIVERSITY and AGENCY representatives to discuss problems and plans and to insure the effective functioning of both institutions with regard to the matters covered by this Agreement; which committee shall meet when necessary.

12. The UNIVERSITY and AGENCY agree that discrimination against any student or faculty member on the basis of race, creed, national origin, age, handicap, or sex will not be tolerated. Consistent therewith, each of the parties affirms positively hereby that its policies preclude discrimination.

13. If a change in the learning environment of the AGENCY should occur that would be disruptive, or that might interfere with the achievement of the objectives of the experience, the UNIVERSITY, after consultation with the representatives of the AGENCY, reserves the right to temporarily withdraw student from the agency.

14. Each of the parties hereto reserves the right to discontinue this Agreement upon six months notice in writing to the other.

IN WITNESS WHEREOF, the parties hereto have hereunto respectively caused their common or corporate seals to be affixed duly attested by their proper officers, the date and year first above written.

VILLANOVA UNIVERSITY

BY: _____
President

_____
Dean, College of Nursing

AGENCY

BY: _____

ATTEST: _____

Reprinted by permission.

Exhibit 32-7.

AGREEMENT OF OBSERVATION
between
VISITING NURSE ASSOCIATION
OF EASTERN MONTGOMERY COUNTY, INC.
and
TEMPLE UNIVERSITY FAMILY PRACTICE RESIDENCY PROGRAM

It is hereby agreed that the *Visiting Nurse Association of Eastern Montgomery County*, hereafter referred to as *Agency*, shall provide and the *Temple University Family Practice Residency Program*, hereafter referred to as *Program*, shall obtain for its family practice residents a clinical facility for observation of skills required in providing home health services and the necessity for discharge planning in the institutional setting for the provision of continuity of care. The above described observational experience shall be limited to one day per resident and subject to conditions hereby given for the year ending June 30, 1986.

Conditions

1. The number of residents sent to the *Agency* by the *Program* shall be mutually agreeable to both parties.

2. The *Agency* will provide each resident with orientation and observation under the direction of a registered nurse.

3. The *Program* will provide the *Agency* with a master schedule listing names of residents and dates of the planned experience prior to beginning of observation. In the event of any change in schedule, either party may notify the other of the change in writing.

4. The *Program* agrees to have its residents:

    a. abide by general policies of the *Agency*, to be given in writing to the *Program*, when visiting patients by direction of registered nurse with whom residents are observing.
    b. keep confidential all knowledge and records of patients.

5. The *Agency* will make available to residents and faculty all pertinent educational material during period of observation.

6. The *Program* will provide Professional Liability Insurance Coverage and Worker's Compensation Insurance for residents representing the *Program* under this agreement.

7. In the event of accident, injury or illness of resident on observation experience, *Agency* will notify *Program* .

Exhibit 32-7, continued.

8. The Faculty of the *Program* agrees to present the terminal evaluation of the observation experience to the Executive Director or Educational Supervisor of the *Agency* within 30 days of its completion.

9. The Agreement will be reviewed and evaluated on an annual basis.

10. Renewal of Agreement will be negotiable on application of *Program* to *Agency* at least 30 days prior to first date scheduled for observation experience.

SIGNATURES OF AGREEMENT

Temple University
Family Practice Residency Program

BY: _James R. MacBride MD_

WITNESS _____

DATE: _11/22/85_

Visiting Nurse Association
of Eastern Montgomery County, Inc.

BY: _____

WITNESS _____

DATE: _11/25/85_

Reprinted by permission.

Finances. To date, there is minimal to no financial compensation to agencies who cooperate in student programs. Financial consideration for clinical experience should be discussed with each institution and included in the agreement whenever this can be negotiated. Compensation could be in the form of actual dollars or free attendance for a specific number of staff from the cooperating agency at continuing education programs. Another form of payment could be the free use of audiovisual equipment. This matter should be discussed each time the contract is renewed.

In spite of all of these considerations, I believe that student programs are beneficial for home health agencies, staff, patients, and students.

Exhibit 32-8.

Guidelines for Cooperative Relationships
Between Clinical Settings and Graduate Program,
College of Nursing, Villanova University

1) Selection of Agency:
   a) Contract and/or letter of agreement with Villanova University with concomitant *Criteria for Selection of Agencies.*
   b) Willingness to cooperate with the University in providing resources for advanced clinical practice.
   c) Willingness to offer opportunities to students to implement advanced clinical concepts.

2) Qualifications of Agency Preceptor:
   a) Delegated as preceptor by nursing service administration of agency.
   b) Demonstrated clinical expertise with a minimum of master's degree in nursing.
   c) Willingness to be clinical resource for student and faculty preceptor, based on same position in agency.
   d) Willingness to be graduate student's role model.

3) Functions of Agency Preceptor:
   a) Participate with student and faculty preceptor in planning for practicum.
   b) Assist student implementation of practicum through facilitating movement in the clinical environment.
   c) Provide a liaison role between expectations of a service agency and a learning agency.
   d) Participate in evaluation of practicum process and preceptorship program.

4) Expectations of Graduate Students:
   a) Minimal expectations of current P.A., R.N. license; current malpractice and liability insurance; health examination and a CPR (Basic Life Support) certificate. Agencies outside Pennsylvania will require a current license in that state. Some agencies may require a student resume. Students should prepare one prior to the practicum.
   b) Written practicum plan including objectives, process and outcomes, activities, time frame, and agency compliance expectations.
   c) Responsibility for faculty preceptor and agency preceptor.
   d) Participation in bimonthly seminars, or in the case of summer term, weekly seminars.
   e) Accountability to client for independent practice.

5) Responsibilities of Faculty Preceptor:
   a) Accountable for planning, implementing, and evaluating clinical practicum.
   b) Periodic on-site supervision/teaching/consultation.
   c) Availability for interim consultation.
   d) Conduct bimonthly clinical seminars.
   e) Participation in evaluation process, e.g., student, peer, preceptorship. In addition to the evaluative processes, the faculty preceptor is responsible for grading the student's practicum.
   f) Assist student to reorder and reorganize current knowledge and apply new knowledge of nursing models to clinical practice.

Exhibit 32-8, continued.

6) Placement Process:
   a) The Director of the Graduate Program is responsible for initiating agency contacts for placement of students and determining feasibility in any given academic term.
   b) The faculty preceptor is responsible for initiating agency preceptor contacts for specific practicum planning.
   c) The Assistant to the Dean is responsible for initiating interagency contracts.

Reprinted by permission.

References

Androwich, I. M. In press. Creative utilization of staff. In *Home Health Agency Management*, by L. Benefield. Brady and Co.: Englewood Cliffs.

Androwich, I. M., and P. Andresen. 1986. Student placements in home health care agencies: Boost or barrier to quality patient care? Poster presented at Second National Symposium of Home Health Nursing, Ann Arbor, MI, May 14-16, 1986.

Harris, M. 1984. Student programs benefit nursing service agencies. *Home Health Care Nurse*. November/December 1984: 34-35.

Van Biervliet, A., & J. Sheldon-Wildgen. 1981. *Liability issues in community-based programs*. Baltimore: Brooks Publishing Company.

Chapter Thirty-Three

The Physician's Role in Home Care

Mary Jane Koren

Home Care and Doctors — Water and Oil?

Home health administrators ask two questions when trying to reconcile these two elements which are thought often to be antithetical:

1. What should our relationship with physicians be? and the corrollary question —

2. How can we improve the relationship between physicians and home health agencies?

There are several reasons why finding answers has been so difficult. First is the assumption that all individuals subsumed under the heading "physician" are homogeneous and interchangeable. Second, there is a recognition that tensions, which need resolution, exist between home health agencies and physicians. Finally, and perhaps most important, there is an implied presumption that there is a single correct or appropriate relationship toward which to strive. These three points will form the framework for this chapter.

Who Are These Physicians?

Physicians are often presumed to share characteristics and motivations and to respond in a uniform and predictable manner to given situations. When they don't, frustration, anger, disappointment, and distrust ensue, and further interactions may be hampered by previous negative experiences. Because medicine today is in such ferment, however, many of the old stereotypes of what doctors are and what they do are being swept away and replaced by an infinitely more diverse and complex system of health care delivery. As a way of organizing this diversity and beginning to appreciate home care and doctor relationships, a spectrum of direct patient care activities can be envisioned, which ranges from those who do nothing but provide care to patients, to those whose activities are completely removed from patient care.

Thus:

| 100% time spent in direct patient care | 0% time spent in patient care |

In the past, most doctors occupied the left-hand side of the above continuum, largely in the context of solo or small group private practice.

This is the model that is presumed by many home care staff to still predominate. However, groups are getting larger and even solo practitioners may belong to Independent Practice Associations (IPAs) or Preferred Provider Organizations (PPOs), which not only direct certain types of patients into a practice but place constraints on physician behavior.

Another change which has affected physician practice patterns is the shift away from primary care (usually thought of as general practice, family practice, pediatrics, or general internal medicine) into subspecialty practice, a shift which has gained momentum over the past 20 years. If one remembers that subspecialists have received intensive training focused on one small part of a broader field, training which largely has stressed the technology and resources available in hospitals, it is not surprising to find them approaching the multiple problems of home care patients with tunnel vision, often unaware or even puzzled by what home care staff are trying to tell them about patients. This miscommunication can be frustrating to both parties.

There are many patients today, however, who are being cared for in settings far removed from the specialty or general office practices familiar from the past. They are receiving care through organizations which employ doctors in the same way as any other staff members. The federal government provides care directly through the Civilian Health and Medical Program for the Uniformed Services (CHAMPUS), and the Veteran's Administration, which runs the largest hospital "chain" in the United States. Cities, counties, and states also operate hospitals and clinics. Many voluntary and some proprietary hospitals also run clinics and medical practices. Any or all of these facilities may operate training programs for interns, residents, and fellows, in addition to having full-time attending physicians who provide care, as well as teach and supervise house staff. How all these doctors with their multiple agendas interact with patients may range from long-term to episodic, from primary care to consultative. Health maintenance organizations, which emphasize low-cost primary care may also have less physician and patient continuity than older practice modalities. All of these developments mean that even in those groups of doctors whose sole or primary work is patient care, enormous variation may exist in the level of commitment to and knowledge about individual patients. This variation is an issue with which administrators in home health must learn to cope.

There is an increasing number of teaching, research, and administrative physicians who spend little or no time caring for patients. They are nevertheless a group which needs to be included in the awareness that home health agency personnel have of physicians. Health policy and cost containment analysts and clinical researchers currently are examining home care with great interest. Medical schools are beginning to acknowledge the need to acquaint students with home care, and faculty have started coming to agencies with requests to permit students to accompany staff on home visits. Physicians also are becoming administrators and health policy advisors, often with advanced degrees in health administration or public health. Given the role that they play in both government and the private sector, they occupy extremely influential positions in health care which ought not to be ignored when trying to set up relations with physicians.

It is evident, therefore, that a more focused appraisal must be made with regard to which type of physician an agency wishes to interact; the solutions developed must be appropriate to the group with which they are dealing. It would simplify things if all of an agency's patients had true primary care physicians but, in fact, an agency's patients may be cared for by an orthopedist, an endocrinologist, an intern, an unlicensed foreign medical graduate, or a professor of medicine to name but a few. The problems which arise will be unique to each, so the solutions will have to be creative and thoughtful if patients are to receive full benefit from their home care stay.

What's The Problem?

The second point to be made when examining the interaction between physicians and home health agencies is to recognize that tensions do exist. Many of them, either real or imagined, probably have a historical base. For centuries, physicians have been involved in home care every bit as much as agency personnel are today. It is only recently that this involvement with patients in their homes has ceased to be common. Until the mid-1950s and, in some areas, the early 1960s, a busy practitioner's day included visiting ill patients in their homes, as well as office and hospital work. The majority of physicians were what we now call primary care physicians. Subspecialization did of course exist, but the diagnostic, technologic, and therapeutic sophistication, which grew exponentially in the years following World War II, provided a major impetus to the growth of subspecialty practice. Devices and services available only in hospitals began to exert a strong influence to keep physician practice in institutions. The public itself, reinforced perhaps by legal opinion, began to expect hospitalization as a right and as an indication that they were receiving the best that could be had. Gradually, it became more fashionable to be seen by a specialist than by a general practitioner, and doctors, who made house calls and didn't rely on high-technology treatment, were held in lower esteem than their ivory tower colleagues.

During the eighteenth, nineteenth and early twentieth centuries, as visiting nurse associations evolved into today's multidisciplinary home health agencies, physicians were actually out in the field and knew about the patient, his family, and his home environment from firsthand experience. In some instances, progressive leaders in health care, such as Dr. E. M. Bluestone and Dr. Martin Cherkasky at Montefiore Hospital in New York, linked the nursing and physician services into a team, which operated not in parallel, but collaboratively. Other hospitals also used this model; however, because of the constraints imposed by physician shortages and burgeoning technology, it never became widespread.

In the minds of those who drafted the Medicare and Medicaid legislation of the mid-1960s, it was taken as a given, however, that physicians were still involved with their patients in their homes. Another prevailing belief was that nurses and other health professionals followed orders and were permitted to exercise independent judgment only in a circumscribed fashion. Without debating either the origin or the illogic of these views, it must be recognized that they were written into the Conditions of Participation in federal home care legislation. Consequently, many of the constraints under which home health agencies currently chafe have been and continue to be upheld by the fiscal intermediaries who approve reimbursement. This of course flies in the face of the current reality that doctors, except in certain instances, no longer make home visits and are therefore usually not aware of the nuances of providing care to patients in their homes. Initially, experience making house calls, common sense, and some reasonable suggestions regarding a care plan were sufficient. Recently, however, reimbursement claim forms have become so exacting and terminology must be so precise that most home health agencies have had to devise and rely on their own carefully worded care plan and documentation, since physician plans may be denied even if they are completely appropriate.

These circumstances lead directly to one of the most prevalent difficulties that agencies have with doctors. It is, by and large, an issue of turf and of control. Whose patient is it? Who is in charge? Who is responsible? Looking at this from a practitioner's perspective, there is little wonder that he may resent an agency for "taking over" a patient. The physician may or may not have actively suggested home care to his patient. (In some areas, it may be a discharge planner who advises the patient to accept home care.) Suddenly, the physician is expected to sign "orders" for services to his patient which he may not understand fully, and about which he hasn't been consulted. Further, he is not permitted to modify the care plan to reflect his own perceptions of what the patient needs. Additionally, the services will be delivered by staff with whom he has never met or worked, in a place, the patient's home, that he has never seen. He has very little way of knowing the competence of the staff, the safety of the home, or the appropriateness of the services being given. He is essentially being asked to sign a blank check for them to act, and yet to accept full responsibility should something go awry. Given today's medico-legal climate, if doctors did not react to all of this with some degree of paranoia it would be unrealistic and abnormal.

Having a patient on home care may well be seen by a physician as being expensive to him also. He cannot, as other professionals, such as lawyers, charge for telephone time, nor can he bill for time spent reviewing or revising care plans. If he is in solo practice, it is hardly surprising that, as a businessman, he is less than pleased to be using his time for uncompensated activities; and if he works for an HMO or clinic, his expected productivity may not take into account these extraneous activities.

Using home care for his patients, therefore, becomes time-consuming and costly and may be a potentially perilous activity. Agencies who push him to do so ought not to be surprised if hostility or reluctance are present. These feelings can, of course, be allayed, but they are neither totally unfounded nor unreasonable. Home health agency administrators must be aware that these problems exist, at least from the physician's perspective, and be willing to deal with them and to try to solve some of the strong disincentives to using home care.

On the other hand, home health agencies, while often willing to humor physicians because they are a potential market and the key to reimbursement, have strong feelings about maintaining the autonomy they have always enjoyed. This is one health delivery service which has grown and prospered away from direct physician input. Many home health agency staff members have come into and have remained in home care because of the enjoyment they derive from working in a setting in which professional judgment can be exercised with relative independence. It is understandable therefore, that feelings of resentment toward the medical establishment may be quickly kindled when the question of permitting doctors to play a more active role in home care is raised.

Two circumstances may help to overcome these concerns. The first is that physicians, especially the younger generation, are now being trained in an environment which recognizes teamwork as essential to patient care in an increasingly complex health care system. They are less and less encouraged to consider themselves the automatic and entitled leaders of any group and are learning the lessons of cooperation. It behooves the leaders in home health to take advantage of that change in attitude and to channel the interest of physicians into home health for the betterment of overall patient care, not just to see them as a "market."

Second, nursing is changing also. There is a growing trend toward collaborative practice, especially in the tertiary care areas. As patients are discharged from hospitals sicker and quicker, possibly with nursing homes as the only viable alternative to home care, the need for closer collaboration is necessary to prevent potentially litigious situations for all parties. The new breed of home health agency (HHA) administrators are more competently trained for their executive functions and are more sensitized to the essential multidisciplinary nature of home care. The hospice movement has not only recognized this but also has incorporated team care into its practice, and might thus serve as a model for the restructuring of more traditional home health agencies.

Home health administrators need to recognize some of the deep-seated fears, which may thwart efforts to bring doctors into the home care fold, especially among older nurses who chose home health because of their desire for greater autonomy. Jealousy, fear, and distrust are all unpleasant emotions. It often is easier to gloss over them or deny their existence. If they are not handled honestly and openly, however, no real or lasting rapprochement can be achieved.

What Relationships Can be Developed?

There are probably three general areas in which doctors can interact with agencies. The first and most familiar is a service connection: that is, the relationship between an agency and a practicing physician whose patient is on home care. The second and less common but slowly emerging type of relationship is an educational one, usually between a medical school or a residency training program and a home health agency. The third is the formal affiliation, either contractual or advisory, which is an area which needs to be strengthened.

Service

The understanding between practicing physicians and home health agencies is and will remain a key one in home care. In many ways, these physicians represent a market which agencies spend a great deal of time trying to attract. By remembering what has been said about the diversity of practice style and specialty needs, an agency can, by studying referral patterns and examining past notable successes or failures, develop service packages which serve special patient populations or address particular patient care needs. Physicians will be more willing to refer and assist home care staff if they feel that the staff is responding to the problems of their patients.

There are certain things an agency can do besides marketing, however, to attract and keep physician referrals. It should simplify the process of doctor-agency interaction, be responsive to physicians' concerns, and maintain high service standards.

Physicians, in whatever type of practice, are busy and often inundated with paperwork of their own. Agencies can use simple techniques, such as batching orders to be signed, prearranging phone calls at convenient times, sending brief, clear instructions on how to fill out forms, or contacting agency staff to expedite the interaction process. Any and all of these procedures would be much appreciated by physicians.

Because of the geographic diffuseness of the typical home health agency, one of the key people in the agency will always be the telephone receptionist. This person often sets the tone for the agency and is in a position to expedite and facilitate resolution of both patient and physician problems. No one likes being put on interminable hold, having messages go astray, or being shunted from one desk to another when trying to resolve a problem, especially if it is felt to be clinically urgent. These small steps may help smooth the flow of information among all concerned parties.

Responsiveness to a physician's concerns may seem an obvious point. Unfortunately, however, difficulty often arises when there is a difference of opinion between the nurse and the physician as to what treatment the patient should be receiving. Although as home health agency staff strongly maintain they know "what's best" for the patient because they have seen the patient in his home environment, this should not blind them to the fact that there are instances when the doctor may have relevant and medically sound opinions which need to be heeded. If these are ignored and the staff simply carries out actions of which the physician is not aware, then the agency places itself at high risk for legal liability, if and when problems occur. For example, a physician visited a patient at home to debride a decubitus and wrote home care orders to use Dakins Solution as a debriding agent on dressings. Three weeks later, he returned and noticed that the ulcer still contained large amounts of slough and wasn't being cleaned out as expected. On questioning the visiting nurse, he was told that they hadn't been able to get Dakins so they had just used normal saline. He had not been informed of the change made to his orders. Should the patient have suffered complications because of this, it would have placed liability squarely on the shoulders of the agency's personnel.

Often, both therapists and nurses have preconceived service packages which they apply to given diagnoses and which tend to fit neatly within a 60-day period. Physicians, who may feel strongly that patient service needs are going to be more frequent and more intense at the beginning of a home care stay, and may well stretch out over a period of several months as the patient slowly improves, are often upset because they are unable to tailor the staff visits to match these needs.

Despite Medicare's restrictions daily visits are permitted, and as long as progress is being made toward a defined goal, patients can remain on programs for over two months. Encourage the physician to help fight retrospective denials; they may be more willing to do this if the denials have come from services they particularly requested, and if they are given a simple format to follow, with names and addresses, of how this can be done.

Although, in many instances doctors do not know how to write orders for rehabilitation, nor may they be aware of the types of skilled nursing functions which may be routinely carried out at home; there needs to be some effort made on the part of agencies to encourage a true collaboration between the case manager at the agency and the private physician. Often the doctor can sketch out what he thinks the plan should be in a general way, discuss with the nurse her recommendation, which can then be transmitted or transcribed into the very carefully worded statement required for retrospective reimbursement by the fiscal intermediaries.

Lastly, attention to high quality care needs to be rigorously maintained by the home health agency. Since physicians feel responsible for their patients, as well as feeling legally liable should complications occur, agencies can best attract doctors by making them feel that what they are ordering is of the highest caliber.

Education

The home health agency is starting to be a training base for doctors as both schools of medicine and residency programs come to realize that more training will have to be done outside the hospital setting. Already there are quite a few home health agencies which permit medical students, as part of their educational program, to make home visits with staff an activity which is usually enthusiastically received by students. To avoid potential problems and enhance the educational experience for visiting learners as well as agency staff, an orientation program for faculty should be developed. This should include, but not necessarily be limited to, the history of home care, the problems which it faces, methods of accessing the system for patients from a physician's perspective, and the type of participation expected of doctors once they have a patient on a program. It is this kind of information which will help students and residents learn to refer patients, and also begin to teach them what their responsibilities are once they do have patients on a program.

Written objectives for student learning experiences also should be developed, along with a protocol in conjunction with faculty for student orientation to the agency. Agency staff should be encouraged to participate in the development and implementation of educational and orientation materials. Finally, staff must have a clear understanding of student and faculty expectations of the learning experience. This will help to reduce, if not eliminate, any misgivings on either side.

There are several problems which agencies must recognize, however, if they are to provide this teaching service. The first is that it does take staff's time away from their normal patient care loads. If requests are too frequent, they may become resentful because it hampers them from meeting productivity standards set by supervisors and increasingly more mandated by Medicare reimbursement standards. In large agencies, this is less of a problem because there are numerous staff and patients over which to spread out medical student visits. However, in smaller agencies or in small population bases, it may become a real problem.

Another activity, which some home health agencies have tried, is to use residents as staff members for 8 to 20 hours per week. This method has been used for providing care and signing orders for those patients who have no identifiable physician but who need home care. They may also assist staff to develop care plans for difficult cases or for clinical problem solving out in the field. Lastly, residents may act as a resource to staff in areas of specialization, such as psychiatry or geriatrics, which might be of great benefit to the agency's patients. These programs show that through this prolonged exposure to the daily workings of a home health agency, residents begin to see not only the advantages of home care for the homebound patient, but also the problems which exist in order to provide needed services. Through their experiences, they then will become referral sources for their own patients in the future and perhaps even more importantly, will be able to act as advocates for the agency with other physicians, both in the hospital and in the community. Thus, by having them participate during their training period not only are they providing a service for patients, but they become enthusiastic, knowledgeable marketing forces in the future.

Formal Affiliations

Physicians may of course be formally affiliated with home health agencies. Agencies usually are most comfortable with this association if doctors act as unpaid advisors on utilization review committees, quality assurance committees, and so forth. Unfortunately, all too often, this relationship is seen primarily from its marketing perspective; i.e., this gives an agency access to the physician referral network which they are trying to reach. Rarely is the clinical expertise of the physician seen as an advantage to the agency itself. This is most unfortunate, since doctors represent more than just a market and are a part of the health care team.

While these part-time advisors are undoubtedly useful, all home health agencies should have a medical director. Obviously, whether or not these individuals are full-time employees at the home health agency will depend mostly on the case and financial mix of patients, as well as the agency's volume of business. However, a medical director can provide liaison to the general medical community, and also participate in in-service education programs for nursing and other staff. In programs having high volumes of patients for whom there is no private physician, the medical director may be able to serve as a primary care physician. Those agencies which are unable to afford full-time medical directors might consider retaining physicians on a limited basis.

Arguments may be made on both sides for the cost of a full-time physician to a home health agency. Some would argue that it is simply a high-priced public relations or marketing ploy, a token physician to lend credibility to the medical community. However, if the medical director is permitted and encouraged to provide leadership along with the other administrators in an agency, he can in fact become a productive member of the management team. Participation in quality assurance or utilization review programs, responsibility for continuing education and in-service, and in-home supervision of service delivery, especially to augment the nursing staff's expertise when delivering high-technology services are all meaningful, necessary tasks suitable for physicians, and most helpful if high quality is to be maintained.

For those agencies providing primarily support services or long-term care, a medical director also can be a valuable asset. By helping to monitor on-going problems similar to a nursing home physician, individuals, who are often thought not to be sick enough (or interesting enough) to be seen in the offices of their private physicians, may benefit most from the consultative home visits of another physician.

In addition to the argument about cost, the issue is often raised that private practitioners in the community will view a home health agency doctor as a competitor and a potential threat to their own practices. If a physician handles him in a tactful manner, it is quickly realized by those in practice that he is not in competition with them;

but rather that it adds a dimension to their own practices having a doctor present on site and readily available to answer questions posed by nursing staff. He can also alert them to potential problems which could complicate their patient's management. In that way much of the agency's time and many unnecessary calls to other physicians can be saved. A close link needs to be maintained with the private physician, and care needs to be taken that no doubts are raised in the minds of patients about who is actually in charge of their cases. It should be made clear to patients, however, that the home health agency's physician acts in a purely consultative role, and that he would call their personal doctors to report any problems before initiating action.

Agencies' staff members, especially nursing administration, are often loath to permit a doctor to be employed by the agency. Physicians are perceived as a direct threat and the turf issues discussed surface quickly. Also, cost is frequently raised as a barrier to this type of relationship; however, the improvements in quality of care, the facilitation of staff accessibility to a doctor for questions and problems to be solved, and the role of preceptor within the agency for any students or residents who are training there, are well worth the cost. Additionally, well-informed, articulate home care physicians can attend medical conferences in the community and nationally and present the case for home care, which often has a greater impact on groups of physicians than similar presentations by nonphysicians.

In conclusion, in order to facilitate good working relationships with physicians in home care, three things must be realized and addressed. First, all physicians are not the same; therefore, any relationships are going to have to take into account individual differences. Second, the fears which agencies have about the role of the physician must be squarely faced and openly discussed, because physicians need to be part of home health agencies. Finally, there are many relationships which agencies can have with physicians, all of them beneficial both for the agency and for patient care. What administrators must do is to look beyond the traditional marketing or referral pattern relationship, which has been the norm in the past, and examine some of the newer and more exciting ways of incorporating physicians into the home health care team.

Chapter Thirty-Four

The Role of the Medicare Fiscal Intermediary

Alan E. Reider

Introduction

The Medicare fiscal intermediary is the federal government's agent for the administration of the Medicare program. Despite the variety of names it may have, Blue Cross, Aetna, Prudential, etc., the entity which serves as fiscal intermediary is the Medicare program's representative, and is responsible for carrying out the Medicare program requirements. This chapter will review the role of the Medicare fiscal intermediary and its relationship to home health agencies in the administration of the Medicare program.

Structure

The fiscal intermediary's authority is based upon a contract with the Health Care Financing Administration (HCFA), the agency responsible for overall administration of the Medicare program. Under the terms of the contract, the fiscal intermediary is required to follow the statutory, regulatory, and program manual provisions promulgated by HCFA. Currently, there are approximately 50 intermediaries throughout the country, serving approximately 6,000 Medicare-certified home health agencies. In an effort to promote economy and consistency in the administration of the program throughout the country, however, HCFA has begun a transition which will result in a total of 10 regional intermediaries and 3 alternates for the entire country.[1] This transition is to be completed by July 1, 1987. The 10 regional intermediaries and the areas for which they are responsible are as follows:

1. Associated Hospital Service of Maine – Connecticut, Maine, Massachusetts, New Hampshire, Rhode Island, and Vermont.

2. The Prudential Insurance Company of America – New Jersey, New York, Puerto Rico, and the Virgin Islands.

3. Blue Cross of Greater Philadelphia – Delaware, District of Columbia, Maryland, Pennsylvania, Virginia, and West Virginia.

4. Blue Cross and Blue Shield of South Carolina – Kentucky, North Carolina, South Carolina, and Tennessee.

5. Aetna Life and Casualty—Alabama, Florida, Georgia, and Mississippi.

6. Blue Cross and Blue Shield United of Wisconsin—Wisconsin, Michigan, and Minnesota.

7. Health Care Service Corporation, Illinois, Indiana, and Ohio.

8. New Mexico Blue Cross and Blue Shield, Inc.—Arkansas, Louisiana, New Mexico, Oklahoma, and Texas.

9. Blue Cross of Iowa, Inc.—Colorado, Iowa, Kansas, Missouri, Montana, Nebraska, North Dakota, South Dakota, Utah, and Wyoming.

10. Blue Cross of California—Alaska, Arizona, California, Hawaii, Idaho, Oregon, Nevada, and Washington.

In addition, the alternate intermediaries and the states where they are available are:

1. The Prudential Insurance Company of America—Alabama, Connecticut, Delaware, District of Columbia, Florida, Georgia, Iowa, Kansas, Kentucky, Maine, Maryland, Massachusetts, Mississippi, Missouri, Nebraska, New Hampshire, North Carolina, Pennsylvania, Rhode Island, South Carolina, Tennessee, Vermont, Virginia, and West Virginia.

2. Blue Cross of Iowa, Inc.—Alaska, Arizona, Arkansas, California, Hawaii, Idaho, Illinois, Indiana, Louisiana, Michigan, Minnesota, Nevada, New Jersey, New Mexico, New York, Ohio, Oklahoma, Oregon, Puerto Rico, Texas, Virgin Islands, Washington, and Wisconsin.

3. Blue Cross of California—Colorado, Montana, North Dakota, South Dakota, Utah, and Wyoming.

As noted above, intermediaries are responsible for the administration of the Medicare program pursuant to regulations and program instructions promulgated from HCFA, whose central office is located in Baltimore, Maryland. Operationally, however, each intermediary responds to the respective HCFA regional office in which the intermediary is located. Only issues requiring significant policy interpretation or clarification, or extraordinary requests for unusual treatment, are forwarded to the central office in Baltimore. In addition, recently there has been established in each HCFA regional office a home health agency liaison, whose function is to address specific home health agency-related concerns which have been ruled on by the intermediary, or which, in the opinion of the agency, the intermediary has failed to address adequately.

Functions of the Fiscal Intermediary

The functions of the fiscal intermediary can be divided into four major areas: (1) education and information dissemination; (2) claims processing; (3) audit; and (4) review and surveillance. Because of the highly technical and somewhat burdensome administrative process associated with both claims processing and audit, it may appear that an undue amount of space has been devoted to those functions. Certainly, they are the predominant functions of the fiscal intermediary, in terms of the allocation of its resources and the impact felt on the home health agency. This should not, however, undermine the importance of the first function, education and information dissemination. Indeed, if the intermediary is effective in fulfilling this responsibility, there will be fewer problems relating to claims processing and auditing, and the need for the review and surveillance function will be minimized.

Education and Information Dissemination

As discussed above, the fiscal intermediary is the agent of HCFA for the administration of the Medicare program. For some agencies, the fiscal intermediary is the only source of information relating to changes and even laws and regulations in Medicare program policies.

The education and information dissemination function of the fiscal intermediary is fulfilled in a number of ways. All intermediaries provide periodic Medicare bulletins to advise agencies about changes in the Medicare program through amendments to laws or regulations, or to advise agencies about the interpretation of a policy which has been particularly troublesome. While this information is generally helpful and often reflects the official policy of HCFA, there have been occasions where intermediaries have promulgated their own interpretations of HCFA policies, and those interpretations may not necessarily represent the views of HCFA. Therefore, if an agency has difficulty with the provisions of an intermediary bulletin, it may wish to pursue the matter further with the intermediary, or, if necessary, with HCFA itself.

Just as important as written bulletins, the intermediary's education function is critical in resolving problems relating to its general claims processing or audit functions. These problems may relate to one or several home health agencies, and may reflect either a lack of understanding on the part of a particular agency, or confusion relating to a particular policy which affects many agencies. For many years, fiscal intermediaries were generally available for on-site consultation tiontiontionwith an individual agency, meetings with state associations, and telephone conferences in order to address specific problems. Recently, however, because of budgetary restrictions, there has been a cutback in the time which intermediaries have been willing to spend with agencies. Unfortunately, cutting back on the education side usually results in increased problems on the claims processing and audit side, thereby creating more overall cost to the program. Home health agencies should not hesitate to approach their respective fiscal intermediary and seek assistance whenever there appears to be a problem. Any resistance to such assistance should be addressed through the agency's state association or the HCFA regional office liaison.

Claims Processing

Review of Claims Submitted. The single largest function in terms of the intermediary's time and resources is claims processing. Periodically, generally every 30 days, home health agencies submit claims to the intermediary reflecting the services rendered to their Medicare patients. Once the intermediary has established that the patient receiving the services is eligible to receive Medicare benefits, it is responsible for reviewing the claim for two additional purposes: (1) to assure that the special requirements for obtaining home health care services were met; and (2) to assure that the services which were provided were medically necessary and appropriate. If the intermediary finds that either one of these requirements is not met, it will deny the claim, which could result in the denial of Medicare payment for the services rendered.

With respect to its review of whether the special requirements for obtaining home health care benefits have been met in a particular case, the intermediary is required to apply the standards set forth in the Medicare statute (Section 1814(a)(2)(C) of the Social Security Act) which provides that Medicare payment will be made for home health services where a physician certifies that "such services are or were required because the individual is or was confined to his home...and needs or needed skilled nursing care on an intermittent basis... ." Therefore, the intermediary will review the claim to assure that: (1) there is proper physician certification; (2) the patient is confined to his home ("homebound"); and (3) the patient requires skilled nursing care on an intermittent basis. If any of these three requirements is not met, the intermediary will deny the claim, and the Medicare program will not pay for services rendered. These denials are generally known as "technical" denials.

With respect to the second element of review, whether the services provided were medically necessary and appropriate, the intermediary may find that some or all of the services provided were not medically necessary for the condition of the patient. In such case, the intermediary will issue a denial, which may or may not have a Medicare reimbursement effect. This denial is known as a "coverage" or "medical necessity" denial. Under a provision known as "waiver of liability," the intermediary may find that although the services provided were not medically necessary, neither the patient nor the agency knew or had reason to know that those services would be denied as medically unnecessary.[2] Under such circumstances, the Medicare program will pay for those services. Alternatively, if the intermediary finds that the patient had no reason to know but that the agency did have reason to know that such services would not be covered, it will deny Medicare payment to the provider and prohibit the provider from billing the patient. Finally, in the rare instance where the intermediary finds that the beneficiary knew or had reason to know that the services would be denied, it will deny Medicare payment, but in this case the agency will be permitted to bill the Medicare patient for services rendered.

Appeal of the Part A Claim Denial. The Medicare program has an elaborate process for appealing the denial of Medicare Part A claims. Under current law, however, access to that process for a home health agency is limited, compared with that of a Medicare patient. Recalling the distinction between the technical denial and the medical necessity denial discussed above, while a Medicare patient has the right to pursue an appeal following a denial under any circumstances, the home health agency may only appeal a medical necessity denial and only when payment under waiver of liability does not apply. In other words, home health agencies may not appeal any technical denials, and may only appeal the medical necessity denial when the agency is fiscally liable.[3]

With respect to the appeal process, the written claim denial (known as an "initial determination"), is sent to both the patient and the agency. Medicare regulations require that the initial determination must state in detail the basis for the denial;[4] too often, however, this requirement is ignored by the intermediary. Agencies should insist on their right to understand fully the reason for the denial. Failure to do so will severely restrict the agency in pursuing a meaningful appeal.

Following receipt of the denial, the Medicare patient (or agency, as appropriate) may request a reconsideration by the intermediary if such request is made in writing within 60 days of receipt of the denial, regardless of the amount in controversy.[5] The request may be submitted either to the intermediary, a Social Security district office, or directly to HCFA. There is no time limit for an intermediary to complete the reconsideration process, and inordinate delays are not uncommon.

Once the reconsideration determination is made, further appeal is available by submitting a request for a hearing before an administrative law judge.[6] This request must be made in writing with 60 days of notice of the reconsideration determination, and may be submitted to the Social Security district office, to HCFA, or to a presiding administrative law judge. For an administrative law judge hearing, there must be at least $100 in controversy, although claims may be aggregated to meet the $100 minimum requirement. The hearing is nonadversarial in nature; that is, the intermediary will not be there to present its position. The home health agency or Medicare patient may appear in person, may have counsel, and may submit evidence or present witnesses.

A party dissatisfied with the decision of an administrative law judge may request review by the Appeals Council, a review body which is located in Arlington, Virginia.[7] Once again, any request for review by the Appeals Council must be made in writing within 60 days of the date of receipt of the administrative law judge's opinion. Unlike the administrative law judge hearing, the Appeals Council may refuse to review the hearing decision. Alternatively, even if not requested, the Appeals Council may review an administrative law judge's hearing decision on its own motion. Generally, Appeals Council decisions are based upon written briefs submitted by the parties.

Finally, a party dissatisfied with the decision of the administrative law judge or Appeals Council may request judicial review in United States District Court in the district in which the agency is located, if the amount in controversy is $1,000 or more.[8] A request for judicial review must be made in writing within 60 days of the date of receipt of the Appeals Council decision or denial of request for review by the Appeals Council. Once a case reaches district court level, it has become adversarial in nature, and the intermediary will be represented by attorneys from the Department of Health and Human Services. The review by the district court will be limited to the question of whether the administrative decision is supported by substantial evidence, and not whether the court would have reached the same result. The decision of the district court is appealable to the appropriate Circuit Court of Appeals, and, finally, to the United States Supreme Court.

In addition to the formal appeal process, the Medicare regulations provide for a discretionary appeal process where a decision may be "reopened" by either the intermediary, the administrative law judge, the Appeals Council, or the district court.[9] A request for reopening must be directed in writing to the highest level which issued a decision. The decision to reopen is purely discretionary, i.e., there is no appeal from a refusal to reopen. Further, the intermediary does not require a request from a party; it has the authority to reopen on its own, as long as an appeal on the claim has not gone beyond the intermediary level. Finally, the regulations provide that a reopening is permitted: (1) within 12 months of the date of notice of the determination or decision, for any reason; (1) within 4 years of notice of the determination or decision, if good cause is shown, which includes submission of new and material evidence, or a finding that a clerical error was made; and (3) at any time, if the original decision was procured by fraud or similar fault, or, in the case of a request by a patient or agency, whether there has been a clerical error or an error on the face of the evidence.

Appeal of the Part B Claim Denial. Although the majority of home health agency claims will likely be submitted under Part A of Medicare, the agency may also submit claims for services rendered under Part B of the Medicare program. The major difference in the intermediary's role, when comparing Part A and Part B claims processing, is in the appeal process. Unlike the Part A side, there is no distinction between the rights of the patient and the rights of the home health agency. Those rights, however, are significantly restricted under Part B.

When the intermediary denies a claim submitted under Part B, both the agency and the patient have the right to request a review of that decision by submitting a request in writing to the intermediary within six months of the date of the decision. There is no minimum dollar amount. If the intermediary's reviewed decision is not favorable, the agency or the patient may request a hearing before an intermediary-appointed hearing officer. Such a request must be made in writing and must be made within six months of the date of the intermediary's notice of review determination. In addition, there must be at least $100 in controversy, although the agency or the patient may aggregate claims to reach the $100 threshold amount.[10]

Here the similarity with the Part A appeal process ends. Unlike the administrative law judge who is completely independent of the intermediary and is bound only by the Medicare statute, regulations, and formal HCFA rulings, the hearing officer is appointed by the intermediary, and is bound by the Medicare program manual provisions and general HCFA instructions.[11] Further, there is no appeal beyond the decision of the hearing officer, either to a higher administrative level or to court.[12] There are, however, provisions for reopening under Part B, similar to those which are provided under Part A.

Audit

Agency Cost Report and Intermediary Audit. Despite the fact that the home health agency submits claims to the fiscal intermediary during the year and is paid either on a claim-by-claim or periodic interim payment (PIP) basis, final Medicare payment to a home health agency is dependent upon resolution of the agency's Medicare Cost Report. The agency is required to submit a cost report to the intermediary within three months following the end of an agency's fiscal year.[13] The Medicare Cost Report sets forth the total cost of the operation of the agency, the allocation of costs between the Medicare program and all non-Medicare payors, and the total amount of Medicare reimbursement claimed by the agency for services rendered to Medicare beneficiaries during the year.

Upon receipt of the cost report, the intermediary will perform what is known as a "desk audit," reviewing the documentation provided by the agency to assure that the calculations are accurate and that only appropriate claims for Medicare-reimbursable costs have been made. Occasionally, the intermediary will settle a cost report without an on-site audit. Generally, however, the intermediary will perform an on-site audit at the agency which may take between two days and two weeks or even longer, depending upon the size of the agency, the complexity of the documentation, and the patience of the auditors. On-site audits may cover more than one cost report year of an agency's operation.

During the on-site audit, the agency must make available to the intermediary auditors any documentation to support the costs claimed on its cost report. The agency should make every effort to provide the auditors with the necessary documentation in order to avoid potential problems which could result in cost disallowances. If such documentation is not immediately available, the agency should arrange to provide the documentation to the auditors following the on-site visit, but prior to the issuance of any formal reimbursement notice.

At the conclusion of the audit, there will be an exit conference at which the auditors will present their findings to the agency. These findings will include the specific disallowances, if any, made to the agency's cost report, as well as any general management findings relating to the operation of the agency. The disallowances may represent reductions of costs claimed by the agency because those costs are determined to be unreasonably high, or may involve the total disallowance of items claimed by the agency which the auditors determine are not related to patient care, or otherwise not covered by the Medicare program. In addition, the auditors may reduce the number of Medicare visits claimed by the agency, based upon their finding that the patients were not Medicare-eligible, or that the services provided were not covered home health services under the Medicare program. This, of course, also affects the total amount of Medicare reimbursement to the agency.

Despite its role as the source of potentially bad news, the exit conference affords a home health agency an excellent opportunity to address and resolve many potential problems at an early stage. Unfortunately, however, most agencies do not take advantage of this opportunity. A home health agency should use the exit conference as an opportunity to clarify the basis for any adjustment proposed by the intermediary, and should attempt to obtain a commitment from the intermediary as to what documentation, if any, is necessary to satisfy the intermediary of the propriety of the costs claimed. Too often, an agency sits politely through the exit conference and awaits the issuance of the intermediary's Notice of Program Reimbursement in which the disallowances are formally issued. At that point, the agency must seek its redress through the administrative appeals process—a long, expensive, and cumbersome road. (The formal appeals process is discussed further below.)

Ideally, if time allows, the agency should try to obtain as much information prior to the exit conference relating to any concerns which the auditors may have raised. The exit conference can then be used to respond to those concerns. Even if this is not possible, if the issues raised by the auditors at the exit conference can be clarified, and it can be agreed by both the agency and the auditors that certain documentation might satisfy the auditors, the agency should do everything possible to provide the documentation as soon as possible in order to avoid the issuance of a formal disallowance. The earlier in the process that a disallowance is addressed, the more likely it will be reversed.

Notice of Program Reimbursement. Following the on-site audit and the exit conference, the intermediary will issue a formal Notice of Program Reimbursement which will delineate all the adjustments to the agency's cost report made by the intermediary on the basis of its audit.[14] Any adjustment must be described adequately, and the basis for the adjustment (that is, a reference to the *Medicare Provider Reimbursement Manual, Home Health Agency Manual,* or program instruction) should be provided by the intermediary. The Notice of Program Reimbursement will also advise the agency that if it is dissatisfied with the results of the intermediary's audit, it may appeal the intermediary's determinations to the Provider Reimbursement Review Board (PRRB) of the Health Care Financing Administration, as long as the amount in controversy is $10,000 or more. If the amount in controversy is between $1,000 and $10,000, the agency may request an intermediary hearing. A request for either a PRRB hearing or an intermediary hearing must be made in writing within 180 days of the issuance date of the Notice of Program Reimbursement.[15]

Intermediary and PRRB Hearing. Once an agency's request for hearing has been acknowledged by an intermediary hearing officer or the PRRB, the agency and intermediary will be instructed to meet and attempt to resolve any of the outstanding issues. Prior to the meeting, the agency should have assembled all documentation to substantiate the costs at issue, and should have researched the issue thoroughly to determine whether there is any precedent either supporting or rejecting its position. In addition, the agency has the right to prehearing discovery, that is, to request all records of the intermediary which relate to the issues subject to the appeal. This information can be very helpful, and may often reveal the real basis for the disallowance. At the meeting with the intermediary, the agency should present its best argument as to why the costs claimed are appropriate. If the agency has appealed several different issues, and some appear to be stronger than others, it may wish to suggest to the intermediary a compromise, which will enable the parties to avoid the necessary time and expense of a formal hearing. This prior meeting serves as an excellent vehicle for negotiating a possible compromise.

Barring complete resolution of the issues subject to appeal, prior to the hearing, the home health agency will be required to submit a formal position paper, which specifies the issues subject to appeal and the reasons that the agency believes it is entitled to the costs claimed. The position paper is a formal document which should review in detail the legal arguments in support of the agency's position. In addition to references to the Medicare statute and regulations, the paper should attempt to address any case law precedent which involves an identical or similar issue. The position paper is the cornerstone of the provider's administrative appeal.

The hearing itself is not as rigid a proceeding as a court hearing. Nevertheless, it is a formal hearing with the opportunity to submit evidence, to present witnesses, and to cross-examine the witnesses of other parties. During the hearing process (as throughout the entire process), agencies may be represented by counsel.[16]

The intermediary hearing represents the agency's only level of appeal when the amount in controversy is less than $10,000. Because the intermediary is bound by contract to enforce the provisions of the Medicare manuals, which represent HCFA's interpretation of the statute and regulations, an agency should pursue an intermediary hearing only when it is apparent that the intermediary has failed clearly to follow program requirements.

The PRRB, however, is not so limited, and further opportunity to appeal PRRB cases is available. Although bound by the Medicare statute, regulations and HCFA rulings, the PRRB is not bound by the Medicare manual provisions, and will not hesitate to reverse an intermediary which has followed the manual when such action is shown to violate the applicable statute or regulations.

For those cases which involve a challenge to the statute, regulations, or to an HCFA ruling, there is a provision for expedited proceedings, whereby the PRRB determines that it does not have the authority to rule in favor of the provider.[17] In such cases, the PRRB will acknowledge its lack of jurisdiction, and the case may proceed directly to district court for review.

One final matter is worth noting with respect to the PRRB hearing. If an agency is one of a group of agencies under common ownership or control, any appeal must be brought as a "group appeal," which involves all the related agencies (as well as other related providers) with respect to any matter involving an issue common to all the providers and for which the amount in controversy is, in the aggregate, $50,000 or more. While this requirement was obviously designed to promote administrative and judicial economy, as well as consistency in the decision-making process, it can lead to a significant administrative burden. For example, for a single cost report year, an individual agency may be involved in a group appeal for one or more issues, as well as individual appeals for issues which do not meet the $50,000 jurisdictional amount, or which are not common to the other related agencies. In this case, an agency must await the resolution of at least two appeals in order to have its cost report finally settled.

Administrator Review. As noted above, there are further appeals available beyond the PRRB level. Following a decision by the PRRB, a dissatisfied agency may request review by the Administrator of the Health Care Financing Administration, or it may appeal directly to district court. In either case, the request for review or appeal must be made within 60 days of receipt of the PRRB decision. The agency should be aware, however, that even if the PRRB decision is favorable, it is possible that the intermediary may request that the Administrator review the PRRB's decision or that the Administrator, on his own motion, may review the decision. Some intermediaries automatically request Administrator review whenever the PRRB issues a decision which is favorable to a provider. If the Administrator agrees to review the case, the Administrator must issue a decision within 60 days of the PRRB decision. In such a case, the agency has 60 days from the date of the Administrator's decision to appeal that decision to district court.[18]

Judicial Review. The role of the district court is to determine whether the administrative decision, that is, the decision of the administrator or the PRRB, was reasonable. Generally, courts will give great deference to a government agency's rulings under its own program. Nevertheless, many providers have successfully challenged PRRB or administrator decisions, where courts have found that the PRRB or administrator had improperly interpreted the Medicare regulations, or, on occasion, that the Medicare regulations were inconsistent with the Medicare statute.

At this level, however, the Department of Health and Human Services will be represented by attorneys, and the controversy may be long, difficult, and expensive. Review beyond the district court may be brought to the appropriate Circuit Court of Appeals, and finally, to the Supreme Court of the United States.[19]

Review and Surveillance

The fourth and final function of the fiscal intermediary is to perform review and surveillance of home health agencies to assure that the program requirements are fulfilled. Generally, this kind of activity focuses in on providers whose statistical data vary somewhat from the norm. This may reflect, for example, high volume providers, providers with a high intensity of services (i.e., a high number of services per patient), an unusual frequency of a particular type of service, such as home health aides, physical therapy, etc., or any other type of activity which suggests that an agency is not performing consistently with its peers. Alternatively, focus may be directed toward agencies based upon allegations from beneficiaries, disgruntled employees, physicians, etc., or findings, made by auditors or medical reviewers, which suggest that the agency is not following program requirements.

The review and surveillance function can be divided into two categories, the compliance audit and program integrity. Each of these is discussed briefly below.

Compliance Audit. Medicare fiscal intermediaries are required to perform on-site medical records reviews for a prescribed number of home health agencies each year. These reviews, known as home health agency coverage compliance reviews, or compliance audits, are designed to assure that home health agencies are providing services consistent with the Medicare program requirements. Agencies are selected on the basis of an annual ranking which considers four factors: (1) the average Medicare cost per Medicare patient; (2) the average number of visits per Medicare patient; (3) the percent of Medicare utilization; and (4) the percent of Medicare visits that are home health aide visits. The intermediary is instructed to review the top 10% of all agencies based on an aggregate ranking of these factors. In addition, any newly participating agency is subject to a compliance audit, at approximately its first anniversary of participation, as is any agency which has lost its favorable waiver of liability presumption (see footnote 2), and any agency which has had an on-site review denial rate of 5% or more on a previous on-site review.

During the compliance audit, the intermediary will randomly select 20 beneficiaries recently served by the agency, and will obtain three months of billings processed within six months of the scheduled review for each beneficiary. Nurse reviewers from the intermediary will perform a record review of all the selected patients; in addition, the reviewers will visit at least five of the selected beneficiaries currently receiving home health services from the agency. While the purpose of the audit is to assure compliance with Medicare requirements, the intermediary is instructed to focus on a number of specific questions, including whether the patient is homebound; whether the services were furnished under a plan of treatment; whether the physician certification requirement was met; and whether the services provided were medically necessary.

At the conclusion of the compliance audit, the nurse reviewers will meet with the agency for an exit conference to discuss the cases reviewed and, specifically, to provide information about the denials which the reviewers propose to make. During the exit conference the home health agency should focus on two concerns: (1) learning the precise basis for the issuance of any proposed denial; and (2) providing as much documentation as possible to the reviewer in order to convince the reviewer that the services provided were appropriate. With respect to collecting information, the agency should ask if it can tape the exit conference. If that request is denied, copious notes should be taken. Further, if there is any question by the agency as to the nature of the denial, the agency should press the nurse reviewers until the basis is absolutely clear. With respect to providing as much information as possible in order to convince the reviewer that the services rendered were appropriate, the agency may be best served by having as many of its own nurses in attendance as possible, particularly those who provided the services. Oftentimes, these nurses can provide the most relevant information and can successfully convince the reviewers that the services rendered were appropriate.

Following the exit conference, the agency has an additional two weeks to provide information to the intermediary. Any proposed denials which remain in place should be addressed at this time, and any additional documentation should be obtained. There is no restriction from providing the intermediary with additional data which was not previously in the medical record. Intermediaries that reject such information are creating unnecessary burdens for all parties, including themselves. Such additional information is clearly allowed during the later stages of the appeal process; it makes no sense for the intermediary to reject it at this early stage. After the intermediary has received whatever additional documentation is provided, it will make its decision on the claims proposed to be denied. Once an intermediary denies a claim, the agency's formal appeal rights begin, identical to those discussed above. Nevertheless, to the extent that an agency can reverse a proposed denial prior to the issuance of a formal denial, it will avoid the long and uncertain formal appeal process.

Program Integrity. The second component of the review and surveillance function of the fiscal intermediary is program integrity. As its name suggests, in this capacity, the intermediary is responsible for assuring the integrity of the Medicare Program with respect to the appropriate payment of claims submitted and costs claimed for reimbursement.

Up until the past few years, the role of the fiscal intermediary in its program integrity function was largely reactive in nature. If a potential problem came to the attention of the intermediary, either through a complaint of the beneficiary, or through irregularities found in the audit process or claims processing system, the intermediary reviewed the matter and determined the nature and extent of the problem. Based on its findings, the intermediary either pursued the matter directly with the home health agency or, if the matter involved a potentially serious fraud issue, the intermediary referred the matter to the regional office of the Health Care Financing Administration for further referral to the Office of Investigations, which is now part of the Office of the Inspector General.

Recently, in light of the increased pressures to control unnecessary program costs, the program integrity function has increased, and the intermediary has taken a more active role. In addition to following up the possible sources for fraud and abuse cases as noted above, intermediaries now perform more intense medical review on claims submitted by home health agencies, participate in audits and inspections sponsored by the Office of the Inspector General in areas where particular program concerns are targeted, and have become generally more aggressive in the conduct of individual case reviews.

Home health agencies, as well as all other providers, physicians, and suppliers under the Medicare program, must be aware that the fiscal agents are under tremendous pressure from HCFA to recover what are generally believed to be significant overpayments in the Medicare program. In fact, among the various basis upon which HCFA evaluates its fiscal agents, a significant portion of the evaluation focuses on the recovery of improper overpayments, as well as the referral of potential fraud cases for investigation. While this will not help to relieve home health agencies of concerns for increased activity in the program integrity area, it is helpful to understand the basis for such increased activity.

Summary and Conclusion

This chapter has attempted to outline the four major functions of the fiscal intermediary in its relationship with the home health agency. A detailed discussion of each element in that relationship and the variety of issues which may arise would take several volumes, let alone a single chapter in a book.

What this chapter has hopefully made clear, however, is that the importance of the fiscal intermediary cannot be overstated in terms of the agency's relationship to the Medicare program. Effectively, the Medicare fiscal intermediary *is* the Medicare program as far as that agency is concerned.

If there is a single message which should be sent to home health agencies, it is the need for a good working relationship with the fiscal intermediary. Ideally, this should be pursued through the intermediary's initial function, that of education and information dissemination. Agencies should do everything possible to encourage free and open communication between themselves and the intermediary. By assuring that the agencies understand the requirements of the Medicare program as perceived by the fiscal intermediary, the risks of problems in the claims processing system, in the audit system, and, most importantly, in the area of review and surveillance, can be minimized.

Postscript

On October 18, 1986, Congress passed the Omnibus Budget Reconciliation Act of 1986 (OBRA) which made several changes to the Medicare program. Among those changes are provisions which will have a direct impact on the home health care industry, particularly on the role of the Medicare fiscal intermediary. Those changes relating to the role of the Medicare fiscal intermediary are as follows:

1. Congress has specifically granted the authority of a provider to represent the beneficiary in an appeal, as long as the provider waives all rights for payment

from the beneficiary for the services involved in the appeal. This directly over-rules a HCFA instruction which prohibited providers from representing beneficiaries in the appeal process.

2. Effective July 1, 1987, the waiver of liability provisions will be extended to include denials for failing to meet the "intermittent" or "homebound" criteria. Under present law, waiver of liability does not apply to any technical denial. This change will remain in effect until October 1, 1989. In addition, the Secretary of Health and Human Services is required to report to Congress in March of 1987 and 1988, concerning denials of claims and payment under waiver of liability, in order that Congress may evaluate the appropriateness of imposing a denial rate standard for the granting of favorable waiver presumptions.

3. With respect to Part B appeals, the entire process has been drastically amended. Effective for services rendered after January 1, 1987, for claims in which more than $500 is at issue, an aggrieved party may obtain a hearing before an administrative law judge, instead of an intermediary fair hearing. Where the amount in dispute is more than $1,000, appeal is available beyond the administrative law judge to district court. Thus, the Part B appeal process is now essentially equivalent to the Part A appeal process. For claims in which there is less than $500 at issue, the fair hearing continues to be available.

4. Finally, OBRA also included a provision which provides beneficiaries with the right to appeal payment denials for services which do not meet the "homebound" or "intermittent care" criteria. Yet, beneficiaries have always had the right to appeal such denials. Until HCFA promulgates regulations relating to this section, it is unclear what change, if any, will result from this section of OBRA.

Endnotes

1. 51 Fed. Reg. 5403 (February 13, 1986).

2. The waiver of liability provisions are based on 1879 of the Social Security Act, and are implemented through Medicare regulations 42 C.F.R. 405.330 405.332. In order to avoid the administrative burden of reviewing each claim for waiver purposes, any home health agency whose denial rate is less than 2.5% is granted a favorable waiver of liability presumption, which means that unless otherwise demonstrated by the intermediary, the agency will be paid for services rendered, even though the intermediary determines that the services were not medically necessary or appropriate. In such a case, it is presumed that the agency did not know or have reason to know that the services would be denied as medically unnecessary. Agencies whose denial rate is above 2.5% during a calendar quarter will not have a favorable waiver of liability presumption, and will have the burden of demonstrating that waiver of liability should apply where the intermediary has denied a particular claim.

3. See Medicare Regulations 42 C.F.R. 405.704.

4. 42 C.F.R. 405.702.

5. 42 C.F.R. 405.710 and 405.711.

6. 42 C.F.R. 405.720 and 405.722.

7. 42 C.F.R. 405.724 and 20 C.F.R. 404.967.

8. 42 C.F.R. 405.730.

9. 42 C.F.R. 405.750.

10. 42 C.F.R. 405.803 405.820.

11. 42 C.F.R. 405.823 and Medicare Carriers Manual, 12016.

12. See United States v. Erika, Inc., 102 S. Ct. 1650 (1982).

13. 42 C.F.R. 405.453(f)(2).

14. 42 C.F.R. 405.1803.

15. 42 C.F.R. 405.1811 and 405.1841.

16. 42 C.F.R. 405.1809 405.1827 and 405.1851 to 405.1865.

17. 42 C.F.R. 405.1842.

18. 42 C.F.R. 405.1875.

19. 42 C.F.R. 405.1877.

20. *See generally Medicare Intermediary Manual*, Part II, 2300-2300.5.

Part X

Putting Things Into Perspective

Chapter Thirty-Five

The Future of Home Care

Val J. Halamandaris

The future of home care in America looks bright. Every year more Americans are living to their 85th birthday and beyond; they are members of the fastest-growing age group in America. Those who survive can expect to be plagued with at least four disabilities. Home health care will be the answer to helping these people live high-quality lives with a maximum of human dignity. It will serve to keep families together and to save the government billions of dollars as compared to the alternative, which is institutionalization.

Several major forces are pushing the American health care system towards home health care. One of these forces is demographics, another is the increasing attention to prevention and wellness, yet another is the trend away from institutionalization toward providing care in the least restrictive environment. Still another factor is the growing need for government and the private sector to solve this riddle: How do you cover the health care needs of more people at less cost? Home care offers a viable answer. Yet another factor is the growing public acceptance and demand for home care. Then there is the not-to-be ignored march of the handicapped and disabled who ask for home care in order that they may lead active and productive lives as full partners in American society.

Another important force dictating the swing back to home care is tradition. Since time immemorial, health care has been given at home. Americans are more and more acting out the dictates of Emerson's essay on self-reliance. A final factor that needs to be mentioned is technology. The same technology that has allowed us to save lives is now being employed to help us care for the survivors. The technology has been miniaturized and made portable so that it can be used not only in the hospital but in the home as well.

It is technology which will allow us to move the 10 million children with birth defects and related chronic problems out of the hospitals back where they belong—at home with their families.

The move toward home care will be rapid and it will be complete. It will be part of the major revolution in the delivery of health care services in America. There is virtually nothing and no one capable of holding back the tide. Those few people who do want to do so work within the Office of Management and Budget.

The concern of critics is that the growing demand for home care and long-term care will be additive—that people will come out of the woodwork to use the services if they are available. They fear that the cost to government programs will increase dramatically, if they ever allow the genie out of the bottle. In the short run, these people have been able to exert their influence on the Department of Health and

Reprinted with permission from the October 1985 issue of *Caring* Magazine, "The Future of Home Care in America," by Val J. Halamandaris.

Human Services to restrict Medicare payment for home health care. The restrictions, which are nothing more than mandated administrative cuts in the Medicare program, have been many. The effect on agencies and beneficiaries who need care has been severed. But these efforts are misguided, grounded in ignorance about what home health care is all about and they will be as effective as building sand castles to hold back the coming tide.

These are the conclusions which evolve from this article. It begins as it must with the primary, unquestionable fact: the greying of America. It ends with the statement that the future of home care lies in the hands of those who are now providing services. The actions they take will determine the shape of events to come. If they continue to spread joy and love along with the highest quality health care services to the needy in their own homes, the number of advocates for home care will multiply by the millions — and home care may just become the primary mode of health care in the 21st century.

Life Expectancy

Throughout history, humanity has been trying to learn the answer to the question of why we must age. Extending the life span was an important goal. At the time of the Emperor Augustus Caesar in Rome, life expectancy was 33 years of age. It was, in the words of a philosopher who came along centuries later, "nasty, brutish, short."

Through the succeeding centuries, every conceivable means was employed to extend the life span. Bloodletting and leeches were one method employed. One of the early Popes of the Catholic Church died as a result of a primitive blood transfusion. The physician of the time took blood from very vigorous young men from the community but they did not allow for differences in blood grouping. Their ignorance of Rh factors proved fatal. Climate and water were explored. The grafting of animal sex glands, the injection of hormones were added to the list. Eating certain foods or abstaining from certain foods were explored by serious medical practitioners who from time to time proclaimed one or another of these as the way to cure illness and disease and help extend the life span. For example, in the 1870s a representative from the world-famous Pasteur Institute in France shouted "Eureka" to the world. He had found the answer which he said was to eat lactobacillus. Unfortunately, eating yogurt has not proven to be the "Fountain of Youth."

Very little progress was made along these lines until the 20th Century. When Claude Pepper and Helen Hayes were born in 1900, life expectancy was 43 years of age. In 1900, only 3% of the population lived to be 65 years of age. The obvious point is that in the 19 centuries following the death of Christ mankind gained only 10 years on average life expectancy.

In the first 85 years of the 20th century, by contrast, life expectancy has increased by 32 years on average. It is now 75 in the United States and as high as 84 in another country. About 12% of the population in the United States is now aged 65 or older and the number is climbing. We have gone beyond the one- and two-generation family to the five-generation family. The greatest increase in longevity is seen among the older members of the senior generation. While the rest of the population increased 9.1% in the past 10 years in the US, those over 85 increased by 56.6%. There are about 15,000 people over 100 alive today. By the year 2000, there will be more than 100,000 centenarians. In the year 2050, there will be more than 16 million people over the age of 85 in the US.

To offer some perspective, Monsignor Charles Fahey once pointed out to me that studies indicate that over two-thirds of the people who ever lived to reach the age of 65 are alive today. He argues that we in the 20th Century have been blessed with a gift of another third of life, a "third age" which was not available to our ancestors.

All the above estimates are conservative they do not take into account the effect of major breakthroughs in medicine, many of which are on the horizon. The revolutionary CAT scan has already yielded to the more advanced NMR (nuclear magnetic resonance), and the capability for gene splicing already exists. It is likely that some modern miracles will continue to evolve. Many scientists believe that we are on the verge of a cure for cancer. With or without such breakthroughs the number of people who live to double the average life expectancy at the time of their birth (like Claude Pepper and Helen Hayes) will continue to multiply. The prospect of thousands of people being born this minute living to age 150 and beyond is truly mind-boggling.

Throughout it all, one thing is certain. As mortality is reduced there is a concomitant increase in disability. This means a greater need for home care and long-term care.

Dollars

It should be no surprise, given all of the above, that American health care expenditures have increased. Health care is the third largest industry in the US costing us $320 billion this year or over 10.5% of the Gross National Product. Health care costs have been increasing at 12% a year, more than double the increase in the consumer price index due to inflation. It is expected that health care costs will reach $1 trillion by 1990—less than 5 years from now.

At the present time 40% of the health care dollar is received by hospitals, 10% by nursing homes, and home care accounts for only one and one-half percent of the total. The home care portion is increasing rapidly and should hit 3% by 1987, 5% by 1990, and exceed 10% in the year 2000.

Government spending accounts for 42 cents of every health care dollar; 12 cents comes from the states, and the federal government pays 30 cents. In 1984, Medicare paid $66 billion for health care, a 17-fold increase since the program started in 1966. Expenditures in fiscal 1985 are estimated at $75 billion. Some 29 million people, including most of the elderly and some individuals who are disabled, qualify for Medicare. Medicare paid about $2 billion for home health care services last year. The Medicaid program—the federal-state partnerhsip for indigent care—paid out of $45 billion last year, some $20 billion of which was federal dollars.

The pressure of ever-increasing health care costs driven by a multiplicity of factors caused the government to move in the direction of prospective payment (DRG reimbursement) for hospitals participating in the Medicare program. The results of this action are noted laster. Cost pressures also fuel the search for alternative systems such as health maintenance organizations and home health care.

The Widening Care Gap

The propaganda is that Medicare covers 44% of the health care costs of the elderly. The truth is a good deal different. In the first place, this estimate includes premiums and co-insurance which are paid into Medicare by beneficiaries. Excluding these taxes which the elderly must pay to unlock Medicare coverage, the percentage coverage drops to 37%. The percentage must be further reduced because millions of dollars are absorbed by the elderly. This is true because they do not know how to navigate in Medicare's insurance-like maze in order to have Medicare reimburse them for money they have advanced.

To be sure, Medicare is a blessing and none would give it up but there are tremendous gaps. There is no coverage for preventive medicine. Physical examinations are not covered, neither are office visits. Such items as eyeglasses, hearing aids, dental care, and out-of-hospital prescription drugs are excluded. Most home care or nursing home care is not covered.

The Medicaid program by contrast is available only to the poor. States set the rules and there is a great deal of variability. Most states have both income and asset tests which limit those who can be helped. Even when individuals can qualify for Medicaid there are tremendous gaps. For example, every state was required in 1967 to cover home health care as a result of an amendment sponsored by Senator Frank E. Moss, but few states have any Medicaid home care program of consequence. New York and California are two exceptions. Total Medicaid payments for home care were in the vicinity of $500 million last year, more than half of this in New York state.

The biggest gap of all is long-term care (as opposed to acute care). What we are talking about here is help for people with multiple and chronic disabilities. A conservative estimate is that 20% of the nation's 26 million elderly need such care. Their needs may be cared for through home care unless they are so acute they require the 24-hour-a-day, round-the-clock care of a nursing home. Add to this number some 10 million children and an equal number of middle-aged individuals, and the magnitude of the problem becomes clear.

Speaking only of the aged, government statistics now show that 5.5 million are going without the home care services that they need. This number will double in the next five years. Most of the 10 million severely disabled and handicapped children can now be cared for at home. Their numbers are expected to expand as well but not so rapidly as the elderly. The handicapped and the middle-aged will likely stay at a level, stable percentage.

After all is said and done, it is estimated that one out of every eight American cannot get the health care he or she needs today. The greatest need is found in the area of long-term care. This unmet need generates pressures on both government and the private sector.

Over the last dozen years, unions have sought to increase the fringe benefit available to their employees more than increasing salaries. Health care is the most popular benefit. Unions are now in the position where they face sharp increases in the cost of providing existing benefits at the same time as demands to expand benefits to cover the every-widening gaps. Home health care is appealing because it allows dollars to be stretched so that the needs of more people can be met at less cost.

The pressures on American business are illustrated by the automobile industry. One would think the biggest cost item for General Motors or Chrysler is the cost of steel. Not so—it is the cost of providing health care to their employees. The cost of health care runs about 10% of total costs. Not surprisingly, major corporations both within and outside of the automobile industry are looking to HMOs, home health, and other cost-saving alternatives.

Fraud, Waste, and Inefficiency

While there is little doubt that Americans have the best quality system of health care on the planet, it is not exactly known for its efficiency. In fact, there is a good deal of inefficiency and waste. America is a wealthy country and we do not always appreciate the value of what we have. And then, too, the American health care system has evolved so rapidly and is in such metamorphosis at present that some inefficiency is predictable.

Here are some examples that I read recently. It is contended that $5-10 billion is wasted on useless medical technology, that there are more than 2 million unnecessary surgical operations in the U.S. every year, costing more than $4 billion a year. Half of the $10 billion Medicare supplementary insurance policy premiums are said to be duplicative, without economic value. Estimates on medical quackery run from $10 to $25 billion a year.

It is alleged that the extent of fraud and abuse in government health care programs runs at a minimum of 5% and may be as high as 30% of these programs. Insurance companies are now willing to admit publicly that similarly sizable ripoffs exists in the private health insurance market. As a matter of fact, many insurance companies have now initiated "fraud squads" to work with investigators to try to plug some of these massive losses.

The Debate in Congress

Having been inundated by all of these factors, the Congress of the United States has been trying to hammer out a health care system to take America through the balance of the 20th century. There is little agreement on what such a system should look like or even on the extent of the role to be played by government. There is, however, the growing consensus that the problem is large and growing—indeed that the problem is and will be so massive that it can only be solved by the federal government

From the point of view of the Congress, the entire issue must be viewed through the prism of the expected $200 billion budget deficits. No nation or private individual can consistently spend 10% to 20% more than they bring in revenues and remain solvent. At the present time, America is already burdened with paying off the debts accumulated from deficit spending in prior years. Interest on the national debt is now the third-largest item in the budget. Of this interest, much is owed to foreign banks that have rushed to bring their capital to America because of the high interest rates they have found here. The Congress can be forgiven for being just a little bit nervous about continuing to run up such deficits.

Once you reach the conclusion that the deficits are too high, the issue becomes: Where do you cut? There is a very sharp division here reflected both in the American public and within the Congress. The Reagan administration has led the parade to cut entitlement programs such as Social Security and Medicare, believing too great a percentage of the budget was spent on these areas and that not enough has been spent on defense. The Democratic-controlled House of Representatives has the opposite view. The battle has raged for five years with the President and his pro-military policymakers winning the day. As a result, the decision has been made to spend beyond our means in order to support the purchase of new military hardware such as a fleet of B-1 bombers, each one of which costs as much as the budget for research on Alzheimer's disease and related problems of aging.

There is no question in my mind how the debate will be resolved in the long run. The growing numbers of older Americans who need health care and supportive services is going to hit like a tidal wave on the beach of America. There is some talk of "senior power" today, but few people really have any idea of the force it will become. By illustration, in the year 2000, the U.S. will have the same percentage of elderly nationally as the state of Florida presently has of its population. You have only to look to Florida to see what that means. The political power of the elderly is enormous there. It will be so throughout America.

The point that is often missed is that it is not only the elderly themselves who will advocate increased home health care and other long-term care benefits. It will be the middle-aged and the middle-class, the so-called "sandwich generation" that is trying to support children in high school or college at the same time as their elderly parents or grandparents — or maybe even great-grandparents — in their long-term care needs.

What remains to be seen, of course, is how the U.S. will handle its increasing federal debt. The most obvious solution is an unpopular one — raise taxes. I suspect that this is what will occur. Here, too, the debate will be whether to use these dollars to pay the debts run up be the previous generations to use the money to meet present needs.

I think a ready solution is at hand in stopping fraud and taxing revenues which are escaping into the underground economy. This will require having our IRS behave more like tax collectors — an unpopular idea perhaps but an increasingly necessary one.

DRGs: The Ripple Effect

In the short run, Congress has made significant changes in the way that Medicare hospitals are to be reimbursed. The increasing dependence of hospitals and the entire health care system on Medicare is illustrated by the ripple effect created when the DRG system was mandated for hospitals in 1983.

What Congress did was to go to a fixed price menu instead of an a la carte menu. The incentives were altered and government placed priority on different values. Gone was the notion of a fair reimbursement for the provision of a service of excellent quality for all. Replace that with the government's new need for certainty of expenditure, to limit overall expenses which became more important than either fairness or quality. DRGs created a discount environment in health care. Competition was encouraged on the theory that it would drive costs down and drive out the inefficient provider — a fanciful notion if there ever was one. There are a million economists on the other side but I contend that in most cases unbridled competition and the unleashing of the free market in health care serves to run overall costs up rather than down.

Another problem that Paul Mass of Florida Home Health in Miami brought to my attention is the collision that is apparent between the statutes of an earlier era to help limit fraud (many of which Senator Moss and I wrote) and the new discount mentality in health care. Government policy now encourages discounts but will put you in jail for paying kickbacks. Government is now more concerned with saving money than stopping fraud.

The ripple effect of DRGs has the entire health care field in disarray. The one central point that should not be lost is this: the major thrust of the DRG system was to move patients out of hospitals sooner. The incentives are stacked that way. The technology has been developed to the point where people can spend less time in the hospital and more time at home. The basic idea was to get people home *and to have their needs met there.* I have found no one who contends that the idea was just to dump people out of hospitals earlier. It is presumed that they will have the care they need at home and, if they so require, that they will be readmitted to the hospital. This being true, one would expect that home health agencies would begin to see an increasing flow of sicker patients — patients with relatively more intensive nursing and medical care needs. Similarly, it follows that the costs of home care would increase and that government would be willing to pay for this.

Some of the results have been predictable, others have not. Hospital inpatients stays have been reduced. The Medicare program has saved millions of dollars. One surprise is the fact that length of stays for non-Medicare patients are also decreasing. Hospitals may be anticipating the adoption of a DRG variation by private health insurance carriers.

There has been an increase in the number of patients discharged into home health agencies. There is no doubt that they have more intensive medical needs and therefore that they are on average more costly to serve. One result has been the tremendous expansion of home health agencies which are attached to hospitals. Another is increased competition for referrals among home health agencies. Another is a sharp increase in average visits and yet another result of all the above is an increase in the aggregate total billed to Medicare by home health agencies. The irony is that through its insurance contractors who pay Medicare bills, HHS sought to reduce the existing level of expenditures for home care or at least to reduce the rate of increase. In effect, HHS has sought to trim the candle at both ends, which is, to a use a kind word, unrealistic.

Hospitals are not the only ones moving into home health. Pharmacists see home care as their top area of expansion. Durable medical goods manufacturers and dealers have moved into the field. Major US corporations, including hotel and motel chains, have begun to acquire agencies. Physicians are eyeing home health care as something they wish to reclaim now that times are changing and a surplus of physicians is looming on the horizon.

Physicians are also feeling the pressure from the Medicare freeze on payment and from so-called "Doc-in-the-Box" operations or ambulatory surgery centers that are popping up like mushrooms all across America.

HMOs and PPOs (preferred provider organizations) are coming into their own as a means of providing an alternative (and usually less expensive) form of care delivery.

There is a great deal of worry that too many patients are being dumped out of hospitals too soon. There is good anecdotal evidence that indicates patients have died unnecessarily because of DRG's fiscal convenience. There is also the fear that the entire experiment may boomerang resulting in the provision of less care to fewer patients, while costs and hospital profits increase. Critics point to this result in New Jersey which set the pace in testing the use of a DRG system. No doubt many hospitals will also be forced into bankruptcy and others will be forced to merge. What is not clear is which ones, and why. Presumably smaller hospitals will have the most problems.

What is likely to happen is the reinstitution of the two-class system of medicine which was renounced in the enactment of Medicare. Medicare said in its preamble that the ability to pay should have nothing to do with the availability of quality medical care in the United States. What seems to be emerging out of the discount environment is First Class for those who can pay, Coach for those who have private insurance, and Standby/Government Rate for those on Medicare. Medicaid corresponds to charter rates. Whether there are two tracks or four, the notion that all Americans have the same *right* to quality health care services seems to have gone by the board. At the very least, it has been limited by a series of exceptions and exclusions that have been added.

Whatever the limitations, the general perception in the Congress at this point is that DRGs have been a success-at least enough of a success that Medicare should continue to move in the direction of prospective payment for nursing homes, home health agencies, and perhaps even for physicians.

Synthesis

After connecting all the dots, what you have is a picture of runaway costs in the health care field in the face of a good deal of inefficiency, coupled with the sharply escalating demand and need for more services, particularly long-term home care. The black frame around the picture represents the looming budget deficits.

The approach that has been tried is one of deregulation. Incentives have been created to stimulate competition and unleash the free market forces. The idea has been that this would cut costs. Government has also reduced costs directly, by paying providers less and less of their costs. This has meant that providers increasingly wind up subsidizing Medicare and Medicaid with dollars gained from treating patients who pay privately.

There is a good deal of cost shifting going on as well. The federal government is increasingly pushing costs off onto private health insurance or the states.

The competitive environment rewards bigness. As a result, major hospital chains have combined with major pharmaceutical chains and suppliers. There is both vertical and horizontal integration. Big fish are continuing to eat little fish until one wonders if we will have more than three or four big whales controlling all of health care. My answer, like my analogy, comes from nature. Whales cannot exist without a tremendous number of smaller fish around them.

In my analysis, there will always be a place for the freestanding, community-based home health agency. In a way, we now have replicated in this century the conditions which led to the creation of VNAs a century ago. I am referring to the tremendous influx of immigrants coming to the US in the past 10 years.

The VNAs were created in response to genuine health crises, the epidemics that swept across America 100 years ago. At this time America was experiencing an influx of new immigrants who sought refuge in whatever housing they could afford within our major cities. The new wave did not know anything much about bacteria and sanitation. They did not understand Western medicine. They did not speak English. The medicine they knew was grounded in folklore and superstition. They could not be relied on to seek out hospitals and physicians when they or their family members became ill. In the first place, there weren't many hospitals and in the second, there were few doctors. It was at this point that Instructive Visiting Nurse organizations were born.

These home health agencies were created by a few public-spirited citizens who devoted themselves body and soul to the task. Nurses were recruited to seek out the sick, the needy, and the children in their homes. Thousands rallied to the call, mostly volunteers. It became the cause with which to be identified at the time of Theodore Roosevelt and Mayor Fiorella LaGuardia. It became an item for the status-conscious wealthy to devote both dollars and time to the care of the sick and needy. The idea was as infectious as Christianity. World War II had a way of rearranging our priorities. The advances in battlefield medicine ushered in the day of the hospital. Wounded soldiers called for a medic and were rushed to a place with bright lighting for surgery and repair. The model took root in civilian soil and for thirty years America has been on a technophilic honeymoon. But the pendulum is swinging back now—going home.

The success of such agencies in the future depends on several factors. First, the extent to which they survive the Medicare roller-coaster until policy is formulated. Right now, accepting a Medicare patient is as risky as putting a quarter in a Las Vegas slot machine. They need to do what they have done so well for so long—involve the community. Get people excited about the cause of home health care and hospice. Bring in the social elite. Give them an opportunity to use their money and their talents to help the truly needy. Second, these agencies need to let go of some things which worked in the past but which do not at the present time. Efficiency and good management are not the exclusive province of the proprietary sector.

For-profit agencies will continue to grow. This is true of large chains, which will have capital with which to expand, and market research to show them where this can be done profitably. Major corporate chains can expect more and more to become part of large entities organized to serve a multiplicity of society's needs. Small for-profit agencies will continue to proliferate. In fact, most of the new jobs in America today are in small business. Home health is attractive because it is labor intensive, only a small amount of capital is required to start one, and there is tremendous demand for services now. The demand can only increase in the future. Family entrepreneurs, particularly in small towns and rural areas, can provide a needed service and make a reasonable return on their dollar.

City and county agencies will either grow dramatically or shrink dramatically depending on available Medicaid coverage for home care. My guess is expansion, once again out of need. Clearly, there will be increased numbers of indigents, many of whom will be elderly. City and county agencies are often places of last resort. It's like the definition someone offered of home: The place where, when you get there, they have to take you in.

I see major changes for those agencies which are incorporated as nonprofits but which subcontract with for-profit subsidiaries. The changes to which I refer are so-called "reforms" in the tax code that will make life difficult for those corporate entities that straddle the line between profit and nonprofit. The IRS seems to want to tidy up the line between the two. My guess is that most agencies will choose to convert to for-profit status while setting up separate nonprofit foundations.

I believe hospital-affiliated home health agencies will continue a rapid growth and the trend will begin to reverse over time. I think hospitals are in the position where they will not be able to afford the luxury of non-profitable cost centers. My feeling is that many hospitals have or will establish their own home health agencies for the wrong reasons: (1) because everyone else is, (2) because they think they can make big profits, and (3) to stake out turf and keep someone else from opening in their area. The right reasons for doing so would be: (1) there is a need in the geographic area which is not being met, (2) the hospital has a volume of referrals sufficient to justify it, and (3) it is in the best interests of both hospital and community that they do so. Generally speaking, what I see is more cooperative joint ventures, subcontracting with the community agency, or exchange of board members with the local freestanding agency. Another model involves several hospitals going together to form one home health agency to which they all make referrals. I believe the present charm of home care will fade for many hospitals when they see losses instead of profits and the amazing amount of red tape associated with the care of relatively few patients for relatively few dollars. And then, too, economic incentive for hospital direct entry will be reduced once home health agencies join hospitals on a prospective payment system.

HMOs and Doctors

It is no great secret that HMOs are looking more and more to the provision of long-term care. In this connection, home health care consistently scores high from the point of need and desirability to the consumer. Consumers can see themselves using home health care. They often cannot see themselves using a nursing home. They don't want to think about what the latter suggests so they deny and block it out of their minds. Moreover, the cost-effectiveness of home care has registered with HMOs. As mentioned above, it is a good way to provide services for many people with a comparatively small outlay of dollars. And then too, it provides HMOs with an outreach into the community and some very positive public relations which are bound to bring in new patients.

My theory is that if you do a good job of taking care of grandmother and make it possible for her to retain her independence at home you will have the everlasting gratitude of the entire family. And will probably get the entire family to enroll in the HMO.

I see HMO involvement in home care increasing. Again, the key question is whether they would provide these services themselves or subcontract. I think this is a decision which will be made on a case-by-case basis after an in-depth economic analysis. My sense is that many of them will want to subcontract with local agencies as a way of limiting their risk, but I may be wrong.

Last and most important of all, I think the future of home care in America is linked inexorably to the future of the medial profession. The manner in which home health agencies work out their relationship with the medical community has far-reaching consequences.

My sense is that there has been an uneasy truce between doctors and home health agencies until recently. If they know of home care at all, physicians see the agencies as nurse-dominated entities that provide custodial care or "maid service." Most physicians have no knowledge of the changes that have taken place in the past 5 years. They do not know that just about any technology they have at the hospital or in their offices is now used at home.

The physicians who know about home care are usually those physicians who are required to sign the orders for such care, and yet they receive no compensation for their services. Many physicians are resentful of the easy access home health agencies have to patients' homes, mourning the loss of territory that once was theirs and was relinquished years ago.

As the surplus of physicians arrives, and given the growing interest in geriatric care, doctors are likely to look more and more closely at home health care. A federal statute now bars them from making referrals to any home care agency in which they have more than a 5% financial interest, and physicians are looking for inventive ways to get around the provision.

Physicians will not be shut out of the growing home care movement. My suggestion is to take them in as partners. Private insurance plans such as Blue Cross provide coverage for physicians' services as part of their home health care benefit. I see no reason why the current Medicare home care benefit could not be amended accordingly. This would allow agencies to send doctors in addition to nurses and therapists, when needed, to a patient's bedside. There would be no increase in costs since this services is now covered by Medicare.

Physicians should also be involved as medical directors, monitoring the quality of care in home health agencies. It seems to me that they are well-suited for the case management function. If home health interests do not reach out to physicians, then I look for physicians to find a way around the current law, starting their own entities or purchasing existing agencies. As is usually the case, the public interest is served better by cooperation rather than competition, which inevitably means duplication and unneeded expenditures increasing overall costs.

Summary

In summary, home care will grow at a meteoric rate through the end of this century. The forces driving it are powerful indeed: tradition, technology, demographics, and public demand.

In the short run, there will continue to be some bumpy air on the journey until OMB, the Congress, and the Department of Health and Human Services agree on a common policy for the Medicare home health benefit.

For a time the debate about growing federal deficits will continue. The most likely result is increased taxes and some reductions in the levels of increase for both defense and entitlement programs.

What appears to be developing is a cafeteria-style plan for health care geared to the ability to pay. For better or for worse, government seems to be backing away from its promise to vouchsafe the equal rights of all Americans to the highest quality health care services that America can offer. This plan will probably continue until exposes in the popular press push for a realignment of values once again. I would expect this to usher in a tide of regulation.

In the foreseeable future, there will be talk of means-testing Medicare and of rationing health care services. Ethical issues will play center stage. I see a vigorous debate revolving around so-called "right to life" issues and the care of chronically disabled children. I look for a debate personified in two individuals. One is Governor Richard Lamm of Colorado, who reportedly made reference to the obligation of the old and sick to die and not be a drain on society. At the other end of the pole is former Senator Jacob Javits, whose dramatic fight with ALS has made national news. He argues that we should provide continuing care. Senator Javits argues that while he cannot move a muscle, his mind is intact. Because of this, he continues to write, to advise, and to contribute and he is a valued member of society. The question is: Which side will we choose in America?

I suspect that we will follow our usual bad habits and not make public policy until we literally have no choice. We are not very good at planning ahead. We deal in stop-gap legislation. When the wave of the aged and increased numbers of the chronically ill hits America later in this century, every effort, public and private, will have to be made to meet their needs. Still, I think there will be a good deal of room left for individual choice as to whether Americans want or do not want heroic measures of care. Choice after all is the American way; choice is the centerpiece of human dignity. Hospice care will become a universally available option. As far as the millions of needy children, I am convinced that we will transfer most of them out of hospitals and care for them where they belong—in their own homes.

While the future looks bright for home health agencies, the final outcome depends on whether caregivers continue to provide quality health care services. The provision of quality services to the most needy members of society is and will continue to be the best advertisement of all. I have no doubt but that they will do so and, because of this, the future is assured.

Chapter Thirty-Six

Surviving the Present and Coping With the Future: A Personal Viewpoint

Marilyn D. Harris

Introduction

There are times when I feel that I know what a swimmer experiences when being pounded by unrelenting waves in a rough surf. During the past year there has been one wave after the other hitting home health administrators. There is hardly time to catch your breath before the next wave hits. These waves have names: DRG aftermath; waiver consideration; Forms 485, 486, and 487; Uniform Bill 82; Gramm-Rudman-Hollings; technical denials; medical denials; discipline rather than aggregate costs; the list seems endless.

In spite of these rough times in 1986, I, as a home health agency administrator, expect to survive the present and cope, and possibly thrive, in the future. In order to accomplish this goal, both long- and short-range strategies must be in place and utilized.

References to the current reimbursement climate appear in various places. A recent cartoon on an editorial page showed a patient lying in a hospital bed with an intravenous line and oxygen in place. The physician, standing at the foot of the bed, said: "Your blood pressure and temperature are way up, but your Medicare coverage is way down. Looks as if you can go home today, Mrs. Fitch."

"Letters to the Editor" in recent nursing journals carried comments from home care nurses who shared their opinions about overtaxing assignments, paperwork, and the negative effects of DRGs.

Eight years ago, Partridge (1978,10) said: "In the face of mushrooming pressures, constituencies, and complexities, we have but three alternatives: we can muddle on with our unsatisfying, uneven national performance; we can succumb; or we can emerge into a tomorrow we helped fashion. The latter choice is within our grasp." Home health administrators can help shape the future of this industry.

Today's Health Care Climate

The changes in acute health care financing methods have had an impact on in-home services. One of the most obvious ones is that patients are being discharged quicker and in need of more intensive levels of service. From the patient's and family's viewpoints, patients require skilled and supportive services, many of which they expect will be paid by Medicare or another third-party payor. This is not necessarily the case. For the administrator, more intensive levels of care may equal longer visits, decreased productivity for staff, and increased costs that present the potential for exceeding cost caps.

At the same time, the interpretations of the regulations for in-home services are becoming more restrictive. Fiscal intermediaries and private insurance carriers are questioning with increased frequency, bills that reflect what they consider to be over-utilization of services, physician's orders that they do not consider to be medically necessary, or clinical documentation of care that they do not consider appropriate for reimbursement. An increase in both medical and technical denials during 1986 has presented new concerns for administrators as well as staff and patients.

Also, patients must be sick enough to need skilled care, but not too sick; i.e., they should not require daily visits for more than three weeks or hire help that is not paid under the Medicare program. The rationale is that if the patients must have extended coverage, regardless of who is paying, they should be in a nursing home. Senator John Heinz of Pennsylvania has referred to this as the "no-care" zone.

More frequent admissions and discharges to home care services result from this change in hospital reimbursement. This results in additional time and paperwork for the visiting staff on admissions but shorter lengths of stay on service.

The administrator faces several challenges:

- Provide quality care in a changing economic and regulatory climate.

- Keep the agency fiscally sound and solvent.

- Maintain budgeted number of staff visits per day.

- Keep staff and supervisors happy and sane.

- Maintain sense of humor and perspective.

- Maintain timely billing to maintain short-term cash flow. This is true for manual billing or for agencies on periodic interim payments (PIP). Failure to maintain this time frame may result in the loss of PIP status.

Section 474 of the Medicare manual states that an agency must submit 85% of their bills promptly and accurately. Eighty-five percent must be submitted within 30 days of the through date on a bill and must pass the intermediary's front-end edit for consistency and completeness. A bill is not received unless it has passed the edit. Bills must now be accompanied by signed physicians' orders. This requirement leaves a short turnaround time when admissions occur close to billing dates. A cooperative team effort throughout the agency is necessary to meet this requirement.

- Maintain Waiver of Liability Presumptive Status based on appropriate determinations of coverage. An agency's denial rate must be less than 2.5% to maintain this status. This is a constant challenge in this time of increased denials for service.

- Consideration of the ethical issues that affect patients, families, and staff. These include the increased responsibilities placed on families as a result of high-tech procedures in the home as well as administrative issues; i.e., who shall receive care in light of shrinking financial resources? How shall this care be distributed?

The staff faces still other dilemmas:

- Provide quality care to patients under increased pressures from internal and external sources.

- Be aware of all regulations regarding care and ongoing changes in coverage.

- Document care for reimbursement purposes, not only clinical and legal purposes.

- Maintain productivity standards established by and communicated to staff by administration to retain financial solvency.

- Maintain sanity and proper perspective amidst all the internal and external demands placed upon them.

Patients and families face still other issues. These include an increased responsibility to care for acutely ill individuals in the home, lack of financial resources to pay for needed services, and a corresponding lack of public funds to pay for long-term care.

Strategies for Survival

Given the assumption that administrators want to survive today and cope with tomorrow, I believe that the following strategies must be utilized. These are not listed in priority order.

1. Establish and improve methods to maintain fiscal stability.

    a. Have a sound and functioning computerized management information system (MIS) to monitor the myriad activities. I believe this is important because of the pending change from a fee-for-service to a prospective payment system in the future. Types of data to be monitored seem endless but are most important in today's economic and political climate.

    b. Manage a fluctuating caseload. A fluctuation of several hundred visits per month can be financially and psychologically devastating to administration and staff. The use of per diem and part-time nurses, who work when work is available, allows flexibility in staffing. But, it also presents new problems related to continuity of care for patients and availability of staff. In addition to flexible staff patterns, there may also have to be a consolidation of staff at all levels, including the office and supervisory staff while the current climate is evaluated.

c.   Establish timely billing procedures. There may be a need for more support staff even though visits are decreasing due to the complexities associated with the billing procedure.

d.   Diversify into one or more of the following areas: chore services; transportation; dental or eye care in the home; podiatry; beautician or barber services; financial counseling; translation; pet and plant care; day care. Other possibilities include wellness programs such as participation in retirement seminars, hypertension screening, exercise, stop smoking, stress management or weight loss programs, and well-child clinics.

2. Maintain productivity.

a.   Several years ago, this agency received a grant to develop a tape recording and transcribing system for clinical records (Harris 1984). The goals were to reduce the amount of time professional staff spent on patient's recordkeeping duties (office time); increase the number of patients the staff would be able to visit in a day (productivity); and increase the amount of time the personnel spend in direct patient care, i.e., less office time equals more time for patient care. Five of the original nurses are still in this six-year study. The visits per day and the office time of these five nurses were compared with five nurses who had less than two years of service. Data from April 1985 were used to determine baseline statistics. There was a drop in the number of visits per day and a corresponding increase in office time in September 1985 with the inception of Forms 485-87. As of September 1986, this lost productivity has not been fully regained.

b.   Develop standardized care plans and flow sheets. The use of standardized flow sheets makes it possible for staff to address all the parameters for a specific nursing diagnosis and classification system without having to do the manual writing of these details. I believe these standardized plans also contribute to quality care; i.e., staff knows what parameters have to be addressed in order to meet the outcome criteria of the agency's Quality Assurance Program.

3. Provide quality care — ever mindful that the main reason we exist is because there are patients who need the services that the agency's staff can provide. Flexibility is needed to meet the individualized needs of each patient. This may impact on productivity! An agency must measure its performance, staff qualifications, outcomes of programs and services, costs of providing services, and fiscal stability. This is done through formal reviews and through patient responses to care.

The provision of quality care also requires that staff either acquire or maintain nursing skills that were once confined to the acute care facilities. High-tech care is a daily occurrence.

4. Be alert to legislative and regulatory issues that affect home care. DRGs, Gramm-Rudman, copayment proposals, 485-88s, loss of waiver of liability

status, different interpretations of existing regulations, etc. These issues have been described in detail in other chapters. It is most important to keep in contact with local, state, and national elected officials through letters and personal visits. It is also important to establish a "hot line" communication network through local or state organizations to address pertinent issues on a timely basis.

5. Recognize the need for research in the administrative and clinical aspects of home health care. The Visiting Nurse Association (VNA) of Eastern Montgomery County has been actively involved in several such projects. An example of clinical research is "Medication Usage Among the Homebound Elderly" (Harris and Lavizzo-Mourey 1985). An example of administrative research is "Cost of Home Care by Nursing Diagnosis" (Harris et al. 1986). These studies provide useful information for staff and administration to maintain or improve the quality of care for patients.

6. Also recognize the need for patient education materials to increase the quality of care given to patients when future reimbursement methods dictate that administrators limit either the number of visits or length of visits based on a yet undetermined method of prospective payment for home care. The VNA is currently involved in such a project with two other organizations. Our first project is the development of educational tapes for our patients with diabetes. These tapes, as well as other tapes which are in the planning phase, will be available to supplement, not replace, teaching done by the nurse.

7. Be aware of the need for careful selection of other providers, such as durable medical equipment (DME) and high-tech companies. Home care staff need good equipment and services to meet patient and staff needs. The nurse needs only one "bad experience," such as not having the proper equipment in the home or not having all of the supplies necessary for a specific procedure, as reason enough not to use a specific company in the future. Waiting for equipment impacts on public relations, productivity, and everyone's satisfaction with the home care services.

8. Be especially cognizant of the importance of marketing home care services in this era of competition.

9. Network with other home care providers. This is accomplished through attendance at local, regional, state, and national conferences. This is also accomplished through sharing of information on successes and failures, development of useful tools, research findings, suggestions for improvements in the delivery of services, and publication of these results in professional journals.

10. Realize that the importance of the educational preparation of the administrative and supervisory staff of the home health agency cannot be overemphasized. Clinical staff must be skilled in providing needed services.

In today's financial health care climate, the role of the administrator is never dull. The National League for Nursing (NLN) Accreditation Manual (1986, 17) indicates that the director should implement board policy; manage the agency; do community assessment; plan, develop, administer, and evaluate agency programs; oversee fiscal management; and work with other organizations to improve the health of the community.

Graduate textbooks state that a nurse administrator should be: a leader of a clinical discipline; problem solver; facilitator; teacher; scholar; manager; be able to do budgeting, staffing, labor relations, and meet regulatory demands.

The basic attributes desirable in an administrator are listed in *Characteristics of the Home Health Agency Administrator* (NLN 1977,3). Included are personal characteristics such as: exhibits a strong commitment and abundant energy for the task — "that extra something" required to achieve goals; shows emotional stability; possesses the ability to operate under pressure; and shows initiative, enthusiasm, pragmatism, and creativity. These attributes are certainly appropriate in the 1980s.

In reality, administration includes varying percentages of all of the above. The stress level is often high for administrators, supervisors, and staff. The important thing to remember is that the administration of health care services is a team effort. Staff must hear about those issues which could and probably will affect their workload and stress level. Administrators must be aware of multiple issues as they affect staff and the agency. Working together as a team, we will be able to survive the current status and progress into the future which we helped to shape.

In 1600 B.C., King Solomon said, "Have two goals, wisdom that is knowing and doing right and common sense. Don't let them slip away for they will fill you with living energy and bring you honor and respect." (Proverbs 3: 21-26) These two goals, wisdom and common sense, are important to me as an administrator of home health services today.

Summary

Administrators must manage the agency in an effective and efficient manner in spite of multiple internal and external changes, current economic conditions, regulations, and budget constraints. The information presented in this book should help both students and practitioners to deal with the multifaceted responsibilities involved with home health administration.

Reference

Harris, M. 1984. A tape recording and transcribing system to maintain patients' clinical records. *Nursing and Health Care.* 5(9): 503-507.

Harris, M. and R. Lavizzo-Mourey. 1985. Medication usage among the elderly requiring home care services. Presented at the Fourth Annual Meeting and Homecare Exhibition of the National Association for Home Care, Las Vegas, NV, 15 October.

Harris, M., D. Peters, C. Parente, and J. Smith. 1986. Cost of home care by nursing diagnosis. Presented at the Second National Nursing Symposium on Home Health Care, University of Michigan School of Nursing, Ann Arbor, MI, 15-16 May. Also presented at the National Association for Home Care Annual Meeting in New Orleans, LA, 10 September.

National League for Nursing. 1977. *Characteristics of the home health agency administrator.* New York: National League for Nursing. Publication No. 21-1681.

National League for Nursing. 1986. *Accreditation program for home care and community health. 1986 Revisions.* New York: National League for Nursing.

Partridge, K. 1978. *Community health administration in a cost-containment era.* New York: National League for Nursing. Publication No. 21-743.

Glossary of Abbreviations

American Nurses Association	ANA
American Federation of Home Health Agencies	AFHHA
Average visits per day	AVD
Bachelor of Science in Nursing	BSN
Conditions of Participation	COP
Cardio Pulmonary Resuscitation	CPR
Certified Nurse Administrator	CNA
Certified Nurse Administrator - Advanced	CNAA
Continuous abdominal peritoneal dialysis	CAPD
Durable Medical Equipment	DME
Diagnosis Related Group	DRG
Full time equivalent	FTE
Home health aide	HHA
Home health agency	HHA
Health Care Financing Administration	HCFA
Health Maintenance Organization	HMO
International Classification of Disease - 9	ICD-9
Intravenous	IV
Joint Commission on Accreditation of Hospitals	JCAH
Licensed practical nurse	LPN
Master of Science in Nursing	MSN
Medical Social Work	MSW
Medicare	Title XVIII
Medicaid	Title XIX
Management Information System See Chapter 23 for specific glossary	MIS
Maternal Child Health	MCH
Nursing Diagnosis	ND
National League for Nursing	NLN
National Association for Home Care	NAHC

Occupational therapy	OT
Patient Classification System	PCS
Physical therapy	PT
Preferred Provider Organization	PPO
Problem Oriented Record	POR
Quarterly Record Review	QRR
Quality Assurance	QA
Registered nurse	RN
Social Health Maintenance Organization	SHMO
Skilled nursing	SN
Speech pathology	SP
Subjective, objective, assessment, plan	SOAP
Supplemental Security Income	SSI
Utilization Review	UR
United States Dept. of Health, Education, Welfare	USDHEW
Uniform bill- 82	UB-82
Visiting Nurse Association	VNA
Visiting Nurse Association of America	VNAA

Bibliography

Allison, S. E. 1973. A framework for nursing action in a nurse-conducted diabetic management clinic. *Journal of Nursing Administration* 3:53-60.

Alutto, J. A., and J. A. Belasco. 1972. *Determinants of attitudinal militancy among nurses and teachers*. Bethesda, MD:ERIC Document Service, ED 063-635.

American Nurses' Association. 1973. *Standards of community health nursing practice*. Kansas City, MO:ANA.

American Nurses' Association. 1973. *Standards*. Kansas City, MO:ANA.

American Nurses' Association. 1978. *Continuing education in nursing guidelines for staff development*. Revised. Kansas City, MO:ANA.

American Nurses' Association. 1978. *Self-directed continuing education in nursing*. Kansas City, MO:ANA.

American Nurses' Association. 1979. *Continuing education in nursing: An overview*. Kansas City, MO:ANA.

American Nurses' Association. 1980. *A conceptual model of community health nursing*. Kansas City, MO:ANA.

American Nurses' Association. 1980. *Nursing: A social policy statement*. Kansas City, MO:ANA.

American Nurses' Association. 1980. A conceptual model of community health nursing. Kansas City, MO:ANA.

American Nurses' Association. 1984. *Standards for continuing education in nursing*. Kansas City, MO:ANA.

American Nurses' Association. 1985. *A guide for community-based nursing services*. Kansas City, MO:ANA.

American Nurses' Association. 1985. *A guide for community-based nursing services*. Kansas City, MO:ANA.

American Public Health Association. 1982. The definition and role of public health nursing practice in the delivery of health care. *American Journal of Public Health* 72:210-212.

American Society of Association Executives and The Chamber of Commerce of the United States. 1975. *Principles of association management*. Washington DC:American Society of Association Executives.

American Society of Association Executives. 1982. *Fundamentals of association management: The volunteer*. Washington, DC:American Society of Association Executives.

American Society of Association Executives. 1984. *ASAE and Annual Management Conference Proceedings Volume II.* Washington, DC.

Anderson, E. T. 1983. Community focus in public health nursing: Whose responsibility? *Nursing Outlook* 31:44-48.

Anderson, H. J. 1986. Two recent home healthcare mergers may signal industry consolidation. *Modern Healthcare* 16 (26 Sept.):118.

Anderson, L. and M. Thobaben. 1984. Clients in crisis: When should the nurse step in? *Journal of Gerontological Nursing* 10:6-10.

Angell, M. 1984. Respecting the autonomy of competent patients. *New England Journal of Medicine* 310:1115-1116.

Anna, D. J. et al. 1978. Implementing Orem's conceptual framework. *Journal of Nursing Administration* 8:8-11.

Archer, S. E. and R. P. Fleshman. 1985. *Community health nursing,* 3rd ed. Monterey, CA:Wadsworth Health Sciences.

Ballard, S. and R. McNamara. 1983. Quantifying nursing needs in home health care. *Nursing Research* 32:236-241.

Bayer, R. 1984. Ethical challenges of the movement for home care. *Caring* 2(10):57-62.

Bayer, R. 1986. Ethics in home care and quality assurance. *Caring* 4(1):50-56.

Bayer, R. 1986. Ethics in home care and quality assurance. *Caring* 5:50-56.

Benton, R. 1978. *Death and dying: Principles and practices in patient care.* New York:D. Van Nostrand.

Bircher, A. U. 1975. On the development and classification of diagnosis. *Nursing Forum* 14(1):11-29.

Bloom, P. 1984. Effective marketing for professional services. *Harvard Business Review.* 62 (Sept./Oct.) 104.

Bloom, P. 1984. Effective marketing for professional services. *Harvard Business Review* 62 (Sept./Oct.):104.

Bonstein, R. G. and J. Mueller, 1985. Improving agency productivity. *Caring* 4(11):4-9.

Boszoimenyi-Nagy, I. and B. Krasner. 1986. *Between give and take.* New York:Brunner/Mazel.

Brickner, P. W. 1978. *Home health care for the aged: How to help older people stay in their own homes and out of institutions.* New York:Appleton-Century-Crofts.

Bromley, B. 1980. Applying Orem's self-care theory in enterostomal therapy. *American Journal of Nursing* 80:245-249.

Brown, B. I. 1980. Realistic workloads for community health nurses. *Nursing Outlook* 23:233-237.

Buhler-Wilkerson, K. 1983. False dawn: The rise and decline of public health nursing in America, 1900-1930. In *Nursing history: New perspectives, new possibilities*, ed. by E. G. Lagemann, 39-106. New York:Teachers College Press.

Buhler-Wilkerson, K. 1985. Public health nursing: In sickness or in health? *American Journal of Public Health* 75:1155-1161

Bulaw, J. M. 1986. *Administrative policies and procedures for home health care.* Rockville, MD:Aspen Systems Corp.

Bullough, V., and B. Bullough. 1978. *The care of the sick: The emergence of modern nursing.* New York:Prodicst.

Callahan, D. 1985. What do children owe elderly parents? *The Hastings Center Report* (April):32-37.

Cangemi, J. P., L. Clark, and E. Harryman. 1980. Differences between pro-union and pro-company employees. In *Labor relations in nursing.* by C. A. Lockhart and W. B. Werther, Jr. Wakefield, MA:Nursing Resources.

Centre County Home Health Service Labor Management Committee. 1984. Minutes of Meeting, 23 May 1984.

Chapman, J. and H. Chapman. 1975. *Behavior and health care: A humanistic helping process.* Saint Louis:C.V. Mosby.

Cherkasky, M. 1949. The Montefiore Hospital home care program. *American Journal of Public Health* 39:163-166.

Chinn, L. 1986. *Ethical issues in nursing.* Rockville, MD:Aspen Systems Corp.

Clark, M. J. 1984. *Community nursing: Health care for today and tomorrow.* Reston, VA:Reston Hall Publishing Co.

Clemen-Stone, S., E. G. Eigsti and S. L. McGuire. 1987. *Comprehensive family and community health nursing*, 2nd ed. New York:McGraw-Hill Book Company.

Colosi, T. R. and A. E. Berkely. 1986. *Collective bargaining: How it works and why.* New York:American Arbitration Association.

Cornell, W. A. 1985. *Understanding Pennsylvania Civics.* Harrisburg, PA:Penns Valley.

Cronbach, L. J. 1983. *Designing evaluations of educational and social programs* San Francisco:Jossey-Bass Publishers.

Cross, J. et al. 1983. How community health nurses spend their time: A study report. *Nursing and Health Care* 4:314-317.

Cunningham, M., Jr. 1985. The evolution of hospice. *Hospitals* 59 (Part 1):124-126.

Curran, C. R. 1985. Sabbaticals: Not for teachers only! *Nursing Outlook* 33:92-94.

Cushman, D. 1980. Organizing campaigns: An analysis of management's use of communication techniques, suggestions for union strategy. In *Unionization and the health care industry: Hospital and nursing home employee union leaders conference report, Nov. 29-Dec. 1, 1978*, ed. by R. J. Peter et al. University of Illinois at Urbana-Campaign:Institute of Labor and Industrial Relations.

Daubert, E. A. 1979. Patient classification system and outcome criteria. *Nursing Outlook* 27:450-454.

Davis, K. 1958. *Human relations in business*. New York:McGraw-Hill Book Co.

DeLozier, M. W. *The marketing communications process*. New York:McGraw-Hill.

DeLozier, M. W. 1976. *The marketing communications process*. New York:McGraw-Hill Book Co.

Division of Nursing, Bureau of Health Professions, Health Resources and Services Administration, Public Health Service. 1985. Consensus conference on the essentials of public health nursing practice and education. Washington, DC:U.S. Department of Health and Human Services.

Dock, L. L., and A. M. Stewart. *A short history of nursing: From the earliest times to the present day*, 2nd ed. New York:G. P. Putnam's Sons.

Easley, C. and C. Storfjell. 1979. *The Easley-Storfjell instruments for caseload/workload analysis*. Ann Arbor, MI:University of Michigan Press.

Elkins, C. P. 1984. *Community health nursing: Skills and strategies*. Bowie, MD:Robert J. Brady Co.

Etzioni, A. 1969. *A sociological reader on complex organizations*. New York:Holt Rinehart Winston.

Fenner, K. 1979. Developing a conceptual framework. *Nursing Outlook* 27:122-126.

Feuer, L. 1985. Ethical issues in health care. *FOCUS: Home health care in the 80's*. 5(1) Winter:1-4. Conshohocken, PA:Foster Medical Corporation.

Fink, A. 1977. *An evaluation primer*. Washington, DC:Capital Publications.

Fitzpatrick, M. L. 1975. *The national organization for public health nursing, 1912-1952: Development of a practice field*. New York:National League for Nursing.

Foundation center annual report. 1984. New York:Foundation Center.

Foundation center catalog - Summer. 1985. New York:Foundation Center.

Freedman, A. E. and P. E. Freedman. 1975. *The psychology of political control*. New York:St. Martins Press.

Freeman, L. H., and P. F. Adams. 1984. A way to provide continuing education. *Nursing & Health Care* 5:34-36.

Freeman, L. H. et al. 1984. Product development and marketing in continuing education. *Nursing Economics* 2:336-340.

Freeman, R. B. and J. Heinrich. 1981. *Community health nursing practice*, 2nd ed. Philadelphia, PA:W. B. Saunders Company.

Fry, S. T. 1983. Dilemma in community health ethics. *Nursing Outlook*. 31:176-179.

Fulmer, T. and T. Wetle. 1986. Elder abuse: Screening and intervention. *Nurse Practitioner* 11:33-38.

Gardner, M. S. 1932. *Public health nursing.* New York:Macmillan Publishing.

Genovich-Richards, J. and D. C. Carissimi. Developing nurses' managerial competence. *Nursing Management* 17:36-38.

Gerrard, B. A. et al. 1980. *Interpersonal skills for health professionals.* Reston, VA:Reston Hall Publishing Co.

Ginzberg, E. 1966. *The development of human resources.* New York:McGraw-Hill Book Co.

Ginzberg, E., W. Balinsky and M. Ostow. 1984. *Home Health Care.* Totawa, NJ:Rowman and Allanheld.

Giovannetti, P. 1979. Understanding patient classification systems. *Journal of Nursing Administration* 9(2):4-8.

Giovannetti, P. and G. C. Mayer. 1984. Building confidence in patient classification systems. *Nursing Management* 15(8):31-34.

Giving USA. 1986. New York:American Association of Fund-Raising Council, Inc.

Goertzen, I. 1980. A nursing administrator's view of ethics in practice. In *Ethics in nursing practice and education.* Kansas City, MO:American Nurses Association.

Golightly, C. K. 1981. *Creative problem solving for health care professionals.* Rockville, MD:Aspen Systems Corp.

Gordon, M. 1982. *Nursing diagnosis process and application.* New York:McGraw-Hill Book Co.

Gregorich, P. and J. W. Long. 1980. Responsive management fosters cooperative environment. In *Labor relations in nursing,* ed. by C. A. Lockhart and W. B. Werther, Jr. Wakefield, MA:Nursing Resources.

Griff, S. 1981. Marketing to expand a home care service. *Home Health Review* 4(1):29-31.

Griff, S. 1981. Marketing to expand a home care service. *Home health review* 4(1):29-31.

Gross, M. J. Jr., and W. Warshauer, Jr. April 1980. *The basics of budgeting.* Association Management.

Guthrie, M. et al. 1985. Productivity: How much does this job mean? *Nursing Management* 16(2):116-120.

Harbert, A. and L. Ginsberg. 1979. *Human services for older adults: Concepts and skills.* Belmont, CA:Wadsworth Publishing.

Hardy, J. A. 1984. A patient classification system for home health patients. *Caring* 3(9):26-27.

Harris, M. et al. 1985. Patient classification systems—A management tool. *Nursing Economics* 3:276-282.

Heinrich, J. 1983. Historical perspectives on public health nursing. *Nursing Outlook* 31:317-320.

Hemsworth, M. J. 1978. *Nurses in collective bargaining*. Ann Arbor, MI:University Microfilms International.

Herrington, J. V. and S. Houston. 1984. Using Orem's theory: A plan for all seasons. *Nursing and Health Care* 5:45-47.

Hillestad, S. G. and E. N. Berkowitz. 1984. *Health care marketing plans: From strategy to action*. Irwin, IL:Dow Jones.

Hillestad, S. G. and E. N. Berkowitz. 1984. *Health care marketing plans: From strategy to action*. Homewood, IL:Richard D. Irwin, Inc.

Hogstel, M. O. 1985. *Home nursing care for the elderly*. Bowie, MD:Brady Communications Co., Inc.

Home health care market trends. 1984 *Caring* 111(6):26-29.

Jackson, B. S. and J. Resnick. Comparing classification systems. *Nursing Management* 13(11):13-19.

Jarvis, L. L. 1985. *Community health nursing: Keeping the public healthy*, 2nd ed. Philadelphia:F. A. Davis, Inc.

Jelinek, R. and D. Lyman. 1976 *A review and evaluation of nursing productivity*. Washington, DC:Government Printing Office DHEW Publication HHR 77-15.

Joint Commission on Accreditation of Hospitals (JCAH). 1986. *Accreditation manual for hospitals*. pp. 47-55. Chicago:The Commission 1986.

Kaluzny, A. and V. James. 1980. *Health services organizations*. Berkeley, CA:McCutchan Publishing Corp.

Kelly, L. Y. *Dimensions of professional nursing*, 4th ed. New York:Macmillan Publishing Co., Inc.

Kissinger, C. 1973. Community nursing administration: Quantifying nursing utilization. *Journal of Nursing Administration* 3(5):113-120.

Kissinger, C. L. 1973. Community nursing administration: Quantifying nursing utilization. *Journal of Nursing Administration* 3(5):42-48.

Kleffel, D. and E. Wilson. 1975. *Evaluation handbook for home health agencies*. Washington, DC:Government Printing Office. DHEW Pub. No. 76-3003.

Koerner, B. L. 1981. Selected correlates of job performance of community health nurses. *Nursing Research*. 30(1):43-48.

Kotler, P. 1980. *Marketing management: Analysis, planning and control*, 4th Ed. Englewood Cliffs, NJ:Prentice-Hall.

Kotler, P. 1980. *Marketing management: Analysis, planning and control*, 4th ed. Englewood Cliffs, NJ:Prentice-Hall, Inc.

Kotler, P. 1982. *Marketing for non-profit organizations*. Englewood Cliffs, NJ:Prentice-Hall, Inc.

Kotler, P. and K. Cox Eds. 1980. *Marketing management and strategy: A reader*. Englewood Cliffs, NJ:Prentice-Hall, Inc.

Kotler, P. and K. Cox. Ed. 1980. *Marketing management and strategy: A reader*. Englewood Cliffs, NJ:Prentice-Hall, Inc.

Krayne, L. 1982. *Home health agency staff survey of variables affecting number of visits per day.* Sewickley, PA:Sewickley Home Health Agency.

Kruger, D. H. 1961. Bargaining and the nursing profession. *Monthly Labor Review* 84 (July):699.

Larson, E. et al. 1984. Job satisfaction, assumptions, and complexities. *Journal of Nursing Administration* 14(1):31-38.

Lazer, W. 1971. *Marketing management: A systems perspective*. New York:John Wiley & Sons.

Lazer, W. 1971. *Marketing management: A systems perspective*. New York:John Wiley & Sons.

Leahy, K. N., M. M. Cobb and M. C. Jones. 1982. *Community health nursing*, 4th ed. New York:McGraw-Hill Book Co.

Levitan, S. A. et al. 1981. *Human resources and labor markets: Employment and training in the american economy*, 3rd ed. New York:Harper & Row.

Levitt, T. 1985. Marketing myopia. *Harvard Business Review*, 53(5).

Levitt, T. 1985. Marketing myopia. *Harvard Business Review*. 53(5).

Lockhart, C. A. and W. B. Werther, Jr. 1980. *Labor relations in nursing.* Wakefield, MA:Nursing Resources.

Logan, M. and E. Hunt. 1978. *Death and the Human Condition*. North Scituate, MA:Duxbury Press.

Loria. L. S. February 1982. Cultivating long-range philanthropy. *Hospital Financial Management*.

Loughron, C. S. 1984. *Negotiating a labor contract: A management handbook*. Washington, D.C.:The Bureau of National Affairs,Inc.

Lustberg, A. 1983. *Testifying with impact* rev. ed. Washington, DC:Association Division U. S. Chamber of Commerce.

Mann, R. 1967. *Interpersonal styles and group development: An analysis of the member-leader relationship*. New York:Wiley.

Mason, D. J. and S. W. Talbott. 1985. *Political action handbook for nurses*. Reading, MA:Addison-Wesley.

Mason, E. and J. Daughtery. 1984. Nursing standards should determine nursing's price. *Nursing Management* 15(9).

Mattson, M. R. 1984. Quality assurance: A literature review of a changing field. *Hospital and Community Psychiatry* 35(6):605-616.

Matz, A. and O. J. Curry. 1972. *Cost accounting: Planning and control.* Cincinnati, OH:South-Western Publishing Co.

McCarthy, E. 1978. *Basic marketing,* 6th ed. Homewood, IL:Richard D. Irwin, Inc.

McIntyre, R. L. 1985. Changing the rules on dying. *New Jersey Medicine* 82:945-948.

McNamara, E. 1982. Home care: Hospitals rediscover comprehensive home care. *Hospitals* 56(21):60-66.

Melosh, B. 1982. *"The physician's hand": Work culture and conflict in American nursing.* Philadelphia:Temple University Press.

Meyer, G. D. 1970. *Determinants of collective action attitudes among hospital nurses: An empirical test.* Ph.D. Dissertation, The University of Iowa.

Milio, N. 1981. *Promoting health through public policy.* Philadelphia:F. A. Davis Co.

Miller, M. A. 1980. Staff evaluation. In *Nursing administration: Theory for practice with a systems approach* ed. by C. Arndt and L. Huckabay. pp. 96-100. St. Louis:C. V. Mosby Co.

Monterior, L. A. 1985. Florence Nightingale on public health nursing. *American Journal of Public Health* 75:181-186.

Morris, L. and C. Fitz-Gibbon. 1978. *Program evaluation kit.* Beverly Hills, CA:Sage Publishers.

Moyer, N. 1986. Public policy politics, and home health care. *Home Healthcare Nurse* 4:7-12.

Moyer, N. 1986. Public policy, politics, and home health care. *Home Healthcare Nurse* 4(5):7-12.

Mundinger, M. O. 1983. *Home care controversy: Two little, too late, too costly.* Rockville, MD:Aspen Systems Corp.

National Hospice Organization. 1984. The basics of hospice. Pamphlet.

National League for Nursing and Council of Home Health Agencies and Community Health Services. 1979. *Productivity (home visits per day per employee).* New York, NY:National League For Nursing.

National League for Nursing. 1979. *Community health: Today and tomorrow.* New York:National League for Nursing.

National League for Nursing. 1984. *Administrator's handbook for community health and home care services.* New York:NLN. Pub. No. 21-1943.

National League for Nursing. 1985. *Accreditation program for home care and community health.* New York:NLN.

Nightingale, F. *Florence Nightingale to her nurses*. London:MacMillan & Co.

Norris, C. M. 1979. Self-care. *American Journal of Nursing* 79:486-489.

O'Connor, A. B. 1986. *Nursing staff development and continuing education*. Boston:Little, Brown and Company.

O'Malley, S. T. 1986. Reimbursement issues. In *Home health care nursing: Administrative and clinical perspectives*, Ed. by S. Stuart-Siddal. Rockville, MD:Aspen Systems Corp. 23-82.

O'Malley, T. 1986. Identifying and preventing family-mediated abuse and neglect. *Caring* 5:28-34.

Olins, N. J. 1986. Feeding decisions for incompetent patients. *Medical Ethics* 34:313-317.

Orem, D. E. 1980. *Nursing: Concepts of practice* 2nd ed. New York:McGraw-Hill Book Co.

Pappas, J. Notes on board-staff relations in associations. Presented at the Presession of the NAHC Legislative Conference, Washington, DC, March 1985.

Pennsylvania Association of Home Health Agencies. 1986. *Home health service provider standards*. Harrisburg, PA: The Association.

Phillips, L. and V. Rempusheski. 1986. Caring for the frail elderly at home: Toward a theoretical explanation of the dynamics of poor quality family caregiving. *Advances in Nursing Science* 8:62-86.

Pirovano, D. O. 1986. The buck stops on health care ethics. *Coordinator* Feb.:28-29.

Polit, D. and B. Hungler. 1978. *Nursing research: Principles and methods*. Philadelphia:J. B. Lippincott Co.

Price, W. M. and O. C. Ferrell. 1980. *Marketing: Basic concepts and decisions*. 2nd ed. Boston, MA:Houghton-Mifflin.

Pride, W. M. and O. C. Ferrell. 1980. *Marketing: Basic concepts and decisions*, 2nd Ed. Boston, MA:Houghton-Mifflin.

Redman, E. 1973. *The dance of legislation*. New York:Simon and Schuster.

Reif, L. 1984. Making dollars and sense of home health policy. *Nursing Economics*. 2(6):382-388.

Reif, L. 1984. Making dollars and sense of home health policy. *Nursing Economics* 2(6):382-388.

Roberts, D. E. and J. Heinrich. 1985. Public health nursing comes of age. *American Journal of Public Health* 75:1162-1172.

Rosen, G. 1958. *A history of public health*. New York:MD Publications, Inc.

Rothstein, J. 1958. *Communication, organization and science*. Indian Hills, CO:Falcon's Wing Press.

Rowland, H. S. and B. L. Rowland. *Nursing administration handbook*. Germantown, MD:Aspen Systems Corp.

Rowland, K. M., and G. R. Ferris. 1982. *Personnel management*. Boston:Allyn and Bacon, Inc.

Runner-Heidt, C. M. 1984. Where does the hospital discharge planner go from here? *Home Healthcare Nurse*. 2(4):30-34.

Runner-Heidt, C. M. 1984. Where does the hospital discharge planner go from here? *Home Healthcare Nurse* 2(4):30-34.

Schein, E. and W. Bennis. 1965. *Personal and organizational change through group methods*. New York:Wiley and Sons.

Scott, R. S. 1985. When it isn't life or death. *American Journal of Nursing* Jan.:19-20.

Scott, W. G. 1962. *Human relations in management: A behavioral science approach*. Homewood, IL:Richard D. Irwin, Inc.

Serluco, R. J. and Institute of Public and Private Service - Trenton State College. 1984. *Innovative financial management and reimbursement strategies for the home health care agency*. Trenton, NJ:Institute of Public and Private Service.

Shapiro, B. P. 1985. Getting things done, rejuvenating the marketing mix. *Harvard Business Review* 63(5):28-34.

Shapiro, P. 1985. Getting things done, rejuvenating the marketing mix. *Harvard Business Review*. 63(5):28-34.

Sienkiewicz, J. I. 1984. Patient classification in community health nursing. *Nursing Outlook* 32:319-321.

Simmons, D. A. 1980. *A classification scheme for client problems in community health nursing*. Washington, DC:Government Printing Office. DHHS Publication No. HRA 80-16.

Smith, C. 1979. Proposed metaparadigm for nursing research and theory development: An analysis of Orem's self-care theory. *Image* 75-80.

Smith, J. A. 1983. *The idea of health: Implications for the nursing professional*. New York:Teachers College Press.

Smith, J. A. 1983. *The idea of health*. New York:Teachers College Press.

Sommers, T. 1985. Long-term care: Biggest dilemma, toughest problem, greatest challenge. *Perspective on Aging* July/August:9-11, 20.

Sorenson, R. 1950. *The art of board membership*. New York:Association Press.

Special Issue On Hospital/HHA Relations. 1984. *Caring* 111(7).

Spradley, B. W. 1985. *Community health nursing: Concepts and practice*, 2nd ed. Boston:Little, Brown & Co.

Stanhope, M. and J. Lancaster. 1984. *Community health nursing: Process and practice for promoting health*. St. Louis:C. V. Mosby.

Stanhope, M. and J. Lancaster. 1984. *Community health nursing.* St. Louis:C. V. Mosby Co.

Stevens, B. J. 1980. *The nurse as executive.* 2nd Ed. Wakefield, MA:Nursing Resources, Inc.

Stewart, J. E. 1979. *Home health care.* St. Louis:C. V. Mosby Co.

Stuart-Siddall, S. A. *Home health care nursing administrative and clinical perspectives.* Rockville, MD:Aspen Systems Corp.

Sweeny, H. W. and R. Rachlin. 1981. *Handbook of budgeting.* New York, NY:Wiley and Sons, Inc.

The Nursing Theory Conference Group. 1980. *Nursing theories: The base for professional nursing practices.* Englewood Cliffs, NJ:Prentice Hall, Inc.

Tilden, V. 1985. Development and use of computer managed instruction. *Computers in Nursing* 3:207-211.

Ting, H. M. 1984. New directions in nursing home and home health care marketing. *Healthcare Financial Management.* 38(5):62-664.

U.S. Department of Health, Education, and Welfare. Social Security Administration. 1967. *Medicare provider reimbursement manual - HIM15.* Washington, DC.Government Printing Office.

United Way of America. 1974. *Accounting and financial reporting: A guide for united ways and not-for-profit human service organizations.* Alexandria, VA:United Way of America, Systems Planning Allocation Division.

Vaughan, R. G. and U. Macleod. Nursing staffing studies: No need to reinvent the wheel. *Journal of Nursing Administration* 10(3):9-15.

Veatch, R. M. 1984. An ethical framework for terminal care decisions: A new classification of patients. *Journal of the American Geriatrics Society* 32:665-669.

Verwoerdt, A. 1966. *Communications with the fatally ill.* Springfield, IL:Charles C. Thomas.

Vroom, V. H. and P. W. Yetton. 1976. Leadership and decision-making: Basic considerations underlying and normative model. In *Concepts and controversy in organizational behavior* ed. by W. R. Nord, 2nd ed. Pacific Palisades, CA:Goodyear Publishing Co.

Wagner, D. M. and D. S. Cosgrove. 1986. Quality assurance: A professional responsibility. *Caring* 4(1):46-49.

Wald, L. D. 1915. *The house on Henry Street.* New York:Henry Holt and Co.

Wanzer, S. et al. The physician's responsibility toward hopelessly ill patients. *New England Journal of Medicine* 310:955-959.

Werther, W. B., Jr. and C. A. Lockhart, ed. 1980. Collective action and cooperation in the health professions. In *Labor relations in nursing.* Wakefield, MA:Nursing resources.

White, M. S. 1982. Construct for public health nursing. *Nursing Outlook* 30:527-530.

Williams, C. A. 1977. Community health nursing—What is it? *Nursing Outlook* 25:250-254.

Williams, M. A. 1977. Quantification of direct nursing care activities. *Journal of Nursing Administration* 7(8):15-18.

Wood, J. B. 1985. Home care agencies and health care competition. *Home Healthcare Nurse*. 3(1):22-24.

Woodham-Smith, C. 1970. *Florence Nightingale: 1820-1910*. London & Glasgow:Fontana Books.

Yarling, R. R. and McElmurry, B. J. 1983. Rethinking the nurse's role in do not resuscitate orders: A clinical policy proposal in nursing ethics. *Advances in Nursing Science* 5:1-11.

Zacur, S. 1982. *Health care labor relations: The nursing perspective*. Ann Arbor:University of Microfilms International.

Index